Ambulatory Surgical Nursing Core Curriculum

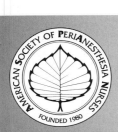

AMERICAN SOCIETY OF PeriAnesthesia NURSES

Ambulatory Surgical Nursing Core Curriculum

Donna M. DeFazio Quinn, BSN, MBA, RN, CPAN, CAPA
Director
Elliot 1-Day Surgery Center
Manchester, New Hampshire

W.B. SAUNDERS COMPANY
A Division of Harcourt Brace & Company
Philadelphia London Toronto Montreal Sydney Tokyo

W.B. SAUNDERS COMPANY

A Divison of Harcourt Brace & Company

The Curtis Center
Independence Square West
Philadelphia, Pennsylvania 19106

Library of Congress Cataloging-in-Publication Data

Ambulatory surgical nursing core curriculum / American Society of
PeriAnesthesia Nurses : editor, Donna M. DeFazio Quinn.
   p.   cm.
  ISBN 0-7216-6522-5
  1. Ambulatory surgical nursing. 2. Operating room nursing.
I. Quinn, Donna M. DeFazio. II. American Society of PeriAnesthesia
Nurses.
  [DNLM: 1. Perioperative Nursing. WY 161A4974 1999]
RD110.5.A53 1999
610.73′677—dc21
DNLM/DLC   98-34732

AMBULATORY SURGICAL NURSING CORE CURRICULUM   ISBN 0–7216–6522–5

Printed in the United States of America

Last digit is the print number: 9   8   7   6   5   4   3   2   1

DEDICATION

To my daughter, Gia Elizabeth Quinn

Foreword

It is essential to provide resource material to meet the particular learning needs of perianesthesia nurses in ambulatory settings. Health care delivery systems are redeveloped and redefined with increased speed. The practice settings we are familiar with today will continue to change as technological and pharmaceutical advances are assimilated. Nurses will provide perianesthesia care for patients in surgery centers, pain management centers, office-based practice, and in remote locations we have yet to imagine. This text was developed to address the core of specialized knowledge utilized by ambulatory perianesthesia nurses. These nurses develop plans of care by identifying and prioritizing patient needs, especially related to the impact of anesthesia, the surgical intervention and discharge needs. They prepare patients both physically and emotionally for surgery and its outcomes with astute skills, continuous reevaluation, and ongoing education.

This Core Curriculum will be an essential resource for ambulatory nurses. It will serve as an excellent guide to assist in orientation of new staff, as well as a resource for study in preparation for the national perianesthesia ambulatory certification examination. As you learn from this text, my hope is that your knowledge base of ambulatory surgery nursing practice will be enhanced, and new questions will emerge for you to generate further study.

Maureen V. Iacono, BSN, RN, CPAN
President, American Society of PeriAnesthesia Nurses

Preface

The specialty of ambulatory surgery has grown tremendously during the past decade. Procedures once performed only on an inpatient basis are now being done in the outpatient arena. Additionally, the advent of recovery care centers has created the opportunity for even more complex surgical procedures to be performed in ambulatory surgery centers that provide overnight care.

As procedures shifted from the inpatient side to outpatients, another shift also occurred. Procedures once performed in the ambulatory surgery center are now being moved to the physician's office. It is expected that this shifting of procedures will continue as third party payers demand procedures be performed in low-cost settings and as technological and pharmacological advances continue.

With the rapid progression of ambulatory surgery, perianesthesia nursing has evolved into a specialty of its own. Ambulatory surgery nursing involves not only the nurses caring for the patient pre- and postoperatively, but also can encompass nurses working in preoperative holding units, endoscopy, radiology, physician's offices, and specialty clinics. Any time the patient is prepared to undergo either an invasive or noninvasive procedure, nurses skilled in caring for the needs of this specific patient population must be available.

This text has been designed to assist the nurse working in the ambulatory surgery setting prepare for the CAPA examination. Certification in one's specialty is a means to promote quality of care to the general public, the nursing profession, and the individual nurse. When a nurse involved in ambulatory surgery achieves certification, this demonstrates commitment to his or her nursing career, provides tremendous personal satisfaction, and can provide opportunities for career advancement.

The text utilizes on outline format to delineate areas of ambulatory perianesthesia nursing practice. The text is not designed to be a complete study guide. The nurse must identify his or her own areas of weakness, seek out additional information from other sources, and develop an individualized study plan that will meet one's needs.

Based on the domains of the CAPA exam as identified by the American Board of PeriAnesthesia Nursing Certification (ABPANC), the book is designed to cover the following:

- Direct care
- Education
- Leadership

The text is divided into sections that will assist the nurse in planning, organizing, and developing a strategy to study for the examination. Included in the text are chapters related to the profession of ambulatory surgery, basic competencies, lifespan considerations, anesthesia, surgical specialties, and management. Each chapter contains objectives, review questions, and a bibliography. The surgical specialty chapters also contain "key patient educational outcomes" to assist the nurse in developing the plan of care. Review questions at the end of each chapter are designed to allow the nurse to reevaluate the material presented. They are in no way intended to replicate the actual CAPA examination.

Although designed to assist nurses in preparation of the CAPA examination, this book can also be used for other purposes such as:

- A study guide for nurses new to the ambulatory surgery setting
- Development of an orientation plan for the ambulatory surgery unit (ASU)
- Development of ambulatory surgical nursing competencies
- A reference guide for student nurses rotating through the ASU

Chapter authors are experts in their field of practice. The information presented is as current and as accurate as possible. All chapters were reviewed multiple times to ensure accuracy.

The development of this Core Curriculum was sponsored by and supported by the American Society of PeriAnesthesia Nurses (ASPAN).

Donna M. DeFazio Quinn, Editor

Acknowledgments

This Core Curriculum brings together the works of many talented individuals. I wish to thank the authors who contributed chapters to this book. The time, dedication, and energy expended was truly an act of love for their profession. Also, I wish to thank the reviewers who assisted by reviewing manuscripts, making recommendations, and sharing their knowledge and expertise. The hard work and dedication to the specialty of ambulatory surgery by both the authors and reviewers is evident throughout this text.

I wish to extend my gratitude to Joan Sinclair from the production department at W. B. Saunders for her expertise in coordinating this project and to Tony Caruso who worked diligently to produce the final product.

My sincere appreciation also goes to Victoria Legnini at W. B. Saunders who always managed to make me smile, and always got me through every crisis unscathed.

From the moment I first had contact with Maura Connor, W. B. Saunders, I knew I had an editor who would champion and support this project wholeheartedly. I thank her for her patience and understanding, and most of all for her support during some difficult times. She gave me time to travel to China to adopt a daughter and then understood my sudden realignment of responsibilities. Her encouragement and kind words were always welcome.

To my coworkers and colleagues at Elliot 1-Day Surgery Center I owe a big "thank you" for putting up with my craziness, forgetfulness, and preoccupation during the past 2 years. On days when I appeared quite "brain dead" you always brought me back to life.

Lastly, I wish to acknowledge the support of my family. To my husband Stephen, who pre-fatherhood played a lot of golf and did a lot of skiing, and post-fatherhood did a great job keeping Gia busy so I could accomplish some work, thanks for your support, understanding, and love; and to Gia Elizabeth, my angel from above, who grew tall enough during this project to open the door of my office to make her presence known, thanks for helping me see the lighter side of life and for sharing your life with me.

Contributors List

Joan Bauer, MS, RN, CPAN
Staff Nurse Phase I PACU
St. Marys Hospital Medical Center
Madison, WI

Evolution of Ambulatory Surgery

Linda Boyum, BSN, RN, CPAN
Nurse Manager
The Outpatient Center of Boynton
  Beach, LTD
Boynton Beach, FL

Special Procedures

Kathy Carlson, BSN, MA, CPAN
Staff Registor Nurse, Surgical Services
Abbott Northwestern Hospital
Minneapolis, MN

*Certification Concepts and Testing Strategies;
Fluid and Electrolyte Balance and Hematologic
Considerations*

Serina Carpenter, MSN
Adjunct Instructor, Neuroscience Clinical
  Nurse Specialist
William Carey College
Forrest General Hospital
Hattiesburg, MS

Neurosurgery/Neurologic Procedures

**Brenda S. Gregory Dawes, RN, MSN,
  CNOR**
Editor, AORN Journal
AORN
Denver, CO

Podiatric Surgery

**Rose Ferrara-Love, MSN, BN, CPAN,
  CAPA**
Clinical Instructor, Clinical Nursing
  Supervisor
Duquesne University
Mercy Providence Hospital
Pittsburgh, PA

*Preoperative Patient Assessment and
Preparation; Postoperative Patient Assessment
and Discharge Criteria—Phases I and II*

Susan Jane Fetzer, PhD, MBA, CCRN
Assistant Professor, PACU Nurse
University of New Hampshire
Elliot Hospital
Manchester, NH

The Nursing Process; Nursing Research

Beverly George-Gay, RN, MSN
Assistant Professor, School of Nursing
Medical College of Georgia
Augusta, GA

Cardiovascular Surgery

Lisa Peck Glazier, BSN, RN, CPAN
Nurse Manager, Ambulatory Care Unit,
  Pain Clinic, Diagnostics
Mercy Hospital
Portland, ME

Plastic and Reconstructive Surgery

Joyce C. Hadley, BA, RN, CPAN
Clinical Instructor
Inova Health Systems
Falls Church, VA

*The Elderly Patient; Patient and Family
Education*

Melody Heffline, RN, MSN, CS-ACNP, CPAN
Acute Care Nurse Practitioner
Southern Surgical Group, LLC
West Columbia, SC

Cardiopulmonary Care and Emergency Support

Vallire D. Hooper, MSN, RN, CPAN
Instructor, School of Nursing
Medical College of Georgia
Augusta, GA

The Adult Patient; Cardiovascular Surgery

Christine Kelley, RN, BSN, CNOR
Clinical Leader
Elliot 1-Day Surgery Center
Manchester, NH

Laparoscopic and Minimally Invasive Surgery; Transcultural Nursing

Nancy K. King, RN, CAPA
TQM Coordinator, ASPAN
The Surgery Centers
Cleveland, OH

Total Quality Management in the Ambulatory Setting

Lonnie Lane, RN, RMT
Nurse Manager, Registered Massage Therapist
Columbia Physicians Daysurgery Center
Dallax, TX

General Surgery

Kim Litwack, PhD, RN, FAAN, CPAN, CAPN, FNP
Associate Professor
University of New Mexico
College of Nursing
Albuquerque, NM

Pre-Existing Medical Conditions

Gayle Miller, MS, MBA, RN, CPAN
Director, Surgical Services
St. Luke's Hospital
Jacksonville, FL

Laparoscopic and Minimally Invasive Surgery; Orthopedic Surgery; Otorhinolaryngologic Surgery; Special Procedures; Urologic Surgery

Cheryl Mullen, BS, RN, CPAN
Director, PACU
Bedford Ambulatory Surgical Center
Bedford, NH

Environmental and Equipment Management

Patricia Muller-Smith, BSN, MA, EdD
Adjunct Faculty, Director, Department
  of Education
University of Tulsa, Tulsa, OK
Northeastern State University,
  Talequah, OK
University of Oklahoma,
  Oklahoma City, OK
Saint Francis Health System
Tulsa, OK

Conflict Management and Team-Building

Debby Niehaus, RN, BS, CPAN
Clinical Nurse III
Bethesda North Ambulatory Surgery
  Center
Cincinnati, OH

Environmental and Equipment Management

Denise O'Brien, BSN, RN, CPAN, CAPA
Clinical Nurse III, Ambulatory Surgery
  Unit, Department of Operating Rooms/
  PACU
University of Michigan Health System
Ann Arbor, MI

Dental/Oral and Maxillofacial Surgery; Gynecologic and Reproductive Surgery

Jan Odom, BSN, MS
Clinical Nurse Specialist, Surgical Services
Forrest General Hospital
Hattiesburg, MS

*Implementation of Nursing Standards; Legal
and Ethical Issues*

Judy Ontiveros, BSN, RN, CPAN, CAPA
Clinical Coordinator PACU/OPS, Facility
  Educational Coordinator
St. Luke Medical Center
Pasadena, CA

Home Support Network

**Donna M. DeFazio Quinn, BSN, MBA,
  RN, CPAN, CAPA**
Director
Elliot 1-Day Surgery Center
Manchester, NH

*The Adolescent Patient: Clinical/Critical Paths
and Case Management; Human Growth and
Development; The Pediatric Patient; Personnel
Selection, Management, and Staff Development;
Policies and Procedures*

Janet L. Ridder, RN, MS, CPAN (late)
Coordinator for Case Management
Hinsdale Hospital
Hinsdale, IL

Patient and Family Education

Nancy Saufl, BSN, MS, RN, CPAN, CAPA
Manager
Port Orange Day Surgery
Halifax Medical Center
Daytona Beach, FL

Ophthalmologic Procedures

Lois Schick, MN, MBA, RN, CPAN, CAPA
Director Emergency Department, Clinical
  Decision Unit, Occupational Health
Exampla Healthcare, Saint Joseph Hospital
Denver, CO

*Anesthetic Agents for Ambulatory Surgery
(Adults and Pediatrics); Anesthetic
Complications; Malignant Hyperthermia;
Pain Management*

Gwen D. Williams, RN
Staff Nurse, Preadmission Department
Our Lady of Lourdes Regional Medical
  Center
Lafayette, LA

*The Mentally and Physically Challenged
Patient*

Reviewer List

Eleanore McGowan Adelman, MEd, RN
Outpatient Surgery Center
Pre-Admission Testing Center
Tucson, Arizona

Sandra Aspacher, RN, CAPA
Eye Institute of Southern Arizona
Tucson, Arizona

Christine C. Beechner, BSN, RN, CAPA
Northern Westchester Hospital Center
Mount Kisco, New York

Mary C. Betz, BSHA, RN, CPAN, CAPA
Holy Redeemer Hospital & Medical Center
Meadowbrook, Pennsylvania

Nancy J. Brent, MS, RN, JD
Attorney at Law
Chicago, Illinois

Jane E. Coyle, MS, RN, CPAN, CNOR,
    CNA
New Britain General Hospital
New Britain, Connecticut

Barbara Waynick Davis, BSN, RN, CPAN
Lexington Medical Center
West Columbia, South Carolina

Linda Elmquist, BSN, RN, CPAN
Clinical Educator, Post Anesthesia Care
    Units
Tucson Medical Center
Tucson, Arizona

Rose Ferrara-Love, MSN, RN, CPAN,
    CAPA
Mercy Providence Hospital
Duquesne University
Pittsburgh, Pennsylvania

Sally J. Foix, RN, CPAN
Nebraska Methodist Hospital
Omaha, Nebraska

Joyce C. Hadley, BA, RN, CPAN
Inova Fairfax Hospital
Falls Church, Virginia

Delores Ireland, RN, CAPA
William Beaumont Hospital-Troy
Troy, Michigan

Pamela B. Kaufmann, BSN, RN
Staff Nurse
Tucson Medical Center
Tucson, Arizona

Jeanne Kozyra, RN, CPAN, CAPA
St. Charles Hospital and Rehabilitation
    Center
Port Jefferson, New York

Susan Letvak, PhD, RN
University of North Carolina-Chapel Hill
Chapel Hill, North Carolina

Ann Butler Maher, MS, RN, NPC, ONC
County College of Morris
Randolph, New Jersey
    and
Jersey Battered Women's Service
Morris Plains, New Jersey

Ellen Manieri, MN, RN, CAPA
Charity School of Nursing
Delgado Community College
New Orleans, Louisiana

Geraldine Maixner, RN, CPAN
Colorado Springs, Colorado

Lila Berry Martin, BSN, RN, CCRN, CPAN
University of Kansas Hospital
Kansas City, Kansas

Candice Murcek, RN, CPAN
American Red Cross
Omaha, Nebraska

Debby Niehaus, BS, RN, CPAN
Bethesda North Ambulatory Surgery
    Center
Cincinnati, Ohio

Judy Ontiveros, BSN, RN, CPAN, CAPA
St. Luke Medical Center
Pasadena, California

Patricia J. Pernes, BS, RN, CPAN
Desert Samaritan Medical Center
Mesa, Arizona

Lynn A. Sekeres, BSN, RN, CCRN, CPAN
University of Pittsburgh Medical Center
Pittsburgh, Pennsylvania

Dorothy J. Stuppy, PhD, RN
School of Nursing
University of Texas at Arlington
Arlington, Texas

David Tilton, BSN, RN
Harrison Hospital
Bremerton, Washington

Grace Walke, BSN, RN, CPAN
Indiana University Hospital
Indianapolis, Indiana

Glenda Wilkinson, BS, RN, CRLS, CURN
Piedmont Stone Center
Winston-Salem, North Carolina

Deanna Wilson, RN
Tucson Medical Center
Tucson, Arizona

Linda B. Wilson, MSN, RN, CPAN, CAPA
Thomas Jefferson University Hospital
Philadelphia, Pennsylvania

Marie Wilson, RN, CURN, CNOR
Louisiana State University Medical Center
Shreveport, Louisiana

Maria T. Zickuhr, MSN, RN, CPAN
Johns Hopkins Outpatient Center
Baltimore, Maryland

Linda Ziolkowski, BSN, RN, CPAN
Henry Ford Hospital
Detroit, Michigan

Contents

NOTICE

Nursing is an ever-changing field. Standard safety precautions must be followed, but as new research and clinical experience broaden our knowledge, changes in treatment and drug therapy become necessary or appropriate. Readers are advised to check the product information currently provided by the manufacturer of each drug to be administered to verify the recommended dose, the method and duration of administration, and the contraindications. It is the responsibility of the treating physician, relying on experience and knowledge of the patient, to determine dosages and the best treatment for the patient. Neither the publisher nor the editor assumes any responsibility for any injury and/or damage to persons or property.

The Publisher

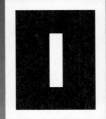

P A R T

I

The Profession of Ambulatory Surgical Nursing

1

Evolution of Ambulatory Surgery

Joan Bauer
St. Marys Hospital Medical Center
Madison, Wisconsin

BEGINNINGS OF AMBULATORY SURGERY

I. Early Beginnings
  A. Trephining of the skull and amputations identified in the year 3500 B.C. as evidenced by cave drawings
  B. Ambulatory surgeries performed at Glasgow Royal Hospital for Sick Children in Scotland from 1898 to 1908
     1. Surgeries performed on 8,988 children
     2. Surgeries included orthopedic problems, hare lip and cleft palate, spina bifida, skull fracture, hernias and others
     3. None of the children required hospital admission
  C. Information from Glasgow Hospital presented at a meeting of the British Medical Association in 1909

II. General Anesthesia in Ambulatory Surgery
  A. First reported in Sioux City, Iowa in 1918
  B. Anesthesia provided by Dr. Ralph D. Waters at the Down-Town Anesthesia Clinic in Sioux City
  C. In 1937, Hertzfeld reported in the *American Journal of Surgery* on over 1,000 outpatient pediatric hernia surgeries performed under general anesthesia
  D. Early ambulation after surgery came into acceptance in the 1940s and 1950s

III. Ambulatory Surgery Programs Established
  A. The nation's first ambulatory surgery program opened at Butterworth Hospital in Grand Rapids, Michigan in 1961, and staff performed 879 ambulatory surgeries between 1963 and 1964

Objectives

1. Explain the early beginnings of ambulatory surgery.
2. Name two associations dedicated to ambulatory surgery and anesthesia.
3. Name three advances in medical technology that led to an increase in ambulatory surgeries.
4. Explain how new anesthetic drugs facilitated surgery in the ambulatory setting.
5. List three reasons for consumer acceptance of ambulatory surgery.

    B. A formal ambulatory surgery program was begun at UCLA in 1962

    C. In 1968, the Dudley Street Ambulatory Surgery Center opened in Providence, Rhode Island

    D. The nation's first freestanding surgery facility was opened in 1970 by Dr. Wallace Reed and Dr. John Ford in Phoenix, Arizona

        1. In 1971, the American Medical Association endorsed the use of surgicenters

        2. In 1974, the Society for the Advancement of Freestanding Ambulatory Surgery (FASC) was formed, which was the precursor for the current Federated Ambulatory Surgery Association (FASA)

    E. The American Society for Outpatient Surgeons (ASOS) was formed in 1978, paving the way for surgery being performed in doctors' offices (now known as American Association of Ambulatory Surgery Centers)

        1. The 1980s brought a shortage of inpatient hospital beds

        2. In 1980, the Omnibus Budget Reconciliation Act (OBRA) authorized reimbursement for outpatient surgery

        3. In 1981, the American College of Surgeons (ACS) approved the concept of ambulatory surgery units as preadmission units for scheduled inpatients

        4. In 1983, Porterfield and Franklin advocated for office outpatient surgery

        5. The Society for Ambulatory Anesthesia (SAMBA) was formed in 1984

IV. The Ambulatory Surgery Concept Proliferated in 1980s

    A. Hospital-affiliated ambulatory surgery accounted for 9.8 million operations (45%) performed within hospital settings by 1987

    B. By 1988, 984 freestanding outpatient surgery centers performed over 1.5 million surgical operations

    C. By 1989, there were 984 Medicare-participating freestanding ambulatory surgery centers in the United States

    D. The list of approved procedures that can be conducted in surgery centers was expanded in 1987 by the Health Care Financing Administration (HCFA)

    E. In 1989, HCFA revised the payment schedule for outpatient surgeries performed on Medicare patients

V. Freestanding Recovery Sites

    A. In 1979, the first freestanding recovery center opened in Phoenix, Arizona

        1. Patients were transported directly to the recovery center from hospital PACUs, from ASUs, and from physicians' offices

        2. Some patients were transferred there from hospitals on their second or third postoperative day

    B. In California, patients may stay in recovery centers up to three days after their surgical procedures

    C. In the 1980s, the concept of 23-hour units led to guest services being developed for patients living more than one hour away from the site where the surgery was to be performed (Hospital Hotels; Medical Motels)

        1. Freestanding medical motels are considered a comfortable, affordable, convenient place to recuperate

        2. Patients are cared for by family members

        3. Home health nurses make visits

    D. Most recent figures (1994) from the National Center for Health Statistics (NCHS) Data Center

        1. An estimated 28.3 million surgical and nonsurgical procedures were performed during 18.8 million ambulatory visits

        2. An estimated 16.0 million (85%) of the ambulatory surgery visits were in hospitals and 2.9 million (15%) were in freestanding centers

        3. Almost 90% of ambulatory surgery patients were discharged to home; 3.1% went to observation units and 1.6% were admitted to hospitals as inpatients

ECONOMICS OF AMBULATORY SURGERY

I. Cost Control a Primary Force in the Development of Ambulatory Surgery
  A. In 1988, 58% of surgery centers contracted with Health Maintenance Organizations (HMOs) and 52% with Preferred Provider Organizations (PPOs)
  B. In 1990, the American Hospital Association (AHA) reported that greater than 50% of all hospital-based surgical procedures were done on an outpatient basis
    1. This amounted to greater than 22 million surgeries
    2. 13.3 million of them in hospitals
    3. 2.3 million in other types of affiliated facilities
  C. In the 1990s, 23 home observation units (recovery centers) were established in the United States
  D. Percent of outpatient procedures approved for payment under Medicare increased
    1. 450 procedures approved in 1982
    2. 2,500 approved procedures by the early 1990s
  E. Medicare reimbursement for physician fees in surgery centers: 100%; Medicare reimbursement for physician fees in offices: 80%
  F. Third-party payers require many surgeries to be performed in an ambulatory setting to avoid the cost of hospitalization
  G. Many freestanding centers have contractual arrangements with managed care plans and nursing homes
  H. Outpatient facilities eliminate the costs of cafeteria, laundry, and the need for 24-hour staffing
  I. Outpatient procedures eliminate unnecessary lab, X-ray, and ECG services
  J. Patients recovering in 23-hour units are considered not hospitalized for purposes of reimbursement by Medicare and third-party payers

TECHNOLOGICAL ADVANCES LED TO MORE OUTPATIENT SURGERIES

I. Expanding Technology Led to More Complex Surgeries Being Performed in Outpatient Settings
  A. Microscopic surgeries abounded
  B. New lasers were developed (Yag, Argon, CO_2)
  C. New laparoscopic instruments facilitated shorter, less invasive laparoscopic procedures
  D. More endoscopic procedures were being performed as outpatient procedures
  E. Video equipment and computer-assisted surgeries were now being performed
  F. Fiber optics led to advances in ophthalmic surgeries, most of which are performed in outpatient settings
II. Many Diagnostic Procedures Done in Ambulatory Settings
  A. X-ray procedures
  B. Laboratory tests
  C. Physical therapy
  D. Cardiopulmonary tests
  E. Pain blocks

LEGISLATION ENCOURAGED GROWTH OF AMBULATORY CENTERS

I. Relaxation of Legislation Concerning Ambulatory Surgery
  A. Relaxation of legislation began to occur in the 1980s
  B. By 1987, the Omnibus Budget Reconciliation Act provided for less reimbursement to hospitals, providing rates equal to those for ambulatory surgery centers

C. The Omnibus Budget Reconciliation Act of 1989 again increased the reimbursement rates for assigned surgical procedures in ambulatory centers

II. **Ambulatory Centers Became Certified**
   A. 90% of freestanding surgery centers were certified by Medicare in 1988
   B. 80% of these centers were certified by state governments

ANESTHESIA ADVANCES LED TO MORE AMBULATORY SURGERIES

I. **Anesthesia Techniques Changed**
   A. Less use of premedications
      1. New agents used
      2. Anticholinergics such as atropine and glycopyrrolate decrease secretions
         a. Premedications may be given IV after patient asleep
   B. Local procedures performed; local infiltration of the operative site facilitated postoperative pain relief
   C. Regional blocks facilitated surgery in ambulatory settings
   D. More procedures were performed with IV conscious sedation and monitored anesthesia care
      1. Provides adequate sedation
      2. Relieves anxiety and causes amnesia
      3. Provides relief from pain
      4. Alters mood but patient remains conscious and cooperative
      5. Protective reflexes remain intact
      6. Shortened recovery time

II. **General Anesthesia Performed in Outpatient Settings**
   A. Barbiturates used less frequently due to their long duration of action and slow elimination
   B. Benzodiazepines such as diazepam (Valium), lorazepam (Ativan) and midazolam (Versed) used to decrease anxiety
      1. These drugs don't ease pain
      2. Can cause restlessness and delirium
      3. Flumazenil (Romazicon) effectively reverses the sedative effects, amnesic affects, and psychomotor effects of benzodiazepines
   C. Newer antiemetics such as droperidol (Inapsine) and ondansetron (Zofran)
      1. Provides sedation, calmness, tranquility
      2. May lead to dysphoria, restlessness, fear
      3. Used because of the potent antiemetic property
   D. Opioid IV agents developed such as fentanyl (Sublimaze), sufentanil (Sufenta), and alfentanil (Alfenta) suitable for ambulatory surgery
      1. Sufentanil 5 to 10 times more potent than fentanyl and has a more rapid onset than fentanyl
      2. Alfentanil less potent than fentanyl and has a more rapid onset with a shorter duration of action
   E. Intraoperative opioids given IV
      1. Morphine, hydromorphone (Dilaudid)
   F. Non-opioid (non-narcotic) pain medication such as ketorolac (Toradol) given intraoperatively or postoperatively
   G. Non-opioid IV agents in ambulatory settings
      1. Thiopental sodium (Pentothal) and methohexital (Brevital) are short-acting barbiturates; Brevital can be administered rectally to children, making it an attractive choice when parents can be present for induction

2. The newer drug propofol (Diprivan) has rapid onset and rapid emergence with low incidence of nausea and vomiting, making it appropriate for ambulatory surgery
3. Etomidate (Amidate) produces minimal cardiovascular effects and decreases intraophthalmic pressure

H. Neuromuscular blocking agents
  1. Depolarizing agent succinylcholine (Anectine)
    a. Used for rapid onset
    b. Has short duration of action
  2. Non-depolarizing agents
    a. Atracurium (Tracrium)
      i. Rapid onset with duration of 30 to 45 minutes
      ii. Little or no cumulative effect
    b. Vecuronium (Norcuron)
      i. Rapid onset of action
      ii. Little or no cumulative effect
    c. Mivacurium (Mivacron)
      i. Shortest duration of action
      ii. Recovery within 12 to 17 minutes

I. Inhalation agents may be used in conjunction with nitrous oxide to provide rapid, safe, adequate anesthetic
  1. Halothane (Fluothane)
    a. Frequently used with pediatric patients
    b. Provides rapid recovery and low incidence of nausea and vomiting
  2. Enflurane (Ethrane)
    a. Provides sufficient muscle relaxation
    b. Patients regain consciousness quickly
    c. Low incidence of nausea and vomiting
  3. Isoflurane (Forane)
    a. Provides rapid induction
    b. Rapid recovery phase
  4. Desflurane (Suprane)
    a. Rapid induction and emergence

J. Antacids and H_2 antagonists such as cimetidine (Tagamet) and ranitidine (Zantac) developed which decrease risk for acid aspiration
  1. Outpatient risk is high but incidence is low
  2. Ranitidine has a longer duration of action than cimetadine
  3. These drugs often given with metaclopramide (Reglan) which increases lower esophageal tone and facilitates gastric emptying

For complete review of anesthetic agents, refer to Chapter 22.

CONSUMER ACCEPTANCE OF AMBULATORY SURGERY

I. **Awareness**
  A. Increased marketing led to increased consumer awareness
  B. Greater awareness led to greater demand for surgery in ambulatory settings
  C. Consumers saw more physician involvement in ambulatory settings
  D. Patient consumers felt more involved and took part in decisions
  E. Few problems were seen with quality of care
II. **Convenience**
  A. Flexible hours

    B. Early admission and same-day discharge

    C. Less time lost from work

    D. Units easily accessible

III. **Wellness Philosophy Well Accepted**

    A. Patients could walk to the operating room

    B. Patients could recover on stretchers or in recliners

    C. Parents could remain with children during induction; parents, and sometimes families, could be present postoperatively

    D. Patients were able to keep dentures, eyeglasses, hearing aids with them

    E. Patients felt more self-responsibility for their care

IV. **Reimbursement**

    A. Reimbursement provided by Medicare for outpatient procedures for the elderly made ambulatory surgery a viable alternative

    B. Employers were paying less and consumers found ambulatory settings less expensive, making outpatient surgery an attractive option

Bibliography

1. American Society of Post Anesthesia Nurses (1994). *Ambulatory Post Anesthesia Nursing Outline: Content for Certification.* Thorofare, NJ: ASPAN.
2. American Society of Post Anesthesia Nurses (1995). *Standards for Perianesthesia Nursing Practice.* Thorofare, NJ: ASPAN.
3. Aquavella, J.V. (1990). Ambulatory surgery in the 1990s. *J Ambulatory Care Manage,* 13(1):21–24.
4. Burden, N. (1993). *Ambulatory Surgical Nursing.* Philadelphia: Saunders.
5. Drain, C.B. (1994). *The Post Anesthesia Care Unit,* 3rd ed. Philadelphia: Saunders.
6. Henderson, J.M. (1990). Ambulatory surgery: Past, present and future. In *Anesthesia for Ambulatory Surgery,* 2nd ed, Wetchler, B.V. (ed.). Philadelphia: Lippincott.
7. Kozak, L.J., Hall, R.P., Lawrence, L. (1997). Ambulatory surgery in the United States, 1994. In *Advance Data,* Centers for Disease Control and Prevention, National Center of Health Care Statistics, March 14.
8. Wetchler, B.V. (1990). *Anesthesia for Ambulatory Surgery,* 2nd ed. Philadelphia: Lippincott.
9. White, P.F. (1990). *Outpatient Anesthesia.* New York: Churchill Livingstone.

REVIEW QUESTIONS

1. In which of the following cities was the nation's first hospital-based ambulatory surgery center established?

    A. Grand Rapids, Michigan

    B. Sioux City, Iowa

    C. Phoenix, Arizona

    D. Los Angeles, California

2. In which of the following cities was the nation's first freestanding surgery center established?

    A. Grand Rapids, Michigan

    B. Sioux City, Iowa

    C. Phoenix, Arizona

    D. Los Angeles, California

3. In 1987, which of the following agencies increased the approved procedure list for surgeries performed in the outpatient setting?

    A. FASA

    B. HCFA

    C. OCS

    D. SAMBA

4. Which of the following drugs is a benzodiazepine used to provide sedation and decrease anxiety?

    A. Midazolam (Versed)

    B. Alfentanil (Alfenta)

    C. Atropine

    D. Thiopental (Pentothal)

5. Which of the following actions is **not** a characteristic of IV conscious sedation with midazolam (Versed)?

   A. Rapid onset of sedation
   B. Causes amnesia
   C. Relieves anxiety
   D. Long duration of action

6. Which of the following is **not** a characteristic of droperidol (Inapsine)?

   A. Does not potentiate narcotics
   B. Provides calmness, tranquility
   C. Has potent antiemetic properties
   D. May lead to dysphoria

7. Anesthetics are being used routinely in ambulatory surgery settings **except** for which of the following?

   A. Methohexital (Brevital)
   B. Propofol (Diprivan)
   C. Ketamine (Ketolar)
   D. Etomidate (Amidate)

8. Which of the following drugs reverses the effects of the benzodiazepines?

   A. Diazepam (Valium)
   B. Midazolam (Versed)
   C. Iorazepam (Ativan)
   D. Flumazenil (Romazicon)

9. Which of the following is **not** a narcotic pain reliever?

   A. Morphine sulfate
   B. Ketorolac (Toradol)
   C. Hydromorphone (Dilaudid)
   D. Meperdine (Demerol)

10. Which of the following induction agents can be administered rectally to children, making its use feasible in ambulatory surgery?

    A. Ketamine (Ketalar)
    B. Methohexital sodium (Brevital)
    C. Propofol (Diprivan)
    D. Etomidate (Amidate)

ANSWERS TO QUESTIONS

1. A
2. C
3. B
4. A
5. D

6. A
7. C
8. D
9. B
10. B

2

Implementation of Nursing Standards

Jan Odom
Forrest General Hospital
Hattiesburg, Mississippi

Objectives

1. Define the term "standard" and identify standards applicable to the ambulatory surgery setting.
2. Explain the three types of standards.
3. Describe the ASPAN Standards of Perianesthesia Nursing Practice.
4. Discuss the Perianesthesia Scope of Practice and how it relates to the perianesthesia nurse in the ambulatory surgery setting.

I. **Definition of Standard**
   A. Established by authority, custom, or general consent as a model or example for measuring quality or quantity
   B. Must be the same for all persons
   C. Standard of care is determined by what a reasonably prudent nurse acting under the same circumstances would do
II. **Evolution of Nursing Standards**
   A. Before 1950
      1. Florence Nightingale
      2. Reports of court cases
   B. Code of Ethics published by American Nurses Association (ANA) in 1950—nurses offer care without prejudice and in a confidential and safe manner
   C. First generic standards for the profession established in 1973 by the ANA Congress for Nursing Practice
   D. Specialty standards followed beginning in 1974
III. **Sources of Standards**
   A. Accrediting organizations
      1. Joint Commission on Accreditation of Healthcare Organizations (JCAHO)
      2. Accreditation Association for Ambulatory Health Care (AAAHC)
   B. American Nurses Association (ANA)
   C. Hospital policies and procedures
   D. Specialty organizations
   E. Nursing texts and articles
   F. Common practice

IV. **Standard Criteria**
   A. Structure—designed to identify the administrative processes that need to be in existence and the framework that is required for an activity to take place (*example:* "Phase I and Phase II are separate and distinct areas.")
   B. Process—designed to reflect the actual activities that take place to assure that the standard is met (*example:* "Professional nurse—Phase II—assures the availability of safe transport of the patient to his/her home.")
   C. Outcome—designed to measure the results of activity (*example:* "Care meets the same standards of practice wherever the care is provided in the health-care organization.")
V. **ANA Standards of Clinical Practice** (generic in nature and apply to all registered nurses engaged in clinical practice)
   A. Standards of Care—describe a competent level of nursing care and delineate care that is provided to all patients
      1. Assessment—the process by which the nurse collects and analyzes data about the patient
      2. Diagnosis—a clinical judgment about a patient's response to actual or potential health conditions/needs
      3. Outcome Identification—measurable and expected, patient-focused goals
      4. Planning—outline of care to be delivered
      5. Implementation—implementation of intervention within the plan of care
      6. Evaluation—process of determining the patient's progress toward attaining goals and effectiveness of nursing care
   B. Standards of Professional Performance—describe a competent level of behavior in the professional role
      1. Quality of Care—evaluation of quality and effectiveness of nursing practice
      2. Performance Appraisal—nurse evaluates own nursing practice in relation to professional standards and regulations
      3. Education—nurse's current knowledge of nursing practice
      4. Collegiality—contributes to professional development of peers, colleagues, and others
      5. Ethics—nurse's decisions and actions determined in ethical manner
      6. Collaboration—nurse collaborates with patient, significant other, and health-care providers in providing care
      7. Research—nurse uses research findings in practice
      8. Resource Utilization—considers issues of safety, effectiveness, and cost in planning and delivering care
VI. **Agency for Health-Care Policy and Research (AHCPR)**
   A. Established in 1989 to enhance the quality, appropriateness, and effectiveness of health-care services and access to those services
   B. In 1992, released the first of a series of clinical practice guidelines: *Acute Pain Management: Operative Procedures*
   C. Standard of practice—implies that patients will receive care according to standard
   D. Guideline—designed to guide practitioners, patients, and consumers in decisions regarding health care
   E. For more information, write or call: AHCPR Publications Clearinghouse, P.O. Box 8547, Silver Springs, Maryland 20907; 1-800-358-9295
VII. **Standards of Perianesthesia Nursing Practice—1998**
   A. ASPAN history of standards
      1. 1983—*Guidelines for Standards of Care* published
      2. 1986—*Standards of Nursing Practice* published

    3. 1989—Definition of immediate postanesthesia nursing expanded to include preoperative and Phase II areas to incorporate ambulatory nurses working only in those areas

    4. 1991—*Standards of Post Anesthesia Nursing Practice* published; included data for initial, ongoing, and discharge assessment (Phase I and Phase II)

    5. 1992—*Standards of Post Anesthesia Nursing Practice* published

    6. 1995—*Standards of Perianesthesia Nursing Practice* published; included preanesthesia and postanesthesia information (preanesthesia or preprocedural, Phase I, and Phase II)

    7. 1998—*Standards of Perianesthesia Nursing Practice* revised

B. Perianesthesia Nursing Scope of Practice—defines perianesthesia scope of practice and identifies the characteristics within the unique specialty area; the ASPAN Scope of Practice uses the following framework:

    1. Core—addresses the essence of pre- and postanesthesia practice, the environment in which it occurs, and the consumers (*example:* environment includes PACUs, ambulatory care settings, preadmission testing, special procedures, dental offices, labor and delivery suites, and pain-management services)

    2. Dimensions—specify roles, behaviors, and processes inherent in perianesthesia practice and identify those characteristics unique to the specialty (*example:* characteristics unique to postanesthesia Phase II include a focus on preparing the patient to care for self or be cared for in an extended care facility)

    3. Boundaries—include those internal and external limits with sufficient flexibility and resilience to change in response to societal needs and demands (*example:* external boundaries include federal and state health codes and the Joint Commission for Accreditation of Healthcare Organizations; internal boundaries include ANA guidelines for practice and institutional policies and procedures)

    4. Intersections—describe the interface of perianesthesia nursing with other professional groups for the improvement of health care (*example:* American Board of PeriAnesthesia Nursing Certification (ABPANC), American Nurses Association (ANA), Association of Operating Room Nurses (AORN), American Society of Anesthesiologists (ASA), and American College of Surgeons (ACS)

C. Standards

    1. Standard I: Patient Rights and Ethics—"Perianesthesia nursing practice is based on philosophic and ethical concepts that recognize and maintain the autonomy, confidentiality, dignity and worth of individuals"

    2. Standard II: Environment—"Perianesthesia nursing practice promotes and maintains a safe, comfortable and therapeutic environment for patients, staff and visitors"

    3. Standard III: Personnel Management—"A sufficient number of qualified nursing staff with demonstrated competency in the provision of nursing care . . . are available to meet the individual needs of patients and families"

    4. Standard IV: Continuous Quality Improvement—"Perianesthesia nursing practice is monitored and evaluated on an ongoing basis"

    5. Standard V: Research—"Perianesthesia nurses participate in research designed to improve patient care"

    6. Standard VI: Multidisciplinary Collaboration—" . . . [F]acilitate continuity of care by assuring that the needs of patients and families are recognized and addressed through coordination with other health team members"

    7. Standard VII: Assessment—"Perianesthesia nursing practice includes the systematic and continuous assessment of the patient's condition"

8. Standard VIII: Planning and Implementation—"The professional nurse designs and coordinates the implementation of a plan of care to achieve optimal patient outcomes"
9. Standard IX: Evaluation—"The professional nurse continuously measures the patient's progress toward the desired outcomes and revises the plan of care and interventions as necessary"
10. Standard X: Advanced Cardiac Life Support (ACLS)—"Perianesthesia nursing practice involves autonomous decision-making and implementation of interventions in a crisis situation . . . completion of an ACLS course or the equivalent is a necessary component"
11. Standard XI: Pain Management—"Perianesthesia nursing practice utilizes established modalities of pain management to assist the patient toward optimal comfort"

D. Resources
1. American Hospital Association (AHA) *A Patient's Bill of Rights*
2. American Nurses Association (ANA) *Code for Nurses*
3. Patient Classification/Recommended Staffing Guidelines
4. Data Required for Initial, Ongoing, and Discharge Assessment
   a. Preadmission
   b. Day of Surgery/Procedure
   c. Phase I
   d. Initial Assessment: Phase I
   e. Ongoing Assessment: Phase I
   f. Discharge Assessment: Phase I
   g. Initial Assessment Phase II
   h. Ongoing Assessment: Phase II
   i. Discharge Assessment: Phase II
   j. Initial/Ongoing/Discharge Assessment: Phase III
5. Recommended Equipment for Preanesthesia Phase, PACU Phase I, Phase II, and Phase III
6. ACLS/PALS and Equivalent
7. Emergency Drugs and Equipment
8. American Society of Anesthesiologists (ASA) *Standards*
   a. Statement on Routine Preoperative Laboratory and Diagnostic Screening
   b. ASA Basic Standards for Preanesthesia Care
   c. ASA Standards for Postanesthesia Care
9. Latex Allergy
10. Agency for Health Care Policy and Research: *Abbreviated Acute Pain Management Flowchart*
11. Critical Elements for the Competent Perianesthesia RN and LPN
12. Competent Support Staff
13. Joint Statement of ASPAN and ASA: "Use of Support Personnel in the Postanesthesia Care Units and Ambulatory Care Units"
14. ANA Position Statement: "Role of the Registered Nurse in the Management of Analgesia by Catheter Techniques (Epidural, Intrathecal, Intrapleural or Peripheral Nerve Catheters)"
14a. Association of Women's Health, Obstetrics and Neonatal Nurses (AWHONN) Position Statement: "Role of the Registered Nurse (RN) in the Management of the Patient Receiving Analgesia by Catheter Techniques (Epidural, Intrathecal, Intrapleural or Peripheral Nerve Catheters)"

15. ANA Position Statement: "Role of the Registered Nurse in the Management of Patients Receiving IV conscious Sedation for Short-Term, Therapeutic, Diagnostic or Surgical Procedures"

E. Competency Based Practice
   1. Mission Statement
   2. Resources
      a. Competency Based Orientation and Credentialing Program (1997 Edition)
      b. Example: Basic Airway Management Competency
      c. Example: Advanced Airway Management Competency

F. ASPAN Position Statements
   1. A Position Statement on Entry into Nursing Practice
   2. A Position Statement on Air Safety in the Perianesthesia Environment
   3. A Position Statement on the Perianesthesia Patient with a Do-Not-Resuscitate Advanced Directive
   4. A Position Statement on Perianesthesia Advanced Practice Nursing
   5. A Position Statement on Minimum Staffing in Phase I PACU
   6. A Position Statement on Registered Nurse Utilization of Unlicensed Assistive Personnel
   7. A Position Statement on ICU Overflow Patients

G. Obtain a copy of *Standards of Perianesthesia Nursing Practice 1998* by calling or writing: ASPAN, 6900 Grove Road, Thorofare, New Jersey 08086; 609-845-5557; Fax 609-848-5274

Bibliography

1. Accreditation Association for Ambulatory Health Care. (1996). *Accreditation Handbook for Ambulatory Health Care.* Skokie, IL: AAAHC.
2. American Nurses Association. (1991). *Standards of Clinical Nursing Practice.* Kansas City: ANA.
3. American Society of PeriAnesthesia Nurses. (1998). *Standards of PeriAnesthesia Nursing Practice 1998.* Thorofare, NJ: ASPAN.
4. Association of Operating Room Nurses, Inc. (1996). *Standards and Recommended Practices.* Denver: AORN.
5. Brent, N.J. (1997). *Nurses and the Law: A Guide to Principles and Applications.* Philadelphia: Saunders.
6. Buss, H. (1993). Continuous quality improvement: Adaptation of the 10-step model with postanesthesia care unit application. *J Post Anesth Nurs,* 8:238–248.
7. Guido, G.W. (1997). *Legal Issues in Nursing,* 2nd ed. Stanford, CT: Appleton & Lange.
8. Joint Commission for Accreditation of Healthcare Organizations. (1996). *Accreditation Manual for Ambulatory Health Care (AMAHC).* Oakbrook Terrace, IL: JCAHO.
9. Litwack, K. (1995). *Core Curriculum for Post Anesthesia Nursing Practice,* 3rd ed. Philadelphia: Saunders.
10. Mamaril, M. (1993). Standard of care: Legal implications in the postanesthesia care unit. *J Post Anesth Nurs.* 8:13–20.
11. Pritchard, V., Eckard, J.M. (1990). Standards of nursing care in the post anesthesia unit. *J Post Anesth Nurs,* 5:163–167.
12. Springhouse Corporation. (1992). *Nurse's Handbook of Law and Ethics.* Springhouse, PA: Springhouse.

REVIEW QUESTIONS

1. Standards related to the organization of the ambulatory surgery center are:

   A. Structure standards
   B. Process standards
   C. Outcome standards
   D. Care plans

2. An example of a process standard of care for the ambulatory nurse is:

   A. Chain of command
   B. Management of the ambulatory surgery patient
   C. Discharge criteria for the patient
   D. Responsibility for the procurement of equipment

3. Sources of nursing standards of care for the ambulatory patient include all but one of the following:

   A. American Nurses Association
   B. Joint Commission on Accreditation of Healthcare Organizations
   C. American Medical Association
   D. Common practice
   E. Hospital Policy

4. A standard is:

   A. Defined by each hospital's policies
   B. A model that is external and objective that measures quantity or quality
   C. Applied differently to new nurses from experienced nurses
   D. Not often used in a court of law

5. An example of an outcome standard is:

   A. The tympanic thermometer will be calibrated once a month
   B. The patient's temperature upon discharge will be at least 96 degrees Fahrenheit
   C. The patient's temperature will be taken on admission, at 30 minutes, and at discharge
   D. Forced warm air therapy will be instituted on all patients whose temperature is less than 95.5 degrees Fahrenheit

6. ASPAN first published its "Guidelines for Standards of Care" in

   A. 1983
   B. 1980
   C. 1995
   D. 1989
   E. 1986

7. ASPAN's Standards of Perianesthesia Nursing Practice may not apply to the following setting:

   A. PACU
   B. Holding Room
   C. Labor & Delivery
   D. Endoscopy
   E. Oncology unit

8. Standards of Professional Performance include:

   A. Research
   B. Performance appraisal
   C. Education
   D. Ethics
   E. All of the above

9. Standards of Care:

   A. Are implemented daily in all aspects of patient care
   B. Are criteria for determining if less than adequate care was delivered to the patient
   C. Are the minimal level of expertise that must be delivered to the patient
   D. All of the above

10. The Perianesthesia standard that states: "Professional nursing practice in Phase I reflects competency in ACLS or the equivalent educational process" is what kind of standard?

    A. Structure
    B. Process
    C. Professional
    D. Outcome

ANSWERS TO QUESTIONS

1. A
2. B
3. C
4. B
5. B

6. A
7. E
8. E
9. D
10. B

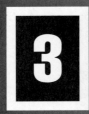

Nursing Research

Susan Jane Fetzer
University of New Hampshire
Elliot Hospital
Manchester, New Hampshire

I. **Purpose of Nursing Research**
   A. Expand the body of nursing knowledge in ambulatory perianesthesia patient care
   B. Validate interventions used by ambulatory perianesthesia nurses
   C. Define the unique contribution of the ambulatory perianesthesia nursing specialty
   D. Uncover perianesthesia phenomenon not previously realized
   E. Develop and test theories able to explain, predict, and control perianesthesia nursing practice and patient outcomes
   F. Substantiate the unique contribution of ambulatory perianesthesia nurses as health-care providers
II. **Goal of Nursing Research**
   A. Maximize patient outcomes from nursing interventions
   B. Establish a unique body of knowledge for ambulatory perianesthesia nursing
   C. Maximize effectiveness and efficiency of ambulatory perianesthesia nursing care delivery
III. **Developing and Planning a Research Study**
   A. Proposal development
      1. A proposal is the plan the researcher intends to implement to answer the research question or support the research hypothesis
      2. Precedes the implementation of a research study
      3. Contains steps listed below

B. Problem statement
1. Dilemma or situation that requires resolution by scientific inquiry and the development of new knowledge
2. Situation that has not been satisfactorily resolved by past research studies or exists as a knowledge gap in the nursing literature
3. One- or two-sentence statement at the beginning of a research report that introduces the topic to the reader
4. Examples of ambulatory perianesthesia nursing problems
   a. Effectiveness of audiovisual preoperative teaching materials
   b. Appropriate scheduling of preadmission visits
   c. Use of unlicensed personnel in freestanding ambulatory centers
   d. Role of registered nurse during conscious sedation
   e. Validity of discharge criteria for regional anesthesia patients
   f. Effectiveness of postoperative telephone calls in measuring patient outcomes
   g. Patient compliance with preoperative fasting guidelines
   h. Effect of the duration of NPO status on discharge guidelines for postoperative voiding
   i. Maintenance of ACLS competency in ambulatory perianesthesia nurses
   j. Cost effectiveness of preoperative pediatric tours on day of surgery anxiety and behaviors
C. Purpose statement
1. The purpose statement provides a direction the researcher will take to solve the research problem
2. Includes the extent of the research project and the clinical context in which the researcher is interested
3. Presents as one sentence that clarifies and provides the specific reason for the research
4. Examples of ambulatory perianesthesia nursing purpose statements
   a. Compare the effectiveness of a preoperative teaching take-home video with face-to-face preoperative teaching in patients who have carpel tunnel surgery
   b. Determine the optimum time for preadmission screening of Type 1 diabetics
   c. Describe elderly patients' attitudes toward care received from unlicensed personnel during the perianesthesia period
   d. Describe the educational requirements for registered nurses administering conscious sedation in a freestanding surgical center
   e. Examine the relationship between preoperative temperature and postoperative temperature in patients receiving intravenous ketorolac
   f. Determine the reasons for lack of contact during postoperative follow-up phone calls
   g. Determine the effect of written instruction on patient compliance with NPO guidelines
   h. Describe the effect of NPO duration and fluid replacement on ability of cystoscopy patients to meet postoperative voiding requirements for discharge
   i. Determine the effect of biannual ACLS reviews on ambulatory perianesthesia nurses' resuscitation self-efficacy
   j. Identify the effect of pediatric preoperative tours on child and parent admission anxiety
D. Review of literature
1. The review of literature presents and clarifies what is known and not known on the research topic
2. The researcher seeks out available solutions to the research problem in the existing literature before planning the study

    3. Includes a written summary of previous research related to the study problem and purpose

    4. Provides the reader with a comprehensive background on the research topic

E. Research question/hypothesis

    1. Research questions and/or hypotheses serve to narrow and focus the study purpose

    2. Research question

       a. An interrogative statement posed by the researcher when little is known about the topic

       b. Question posed when there is insufficient past research to predict a relationship between two characteristics (variables) or an effect of one variable on another

       c. Components of a research question include the group to be studied and the characteristics (variables) under investigation

       d. Examples of ambulatory perianesthesia nursing research questions

         i. What is the best method of delivering preoperative information to cataract patients?

         ii. What is the effect of a greater than three-day delay from preadmission visit to day of surgery on ambulatory surgery patient preoperative anxiety?

         iii. What is the ambulatory patient's perception of competency of unlicensed personnel?

         iv. What are the educational characteristics of RNs administering conscious sedation?

         v. What is the effect of ketorolac on discharge temperature of elderly patients?

         vi. What is the most frequent reason for inability to contact patients by phone for discharge follow-up?

         vii. What are the characteristics of patients who do not comply with fasting limits (e.g., NPO) preoperatively?

         viii. What is the optimum fluid replacement volume to promote postoperative voiding in cystoscopy patients?

         ix. What are the factors associated with ambulatory perianesthesia nurse's proficiency with cardiopulmonary resuscitation?

         x. How do parents describe the effect of pediatric preoperative tours on the child's behavior?

    3. Research hypothesis

       a. A formal declaration of an expected relationship or cause and effect between two characteristics (variables) made by the researcher based on established theory and/or past research

       b. Statement that offers a potential solution to the research problem which can be supported by the existing literature and the researcher's experience

       c. The hypothesis is always determined prior to the study and offers a framework for the research methodology

       d. The hypothesis includes the group being studied, the characteristics (variables) to be studied, and the direction of the expected relationship (e.g., positive, negative, increased, decreased)

       e. Examples of ambulatory perianesthesia nursing research hypotheses

         i. Cataract patients who are provided with face-to-face preoperative education will remember more information than cataract patients who are given an audiovisual preoperative video

    ii. Patients scheduled for breast biopsy will report more anxiety if the time between preadmission interview and day of surgery is longer than three days

    iii. Ambulatory surgery patients will report more satisfaction with care when assigned a registered nurse than those assigned an unlicensed health-care provider

    iv. Ambulatory perianesthesia nurses with critical-care experience will report greater comfort administering conscious sedation than ambulatory perianesthesia nurses with medical-surgical experience

    v. Ambulatory surgery patients who receive ketorolac will have a lower discharge temperature than patients who receive acetaminophen compounds for pain

    vi. Discharge assessment phone calls placed after 5:00 P.M. will be more successful than phone calls placed before 5:00 P.M.

    vii. There is a positive relationship between patient educational level and compliance with NPO guidelines

    viii. There is a negative relationship between duration of preoperative NPO status and ability to void prior to discharge in cystoscopy patients

    ix. Ambulatory perianesthesia nurses who participate in a 6-month ACLS review course will hold greater resuscitation self-efficacy than those who do not participate

    x. Pediatric patients who participate in preoperative pediatric tours will recover faster than patients who do not participate

4. Variables

  a. Any quality or characteristic that is likely to change and/or is observed or measured by the researcher

  b. The independent variable is a characteristic selected by the researcher and believed to effect another characteristic (i.e., dependent variable)

  c. The dependent variable is the characteristic believed by the researcher to change when the independent variable is changed

  d. The independent variable is the cause or antecedent; the dependent variable is the effect or outcome

  e. Demographic variables are characteristics of the group (e.g., patients) being measured (i.e., gender, age, type of anesthesia, type of surgery, height, weight)

  f. The independent, dependent, and demographic variables require definition and measurement by the researcher; other characteristics, which may impact the research study, should be controlled

  g. The independent and dependent variables are found in the purpose statement and the research question or the hypothesis

  h. Examples of ambulatory perianesthesia nursing variables of interest

    i. Type of preoperative teaching strategy (e.g., face to face, video)

    ii. Timing of preadmission visits (e.g., 2 days preop, day of surgery)

    iii. Licensure of health-care providers (e.g., CRNA, RN)

    iv. Educational level of registered nurses (e.g., AD, BSN)

    v. Postoperative temperature (e.g., 36.5°C, 37.0°C)

    vi. Timing of discharge follow-up phone call (e.g., 5:00 P.M., 7:00 P.M.)

    vii. Compliance with NPO guidelines (e.g., NPO after midnight, NPO 4 hours prior to surgery)

    viii. Volume of intraoperative fluid replacement (e.g., 125cc/hr, 100cc/hr)

    ix. Self-efficacy of nurse resuscitation (e.g., novice, competent)

    x. Anxiety behavior of pediatric patients postoperatively (e.g., moderate, extreme)

        i. Examples linking independent (IV) and dependent variables (DV) of interest to ambulatory perianesthesia nursing
- i. Type of teaching strategy (IV) and preoperative knowledge using a posttest score (DV)
- ii. Time of preadmission visit (IV) and anxiety behavior (DV)
- iii. Type of health-care provider (IV) and patient satisfaction (DV)
- iv. Education of RN provider (IV) and amount of conscious sedation administered (DV)
- v. Use of ketorolac (IV) and discharge temperature (DV)
- vi. Postoperative phone call (IV) and patient satisfaction (DV)
- vii. Patient educational level (IV) and compliance with NPO guidelines (DV)
- viii. Volume of intraoperative IV fluids (DV) and time to void postoperatively (DV)
- ix. Frequency of ACLS education programs (IV) and nurse self-efficacy of resuscitation (DV)
- x. Use of pediatric tours (IV) and child anxiety behavior upon discharge (DV)

IV. Conducting a Research Project
  A. Methodology
1. Research methodology is the blueprint or plan taken by the researcher to collect the data required to answer the research question or support the research hypothesis
2. Research procedures requires decisions by the researcher that may affect the research results
3. The researcher seeks to design the methodology so that the findings will have implications for nursing in general, not just the group being studied (e.g., generalizability)

  B. Research design
1. The research design selected by the researcher depends on the purpose of the study and the research question or hypothesis
   - a. A qualitative research design focuses on the perianesthesia experience from the perspective of the patient
     - i. Emphasis is on the holistic approach to the patient
     - ii. Seeks to examine meaning and insight into a patient's experience
     - iii. Used when previous research on the topic is limited or absent
     - iv. Data is collected using words and narratives of patients
     - v. Examples of topics using qualitative research designs in ambulatory perianesthesia nursing
       - (a) Patient's account of the experience of postanesthetic shivering
       - (b) A narrative response to inquiry about satisfaction with caregivers
       - (c) Experience of parents during the child's surgery
       - (d) One patient's account of midazolam-induced amnesia
       - (e) Nurse's feelings about resuscitation failures
   - b. A quantitative research design focuses on one part of the patient's experience
     - i. Emphasis is placed on one or two selected variables of interest to the researcher
     - ii. Used when a variable is in need of description (e.g., Descriptive Research), a relationship is being examined (e.g., Correlational Research), or cause and effect is being tested (e.g., Experimental Research)
     - iii. Data collected for quantitative research can be reduced to numbers for statistical analysis

iv. Examples of topics using quantitative research designs in ambulatory perianesthesia nursing
   (a) Characteristics of patients who fail to follow preoperative instructions (Descriptive Research)
   (b) Relationship between fluid volume replacement intraoperatively and incidence of postoperative nausea (Correlational Research)
   (c) Effect of pediatric tours on parental anxiety (Experimental Research)
   (d) Effect of ketorolac on discharge temperature (Experimental Research)
   (e) Effect of surgery facility (freestanding versus hospital based) on patient satisfaction (Experimental Research)

C. Research sample
   1. Is composed of individuals (i.e., patients, nurses, and family members) who agree to participate in a research study
   2. Is selected so that the individuals are representative of all the individuals who are known to have the variable(s) of interest to the researcher
   3. The size of the sample, or number of individuals included, depends on
      a. The research design used
      b. Number of variables being studied
      c. The type of variables being studied
      d. The statistical analysis selected
   4. Examples of selection criteria for an ambulatory perianesthesia nursing research sample
      a. 50 male patients having regional anesthesia for hernioraphy
      b. All cataract patients requiring conscious sedation during the month of June
      c. Every other adult patient on the ambulatory surgical schedule who is not allergic to aspirin
      d. Children from 3 to 7 years old who are accompanied by a parent
      e. Registered nurses, certified in ambulatory perianesthesia nursing (CAPA), who work full time in a freestanding surgical center in New Hampshire

D. Research setting
   1. Represents the environment where the data for the study will be collected
   2. A detailed description of the setting allows the reader to determine if the research environment is similar to the reader's environment and the findings are applicable to the reader's practice
   3. Examples of an ambulatory perianesthesia nursing research setting
      a. Waiting area of preadmission testing department
      b. Phase I PACU of a freestanding ambulatory facility with four operating suites
      c. Hospital-based surgery center caring for 30 pediatric surgical cases per week
      d. Operating room with temperature controlled at 60 degrees and humidity of 75%
      e. Waiting area of the surgeon's office

E. Research instrument
   1. Is any device (e.g., monitor, questionnaire, interview) that produces or records data required by the research project
   2. Selection of the instrument depends on the variable being studied, the availability of the instrument, the expertise of the researcher, and the subject's capabilities
   3. The instrument should be able to actually measure what the researcher intends (i.e., be a valid representation of the variable)
   4. The instrument should be able to collect consistent measurements of the variable being studied (i.e., be a reliable representation of the variable)

      5. The researcher must establish the instrument's reliability and validity for the study before data is collected

      6. Examples of ambulatory perianesthesia nursing research instruments

        a. Visual Analog Pain Scale (VAS)

        b. Tympanic thermometer in core mode

        c. Speilberger's State-Trait Anxiety Questionnaire

        d. Anesthesia Record of the Ambulatory Surgery Center

        e. Postanesthesia discharge criteria modified by Aldrete

  F. Research procedure

    1. Consists of a description of the steps taken to implement research data collection including the selection of the sample, the identification of the setting, the administration of the research instrument, and any protocols for the independent variable

    2. Is provided in sufficient detail to allow the study to be replicated (repeated with a different group of participants) by other researchers

  G. Data analysis methods

    1. Data analyses are the procedures used to analyze the data

      a. Statistical analysis can include descriptive procedures, correlational procedures, or tests of hypotheses

      b. The statistical procedure selected is based on the type of data collected and the format of hypothesis

      c. Statistical experts are consulted to determine the appropriate statistical procedures

V. Reporting the Results of a Research Project

  A. Discussion of research findings

    1. The results of the data analysis are provided with an interpretation of their meaning

    2. The findings are presented in the order of the research questions or hypotheses

    3. Findings are presented that answer the research question or support/reject the hypothesis

    4. Other research that supports or refutes the study results is discussed from the perspective of the researcher's findings

    5. Examples of ambulatory perianesthesia nursing research findings

      a. Findings from this study indicated that face-to-face preoperative instructions improve posttest scores significantly more than video teaching

      b. Findings of this study revealed that two days prior to surgical intervention is the appropriate time for a preadmission interview

      c. Findings from this study did not identify a difference in patient satisfaction between care delivered by unlicensed providers and licensed providers

      d. Findings from this study indicated no difference in postoperative temperature between patients who received ketorolac and patients who received acetaminophen

      e. Findings from this study showed that postoperative follow-up phone calls made in the afternoon were more successful than those made in the morning

  B. Conclusions

    1. New knowledge revealed by the research findings is summarized into one or two specific statements in the conclusion

    2. The conclusion attempts to answer the research problem presented at the beginning of the study

    3. Examples of ambulatory perianesthesia nursing research conclusions

      a. The findings of the study support the conclusion that patients who receive face-to-face preoperative teaching learn better

     b. The conclusion of this study is that the timing of preoperative visits can impact patient anxiety related to their surgical experience

     c. The conclusion of this study is that level of patient education is a predictor of compliance with NPO guidelines

     d. The research findings support the conclusion that pediatric preoperative tours reduce parental anxiety but have no affect on child anxiety prior to discharge

     e. The findings of the study support the conclusion that a nurse's education is related to the amount and type of drugs administered during conscious sedation

  C. Implications for practice

    1. The researcher suggests ways the research conclusions could be utilized in nursing practice, nursing education, nursing administration, or by future researchers

    2. Implications for practice translate the research findings into usable interventions to improve patient outcomes

    3. At least one implication is reported for each research conclusion

    4. Examples of ambulatory perianesthesia nursing research implications

     a. The study suggests that preoperative teaching be conducted by trained ambulatory surgical nurses during individualized face-to-face sessions

     b. The study findings suggest that preadmission visits should be scheduled a maximum of two days before the day of surgery

     c. The study findings recommend that NPO guidelines be explained based on the patient's educational level

     d. The study findings suggest that parental tours may be just as effective as pediatric tours in reducing postoperative anxiety behaviors of children

     e. The researcher recommends that the study be repeated using male and female patients of a wide range of ages

VI. Ethical Issues in Nursing Research

  A. The researcher is required to protect the vulnerable patient from harmful effects and to ensure that participant benefits outweigh risks of participating in the research

  B. Ethical research behaviors include objectivity, cooperation with institutional guidelines, integrity, and honesty

  C. Any research on human subjects requires review and approval by an Institutional Review Board (IRB) or Human Subjects Committee

    1. Composition of the IRB includes nurses, physicians, and other health-care professionals; clergy, community members, attorneys, and ethicists also participate on the IRB

    2. The IRB independently determines the ethical implications of the research methodology

  D. The research methodology provides for participant's informed consent either in writing or verbally

  E. Ambulatory perianesthesia nurses participating in nursing research are responsible for:

    1. Being aware of the research purpose and methodology

    2. Validating that the research project has undergone independent review

    3. Advocating for the participant's informed consent

    4. Supporting the research method where possible

VII. Quality Improvement and the Research Process

  A. Quality improvement (i.e., QA, TQI, and TQM) projects are designed to measure performance against pre-established criteria

    1. Permission for project is granted by institution's administration

      2. Purpose is to solve problem or improve current practice

      3. Does not use research questions or hypotheses

      4. Does not require a review of literature

      5. Sample is not representative of entire population

      6. Setting may not be representative of other facilities

      7. Instrument can be a questionnaire or data-collection device developed by the project coordinators

      8. Methodology is not controlled for influencing variables

      9. Reliability and validity of instrument is not required

     10. Conclusions are pertinent to the institution being monitored

     11. Findings will not be published in research journals

  B. Nursing research is the process of applying the scientific method to answer questions of interest about nursing practice, nursing education, and nursing administration

      1. Approval from the IRB to conduct the nursing research is required

      2. Purpose of research is to solve a problem by discovering new knowledge

      3. A research question or hypothesis is proposed that directs the study

      4. Review of literature is conducted to place study within existing knowledge

      5. Selection of sample requires consideration of characteristics of the entire population

      6. Selection of setting requires consideration of characteristics of similar settings

      7. Instrument is tested for reliability and validity before collecting data

      8. Methodology is clearly explained so that it can be replicated by future researchers

      9. Discussion of data includes reference to the literature and knowledge already available

     10. Conclusions represent the generation of new knowledge

VIII. Utilization of Research Findings

  A. Research findings can be located in a variety of sources

  B. Sources of ambulatory perianesthesia nursing research include:

      1. Poster displays at national and local conferences and meetings of professional organizations

      2. Oral presentations at continuing education meetings

      3. Local and national publications

         a. *Journal of PeriAnesthesia Nursing (JOPAN)*

         b. *Breathline*

         c. *AORN Journal*

         d. *Perianesthesia and Ambulatory Surgical Nursing Update*

  C. Communicating research to colleagues

      1. An Ambulatory Surgical Nursing Journal Club can be used to communicate findings to colleagues

         a. A journal club is composed of a group of nurses who meet regularly to discuss and analyze research related to their practice

         b. Familiarizes colleagues with a wide variety of publications and research issues

      2. Policy and Procedure Committee utilizes research findings

         a. Applies research conclusions to standard of care in the institution

         b. Notes procedures that are research based by including references of research studies

         c. Revises policies and procedures as new knowledge is discovered by nurse researchers

D. Professional responsibility
  1. Nurses have a professional responsibility to maintain practice currency by reading, discussing, and participating in ambulatory perianesthesia nursing research
  2. Research utilization should be included in all professional job descriptions

Bibliography

1. Burns, N., Grove, S.K. (1996). *The Practice of Nursing Research: Conduct Critique and Utilization*, 2nd ed. Philadelphia: Saunders.
2. Fetzer, S.J., Vogelsang, J. (1996). *Research Primer for Perianesthesia Nurses*. Thorofare, NJ: ASPAN.
3. Grant, J.S., Davis, L.L., Kinney, M.R. (1993). Criteria for critiquing clinical nursing research reports. *JOPAN*, 8:163–171.
4. Massey, V.H. (1995). *Nursing Research: A Study and Learning Tool*. Springhouse, PA: Springhouse.
5. Tournquist, E.M., Funk, S.G., Champagne, M.T., Wise, R.A. (1993). Advice on reading research: Overcoming the barriers. *Applied Nursing Research*, 6:177–183.

REVIEW QUESTIONS

1. The first step in developing a research proposal is to:

   A. Conduct a library review of literature
   B. Determine the situation requiring scientific inquiry
   C. State a research question
   D. Select a group of patients to study

2. In order to narrow the research study purpose, the researcher develops a:

   A. Problem statement
   B. Data questionnaire
   C. Research methodology
   D. Research question

3. Which of the following is **not** an example of a variable?

   A. Amount of narcotic used
   B. Body surface area
   C. Type of surgery
   D. Anesthesia flow sheet

4. When participating as a data collector for an ambulatory perianesthesia nursing research study, the nurse should:

   A. Provide the patient with informed consent
   B. Change the study protocol if necessary
   C. Verify that IRB approval has been obtained
   D. Question the selection of the sample participants

5. The purpose of an Ambulatory Surgical Nursing Journal Club is to:

   A. Produce manuscripts for journal publication
   B. Review published research pertinent to the specialty
   C. Revise procedures to reflect published research findings
   D. Critique publications for institutional purchase

6. A research hypothesis is proposed when the researcher:

   A. Has support from the existing literature
   B. Has little information on the research problem
   C. Seeks IRB approval for the study
   D. Wishes to expand the purpose of the study

7. Quality-improvement projects differ from nursing research projects because quality-improvement projects:

   A. Are conducted in several units simultaneously
   B. Do not require control of all variables
   C. Require a smaller sample
   D. Use reliable questionnaires

8. Institutional review and approval of a research study assures that the:

   A. Nurse researcher is honest and ethical
   B. Participant benefits outweigh the risks
   C. Study will develop new knowledge
   D. Study will adhere to current policies

9. Which step of the research process is **not** found in a quality-improvement project?

   A. Conclusion
   B. Data analysis
   C. IRB approval
   D. Purpose statement

10. Which of the following is an example of a quality-improvement project?

    A. Description of patient's response to spinal anesthesia
    B. Compliance with temperature documentation at Doctor's Regional Surgical Center
    C. Relationship between ketorolac and nausea in laproscopic patients
    D. Effect of music on preoperative anxiety

ANSWERS TO QUESTIONS

1. B
2. D
3. D
4. C
5. B

6. A
7. B
8. B
9. C
10. B

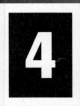

4

Legal and Ethical Issues

Jan Odom
Forrest General Hospital
Hattiesburg, Mississippi

1. Identify at least five common causes of nursing liability.
2. Discuss methods for prevention of a malpractice suit.
3. List and describe the four elements of negligence.
4. Discuss phases of litigation that can occur with a malpractice suit.
5. Identify four important ethical principles.
6. Discuss the steps applicable to an ethical decision-making process.

LEGAL TERMINOLOGY

Assault   An attempt or threat that causes a person to fear physical touch or injury

Battery   The unauthorized touching of an individual's body, any extension of it, or anything attached to it in an offensive or injurious manner

Defendant   Person or entity against whom plaintiff's allegations are made

Expert Witness   A person who serves to educate the court and jury about the subject under consideration, including the appropriate standard of care

Malpractice (Professional Negligence)   A type of negligence that involves a standard of care that can be reasonably expected from professionals, e.g., attorneys, nurses, physicians, accountants; failure to act as a reasonably prudent nurse would act under similar circumstances

Negligence   Deviation from the standard of care that a reasonable person would use in a certain set of circumstances

Plaintiff   The person or party who brings the lawsuit and alleges harm

LEGAL CONCEPTS

I. **Sources of Law**
   A. Constitutional—system of laws for governance of a nation; may be federal or state
   B. Statutory—made by the legislative branch of the government

   C. Administrative—laws enacted by administrative agencies charged with implementing particular legislation
   D. Judicial—laws made by the courts that interpret legal issues that are in dispute

II. **Types of Law**
   A. Common law—derived from principles rather than rules and regulations
   B. Civil law—based on rules and regulations
      1. Administered through courts as damages or money compensation
      2. Most important area is *tort* law which involves compensation to those wrongfully injured
   C. Criminal law—conduct that is offensive or harmful to society as a whole
   D. Substantive law—concerns the wrong, harm, or duty that caused the lawsuit
   E. Procedural law—concerns the process and rights of the individual charged with violating substantive law

III. **Negligence Law**
   A. Tort law—a civil wrong that allows the injured party to seek reparation; concerns any action or omission that harms someone
      1. Negligence
      2. Malpractice
      3. Assault and battery
      4. Invasion of privacy
      5. False imprisonment
      6. Defamation
   B. Essential elements of professional negligence (malpractice)
      1. Duty—once you, as a nurse, undertake the care of a patient, you are under a duty to act in accordance with the standard of care
      2. Breach of Duty—failure to act in accordance with the standard of care
         a. May be an act of omission
         b. May be an act of commission
      3. Causation—plaintiff must prove that the breach of duty was the cause of damages
         a. Most difficult element to prove
      4. Damages—actual loss or damages must be established
   C. Employer liability
      1. Respondant superior—employer is vicariously liable for negligent acts of employee if the act occurred during an employment relationship and within part of the employee's job responsibilities
      2. Corporate liability—health-care delivery system can be sued when it breaches any direct duty to the patient
   D. *Res ipsa loquitur*—"the thing speaks for itself"; a rule of evidence that allows a supposition of negligence on the part of the defendant
      1. Defendant must be solely in control at the time injury occurred and injury would not have occurred if defendant had exercised due care
      2. Plaintiff must have done nothing to contribute to negligence, e.g., foreign object left inside patient after surgery
   E. Intentional torts—intent is necessary and there must be a willful action against the injured person
      1. Assault—an action that causes apprehension or unwarranted touching
      2. Battery—unauthorized touching of one person by another, e.g., lack of consent for treatment
      3. False imprisonment—unjustifiable detention of a person without a legal warrant
   F. Quasi-intentional torts
      1. Invasion of privacy—patient's right to privacy is recognized
      2. Defamation—wrongful injury to another's reputation

G. Standards of care—minimal requirements that define an acceptable level of care
   1. May be established by:
      a. State Nurse Practice Act
      b. Federal agency guidelines and regulations
      c. American Nurses Association (ANA)
      d. American Society of PeriAnesthesia Nurses (ASPAN) or other national specialty organization
      e. Joint Commission on Accreditation of Healthcare Organizations (JCAHO) or other accrediting bodies, such as Accreditation Association for Ambulatory Health Care (AAAHC)
      f. Hospital or ambulatory surgery facility rules and procedures
      g. State Board of Nursing
      h. Common practice
      i. Nursing texts and articles
   2. Determined by expert witnesses for judicial system
      a. Essential in professional negligence cases

LIABILITY ISSUES

I. **Possible Causes of Nursing Liability for the Ambulatory Surgical Nurse**
   A. Failure to adequately monitor a patient
   B. Errors in the use of equipment
   C. Errors in medication or treatment
   D. Failure to communicate
      1. To another nurse
      2. Changes in patient condition to a physician
   E. Patient falls
   F. Operating Room errors (*example:* sponges/instruments left inside patient)
   G. Mix-ups during patient transfers (*example:* wrong surgery on patient)
   H. Failure to report or act on deviations from accepted practice
      1. Nurses expected to exercise independent judgment and object when physician's orders are inappropriate
      2. Report facts to manager or otherwise follow chain-of-command
   I. Failure to follow a physician's order promptly and accurately
   J. Failure to follow institutional/facility procedures
   K. Patients who are HIV positive
      1. Discrimination in treatment
      2. Nosocomial transmission
      3. Breach of confidentiality
      4. Participation in testing without informed consent
   L. Failure to properly teach patient or caregiver accurate and appropriate discharge instructions
      1. Should receive discharge instructions before admission/surgery
      2. Use preprinted discharge instructions
      3. Give verbal and written instructions
   M. Premature discharge for the ambulatory surgery patient
   N. Failure to ensure the presence of an informed caregiver (responsible adult)
   O. Failure to assess the ambulatory surgery patient on admission, e.g., NPO status, any signs or symptoms that might affect reaction to anesthesia or surgery, medication use that day

II. Prevention of Liability
  A. Documentation
    1. Accurate and comprehensive documentation essential
    2. Purposes of documentation
      a. To communicate the patient's condition to other health professionals
      b. To obtain reimbursement—from the government and insurance
      c. As a legal record
      d. To use as data for quality-of-care review
    3. Nurses' notes first place an attorney will look
      a. Written with time and date and in chronological order
      b. Contains most detailed information regarding the patient
    4. Rules to follow:
      a. Chart accurately
        i. It is very difficult to prove that something was done if it is not charted
        ii. On the other hand, deliberate inaccuracies can totally destroy defense and expose nurse to criminal charges of fraud
      b. Chart objectively
        i. Describe only what you observe
        ii. Do not use words such as "seems," "apparently," or "appears"
      c. Write legibly and use standard abbreviations adopted by the health-care facility
      d. Do not use the chart to criticize or complain
        i. Use other appropriate avenues if there is criticism of another nurse
      e. Do not destroy or obliterate documentation
        i. Do not use Black-out,™ White-out,™ or any other kind of eradicator
        ii. Draw one line through the error, initial, and date the line
      f. Do not leave vacant lines; sign every entry
      g. Chart as promptly as possible after the care is given
      h. Correct grammar, spelling, and punctuation make a difference
      i. Do not chart for someone else or allow someone else to chart for you
      j. Use appropriate procedure for documenting a late entry
      k. Document patient and/or family teaching
      l. Document disposition of any personal belongings
      m. Document any nursing interventions and patient responses
  B. Electronic documentation guidelines
    1. Protect the user identification code or password given for personal use
      a. No one else should be given access to that password or document for the user
    2. Only access information and document in chart as authorized to do so
    3. Never ignore electronic reminders that information is coded incorrectly, important data overlooked, or flags for critical information about the patient, e.g., labwork
    4. Know the facility procedure for how to handle late entries
    5. Stay updated when changes in documentation format occur
  C. Incident reports
    1. Use has changed from punitive measure to a documentation of unusual events
    2. All actual and potential injuries must be reported
    3. Documentation should be factual and objective
    4. Allows risk manager to assess situation and decide on best corrective action
    5. Record fact about event in nurses' notes, but not fact that incident report filed
  D. Telephone calls
    1. Document any telephone calls made to report changes in patient condition
    2. Important information to include:
      a. Specific time call was made
      b. Who made the call

       c. Who was called
       d. To whom information was given
       e. All information given
       f. All information received
    3. When obtaining consents (and any other time appropriate), have another witness listen in
  E. Personal accountability
    1. Know your state Nurse Practice Act
    2. Know the national standards for ambulatory surgical nursing practice
    3. Continuing education
       a. Read professional journals and books
       b. Attend pertinent seminars
       c. Maintain membership in professional organization pertinent to specialty
    4. Policies and procedures
       a. Will be held accountable for knowing and following hospital or ambulatory facility's policies and procedures
       b. Policies and procedures should not conflict with one another
       c. Policies and procedures should reflect actual practice
    5. Patient relations
       a. Important aspect of prevention of liability
       b. Old adage is true: "Happy patient rarely sues"
       c. Do not criticize other health-care providers in the presence of the family or patient
       d. Maintain good communication and rapport with the patient and family

THE LEGAL PROCESS

I. Phases of Litigation
  A. Evaluation for suit—review of medical record
  B. Pleadings
    1. Complaint—outlines alleged negligence, states the injury, and may indicate an amount of compensation demanded
       a. Notify insurer and hospital after complaint received
    2. Answer—defendant is allowed a certain period of time to respond to allegations
       a. Attorney prepares the answer
  C. Prelitigation panels—required by some states
    1. Medical review panel
    2. Medical tribunal
    3. Arbitration panel
  D. If you've been sued
    1. Don't discuss the case with anyone other than the risk manager or your attorney
    2. Don't talk to the plaintiff, the plaintiff's attorney, or anyone testifying for the plaintiff
    3. Don't discuss with reporters
    4. Don't alter patient's chart or hide any information from your attorney
  E. Discovery (Pretrial phase)—attempts to narrow issues for trial by gathering and clarifying facts
    1. Interrogatories—list of written questions that seeks information to support or refute the complaint
    2. Production of documents—may be requested, e.g., ambulatory surgery facility records, incident reports, anesthesia records, policies and procedures, discharge teaching forms

   3. Deposition—oral testimony of any person thought to have information pertaining to the case
      a. Testimony given under oath
      b. Recorded by court reporter
F. Settlement negotiations—may continue throughout process and occur at any time in the process
G. Trial of lawsuit—may be a judge or jury trial
   1. Jury selection
   2. Opening statements by plaintiff and defendant
   3. Plaintiff presents case—uses expert witnesses
   4. Defendant presents case—uses expert witnesses
   5. Defense may make motion for directed verdict against plaintiff—argues that the plaintiff has not met the burden of proof
   6. Closing statements by plaintiff and defendant
   7. Jury instructions by the judge
   8. Jury deliberations
   9. Verdict
   10. Appeal (optional)

ISSUES OF CONSENT

I. **Informed Consent**
   A. Consent obtained after the patient has been fully informed by the physician or dentist about the risks and benefits of the treatment, alternatives, and consequences of no treatment
   B. Types of consent
      1. Express—given by direct words, either written or oral
      2. Implied—inferred by the patient's conduct or may be legally presumed in emergency situations
   C. If patient not legally competent adult, patient's parents, legal guardian, or—in some states—next of kin or friend can make health-care decisions
   D. Treatment without consent
      1. Assault and/or battery
      2. Negligent failure to obtain consent
   E. Exceptions to duty to disclose
      1. Some emergency situations—life or well-being of the individual is threatened and consent cannot be obtained or would result in a delay of treatment
      2. Therapeutic privilege—physician believes information would be harmful to the patient; very restricted
      3. Patient has waived right to consent—does not want to be informed
      4. Lack of decision-making capacity—information must be shared with proxy decision-maker or guardian
   F. Documentation of consents
      1. Nurses who sign as witnesses are only witnessing signature of person signing consent form
      2. If patient has additional questions, should refer questions to physician
      3. If physician fails to discuss questions further with the patient, nurse must report that information through the appropriate chain of command
      4. If English is not primary language of patient, an interpreter must be used
II. **Advanced Directives**
   A. Living will—directive from competent individual to medical personnel and family

members regarding treatment he/she wishes to receive when he/she can no longer make the decisions him-/herself

B. Natural Death Act
   1. State-legislated legally recognized living wills with statutory enforcement
   2. Protects practitioner and ensures patient's wishes are followed
C. Durable power of attorney for health care—Allows competent patients to appoint an individual to make health-care decisions if they become incompetent to do so
D. Patient Self-Determination Act (PSDA)
   1. Passed in 1990 as part of federal Omnibus Budget Reconciliation Act (OBRA)
   2. Requires hospitals and other facilities on admission to advise all patients of their right to refuse treatment and of any relevant state laws dealing with advanced directives
E. Do-not-resuscitate directives—Require documentation that the patient's decision was made after consultation with physician and understanding of options

ETHICAL ISSUES

I. **Ethics**
   A. The science relating to moral action and moral values
   B. Concerned with motives and attitudes and their relation to the good of the individual
II. **Professional Responsibilities or Duties**
   A. Duty of veracity—a duty to tell the truth
   B. Rule of confidentiality—a duty to control disclosure of personal information about patients to others
   C. Duty of advocacy—nurse supports the best interests of the individual patient
   D. Accountability—answerable to others for one's actions
   E. Duty of fidelity—obligation to be faithful to commitments to self and others
III. **Ethical Theories**
   A. Utilitarianism—defines "good" as happiness or pleasure
      1. Greatest good for the greatest number of people
      2. The end justifies the means
   B. Deontology—system of ethical decision making based on moral obligation or commitment to others; has emphasis on the dignity of human beings
   C. Principalism—an emerging theory that incorporates various existing ethical principles and attempts to resolve conflicts by applying one or more of them
IV. **Ethical Principles**
   A. Beneficence—views the primary goal of health care as doing good for patients
   B. Nonmaleficence—requirement that health-care providers prevent or do no harm to their patients
   C. Autonomy—freedom of action as chosen by an individual
   D. Justice—duty to be fair to all people
V. **Ethical Decision-Making Process** (goal is to determine right from wrong in certain situations in which the lines are unclear)
   A. Decision-making process
      1. Obtain as much information as possible
      2. State the problem or dilemma as clearly as possible
      3. List all possible choices of action
      4. Evaluate the consequences of each choice
      5. Make a decision
   B. MORAL model
      1. **M**assage the dilemma
      2. **O**utline the options

   3. Resolve the dilemma
   4. Act by applying chosen option
   5. Look back and evaluate entire process
VI. **Law and Ethics**
   A. Legal system founded on rules and regulations that are formal and binding; ethical values are subject to philosophical, moral, and individual interpretation
   B. Legal right may or may not be ethical
   C. Moral right may or may not be a legal right
   D. Law influences ethical decision-making and ethics can influence legal decision-making

Bibliography

1. Aiken, T.D. with Catalano, J.T. (1994). *Legal, Ethical, and Political Issues in Nursing.* Philadelphia: Davis.
2. American Society of Post Anesthesia Nurses. (1995). *Standards of Perianesthesia Nursing Practice.* Thorofare, NJ: ASPAN.
3. Berry, F.A. (1992). What to do when sued. *Curr Rev for Post Anesth Nurs,* 14(19):153–160.
4. Brent, N.J. (1997). *Nurses and the Law: A Guide to Principles and Applications.* Philadelphia: Saunders.
5. Brunson, C.D., Eichhorn, J.H. (1997). Risk management—avoiding complications and litigation. In White, P.F., *Ambulatory Anesthesia & Surgery.* Philadelphia: Saunders, pp. 691–699.
6. Calfee, B.E. (1993). Ethics and the law: The common interface. *Revolution,* 3(3):34–37.
7. Calloway, S.D. (1995). Legal issues in post anesthesia care nursing. In Litwack, K (ed.), *Core Curriculum for Post Anesthesia Nursing Practice,* 3rd ed. Philadelphia: Saunders, pp. 25–33.
8. Creighton, H. (1987). Legal significance of charting—part I. *Nurs Manag,* 18(9):17, 20, 22.
9. Creighton, H. (1987). Legal significance of charting—part II. *Nurs Manag,* 18(10):14–15.
10. Creighton, H. (1987). Recovery room nurses: Legal implications. *Nurs Manag,* 18(1):22–23.
11. De Kornfeld, T.J. (1992). Medico-legal considerations in the recovery room. *Curr Rev for Post Anesth Nurs,* 14(3):17–24.
12. Douglas, M.R. (1997). Ethics and nursing practice. In Brent, N.J., *Nurses and the Law: A Guide to Principles and Applications.* Philadelphia: Saunders, pp. 187–210.
13. Ericksen, J.R. (1988). Making choices: The crux of ethical problems in nursing. *AORN J.* 52(2):394–397.
14. Feutz-Harter, S. (1989). Documentation principles and pitfalls. *JONA,* 19(12):7–9.
15. Feutz-Harter, S. (1994). Nursing case law update. *J Nurs Law,* 1(2):57–61.
16. Fiesta, J. (1993). Failure to assess. *Nurs Manag,* 24(9): 16–17.
17. Fowler, M.D.M., Levine-Ariff, J. (1987). *Ethics at the Bedside: A Source Book for the Critical Care Nurse.* Philadelphia: Lippincott.
18. Guido, G.W. (1997). *Legal Issues in Nursing,* 2nd ed. Stamford, CT: Appleton & Lange.
19. Kelly, L.Y., Joel, L.A. (1996). Ethical issues in nursing and nursing practice. In *The Nursing Experience: Trends, Challenges, and Transitions.* New York: McGraw-Hill, pp. 311–347.
20. Kelly, L.Y., Joel, L.A. (1996). Legal aspects of nursing practice. In *The Nursing Experience: Trends, Challenges, and Transitions.* New York: McGraw-Hill, pp. 481–522.
21. Kemmy, J.A. (1993). OR nursing law: Legal implications of perioperative documentation. *AORN J,* 57(4):954, 956, 968.
22. Litwack, K. (1995). Legal and ethical issues in PACU practice. In *Post Anesthesia Care Nursing,* 2nd ed. St. Louis: Mosby–Yearbook, pp. 42–69.
23. Mannino, M.J. (1992). An interesting postanesthesia case presented., *CRNA,* 3(4):197–198.
24. Murphy, E.K. (1991). OR nursing law: Liability exposure in ambulatory surgery settings. *AORN J,* 54(6):1287–1289.
25. Odom, J.L. (1990). The emerging role of risk management. *J Post Anesth Nurs,* 5(2):120–123.
26. Quan, K.P., Gee, D.C. (1997). Legal responsibilities and informed consent—United States and international perspectives. In White, P.F., *Ambulatory Anesthesia & Surgery.* Philadelphia: Saunders, pp. 682–690.
27. Rozovsky, L.E., Rozovsky, F.A. (1990). Legal woes of incomplete intraoperative charting. *Can OR Nurs J,* 8(1):29–30.
28. Schild, S.M. (1991). Negligence in the operating room: Understanding the law. *Today's OR Nurs,* 13(11):11–16.
29. Springhouse Corporation. (1992). *Nurse's Handbook of Law & Ethics.* Springhouse, PA: Springhouse.
30. Tammelleo, A.D. (1993). Patient sues nurse for failure to obtain consent. *Regan Report on Nurs Law,* 33(10):4.
31. Tammelleo A.D. (1991). Recovery room nurse fails to monitor patient. *Regan Report on Nurs Law,* 32(2):2.
32. White, G.B. (1992). *Ethical Dilemmas in Contemporary Nursing Practice.* Washington, DC: American Nurses Association.
33. Zuffoletto, J.M. (1992). OR nursing law: Anatomy of a lawsuit. *AORN J,* 56(5):933–936.
34. Zuffoletto, J.M. (1993). OR nursing law: Proving causation, damages in malpractice cases. *AORN J,* 58(3):589–592.

REVIEW QUESTIONS

1. All the following are elements of negligence except:

   A. Proximate cause
   B. Duty
   C. Injury
   D. Standard
   E. Breach of duty

2. Once a nurse has been sued, he/she should:

   A. Change the patient's chart to improve the nursing notes
   B. Ask the plaintiff to drop the case
   C. Call the newspaper and state his/her side of the case
   D. Not discuss the case with anyone else at the hospital other than the risk manager

3. Negligence is defined as:

   A. A breach of duty causing injury
   B. Leaving a patient unattended
   C. An action that results in complications
   D. Misdiagnosing a patient's illness

4. If, after a doctor has gone, a patient says he doesn't understand the information the doctor gave him for an informed consent, you should:

   A. Answer the patient's questions
   B. Notify your supervisor
   C. Notify the doctor
   D. Do nothing, as the consent is already signed

5. When adding information to a previous day's entry, you should:

   A. Identify it as late and cross-reference it to the appropriate page
   B. Squeeze it in between existing entries
   C. Write it in the margin nearest the appropriate entry
   D. Write it neatly to avoid the inference that a sloppy chart equals a sloppy nurse

6. The main purpose of an incident report is to:

   A. Help the hospital's lawyer prepare a defense in a lawsuit
   B. Apportion blame
   C. Enable the hospital to spot significant trends or problems
   D. Protect those filing the report

ANSWERS TO QUESTIONS

1. D
2. D
3. A

4. C
5. A
6. C

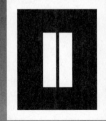

Basic Competencies of Ambulatory Surgical Nursing

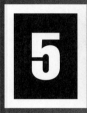

The Nursing Process

Susan Jane Fetzer
University of New Hampshire
Elliot Hospital
Manchester, New Hampshire

I. **Overview of Nursing Process**
   A. Nursing process is a systematic, rational method of providing individualized nursing care
   B. A cyclic process that follows a logical sequence of interrelated phases
   C. Derived from the scientific method of problem-solving and decision-making
   D. Five phases compose the nursing process: assessment, diagnosis, planning, implementation, evaluation
   E. Goals of Nursing Process
      1. Establish a patient data base
      2. Identify health-care needs
      3. Determine goals of care, priorities of care, and expected outcomes
      4. Direct nursing action necessary to meet patient needs
      5. Evaluate effectiveness of nursing systems in achieving patient outcomes

II. **Nursing Process: Assessment**
   A. Information-gathering phase of nursing process
   B. Types of data included in assessment
      1. Subjective data
         a. Primary sources include data obtained from patient reports, descriptions, and perceptions during the:
            i. Preadmission interview with ambulatory surgical patient
            ii. Health history completed by the patient
            iii. Surgical experience under local or regional anesthesia

1. Describe the application of the nursing process to each phase of ambulatory perianesthesia care.
2. List the resources used for data collection during the preadmission assessment.
3. Identify the frequently used diagnostic statements for actual, high-risk, and possible nursing diagnosis during ambulatory surgery and anesthesia.
4. Discuss the role of standards, policies, and procedures in planning ambulatory perianesthesia nursing care.
5. Describe methods used to evaluate ambulatory perianesthesia nursing care.

   iv. Postanesthesia recovery

   v. Prior to discharge

   vi. During postdischarge follow-up interview

  b. Secondary sources include data obtained from family and significant others

   i. Parental reports of child behavior

   ii. Spouse, caretaker report of adult behavior

 2. Objective data

  a. Includes data obtained from nursing observation

   i. Physical appearance during preadmission interview, during surgery, and the postanesthesia phase

   ii. Patient behavior during preoperative and discharge teaching

   iii. Patient behavior during preadmission interview, when experiencing local, or regional anesthesia, and during the postanesthesia phase

  b. Includes data obtained through nursing examination

   i. Preanesthetic physical assessment

    (a) Vital sign measurements

    (b) Systems assessment: skin, respiratory, cardiovascular, musculoskeletal, neurological, psycho-social, hematological

    (c) Assessment related to specific surgical or anesthetic procedure anticipated (e.g., visual acuity for elderly patient scheduled for cataract surgery, assessment of radial pulse in patient scheduled for carpal tunnel release)

   ii. Intraoperative physical assessment

    (a) Vital sign monitoring

    (b) Systems assessment depends on type of anesthesia and surgical procedure: respiratory, cardiovascular, neurological, skin

   iii. Postanesthesia physical assessment

    (a) Vital sign monitoring

    (b) Systems assessment: respiratory, cardiovascular, musculoskeletal, neurological, endocrine, urinary, skin are compared to preanesthetic baseline

    (c) Appearance of surgical site

    (d) Level of pain, nausea, dizziness

 3. Tertiary sources of objective data

  a. Preanesthetic phase

   i. Previous medical records

   ii. Current medical history and physical

   iii. Laboratory, radiology, cardiology, and diagnostic procedure reports

   iv. Information sources can include community health nurses, primary care physicians, physician consultants, physical therapists, dietitians, pharmacists, social workers

  b. Intraoperative phase

   i. Circulating nurse record

   ii. Anesthesia record

   iii. Surgeon operative report or progress note

  c. Postanesthesia phase

   i. Laboratory, radiology, cardiology reports as needed

 4. Specific data to be collected during ambulatory surgery and anesthesia assessment

  a. Contact person in case of emergency

  b. Patient telephone number for discharge follow-up

  c. Past and current medical health responses to treatment

      i.   Allergies to foods (especially milk products, shellfish)
     ii.   Allergies to medications
    iii.   Sensitivities to medications
    iv.   Contact allergies (especially latex, tape, and iodine products)
     v.   Presence of implants or prostheses (e.g., pacemakers, contact lenses, hearing aids)
    vi.   Anesthetic intolerance (e.g., drug intolerance, risk factors for malignant hyperthermia, risk factors for pseudocholinesterase deficiency)
   vii.   Personal habits including frequency and last use of tobacco, alcohol, street drugs, over-the-counter medications
   d. Type, amount, and time of last oral intake

C. Organization of assessment data
   1. Data can be organized and documented using systems or medical model approach (i.e., cardiac, respiratory, neurological, etc.)
   2. Data can be organized and documented using functional health patterns
     a. Health perception–health management pattern
     b. Nutritional–metabolic pattern
     c. Elimination pattern
     d. Activity–exercise pattern
     e. Sleep–rest pattern
     f. Cognitive–perceptual pattern
     g. Self-perception–self concept pattern
     h. Role-relationship pattern
     i. Sexuality–reproductive pattern
     j. Coping–stress tolerance pattern
     k. Value–belief pattern
   3. Data can be organized and documented using a nursing model (e.g., Orem's Self-Care Deficit Theory)

D. Nursing data from multiple sources is analyzed
   1. Data from multiple sources is compared
   2. Data is compared against standards and norms
   3. Data is examined for gaps and inconsistencies

E. Data is organized and documented so that findings are communicated to health-care providers

F. All assessment data is considered confidential and communicated only to health-care providers who have a work-related right to know

III. Nursing Process: Diagnosis

A. A nursing diagnosis is a clinical judgment about the patient's response to actual or potential health problems

B. Nursing diagnosis is derived from an analysis of assessment data

C. Purpose of nursing diagnosis is to communicate nursing judgment using a common and consistent language

D. By clearly identifying the domain of nursing, nursing diagnosis promotes accountability and professional autonomy

E. Components of a nursing diagnosis
   1. Nursing diagnosis incorporates a three-part diagnostic statement referred to as the PES format
   2. P = Problem
     a. Problem is also referred to as a diagnostic label
     b. Concise description of patient's human response for which nursing is needed
     c. Described using North American Nursing Diagnosis Association (NANDA) diagnostic label

      d. Directs the patient outcome criteria
        i.   Outcome may be resolution of problem
        ii.   Outcome may be no change in problem
      e. Examples of ambulatory perianesthesia diagnostic labels
        i.   Preoperative
           (a) Anxiety
           (b) Fear
           (c) Knowledge deficit
           (d) Fluid volume deficit
        ii.   Intraoperative
           (a) High risk for injury
           (b) High risk for altered body temperature
           (c) Ineffective breathing pattern
           (d) Decreased cardiac output
           (e) Altered peripheral tissue perfusion
        iii. Postanesthetic
           (a) Sensory/perceptual alterations (kinesthetic)
           (b) Pain
           (c) Self-care deficit (dressing)
           (d) Altered nutrition: less than body requirements
   3. E = Etiology
      a. Etiology or related factors includes the conditions or circumstances that cause or contribute to the problem
      b. Follows the problem, prefaced by the words *related to*, or *associated with*
      c. Etiology directs the nursing interventions
      d. Categories of etiologies
        i.   Pathophysiologic
        ii.   Treatment related
        iii. Situational (i.e., environmental, personal)
        iv. Maturational
      e. Examples of etiologies in ambulatory perianesthesia
        i.   Environmental temperature (problem of hypothermia)
        ii.   Persistence of regional anesthetic (e.g., spinal, epidural) (problem of sensory/perceptual alteration)
        iii. NPO for past 12 hours (problem of fluid volume deficit)
        iv. Insufficient knowledge of surgical routines (problem of anxiety)
        v.   Side effect of surgical procedure (problem of shoulder pain after diagnostic laparoscopy)
   4. S = Signs and symptoms
      a. Signs and symptoms are also referred to as defining characteristics
      b. Follows the etiology, prefaced by the words *as evidenced by*
      c. Based on findings during nursing assessment
      d. Only identified when an actual nursing diagnosis is made
      e. Risk nursing diagnoses do not have evidence of signs and symptoms
      f. Examples of defining characteristics found in ambulatory perianesthesia patients
        i.   Tympanic temperature of 35°C (problem of hypothermia)
        ii.   Inability to move or stand (problem of sensory/perceptual alteration)
        iii. Orthostatic blood pressure changes, tachycardia (problem of fluid volume deficit)
        iv. Pacing behavior, crying, wringing hands (problem of anxiety)
        v.   Verbal complaint of pain (problem of pain)

F. Types of Nursing Diagnosis
  1. Actual nursing diagnosis
    a. Represents a problem present at the time of the nursing assessment
    b. Patient database contains evidence of defining characteristics
    c. Examples of ambulatory perianesthesia actual nursing diagnoses in PES format
      i. Pain related to surgical incision as evidenced by report of 5/10 on visual analog pain scale
      ii. Hypothermia related to abdominal irrigation during surgery as evidenced by tympanic temperature of 36.5°C
      iii. Acute urinary retention related to spinal anesthetic as evidenced by bladder distention and inability to void
  2. High-risk nursing diagnosis (previously labeled potential nursing diagnosis)
    a. Represents nursing judgment that patient is more vulnerable to develop an actual problem than others in the same situation
    b. Patient database contains evidence of risk factors for the actual diagnosis but no defining characteristics are evident
    c. Examples of ambulatory perianesthesia high-risk nursing diagnoses
      i. High risk for impaired skin integrity
      ii. High risk for aspiration
      iii. High risk for fluid volume deficit
  3. Possible nursing diagnosis
    a. Represents nursing judgment that evidence about a health problem is unclear or causative factors are unknown
    b. A problem is suspected but confirmation requires additional assessment data
    c. Examples of ambulatory perianesthesia possible nursing diagnoses
      i. Ineffective family coping related to surgical findings
      ii. Risk for activity intolerance related to surgical intervention
      iii. Ineffective individual coping
  4. Collaborative problems
    a. Collaborative problems are stated when a nursing diagnosis is not appropriate because definitive interventions are not independent nursing actions
    b. Collaborative problems relates to a specific physiologic complication associated with structure or function of organ or systems that require both physician-prescribed and nurse-prescribed interventions
    c. Goal of nursing in collaborative problems is to minimize complications of the physiological event
    d. The PES format is not used as patient has no signs and symptoms
    e. Uses the diagnostic label of "potential complication" (PC)
    f. Examples of collaborative problems during the ambulatory perianesthesia period
      i. PC: hypoglycemia
      ii. PC: hypoxemia
      iii. PC: laryngospasm
      iv. PC: hypertension
      v. PC: dysrhythmias
      vi. PC: allergic reaction
G. Once identified, nursing diagnoses are prioritized
  1. Life-threatening problems and those interfering with physiological needs
    a. Airway maintenance
    b. Breathing
    c. Circulation temperature regulation

2. Problems interfering with safety and security
   a. Fear
   b. Knowledge deficit
   c. Anxiety
   d. Potential for injury
3. Problems related to general health of patient
   a. Self-care activity deficit
   b. Altered nutrition (less than body requirements)
4. Prioritizing diagnoses includes considering:
   a. Patient's perception of priorities
   b. Completeness of assessment database
   c. Expected length of stay in health-care system
   d. Standards of care
   e. Implementation of critical paths
5. Examples of prioritizing nursing diagnoses in ambulatory perianesthesia nursing
   a. Preadmission priorities
      i.   Anxiety related to planned surgery
      ii. Fear of preoperative testing
      iii. Knowledge deficit of preoperative NPO status
   b. Intraoperative
      i.   Ineffective breathing pattern related to sedation
      ii. Risk of alteration in body temperature related to body cavity irrigation
      iii. Risk for fluid volume excess related to body cavity irrigation
   c. Postanesthetic
      i.   Acute urinary retention
      ii. Acute pain
      iii. Self-care deficit (toileting)

IV. **Nursing Process: Planning**
   A. Planning includes setting goals and expected outcomes of care
   1. Goals (i.e., long-term goals) are broad statements about the effect of nursing interventions
      a. Goals may be achieved after discharge from an ambulatory setting
      b. Goals may be ongoing
      c. Goals are patient-centered and focused on what patient is expected to achieve
      d. Examples of ambulatory perianesthesia goals
         i.   Patient will be free of postoperative infection
         ii. Patient will resume activities of daily living without pain
         iii. Patient will walk unassisted with cane
         iv. Patient's vital signs will be within 20% of preoperative levels
   2. Expected outcomes (i.e., short-term goals, outcome criteria, predicted outcomes, objectives) are specific measurable statements used to evaluate whether a goal has been met
      a. Expected outcome statements include five components
         i.   Subject—who is expected to achieve expected outcome
         ii. Verb—what actions must the person take to achieve the expected outcome
              (a) Measurable verbs should be used (e.g., identify, describe, perform, state, list, verbalize, demonstrate, express, communicate, walk, stand)
         iii. Condition—under what circumstance(s) will the action take place
         iv. Criteria—how well is the action to be performed
         v.   Time—when is the action to be performed
      b. Characteristics of expected outcomes
         i.   Realistic in relation to the patient's preoperative and potential capabilities

        ii. Mutually set with patient or significant others

        iii. Reflect the ASPAN Standards of Practice, state's practice act, and standards of facility

    c. Examples of ambulatory perianesthesia expected outcome statements

        i. The patient *(subject)* will state *(verb)* that pain is less than 5/10 *(criteria)* when asked by the ambulatory perianesthesia nurse *(condition)* one hour before expected discharge *(time)*

        ii. The patient will demonstrate proper instillation of eyedrops prior to home discharge from the surgi-center

        iii. The patient will drink at least 120 cc of clear liquids and deny nausea prior to home discharge

  B. Planning is documented in writing to inform all health-care providers

    1. Preprinted, standardized care plans or critical paths are guides adapted to each patient

    2. Individualized care plans include assessments and diagnoses that are specific to the patient

    3. The care plan usually consists of preprinted document which is individualized as needed

V. Nursing Process: Implementation

  A. Nursing implementation consists of those activities or interventions performed by the nurse or delegated to unlicensed health personnel intended to eliminate or reduce the etiology (cause) of the nursing diagnosis, or reduce the patient's risk factors

  B. Purpose of interventions

    1. Interventions for actual nursing diagnoses

      a. Reduce contributing factors or etiology

      b. Eliminate contributing factors or etiology

      c. Monitor status

      d. Promote wellness

    2. Interventions for high-risk nursing diagnoses

      a. Reduce or eliminate risk factors

      b. Prevent occurrence of problem

      c. Monitor onset of problem

    3. Interventions for possible nursing diagnoses is to collect additional data to confirm or rule out diagnoses

    4. Interventions for collaborative problems

      a. Monitor for change in status

      b. Manage problem with physician-prescribed therapy

      c. Evaluate response of prescribed therapy

  C. Nursing interventions may be selected from the Nursing Interventions Classification (NIC) system

  D. Types of interventions

    1. Independent—activities initiated by the registered nurse on the basis of knowledge and skill (e.g., teaching patient about wound care after discharge)

    2. Dependent—activities carried out under the physician's order (e.g., administer ketorolac for pain)

    3. Collaborative—activities carried out in conjunction with other health team members (e.g., reinforcing crutch walking initiated by physical therapy)

  E. Characteristics of interventions

    1. Consistent with the nursing diagnosis

    2. Implemented safely or delegated appropriately

    3. Documented

F. Interventions include the following actions:
   1. Directly performing an activity
   2. Assisting the patient to perform the activity
   3. Supervising the performance of the activity by patient or caregiver
   4. Teaching patients
   5. Counseling patients about health-care alternatives
   6. Monitoring for potential complications

G. Examples of nursing interventions in ambulatory perianesthesia nursing
   1. Preoperative
      a. Obtain baseline vital signs
      b. Reinforce preoperative teaching
      c. Initiate intravenous access for antibiotic prophylaxis
      d. Measure patient for postoperative sling
   2. Intraoperative
      a. Monitor vital signs
      b. Position patient to maintain skin integrity
      c. Provide emotional support during local anesthetic
      d. Administer conscious sedation
   3. Postoperative
      a. Monitor vital signs
      b. Encourage fluids
      c. Administer pain medication
      d. Reinforce preoperative teaching prior to discharge

VI. **Nursing Process: Evaluation**
   A. Evaluation of the nursing process requires a determination of the achievement of the patient outcomes
   B. Steps in patient outcome evaluation
      1. Perform assessment to determine patient status
      2. Compare assessment findings to expected outcomes
      3. Determine extent of expected outcome achievement
         a. Completely met
         b. Partially met
         c. Not met
      4. Identify variables that have affected achievement of expected outcomes (e.g., unexpected anesthetic technique, development of postoperative nausea, inability to contact adult caregiver)
      5. Decide whether to continue, modify, or terminate the plan of care
         a. Continue plan if outcome not achieved but variables impeding care are not identified
         b. Modify plan if outcome not achieved but variables impeding care have been identified and can be resolved
         c. Terminate plan if outcome achieved

VII. **Communicating the Nursing Process**
   A. Communicating nursing process includes written documentation and oral reporting to health-care providers
   B. All phases of nursing process are communicated
   C. Purpose of communicating nursing process
      1. Informs other health-care providers of patient status
      2. Assists in identifying common response patterns
      3. Provides foundation for evaluation of services (e.g., quality improvement, research)
      4. Creates a legal document
      5. Validates service rendered for reimbursement

   D. Written documentation by ambulatory perianesthesia nurse includes:
1. Patient history
2. Standardized care plan or critical path flow sheet
3. Flow sheet for assessment findings and vital signs
4. Nurses' progress notes for variations from norm
5. Discharge teaching instructions

   E. Oral communication is used when providing change of shift report, or providing report to other health-care providers (e.g., anesthetist, unlicensed caregiver)

   F. Oral communication must be delivered in private environment to ensure patient confidentiality

   G. Oral communication should stress unusual or abnormal findings

VIII. Nursing Process Specific to Ambulatory Perianesthesia Nursing

   A. The steps of the nursing process in the ambulatory environment are accomplished almost simultaneously due to the rapid turnover of cases

   B. Assessment of the patient from the preadmission interview to the postdischarge follow-up is an ongoing process

   C. A strong emphasis is placed on identifying nursing diagnoses concerning knowledge deficits

   D. Evaluations of expected patient outcomes may occur after discharge during follow-up telephone contact

   E. Documentation of instructions for aftercare and the patient's understanding are crucial

   F. Documentation of care must comply with predetermined standards established by third-party payers for reimbursement purposes

Bibliography

1. Alfaro-LeFevre, R. (1994). *Applying nursing process: A step by step guide*, 2nd ed. Philadelphia: Lippincott.
2. Carpenito, L.J. (1995). *Nursing diagnosis: Application for clinical practice*, 6th ed. Philadelphia: Lippincott.
3. Chitty, K.K. (1997). *Professional nursing: Concepts and challenges*, 2nd ed. Philadelphia: Saunders.
4. Kozier, B., Erb, C., Blais, K. (1997). *Professional nursing practice: Concepts and Perspectives*, 3rd ed. San Francisco: Addison Wesley.
5. McCloskey, J.C., Bulecek, G.M. (1996). *Iowa Intervention Project: Nursing Intervention Classification (NIC)*, 2nd ed. St. Louis: Mosby.

REVIEW QUESTIONS

1. Which term best describes the nursing process?

   A. Cyclic
   B. Linear
   C. Includes four phases
   D. Deals with nursing problems

2. A primary source of data during a preadmission interview of an ambulatory surgical patient will include:

   A. ECG and chest X-ray report
   B. Patient-completed health history
   C. Previous anesthesia record written
   D. Report from home health nurse

3. "High risk for injury" is an example of a(n):

   A. Collaborative diagnosis
   B. Expected outcome following anesthesia
   C. Problem statement
   D. Manifestation of a surgical intervention

4. The difference between an actual and a high-risk nursing diagnosis is the:

   A. Description of the problem
   B. Documentation on the database
   C. Lack of etiology
   D. Presence of defining characteristics

5. "Preoperative hypertension related to anxiety" is an example of a(n):

   A. Actual nursing diagnosis
   B. Collaborative problem
   C. High-risk diagnosis
   D. Possible nursing diagnosis

6. "Patient will be free of pain when walking" is an example of a(n):

   A. Expected outcome
   B. Goal
   C. Objective
   D. Outcome criteria

7. Interventions for high-risk nursing diagnoses are intended to:

   A. Eliminate problem etiology
   B. Monitor problem status
   C. Prevent problem occurrence
   D. Reduce contributing factors

8. Demonstrating instillation of eyedrops to a family member of a cataract patient is an example of a(n):

   A. Collaborative intervention
   B. Delegated intervention
   C. Dependent intervention
   D. Independent intervention

9. Which is **not** a characteristic of an expected outcome statement during the planning phase of the nursing process?

   A. Congruent with ASPAN Standards of Practice
   B. Mutually determined
   C. Occurs after discharge
   D. Realistic

10. Which step of the nursing process occurs prior to the preadmission interview?

   A. Assessment
   B. Planning
   C. Intervention
   D. Evaluation

ANSWERS TO QUESTIONS

1. A	6. D
2. B	7. C
3. C	8. D
4. D	9. C
5. B	10. A

6

Clinical/Critical Paths and Case Management

Donna M. DeFazio Quinn
Elliot 1-Day Surgery Center
Manchester, New Hampshire

I. **Case Management** (also known as care management, collaborative management, managed care, collaborative care, outcomes management)
  A. Definition
    1. Multidisciplinary system involving
      a. Health assessment
      b. Planning
      c. Ability to obtain needed services
      d. Delivery of services
      e. Coordination of services
      f. Monitoring of services to ensure multiple needs of the patient are met
    2. Set of logical steps
      a. Involves interaction with service networks
      b. Assures patient receives needed services
        i. Services provided in supportive environment
        ii. Services provided efficiently
        iii. Services provided in a cost-effective manner
  B. History
    1. Model first introduced in inpatient setting
      a. Method of restructuring patient care delivery
        i. Decrease cost
        ii. Improve quality
    2. Reasons for case management development
      a. Implementation of prospective payment system (1982)

Objectives

1. List five benefits of case management.
2. Define case management and clinical pathways.
3. Discuss three benefits to the patient when a case management model of care is implemented.
4. Discuss five benefits of clinical pathways to health-care members.
5. Identify five common causes why clinical pathways may not be used by health-care professionals.
6. Discuss the steps involved in developing a clinical pathway program.

        i. Diagnostic related group (DRG)-based payment for hospitalized Medicare patients

        ii. Need to reduce cost of delivering service

        iii. Optimize patient outcomes

    b. High cost services was due in part to

        i. Variation in physician practices

          (a) Vary due to experience

          (b) Variation in practice styles

        ii. Prolonged length of stay

        iii. High consumption of health-care resources

        iv. Untimely discharge planning

          (a) Usually began the day of discharge

          (b) Resulted in lack of patient teaching

          (c) Could not ensure continuity of care

C. Practice models

  1. Designed to increase nursing involvement in standards of practice

  2. Integrates

    a. Patient satisfaction

    b. Provider satisfaction

    c. Cost-containment strategies

  3. Uses system approach to complete assessment

  4. Identifies specific patient populations

  5. Outcomes are identified with expected time frame for accomplishment

  6. Involves the patient and family in reaching agreement on the plan of care

  7. Implements the plan of care

  8. Monitors and evaluates results

  9. Takes action as needed to redesign the plan of care

  10. Used to manage patient care to ensure optimal outcomes

D. Case managers

  1. Can be nurse, administrator, social worker, independent practitioner, physician, rehabilitation worker, insurance company, health maintenance organization

  2. Nursing case manager

    a. Qualifications

        i. Minimum requirements—baccalaureate prepared (recommended by the American Nurses Association)

        ii. Master's prepared clinical nurse specialist—better suited for complexity of role

  3. Functions of case manager include, but are not limited to:

    a. Coordinating care and services for specific patient population

    b. Assessing needs of patient and family

    c. Collecting all relevant patient information

    d. Assessing patient's ability to cope with illness

    e. Assessing patient's ability to care for self

    f. Identifying appropriateness of patient's formal and informal support systems

    g. Identifying problem areas; intervenes appropriately to correct situation

    h. Acting as a resource to connect the patient to appropriate resources

    i. Facilitating access to health care for the patient

    j. Providing direct patient care as necessary

    k. Educating the patient and family as appropriate

    l. Acting as a liaison to facilitate communication

    m. Monitoring and evaluating care

      n. Monitoring outcomes

      o. Documenting appropriate information

      p. Monitoring the outcome of specific programs

E. Components of case management

    1. Includes a patient care plan (multidisciplinary or interdisciplinary)

    2. Includes a time-specific path (clinical path)

    3. May include financial analysis

    4. May incorporate continuous quality improvement

F. Benefits and advantages of case management

    1. Provides in-depth clinical knowledge

    2. Decreases length of stay (LOS)

    3. Increases customer (patient) satisfaction

      a. Patient and family is aware of timeline for episode of care (i.e., surgical procedure)

      b. Patient and family aware of expectations for discharge from ASC

    4. Increases staff satisfaction

    5. Incorporates nursing diagnosis as a communication pattern

    6. Utilizes product-line management

    7. Provides means to ensure optimal quality care outcomes

    8. Provides for coordination of care utilizing a multidisciplinary team approach which reduces fragmentation of care

    9. Promotes delivery of care in a cost-effective environment

    10. Improves quality

    11. Is responsive to the needs of third-party payers by providing quality care in a cost-effective environment

    12. Improves communication among health team members

    13. Can be used as a marketing tool to tout accomplishments

    14. Is well suited for the perioperative arena due to timing of preoperative, intraoperative, and postoperative periods

      a. Variances are easily identified

      b. Possible causes of variance may be due to:

        i. Patient noncompliance with preoperative instructions

        ii. Missing preoperative laboratory results

        iii. Equipment failure

        iv. Staffing shortage

      c. Quality-improvement activities to correct variances easily identified

G. Disadvantages of case management

    1. May require additional personnel or position

      a. Increased cost

      b. Increased educational requirements

    2. May be viewed as an increase in documentation

    3. Increase in paperwork requirements

    4. Staff members may become frustrated with the case management model

H. Predicaments associated with case management

    1. Which model to use

    2. Appointment of case managers

      a. Registered nurse (degree preferred)

      b. Clinical nurse specialists

      c. Medical record practitioners

    3. How case manager is utilized

      a. Involved in direct patient care or

b. Management responsibilities only
    i. Oversees care provided by others
c. Consultant
4. How to develop and implement clinical pathways

II. **Clinical Pathways** (also known as clinical paths, critical paths, pathways, care maps, collaborative plans of care, multidisciplinary action plans [MAPs], care paths, and anticipated recovery paths)
   A. Clinical pathways
      1. Definition
          a. Interdisciplinary plan of care
              i. Outlines optimal sequencing and timing of interventions for a particular diagnosis, procedure, or symptom
          b. Designed to:
              i. Minimize delays
              ii. Minimize use of resources
              iii. Maximize quality of care
          c. Typically developed for diagnoses, procedures, or symptoms that are:
              i. High volume
              ii. High cost
              iii. High risk
      2. Project management tool
          a. Based on standards of care for a particular case type
          b. Considered "shorthand version" for larger patient case management plan
      3. Components generally include:
          a. Patient outcomes
              i. Typically expected patient outcome prior to discharge
              ii. May include daily outcomes as well as discharge outcomes
          b. Timeline
              i. Timeline for sequencing of interventions
                  (a) May be day by day (hospital setting)
                  (b) May be hour by hour (PACU, Emergency Department)
                  (c) May be week by week (home setting, rehabilitation setting)
          c. Collaboration
              i. Multidisciplinary approach to development of pathway
                  (a) Nurses
                  (b) Physicians
                  (c) Other related health-care professionals (pharmacist, social worker, nutritionist, etc.)
          d. Comprehensive aspects of care
              i. Track aspects of care
              ii. Begins with preadmission
      4. Use of clinical pathways
          a. Complements or replaces nursing care plan
          b. Serves as focal point for change of shift reports, care coordination, or intervention
          c. Nurses use clinical pathway as guide
              i. Nurse assumes case manager role as part of direct patient care responsibilities
              ii. Bedside nurse or case manager monitors patient's progress daily
                  (a) Notes variances, digressions, detours from pathway
      5. Variances
          a. Considered deviations from:
              i. Intermediate goals

        ii. Outcomes

        iii. Staff interventions as outlined on pathway

      b. May alter:

        i. Anticipated discharge date

        ii. Expected cost

        iii. Expected outcomes

    6. Documentation

      a. Clinical pathway can be used as a documentation tool

        i. Record interventions during patient's hospitalization

III. Advantages of Clinical Pathway

  A. Benefits to patient

    1. Involved in planning own care

    2. Patient aware of expectations

    3. Mutual goal setting between health-care members and patient

    4. Teaching tool for patient and family

    5. Increased patient satisfaction

  B. Benefits to health-care members

    1. Reduce variation in patient management practices (standardization)

      a. Minimized range of treatment decisions by:

        i. Physicians

        ii. Nurses

        iii. Other health-care professionals

    2. Increase health-care members' awareness of physician expectations

    3. Force physicians to work in collaboration with other health-care members

    4. Increase communication among all health-care members

    5. Eliminate system breakdowns

    6. Assist in visualizing current practice

      a. Easily identify when nothing is being done

      b. Easily identify if too much is being done

    7. Ability to continuously refine processes of care

      a. Find and eliminate system breakdown

      b. Incorporate new medical knowledge into the treatment plan

    8. Potential for ongoing improvement in patient care

    9. Increase staff satisfaction

    10. Educational tool for students and new graduates

      a. Instills principles of cost effectiveness

      b. Guideline for implementing procedures in a timely manner

  C. Additional benefits

    1. Improve liability management and outcomes by reducing variation in patient management practices

      a. Keeps patient on track

        i. Pathway is explicit and comprehensive

        ii. Covers both timing and elements of care

        iii. Reduces delay in care

        iv. Focuses attention on important steps that may otherwise be lost

    2. Everyone working off "same program" facilitates communication and collaboration

    3. Financial benefits

      a. Reduced length of stay

      b. Decreased patient charges

      c. Improved quality

      d. Increase competitive edge

   4. Ability to integrate quality improvement, utilization management, and risk-management activities
   5. Data easily retrievable for evaluating outcomes

IV. Disadvantages, Deficiencies, and Concerns of Clinical Pathways
   A. May be used by plaintiff's attorney in medical malpractice claim
   B. Represents a standard to which health-care professionals are held accountable
      1. Terms such as "variance" or "deviation" suggest error
      2. Minimize liability by using terminology such as "guideline"
   C. Health-care professionals may be reluctant to use clinical pathways
      1. Common causes
         a. Lack of involvement of physicians and other health-care professionals in design phase
         b. Lack of leadership education
         c. Delegation of program to middle management without active administrative and medical staff leadership involvement
         d. Failure to identify goals
         e. Unrealistic goals
         f. Unnecessary paperwork
         g. Collection of information about variances without regard to what information was really necessary for problem identification
         h. Inability to convince health-care professionals of value of process
   D. Placement in medical record
      1. Most often placed in permanent medical record
         a. Placement within medical record varies by institution
         b. Generally placed in Physician Orders section
      2. May be discarded when patient is discharged
   E. Use as a documentation tool
      1. Should not be viewed as additional paperwork
      2. Should replace existing documentation record
      3. Goal is to streamline documentation while ensuring complete documentation to avoid legal liability

V. Clinical Pathways and Quality Improvement
   A. Clinical pathways
      1. Integral part of clinical process improvement activities
      2. Methodology for describing the processes of patient care
      3. Clinical pathway tool corresponds with the "plan" phase of Deming's plan–do–check–act (PDCA) cycle of continuous improvement
         a. Plan
            i. Evaluate clinical process
            ii. Identify ways to improve process
            iii. Map out using clinical path or algorithm
         b. Do
            i. Use the clinical path to manage patient care
            ii. Keep patient on path to ensure better outcomes, decreased cost, and improved quality
      4. Variance analysis corresponds with "check" phase of cycle
         a. Check
            i. Identify variances
            ii. Evaluate patient outcome data
            iii. Identify system problems that resulted in unnecessary variances from clinical path

Table 6–1 • CLINICAL PATHWAY EDUCATION GUIDE

- Announcement of the project:
  Definition and purpose of clinical pathway
  Why the hospital/ASC will do it
  Who the key players are
- Benefits and disadvantages of pathways for:
  Patients
  Families
  Staff
  Physicians
  Hospital/ASC
  Students
  (NOTE: This information is often presented in an interview format.)
- General status update:
  How staff can get involved
  Roles and responsibilities of the staff
- Which pathway(s) were selected for initial implementation and where it will be piloted
- Format for pathway: call for staff input
- Implementation plan: schedule of inservices
- Evaluation of project:
  Variance analysis
  Outcomes management

From Ignatavicius, D.D., Hausman, K.A. (1995). *Clinical Pathways for Collaborative Practice.* Philadelphia: Saunders.

  b. Act
     i. Resolve any system problems that were identified
     ii. If patient outcome data is positive, promote clinical path as ideal process
     iii. If patient outcome data is negative, change clinical path to reflect the ideal process
     iv. Continuously collect data to ensure positive outcome data; identify system problems and correct immediately to ensure continuous positive outcomes
VI. **Process of Clinical Pathway Development**
  A. Planning
     1. Need to ensure long-term commitment to implement methods to improve clinical processes
     2. Need to change the way patient care is delivered
     3. Need to educate all health-team members involved (Table 6–1)
  B. Steps
     1. Establish multidisciplinary task force (Table 6–2 and Table 6–3)
        a. Charge
           i. Oversee the design and implementation process
        b. Include key administrative personnel, nursing, physician, and information systems
        c. Set goals
        d. Ensure availability of required resources
        e. Provide education and orientation once paths are approved
     2. Set goals
        a. Express in measurable terms
        b. Allow for assessment of goal attainment

3. Goals include:
   a. Quality improvement
   b. Cost reduction
4. Select patient categories for developing first paths
5. Set ground rules
6. Project required resources
   a. Time
   b. Manpower
   c. Financial
7. Educate
   a. Medical staff (Table 6–4)
   b. Middle managers

Table 6–2 • CLINICAL PATHWAY PROGRAM

1. Educate and obtain support from staff and physicians
2. Form the interdisciplinary teams
   a. Steering committee and pathway-specific group
   b. Group to identify potential obstacles to implementation
3. Data collection: determine patient population, DRG, ICD-9 code to focus on those who are:
   a. High volume
   b. High cost
   c. High risk
   d. Difficult to manage
4. Use continuous quality-improvement methods and tools to select:
   a. Pareto charts
   b. Statistical process control charts
5. Determine which ICD-9 code is most predictable
6. Determine staff interest
7. Select pathway to develop
8. Develop format for pathway
9. Select interdisciplinary clinical experts for pathway team
10. Collect clinical pathway data
    a. Medical record review for practice patterns
    b. Literature review
    c. Comparison with other institutions
    d. Practice guidelines
11. Write the pathway
    a. Review by staff
    b. Review as necessary
12. Develop variance analysis system
    a. Information needed to measure compliance with the pathway
    b. Outcomes measurement
    c. Clinical and financial measurements
13. Present pathway to hospital/ASC committees for approval; incorporate revision
14. Develop implementation plan
15. Provide inservice to staff
16. Use pilot pathway for 3 to 6 months; revise as needed
17. Monitor variances
    a. Develop automated data collection if possible
    b. Present variance data to staff and physicians

From Ignatavicius, D.D., Hausman, K.A. (1995). *Clinical Pathways for Collaborative Practice*. Philadelphia: Saunders.

Table 6–3 • STEERING COMMITTEE RESPONSIBILITIES

- Establish format for meetings
    time, place, and need for agenda before meeting
- Review roles of team members
- Identify recorder (writes on board or flip chart)
- Identify secretary (recorder of meeting minutes)
- Articulate purpose, goals, and objectives of the committee
- Integrate continuous quality improvement or total quality management into pathway development
- Obtain information needed to develop the pathway(s)
    length of stay
    cost
    volume
    problem-prone procedures
    high-risk procedures
- Recommend which pathways to develop first and prioritize others
- Develop guideline for the format and use of the clinical pathway
- Determine which departments need to participate or assist in pathway development
- Advise hospital administration/ASC administration and other staff on project progress
- Use practice pattern information, community standards, published guidelines, and comparisons to write pathway
- Develop format to monitor variances
- Develop policies, procedures, and guidelines for use of clinical pathways
- Evaluate the outcome of the project and make recommendations for the future
- Assume accountability for the project

From Ignatavicius, D.D., Hausman, K.A. (1995). *Clinical Pathways for Collaborative Practice.* Philadelphia: Saunders.

Table 6–4 • GUIDELINES TO OBTAIN PHYSICIAN SUPPORT

1. Involve the physician in the process from the beginning:
   a. Clinical pathway to pilot
   b. Format to use
   c. Material to include on pathway
2. Show benefits to patient and family
3. Demonstrate benefits to the physician's personal practice
4. Use objective data to provide the physician with his or her own practice pattern information and how it compares with that of other physicians in the hospital and community
5. As needed, assist the physician to change or modify practice pattern based on community standards, guidelines, etc.
6. Share variance analysis data
7. Elicit the physician's involvement and support to review and revise the pathway based on variance data and changes in practice guidelines or technology
8. Follow-up on agreed action plan or strategies for doing things better
9. *Keep the lines of communication open*

From Ignatavicius, D.D., Hausman, K.A. (1995). *Clinical Pathways for Collaborative Practice.* Philadelphia: Saunders.

8. Provide information
   a. Benefits of adopting clinical paths
   b. Long-range plan
      i. Minimize risk of individual departments developing own
9. Final review
   a. Determine if complete
   b. Assess for additional factors that could decrease cost and LOS without compromising quality
   c. All disciplines review clinical pathway
   d. Identify how variances will be monitored and outcomes evaluated
   e. Develop guidelines, policies, and procedures for the use of the clinical pathway
   f. Prepare action plan
      i. For implementation
      ii. For evaluation
   g. Clinical pathway reviewed by legal counsel
      i. Must be consistent with local, state, and federal regulatory agencies and accreditation bodies

VII. Implementation of Clinical Pathways
   A. Staff awareness
      1. Involve staff as appropriate
      2. Inform staff not involved
      3. Assist staff in gaining awareness of need for change
      4. Provide reassurance
      5. Provide educational opportunities
   B. Educate staff directly involved
      1. Purpose
      2. Correct use of clinical pathway
      3. How pathway improves care of patient and family
   C. Ensure resource staff readily available
      1. Around the clock if appropriate
   D. Start with one or two pathways initially
      1. Pilot on appropriate patient care area
   E. Evaluate effectiveness (ongoing)
   F. Obtain staff input on possible improvements in pathways
   G. Analyze data (3 to 6 months' worth)
      1. Make changes based on the data collected and recommendations from staff

Bibliography

1. Ashwill, J.W., Droske, S.C. (1997). *Nursing Care of Children, Principles and Practice.* Philadelphia: Saunders.
2. Brown, L., Deckers, C., Magallanes, A., et al. (1996). Clinical case management: What works, what doesn't. *Nursing Management,* 27(11):28–30.
3. Everroad, S., Mayo, A. (1996). Clinical Practicum in the Ambulatory Setting. *Nursing Management,* 27(11):33–34.
4. Forkner, D.J. (1996). Clinical pathways: Benefits and liabilities. *Nursing Management,* 27(11):35–38.
5. Fujihara Isozaki, L.F., Fahndrick, J. (1998). Clinical pathways—A perioperative application. *AORN J,* 67(2):376–396.
6. Girard, N. (1994). The case management model of patient care delivery. *AORN J,* 60(3):403–415.
7. Huber, D. (1996). *Leadership and Nursing Care Management.* Philadelphia: Saunders.
8. Ignatavicius, D.D., Hausman, K.A. (1995). *Clinical Pathways for Collaborative Practice.* Philadelphia: Saunders.
9. Moss, M.T., O'Connor, S. (1993). Outcomes management in perioperative services. *Nursing Economics,* 11(6):364–369.
10. Patterson, P. (1997). Pathways: What role do they play in the OR? *OR Manager,* 13(2):1, 14–15.

11. Sohl-Kreiger, R., Lagaard, M.W., Scherrer, J. (1996). Nursing case management: Relationships as a strategy to improve care. *Clinical Nurse Specialist*, 10(2): 107–113.

12. Spath, P.L. (1994). *Clinical Paths Tools for Outcomes Management*. Chicago: American Hospital Publishing.

13. Walrath, J.M., Owens, S., Dziwulski, E. (1996). Case management—A vital link to performance improvement. *Nursing Economics*, 14(2):117–122.

14. Zander, K. (1995). *Managing Outcomes Through Collaborative Care*. Chicago: American Hospital Publishing.

REVIEW QUESTIONS

1. Case Management:

   A. Was developed in response to the implementation of a prospective payment system
   B. Is based on CPT-4 codes
   C. Has no effect on outcomes management
   D. Decreases cost while increasing length of stay

2. Benefits of case management include all except:

   A. Decrease cost
   B. Decreased length of stay
   C. Increase in patient satisfaction
   D. Decrease in staff satisfaction
   E. Improved quality of care

3. The components of case management include all of the following except:

   A. A time-specific path
   B. Financial analysis
   C. Continuous quality improvement
   D. A nursing specific care plan
   E. A multidisciplinary patient care plan

4. Typically, clinical pathways are developed for procedures, diagnoses, or symptoms that are:
   (1) High volume
   (2) Low volume
   (3) High risk
   (4) Low risk
   (5) High cost
   (6) Low cost

   A. 1, 3, 5
   B. 2, 4, 6
   C. 1, 4, 6
   D. 2, 3, 5
   E. None of the above

5. The timeline for sequencing of interventions outlined on the clinical path can be:
   (1) Day by day
   (2) Week by week
   (3) Hour by hour
   (4) Varied according to patient response
   (5) Varied according to resources available

   A. 1, 4
   B. 1, 2, 4
   C. 1, 2, 3
   D. All of the above
   E. None of the above

6. Variations in patient outcomes are considered:

   A. Deviations from the immediate goals
   B. An expected outcome
   C. Unrelated to expected sequencing of timelines
   D. Normal progression towards expected patient outcomes

7. Advantages of clinical pathways include all of the following except:

   A. Ability of the patient to plan his/her own care
   B. Reduction in variation in patient management practices
   C. Ability for physicians to work collaboratively with other healthcare professionals
   D. Increased patient satisfaction
   E. Decrease in competitive edge

8. Common reasons for failure of health-care professionals to use clinical pathways include:
   (1) Lack of education regarding them
   (2) Failure to identify goals
   (3) Unrealistic goals
   (4) Unnecessary paperwork
   (5) Collection of information regarding variances without regard to what was really needed to identify the problem

   A. 1, 3, 4
   B. 1, 2, 3
   C. 2, 3, 5
   D. 1, 4, 5
   E. All of the above

9. Resources required to implement a clinical pathway program include all except:
   A. Time
   B. Manpower
   C. Financial support
   D. Patient need

10. A clinical pathway should be used for what period of time before it is revised?
   A. 1–2 weeks
   B. 1–2 months
   C. 3–6 months
   D. 3–6 weeks
   E. One year

ANSWERS TO QUESTIONS

1. A
2. D
3. D
4. A
5. C

6. A
7. E
8. E
9. D
10. C

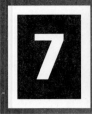

7

Preoperative Patient Assessment and Preparation

Rose Ferrara-Love
Duquesne University
Mercy Providence Hospital
Pittsburgh, Pennsylvania

Objectives

1. State goals of preoperative preparation.
2. Evaluate the alternatives to onsite visit to surgical center.
3. Identify essential components of preadmission assessment.
4. Discuss how the psychological and emotional assessment of a patient will reduce anxiety on day of surgery.
5. Analyze the learning needs of ambulatory surgery patients.

I. **Goals of Preoperative Preparation**
   A. Collection of data through assessment and interview
      1. Nursing process
         a. Essential that initial assessment be complete and accurate
            i. Nursing discharge plan is built on this information
   B. Provision of accurate information to patient and family
      1. Physician and anesthesiologist primary sources of information
   C. Nurse has specific teaching role as a primary "information provider"
      1. Nurse's role is to clarify patient understanding of:
         a. Procedure
         b. Anesthetic approach
         c. Expected outcomes
         d. Personal responsibilities
            i. Comprehensive nursing instructions assist patient and family
               (a) Understand and comply with preoperative preparations
               (b) Allow patient and family to prepare for postoperative home needs
   D. Assurance of appropriate preoperative compliance

    E. Promotion of the wellness concept

    F. Provision of emotional support

       1. Encourage patients and families to express openly and honestly:

          a. Needs

          b. Emotions

          c. Concerns

             i. Often inaccuracies or misinformation causes fear

    G. Reduction of patient anxiety

       1. Done by providing clear explanations

       2. Opportunities for expressions of fears and emotions

          a. Induction of anesthesia smoother in calm persons

          b. Recovery is less stressful

    H. Decreasing potential for complications

       1. Potential problems are identified prior to surgery

       2. Promotes patient safety

       3. Ensures smooth-flowing operative schedule

          a. Fewer cancellations

    I. Provision of smooth flow of the surgery schedule

       1. Initial steps

          a. Selection

             i. Based on

                (a) Type of planned surgery

                    (i) Likelihood of complications

                (b) Potential for more complex surgery

                (c) Third-party reimbursement

          b. Scheduling

             i. Based on comprehensive:

                (a) History and physical

                (b) Emotional attitude

                (c) Available home support

II. Scheduling Concerns

    A. Surgery scheduling

       1. Based upon:

          a. Surgeon

          b. Available time slots on the operative schedule

          c. Patient needs

             i. Emotional

            ii. Physical

            iii. Urgency of surgical procedure

            iv. Personal and familial schedule

                (a) May not want to delay procedure for someone who is extremely apprehensive and nervous

            v. Amount of time needed for day of surgery preparation

                (a) Patients with mobility problems or the elderly need extra time for preparation

                (b) Children and diabetics need to maintain nutrition and medication schedules

                (c) Patients who need extended postoperative observation should be done early in the day

                    (i) Patients undergoing general anesthesia tend to do better physiologically and psychologically when done early in morning

      (d) Hospital-based ambulatory surgery centers must coordinate with main operating room schedule if operating rooms are integrated

      (e) Preoperative policy may indicate time necessary between admission and start of surgery

         (i) Completed preadmission work-up may require arrival time of only one hour prior to surgery

         (ii) Two or more hours may be needed if preoperative work-up has not been completed

III. Preoperative Program Alternatives

  A. On-site preadmission visits

    1. Formal preadmission program

      a. Necessitates extra trip for patient

      b. May be costly

        i. Nursing hours

    2. Necessary space requirements

    3. Advantages

      a. Patient satisfaction

      b. Fewer delays and cancellations

        i. May also meet with anesthesiologist during this visit

         (a) History and physical may be completed by anesthesiologist including:

           (i) ASA status

             a) ASA-1. A normal, healthy patient

             b) ASA-2. A patient with mild systemic disease (chronic bronchitis, moderate obesity, diet-controlled diabetes mellitus, mild hypertension, old MI)

             c) ASA-3. A patient with severe systemic disease (coronary artery disease with angina, insulin-dependent diabetes mellitus, morbid obesity, moderate to severe pulmonary insufficiency)

             d) ASA-4. A patient with severe systemic disease that is a constant threat to life (organic heart disease with marked cardiac insufficiency, persisting angina, intractable dysrhythmias, advanced pulmonary, renal, hepatic, or endocrine insufficiency)

             e) ASA-5. A moribund patient who is not expected to survive without the surgery (ruptured abdominal aortic aneurysm with profound shock)

             f) ASA-6. A declared brain-dead patient whose organs are being removed for donor purposes

             g) E. The suffix E is used to denote an emergency surgical procedure

           (ii) Ambulatory surgery patients usually fall into the first three categories

      c. Allow for adequate preparation

        i. Home

         (a) Caregiver present

         (b) Practice techniques

           (i) Crutch walking

           (ii) Dressing changes

           (iii) Emptying of drains or catheters

       d. Psychosocial
          i.   Address fears
          ii.   Provide for question and answer
          iii. Opportunity to meet staff
              (a) Form relationship with staff
       e. Earlier recognition of potential complications or problems
          i.   Allows time for further evaluation or treatment without altering original surgery schedule
    4. Scheduling issues
       a. Need for flexibility
          i.   Arrange convenient time for patients
          ii.   No need to take extra time off work
       b. Coincide with availability of anesthesiologist and nursing staff
       c. Coordinate diagnostic testing so only one trip is necessary
  B. The telephone interview
    1. Common means of preadmission assessment and instructions
       a. May be screening tool for identifying high-risk patients
          i.   Then requested to make personal visit to ASC for further work-up
       b. Provides emotional and personal contact
          i.   Allows for question-and-answer session
          ii.   Health history can be obtained
               (a) Doesn't replace physical assessment
               (b) Supplies clues to patient's physical status and needs
          iii. Opportunity to provide instructions
               (a) Safety
               (b) Comfort
          iv. Contact day or evening prior to surgery
               (a) Confirm arrival time
               (b) Reinforce NPO status
               (c) Ensure transportation arrangements
               (d) Medication instructions
    2. Disadvantages
       a. Complete physical assessment must be done on day of surgery
       b. Timing of call is important
          i.   Early enough to allow time to follow up on identified problems
          ii.   Not too early that instructions are forgotten
       c. Phone calls may be to patient's place of employment
          i.   Not conducive to teaching as patient may not be able to speak freely
               (a) May not be able to ask needed questions
               (b) Elicit best time to phone patient
    3. Documentation/communication
       a. Information must be forwarded to other members of health team
          i.   Indicates preoperative teaching and preadmission health history has been completed
  C. Preparation of patients at alternate sites
    1. Physician offices may provide ambulatory center with:
       a. History and physical
       b. Diagnostic testing results
       c. Surgical consent
       d. Preoperative orders
       e. Evidence of preoperative teaching completed

D. Admissions coordinator
  1. Responsible for preadmission of ambulatory surgery patients
    a. Securing paperwork and test results
      i. Often from other facilities
    b. Experienced in preoperative preparation
      i. Provides preoperative evaluation and teaching
    c. Liaison among the ASC, physicians, and other departments

IV. **The Nursing History and Physical Examination**
  A. General health
    1. Questions and observations regarding overall health include:
      a. General appearance
      b. Height
      c. Weight
        i. Often converted to kilograms to facilitate rapid calculation of medication doses in mg/kg format
          (a) Weight in pounds ($\div 2.2$ = weight in kilograms)
          (b) Weight in kilograms ($\times 2.2$ = weight in pounds)
        ii. Obesity
          (a) Many freestanding surgical centers enforce weight restrictions due to increased risk of anesthesia complications
            (i) Usually 300 pounds (136.4 kg)
        iii. Recent unplanned weight loss
      d. Recent or current infection
      e. Allergies
      f. Nutrition habits
      g. Physical handicaps
    2. Physical examination includes observation
      a. Skin
        i. Color
        ii. Turgor
        iii. Elasticity
        iv. Presence of bruises
          (a) May necessitate report to authorities if abuse is suspected
        v. Other injuries
        vi. Dryness
        vii. Lesions
          (a) Include mucous membrane
        viii. Cleanliness
        ix. Dental hygiene
      b. Abnormalities
        i. Posture
        ii. Gait
        iii. Mobility
          (a) Use of wheelchair, walker, cane should be noted
        iv. Pain at rest
      c. Physical characteristics
        i. Potential complications
          (a) Short, stocky neck
          (b) Cervical fusion or arthritis
          (c) Thick tongue
          (d) Temporal mandibular joint disease
          (e) Dental or orthopedic abnormalities

    d. Vital signs should be obtained to identify aberrancies and for baseline measurements
- i. Blood pressure
  - (a) Dynamic measurements that change minute to minute
    - (i) Response to
      - a) Environment
      - b) Physiologic demands
  - (b) Average ranges
    - (i) 100–135 mm Hg systolic
    - (ii) 60–80 mm Hg diastolic
- ii. Pulse
  - (a) Average range 60–100 beats per minute
- iii. Respirations
  - (a) Average rate 12–20 breaths per minute
- iv. Temperature
  - (a) Oral temperatures considered normal range from 97.7° F to 99.5° F (36.5° C to 37.5° C)
  - (b) Rectal temperatures average slightly less than one degree Fahrenheit higher
  - (c) Axillary temperatures are approximately ½ to 1 degree lower
  - (d) Tympanic thermometers offer comfortable, rapid, and accurate readings
    - (i) Approximately 1 degree higher than oral readings
  - (e) Variances in normal ranges
    - (i) Normal physiologic status
    - (ii) Extrinsic forces
      - a) Medication
      - b) Recent exercise
      - c) Effort
      - d) Anxiety/fear

B. Medication history
1. Medication protocol affects types of medications and anesthetic agents used
   - a. Helps avoid untoward drug interactions or withdrawal episodes
2. Include in history form:
   - a. Names
   - b. Dosages
   - c. Frequency
   - d. Nonprescription drugs
   - e. Tobacco usage
   - f. Alcohol usage
   - g. Recreational drugs usage
     - i. Especially important to plan appropriate anesthetic course
   - h. Allergic reactions
     - i. Specific drug
       - (a) May know only category of drug, i.e., antibiotic
       - (b) Identify if related categories will be used in the ASC
     - ii. Specific reaction
       - (a) True allergy or expected side effect
     - iii. Usually documented in red
       - (a) Highly visible
         - (i) On medical record
         - (ii) On patient identification band

iv. Environmental and food allergies
  (a) Allergy to eggs may have possible cross-sensitivity with Propofol
  (b) Allergy to bananas, kiwis, peaches, water chestnuts may have link with latex allergies
    (i) Cutaneous exposure
      a) Anesthesia masks, head straps, rebreathing masks, tourniquets, ECG patches, adhesive tape, surgical gloves
      b) Other sources include elastic bandages, rubber positioning rings, rubber shoes, elastic clothing, balloons, Koosh balls, sporting equipment
    (ii) Mucous membrane
      a) Nasogastric tubes, balloons, nipples, pacifiers, products used in dentistry, urinary catheters, glove contact with vaginal mucosa, enema kits, rectal pressure catheters (especially in patients with spina bifida and impaired bowel control)
      b) Other sources include condoms
    (iii) Inhalation
      a) Often associated with glove powder
    (iv) Internal tissue
      a) Intraoperative resulting from surgical gloves contacting the peritoneum or internal organs
    (v) Intravascular
      a) Disposable syringes, medication aspirated from vials with latex stoppers, injection of medication via ports of intravenous tubing (latex can leech into solutions injected)
C. Nutrition status
  1. Physiologic processes dependent upon proper nutrition
    a. Wound healing
    b. Oxygen transport
    c. Enzymes synthesis
    d. Clotting factors
    e. Resistance to infection
  2. Diseases associated with poor nutrition
    a. Crohn's disease
    b. Malignancies
    c. Chronic obstructive pulmonary disease (COPD)
    d. Ulcerative colitis
  3. Indications of malnutrition
    a. Anorexia
    b. Recent weight loss
    c. Dull hair
    d. Brittle nails
    e. Diagnostic tests
      i. Decreased lymphocytes
      ii. Decreased serum albumin and transferrin levels
  4. Obesity complicates
    a. Administration of anesthesia
      i. Requires higher-than-normal levels of anesthetic agents
        (a) Fat-soluble agents tend to prolong effects
      ii. Increased stress on cardiovascular system
        (a) Increased oxygen needs

        (b) Increased carbon dioxide production
           (i)   Associated with increased body mass

  b. Technical aspects of performing procedure
      i.   Often difficult to intubate
          (a) Difficult to maintain airway
            (i)   Increased risk of aspiration
               a) Increased intra-abdominal pressures
               b) Gastric contents higher in volume and more acidic
      ii.   Problems with positioning
          (a) Weight of abdominal and chest contents can cause respiratory embarrassment when in Trendelenburg position
      iii. Difficult to perform venipuncture

  c. Patient's recovery
      i.   Electrolyte and fluid balance essential for homeostasis
          (a) Regulates cardiac rhythm
          (b) Muscle strength
          (c) Distribution and metabolism of drugs
            (i)   Mental alertness
            (ii)   Table 7–1 highlights signs and symptoms of electrolyte imbalances
      ii.   Signs of dehydration
          (a) Loss of skin turgor
          (b) Listlessness
          (c) Orthostatic hypotension
          (d) Rapid and thready pulse
          (e) Dryness of mucous membranes
          (f) Thirst
      iii. Cardiovascular
          (a) Symptoms of cardiac disease
            (i)   Chest pain/tightness
            (ii)   Palpitations
            (iii)   Chronic fatigue
            (iv)   Loss of appetite
            (v)   Angina
            (vi)   Swelling of the ankles
            (vii) Paroxysmal nocturnal dyspnea (PND)
            (viii) Exhaustion
      iv.   Particular importance
          (a) Recent cardiac surgery
          (b) Myocardial infarction (MI)
            (i)   Considered most important indicator of anesthesia morbidity
            (ii)   Generally elective, non-urgent surgery postponed for at least 6 months after an MI
          (c) Angina
          (d) Aortic stenosis
          (e) Poorly controlled dysrhythmias
          (f) Congestive heart failure
          (g) Extremes in blood pressure
          (h) Presence of pacemaker
      v.   Physical examination parameters
          (a) Apical pulse
            (i)   Rate

Table 7–1 • SIGNS AND SYMPTOMS OF ELECTROLYTE IMBALANCE

ELECTROLYTE NORMAL VALUE	PHYSIOLOGIC FUNCTIONS	EXCESS	DEFICIENCY
Potassium (K) 3.5–5.0 mEq/L	• Nerve conduction • Muscle contraction • Enzyme action for cellular energy production • Regulates intracellular osmolality	• Generalized muscle weakness and flaccidity; can affect respiratory muscles, paresthesia • **Cardiac:** bradycardia, ventricular ectopy and fibrillation, 3° heart block, asystole (>7.0 mEq/L) • **ECG Changes:** flat or absent P wave, wide QRS, peaked T wave, prolonged PR interval	• Muscle weakness, flaccidity, fatigue, leg cramps, ↓ deep tendon reflexes, shallow respirations, weak, thready pulse, hypotension • **Cardiac:** atrial dysrhythmias, PVCs, AV blocks, cardiac arrest (<2.5 mEq/L) • **ECG Changes:** flat or inverted T wave, depressed ST segment, U wave present, potentates digitalis toxicity, PACs or PVCs
Sodium (Na) 135–145 mEq/L	• Transmission and conduction of nerve impulses • Regulates vascular osmolality • Regulates body fluids and acid/base balance • Regulates neuromuscular activity via sodium pump	• Excitement; thirst; dry, sticky tongue and mucous membranes; oliguria; flushed skin; confusion; lethargy; coma; convulsions; hypo- or hypertension; elevated temperature	• Abdominal cramping, anorexia, malaise, nausea and vomiting, muscle weakness, headache, confusion, lethargy, convulsions, coma
Calcium (Ca) 9–11 mg/dl	• Nerve and muscle activity • Myocardial contractility • Maintains cell permeability • Converts prothrombin to thrombin • Formation of teeth and bones	• Lethargy, depression, apathy, anorexia, nausea and vomiting, muscle weakness, headache, confusion, decreased attention span, slurred speech, hypertension • **Cardiac:** heart block, PVCs, idioventricular rhythms, cardiac arrest • **ECG Changes:** shortened QT interval	• Anxiety, excitement, hyperreflexia, grimacing, numbness and tingling of lips or fingers, muscle cramps and spasms, laryngospasm, convulsions, tetany, dysrhythmias including VT • **Positive Trousseau's Sign:** Carpal spasm after inflation of BP cuff on upper arm to 20 mm Hg over systolic for 3 minutes, shows tetany • **Positive Chevostk's Sign:** abnormal facial spasm when facial nerve in front of ear is tapped • **ECG Changes:** prolonged QT interval

(ii)   Rhythm
(iii) Quality
(b) At least one blood pressure reading
(c) Palpation of peripheral pulses
(d) Observation for edema
(e) Clubbing of fingers
(f) Cyanosis
(g) Distention of neck veins
(h) General energy level
(i) Respiratory ease
(j) Auscultation of heart for murmurs
(i)   Systolic murmur over right sternal border, second intercostal space may indicate presence of aortic stenosis
a) Associated with unexpected dysrhythmias
b) Diminished stroke volume
5. Cardiac drugs
a. Maintain normal routine preoperatively
i.   Do not skip doses
(a) Beta blockers
(b) Calcium channel blockers
(c) Antihypertensives
D. Peripheral vascular disease
1. Occlusive
2. Spastic
3. Thrombolytic
4. Symptoms
a. Peripheral cyanosis
b. Pain
c. Cold
d. Intermittent claudication
e. Central vessel involvement
i.   Confusion
ii.   Transient blindness
iii. Hemiparesis
5. Nursing interventions
a. Intraoperative passive range of motion
b. Use of padding of bony prominences intraoperatively
i.   Heels
ii.   Elbows
iii. Shoulders
iv. Hips
v.   Coccyx
c. Encouragement of active exercises before and after surgery
d. Use of antiembolism stockings
e. Explanation of symptoms of thrombophlebitis
f. Encouragement of adequate fluid intake
g. Have patient immediately report any of the following symptoms postoperatively
i.   Pain in the leg, especially increased calf pain when foot is dorsiflexed (positive Homan's sign)
ii.   Fever
iii. Chills

        iv. Swelling
        v. Redness
        vi. Heat
        vii. Tenderness in leg
  E. Respiratory
      1. History
          a. Infectious or chemical influences
          b. Smoking habits
          c. Chronic cough
          d. Previous lung surgery
          e. Emphysema
              i. Patients may not admit to emphysema as a disease
              ii. Look for symptomatology
                  (a) Dyspnea
                      (i) Minimal exertion
                      (ii) Rest
                  (b) Chronic cough
                  (c) Barrel chest
                  (d) Elevation of shoulders
                  (e) Pursed-lip breathing
                  (f) Cyanosis
                  (g) Clubbing of fingers
                  (h) Tachypnea
                  (i) Predisposition to respiratory infections
              iii. Shortness of breath
              iv. Current or past episodes of:
                  (a) Pneumonia
                  (b) Tuberculosis
                  (c) Bronchitis
                  (d) Asthma
      2. Physical examination
          a. Auscultation of the chest
              i. Crackles
                  (a) Typically short, explosive, discontinuous sounds
                  (b) May be heard in patients with:
                      (i) Pulmonary emphysema
                      (ii) Bronchitis
                      (iii) Asthma
                      (iv) Pulmonary congestion
                          a) Due to CHF
              ii. Rhonchi
                  (a) Coarser, rattling sounds with lower pitch
                      (i) Generally heard over large airways
              iii. Wheezes
                  (a) Continuous, musical sound
                      (i) Asthma or emphysema
                      (ii) Particularly expiration
          b. Baseline breath sounds
              i. Comparison for postanesthetic findings
                  (a) Aspiration
                  (b) Fluid overload
                  (c) Bronchospasm

     c. Baseline oximetry readings
- i. Observation of:
  - (a) Rate
  - (b) Depth
  - (c) Ease of breathing

     d. Cyanosis
     e. Symmetry of chest movements
     f. Use of accessory muscles
     g. Production of sputum
     h. Upper airway including anatomic structures
- i. Short, stocky neck
- ii. Excessive skin or fat on back of neck
- iii. Thick tongue
- iv. Previous cervical fusion
- v. Temporal mandibular joint disease
- vi. Down syndrome
  - (a) Thick, protruding tongue
  - (b) Skin folds on posterior neck
  - (c) Instability of atlantalaxial joint in cervical spine
    - (i) Found in approximately 10–20% of persons with Down syndrome
      - a) Dislocation or subluxation of this joint can occur with hyperextension of neck
      - b) Cervical cord compression with nerve damage and possible death in 5–10% of those predisposed

F. Neurologic
  1. Assessment
     a. General affect
- i. Behavior
- ii. Speech patterns
- iii. Orientation
- iv. Gait

     b. Fine motor movements
- i. Writing
- ii. Cough
- iii. Blink
- iv. Swallow
- v. Pupil reflexes

     c. Motor abilities
- i. Muscle strength
- ii. Vision
- iii. Hearing

     d. Presence of:
- i. Headache
- ii. Dizziness
- iii. Paralysis
- iv. Seizures
- v. Loss of motor control

     e. Pre-existing neurologic deficit
- i. More complete examination
  - (a) Cerebral
  - (b) Motor
  - (c) Cranial nerves

        (i)   Table 7–2 describes abnormalities in function of the cranial nerves

    (d) Reflex functions

G. Sensory and prosthetic
   1. Patients may not provide accurate information about sensory deficits
      a. Embarrassment
      b. Vanity
      c. Assessment skills
         i. Hearing loss
           (a) Patient may lean or turn toward conversation
           (b) Answer questions inappropriately or not at all
           (c) Watch interviewer's lips
           (d) Provide interpreter in American Sign Language if patient is knowledgeable in use
              (i)   Provide information and answers to questions that patient can understand
        ii. Visual impairment
           (a) Difficulty seeing documents

Table 7–2 • ABNORMALITIES IN CRANIAL NERVE FUNCTION

NAME	TYPE	FUNCTION	TEST ABNORMALITY
I. Olfactory	S	Smell	Coffee, tobacco
II. Optic	S	Vision	Visual acuity; Pupillary reaction, visual fields
III. Oculomotor	M	Eye movement	Ptosis; lateral and downward deviation of eye
IV. Trochlear	M	Eye movement	Medial and upper deviation of eye
V. Trigeminal (3 branches—opthalmic, maxillary, mandibular)	S	From skin of face and cornea	Loss of sensation on one side of face
VI. Abducens	M	Eye movement	Medial deviation of eyeball
VII. Facial	S	Taste—anterior tongue;	Inability to grimace on one side of face
	M	Muscles of facial expression	
VIII. Acoustic auditory vestibulocochlear	S	Hearing	Watch ticking, whispered voice;
	S	Equilibrium	Vertigo, nystagmus
IX. Glossopharyngeal	S	Taste on posterior portion of tongue;	Loss of gag reflex; deviation of uvula toward the unaffected side
	M	Pharyngeal muscles	
X. Vagus	S	From thoracic and abdominal organs;	As with IX plus hoarseness
	M	Pharyngeal and laryngeal muscles plus thoracic and abdominal organs	
XI. Spinal accessory	M	Sternocleidomastoid and trapezius muscles	Inability to shrug one shoulder or to move chin to one side against pressure of examiner's hand
XII. Hypoglossal	M	Tongue movement	Deviation of tongue to affected side

S = Sensory   M = Motor

            (b) Should have instructions, consents, and other forms read to them prior to having them signed
- 2. Note that this occurred on patient record
  - a. Emphasis is to ensure effective communication and understanding between patient and staff throughout surgical experience
  - b. Patient must be able to understand instructions and explanations
    - i.   May need sensory aids such as:
      - (a) Hearing aids
      - (b) Glasses/contact lenses
      - (c) Electronic voice stimulator
      - (d) Historically banned from operating room
        - (i)   Current wellness-centered care approach brings more liberal policy
        - (ii)   As long as there is no threat to patient safety, potential for loss or harm to device, these devices are often allowed to remain with the patient
        - (iii) Decision usually made by anesthesiologist
      - (e) Reassures patients that they may retain these devices and promotes psychological health
      - (f) Same is true for dentures, wigs, prosthetic limbs and breasts
        - (i)   Essential for self image and security
        - (ii)   If they must be moved, reassure patients that they will be returned as soon as possible
        - (iii) Personal privacy and dignity will be maintained
        - (iv) Some ASCs are reevaluating the policy of removing dentures from all patients
          - a) Unless having general anesthesia, usually not necessary
  - c. Documentation of presence of:
    - i.   Loose/chipped teeth
    - ii.   Permanent bridgework
      - (a) Avoid accidental injury during airway or tube insertion
      - (b) Identify potential complications of airway management
      - (c) Establish pre-existing problems for legal reasons
- H. Musculo-skeletal
  - 1. History
    - a. Arthritis
    - b. Scoliosis
    - c. Osteoporosis
    - d. Sciatica
    - e. Vertebral disc problems
    - f. Amputations
    - g. Prior fractures
    - h. Frequent falls
  - 2. Physical assessment
    - a. Muscle strength
    - b. Gait
    - c. Mobility
    - d. Range of motion
    - e. Use of orthopedic appliances/prostheses
    - f. Need for assistive devices
      - i.   Walker
      - ii.   Cane
      - iii. Wheelchair

I. Integumentary
   1. Assessment
      a. Observation
         i. Color
         ii. Temperature
         iii. Texture
         iv. Dryness
         v. Turgor
         vi. Loss of elasticity
            (a) Normal change in aging
            (b) Can also indicate dehydration
         vii. Integrity
            (a) Easy bruising/petechiae
                (i) Could indicate hematologic problems
         viii. Jaundice
            (a) Could indicate history of hepatitis
         ix. Cyanosis or mottling
            (a) May indicate serious vascular or cardiac disease
J. Communicable diseases
   1. Scabies
   2. Pediculosis (lice)
   3. Impetigo
      a. Presence of rash, especially in children
   4. History of:
      a. Recent fever
      b. Upper respiratory symptoms
      c. Measles (rubeola)
      d. German measles (rubella)
      e. Chicken pox (varicella)
         i. Treatment prior to admission to ASC
         ii. Other people, including patients in contact, could contract disease or infestation
         iii. Wound infection potential as result of self-contamination
K. Gastrointestinal
   1. History
      a. Previous surgery
         i. Diversional surgery
         ii. Colostomy
      b. Gastrointestinal bleed
      c. Cancer
      d. Hiatal hernia
      e. Chronic diarrhea or constipation
      f. Presence of postoperative nausea and vomiting (PONV)
         i. If predisposition known, psychological and pharmacological interventions can be initiated to prevent occurrence
         ii. PONV unpleasant but potential for aspiration strong
      g. Aspiration risk
      h. Pyloric obstruction
      i. Intestinal obstruction
      j. Esophageal diverticula
      k. Diminished pharyngeal reflexes
      l. Obesity

      m. Advanced pregnancy

      n. Unknown compliance with NPO requirements

  2. Assessment

      a. Mouth

      b. Pharynx

      c. Esophagus

      d. Stomach

      e. Large intestine

      f. Small intestine

      g. Pancreas

      h. Liver

      i. Gallbladder

L. Renal/Hepatic

  1. Many anesthetic drugs are metabolized in the kidneys and liver

  2. History or presence of renal or hepatic disease is of great concern

      a. Pseudocholinesterase

         i. Enzyme necessary for metabolism of succinylcholine and ester-type local anesthetics

  3. Kidney function

      a. Excretion of urine

      b. Influences fluid and electrolyte and acid-base balance

      c. Nitrogenous wastes from protein metabolism are excreted

      d. Electrolytes are maintained

         i. Sodium, potassium, chloride

         ii. Excretion of some drugs is also dependent on kidney function

  4. Liver function

      a. Metabolism of bilirubin

      b. Byproducts of red blood cell breakdown

      c. Protein synthesis

         i. Particularly albumin

         ii. Chronic liver disease patients have decreased serum protein levels

      d. Drug biotransformation

         i. Protein-bound drugs (thiopental and bupivacaine) have fewer sites to bind

         ii. Unbound portions remain active in bloodstream creating prolonged or enhanced effects

  5. Physical assessment

      a. Renal disease

         i. May not be evident until 50% or more function is lost

      b. Liver disease

         i. Jaundice

         ii. Spider angiomata

         iii. Ecchymosis

         iv. Ascites

         v. Pedal edema

         vi. Scleral icterus

  6. History

      a. Cirrhosis

         i. Chronic alcohol or drug abuse

      b. Hepatitis

      c. Immune disorders

      d. Extreme forms of dieting

Table 7–3 • **ENDOCRINE IMBALANCES**

HORMONE	HYPOSECRETION	HYPERSECRETION
Thyroid Hormone	Children—cretinism Adults—myxedema ↓ BMR, tiredness, mentally slow, bradycardia	Hyperthyroidism, ↑ BMR*, always hungry, irritable, tachycardia, weight loss
Parathyroid Hormone	Spontaneous discharge of nerves, spasms, tetany, death	Weak, brittle bones; kidney stones
Insulin	Diabetes mellitus	Hypoglycemia
Adrenocortical Hormones	Addison's disease (body does not synthesize enough glucose, unable to deal with stress, sodium loss in urine may lead to shock)	Cushing's disease (edema gives full moon face, fat around trunk, ↑ blood glucose levels, depressed immune response)

*BMR = Basal Metabolic Rate

      e. Liver or kidney insufficiency/failure
      f. Extremes in blood pressure
      g. Anemia
      h. Electrolyte imbalance
      i. Depression
  M. Endocrine
    1. Diverse diseases; can affect many processes necessary for tolerance of anesthesia and surgery
    2. Hormones regulate:
      a. Response to stress
      b. Rate of metabolism
      c. Blood pressure
      d. Pulse rates
      e. Blood glucose levels
      f. Urine production
      g. Electrolyte balance
      h. Table 7–3 lists principal hormones and symptoms from imbalances
    3. Diabetes
      a. Complications secondary to diabetic condition
        i. Delayed wound healing
        ii. Retinopathy
        iii. Kidney failure
        iv. Peripheral artery disease
        v. Potential for:
          (a) Ketoacidosis
          (b) MI
          (c) Severe hypoglycemia
      b. Requires special instructions especially with regard to insulin and diet on day of surgery
        i. Often asked to bring own insulin to ASC
        ii. May be asked to bring own food if ASC does not serve food or serves only donuts or sweet rolls for postoperative nourishment
  N. Hematologic
    1. Disorders of the blood may involve:
      a. Red blood cells
        i. Anemia

        ii.   Sickle cell anemia
        iii. Thalassemia
        iv. Polycythemia
    b. Lymphocytes/plasma cells
        i.   Agranulocytosis
        ii. Leukemia
        iii. Multiple myeloma
    c. Lymph nodes/spleen
        i.   Lymphoma
        ii. Infectious mononucleosis
    d. Platelets/clotting factors
        i.   Hemorrhagic disorders
        ii. Purpura
        iii. Coagulation disorders
            (a) Hemophilia
            (b) Hypoprothrombinemia
  2. Physical examination
    a. Observation
        i.   Petechiae/bruising
        ii. Pallor/cyanosis
            (a) Skin and mucus membranes
        iii. Hepatomegaly
        iv. Splenomegaly
  3. History of:
    a. Fatigue
    b. Lassitude
    c. Easy bruising
    d. Frequent nosebleeds
    e. Hematuria
    f. Blood in stools
    g. Excessive bleeding after minor injuries or dental extractions
  4. Leukemia and acquired immunodeficiency syndrome (AIDS)
    a. May be scheduled in ASC to avoid hospitalization and subsequent nosocomial infections

V. Psychosocial Assessment
  A. Evaluation of emotional, cognitive, social, and cultural assessments occurs during physical assessment
  B. Emotional assessment
    1. Most patients express a moderate to high degree of anxiety and fear facing surgery
      a. Patients have a right to feel anxiety
         i.   Placating or belittling the situation is seen as demeaning to the patient
         ii. Credibility of staff is undermined by this approach
    2. Anxiety and fear are similar but different
      a. Anxiety is described as a vague, unknown, or unidentified source evoked by a threat to one's existence or personality
      b. Fear is related to a more specific person or occurrence
         i.   Some common fears related to surgery are:
             (a) Possibility of not waking up after anesthesia
             (b) Having a mask placed on the face
             (c) Regaining consciousness during the surgery
             (d) Making a fool of oneself

          (e) Feeling the operation

          (f) Anticipated postoperative pain

          (g) Outcome of surgery

  c. Ambulatory surgery would seem to provoke less fear and anxiety but this is not the case

      i. Home recuperation can add additional pressure

          (a) Fear of facing emergencies at home without medical attention

          (b) Concern about family members who would have to care for them

          (c) Inadequate pain medication

          (d) Need to have another adult for transportation and home support

             (i)   Threat to independence

             (ii)   Embarrassment at having to ask for help

             (iii) Problems of obtaining other person to provide support

          (e) Pressure of arriving on time

             (i)   Many people do not sleep the night before for fear of not waking in time

             (ii)   May be primary caregiver for spouse

                 a) Concern over their care while in surgery and during recuperation period

3. Preoperative interview important

  a. Assess emotional state

      i. Objective observations

          (a) General appearance

          (b) Nervousness

          (c) Decreased attention span

          (d) Lack of eye contact

          (e) Increase heart rate

          (f) Lack of self-confidence

          (g) Decreased concentration

          (h) Rapid speech patterns

          (i) Diaphoresis

          (j) Dry mouth

          (k) Clammy skin

          (l) Pressure of arriving on time

          (m) Nausea

          (n) Urinary frequency

          (o) Hyperventilation

          (p) Precordial chest pain

      ii. Subjective information

          (a) Patient

          (b) Family

      iii. Provide answers to questions

          (a) Information and support allow patient to gain understanding of upcoming surgery

          (b) Trust develops with surgical staff

          (c) By allowing patient to express feelings, patients can identify coping mechanisms to deal with rational and irrational fears

          (d) Anxiety can influence amount of teaching patients understand

             (i)   Mildly anxious patients receive the most complete instructions

             (ii)   Moderately anxious patients receive less information

                 a) More attention to their specific areas of concern

            (iii)   Severely anxious patients should receive only basic information
                    a) Need encouragement to verbalize fears
                    b) Patients in state of panic are unable to learn
                    c) No instructions should be given
                    d) Physician should be notified of patient's status

      iv.   Cognitive assessment
          (a) Evaluate patient's understanding of procedure
          (b) Ask open-ended questions to elicit and encourage patient's response in own words
          (c) Avoid yes/no answers
          (d) Evaluate prior to having patient sign consent
          (e) Patient and/or family must be sufficiently intelligent and responsible to provide care
          (f) Understand and comply with:
               (i)   Pre- and postoperative instructions
               (ii)   Knowledge of hygiene
               (iii)   Nutrition requirements
               (iv)   Complying with NPO status

C. Illiteracy
    1. Written instructions of no use to person who cannot read or understand what is read
    2. Estimated more than 23 million Americans are illiterate
      a. Cannot read at the level most health-care information is written (fifth-grade level)
         i.   Many may be able to sign name without reading form
           (a) Clear verbal instructions particularly important
      b. Language barrier
         i.   English as a second language
           (a) Need for interpreter to provide information
               (i)   Preferably *not* a family member
                    a) May be protecting patient by withholding information they feel patient should not know

D. Social assessment
    1. Concept of ambulatory surgery is family- and home-based
      a. Patients need strong support system
      b. Equally important is those persons be responsible for after care
    2. Evaluation of home situation important during preoperative planning process
      a. Elderly patients
         i.   Surgical patient may be healthier of couple
           (a) Often require outside help
               (i)   Neighbors
               (ii)   Other family members
               (iii)   Home health provider
           (b) Physical environment of home
               (i)   Number of stairs
               (ii)   Bathroom location
               (iii)   May need to utilize social services to provide discharge planning
          (c) Proximity of home to surgical center

E. Cultural assessment
    1. Cultural and ethnic beliefs play role in patient's attitudes about health care

      a. Difficult to separate beliefs from modern health care

      b. May be considered superstitions by health-care workers

          i. Spiritual control over body

          ii. Faith healing

          iii. Being one with the environment

      c. Health-care workers must respect patient's cultural beliefs

VI. Diagnostic Assessment

  A. 1970s–1980s

    1. Many ambulatory surgery centers cared for essentially healthy individuals

      a. Diagnostic practices were limited to few tests

          i. Fingerstick hemoglobin and hematocrit screen

          ii. Dipstick urinalysis

             (a) Provided sufficient data to safely administer anesthesia

  B. Today—sicker patients having surgery on an outpatient basis

    1. Diagnostic requirements now include a variety of basic and complex testing

      a. Often same requirements as hospitalized counterparts

    2. Preoperative testing is done to reduce risks associated with anesthesia and surgery

      a. Provides information about whether the patient can tolerate surgical procedures

  C. Debate over amount and type of preoperative testing

    1. Cost effectiveness

      a. Current trend is toward ordering only those tests specifically indicated by abnormal clinical symptoms or history

    2. Clinical thoroughness

      a. Diagnostic testing is expensive

          i. Benefit thought to outweigh expense

             (a) Offers early detection of previously undiagnosed diseases

             (b) Provides information regarding general health and ability to tolerate surgery of patient

VII. Documenting the Preoperative Assessment

  A. Format for documenting health history and physical assessment

    1. Completed prior to actual admission to ASC

    2. Differs from center to center

  B. Preanesthesia assessment

    1. May be completed by patient or family member

      a. Nontechnical form

      b. Easy to read, understand, and complete

    2. Allow space for nurse's objective findings

      a. Vital signs

      b. Physical assessment

      c. Emotional assessment

      d. Special instructions given to patient

      e. Name of responsible adult

      f. Time patient told to arrive on day of surgery

      g. Any other pertinent information

          i. Medications to take on morning of surgery

          ii. What to bring to center

             (a) Type of clothing to wear

VIII. Preoperative Instructions

  A. Steps in teaching process

    1. Assessing learning needs

   a. Nurse's ability to teach
   b. Patient's learning needs and readiness to learn
      i.   Patient's interest level
           (a) Attentiveness
      ii. Level of understanding
      iii. Ability to comprehend
      iv. Obstacles to learning
           (a) Language barrier
           (b) Sensory losses
 2. Planning a teaching approach
   a. Content/type of information
      i.   Provided at level of patient understanding
           (a) Avoid use of medical jargon
           (b) Provide easy-to-understand explanations
   b. Type of media
      i.   Learning and retention enhanced with more than one medium
           (a) Verbal and written instructions
               (i)   Verbal instructions more personal and individualized
               (ii) Encourage questions and feedback from patients
               (iii) Written instructions allow for reference later on
           (b) Audio tapes
           (c) Video tapes, slides, films
           (d) Charts
           (e) Hands-on demonstrations
           (f) Tour of facility
               (i)   Especially useful for children
   c. Who will be involved
   d. Environment
   e. Time frame
   f. Group vs. one-on-one teaching
      i.   One-on-one most effective
           (a) More personal
      ii. Group more economical
B. Implementing a teaching plan
 1. General information
   a. Arrival time
      i.   Varies for individual surgical center
   b. Diet
      i.   NPO restrictions
      ii. Smoking
           (a) Refrain from smoking for at least 8 hours or longer before
               surgery/or per facility policy
               (i)   Reduce the amount of carbon monoxide in blood
                     a) Promotes better oxygenation during anesthesia
               (ii) Reduce upper airway irritation
               (iii) Reduce bronchospastic tendency
               (iv) Reduce gastric volumes
 2. Medication protocol
   a. Instructions usually given by surgeon or anesthesiologist regarding
      medications
      i.   Reinforced by nurse
      ii. Patients should follow usual medication routine at least until midnight
           prior to surgery

(a) Some drugs are continued up to the time of surgery
    (i) Cardiac drugs
    (ii) Antihypertensives
    (iii) Beta blockers
    (iv) Calcium channel blockers
    (v) Anticonvulsants
    (vi) Monoamine oxidase inhibitor (MAOI) antidepressants
        (Parnate, Nardil, Eutonyl)
        a) Usually discontinued prior to anesthesia
        b) Interaction between MAOIs and anesthetic drugs can result
           in a release of epinephrine and dopamine stores
    (vii) Anticoagulant therapy
        a) Coumadin is often discontinued 48 hours prior to surgery
        b) Clotting studies done immediately prior to surgery
        c) Patients on long-term therapy must be monitored closely
           for signs of bleeding
        d) Platelet function
        e) Aspirin
            i) Affects platelet adhesiveness for up to one week
            ii) Discontinued 7 days prior to surgery
        f) Dipyridamole (persantine) usually stopped 2 days prior to
           surgery
        g) Indomethacin, vitamin E, tricyclic antidepressants,
           phenothiazines, furosemide, steroids also interfere with
           platelet function

C. Patient participation
    1. Encourage patients to ask questions
    2. Obtain information necessary to personalize care
D. Documenting the teaching
    1. Checklist format is efficient way to identify topics covered and patient's
       response to them
    2. Special needs or problems should be charted to alert health-care workers on day
       of surgery
    3. Appropriate follow-up care can be completed

IX. **Consents**
A. Surgical consents
    1. Must accurately identify procedure being performed
    2. Words and names should be spelled correctly
        a. Avoid abbreviations
        b. No blank areas
        c. No erasures
        d. No obliterations
        e. Language that is understood by patient
            i. Changes or additions to consent should be written or typed clearly
            ii. Person making change should initial change and date it
            iii. Patient should also initial and date area that is changed
                (a) Significant changes are best done with new consent form
    3. Nurse's role in obtaining consent
        a. Actual consent for surgery occurs when the surgeon and patient agree to
           proceed
        b. Explanation of the procedure, including risks, benefits, outcome, and
           potential complications is surgeon's responsibility

   c. Legal responsibility to obtain consent
      i. Many institutions require that the nurse facilitate the process by obtaining patient's signature on consent form as well as witnessing that signature
      ii. The nurse is not legally responsible for obtaining actual consent for surgery or treatment
   d. According to the American Nurses Association:
      i. Moral and ethical obligation to ensure that the patient does not feel forced or pressured into treatment
      ii. Patient receives accurate information that is understood by the patient
      iii. Patient understands that consent can be withdrawn at any time
      iv. Ensure that the patient understands what is being done
         (a) If patient understands, the nurse may obtain signature on consent form and witness that signature
         (b) If patient does not indicate understanding or is unsure about other aspects of the surgery, inform surgeon prior to obtaining signature
         (c) Document incident and subsequent conversation in patient record

  B. Special consents
   1. In some instances, additional consents may be required
     a. Sterilization procedures
     b. Termination of pregnancy
     c. Implantation of investigational devices
     d. Photographing procedure
     e. Exception is procedure done via video
     f. Laparoscopic procedures
     g. Release of information to another physician and/or institution

X. Patient Self-Determination Act
  A. Omnibus Budget Reconciliation Act of 1990
   1. Patient Self-Determination Act
     a. Requires all individuals receiving medical care be given written information about their rights under state law
     b. Decisions regarding medical care
       i. Right to accept or refuse treatment
         (a) Medical or surgical
      ii. Right to initiate advance directives
         (a) Living will
         (b) Durable power of attorney
         (c) Right to direct end-of-life decisions
      iii. Does not require that patients have living will or durable power of attorney, only that they be given this information
         (a) Currently only hospitals, nursing homes, nursing facilities, and home health agencies are required to participate
         (b) Some freestanding surgical centers are supplying this information

XI. A.M. Admissions
  A. Response to increasing costs of hospitalization
   1. Large percentage of surgical patients are having diagnostic testing performed as an outpatient
     a. Patients are then admitted the morning of surgery
       i. Following postanesthesia care, they are admitted to hospital room
   2. Often require extensive preoperative work-up on morning of surgery
     a. May be done as outpatient to facilitate morning admission

3. Preoperative assessment
   a. May be done as outpatient or by telephone interview
      i. History
      ii. Physical
      iii. Preoperative teaching
      iv. Anesthesia evaluation

XII. Immediate Preoperative Preparations
   A. General preparations
      1. Morning of surgery
         a. Physical and emotional support
            i. Ensure privacy
            ii. Family/friends
               (a) Directed to waiting room
               (b) Given approximate length of time for surgery completion
         b. Clothing/valuables
            i. Hospital gowns
               (a) Some surgical centers allow patients to wear undergarments if they don't interfere with surgical site
                  (i) *No* nylon undergarments
            ii. Clothes are kept in patient lockers
               (a) Some surgical centers place clothing in bags to be kept below stretcher and with patient throughout stay
            iii. Women are usually asked not to wear makeup
               (a) Especially mascara due to potential for eye irritation
               (b) Nail polish
                  (i) Nearly all pulse oximeter manufacturers provide information regarding use with nail polish or artificial nails
            iv. Valuables
               (a) Allow family members to keep any valuables
               (b) Sensory aids
                  (i) Beneficial to encourage adequate communication
                  (ii) If glasses, hearing aids, or dentures must be removed, they should be returned as soon as the patient is awake
               (c) Label with patient's name and keep with patient's belongings
   B. Reassess patient's understanding of procedure and preoperative instructions
      1. Medication instructions
      2. NPO status
         a. Specifically water (if not taking medication)
         b. Hard candy
         c. Chewing gum
            i. Many people seem confused about these items and maintaining NPO status
            ii. Chewing gum and hard candy stimulates increased production of stomach juices
      3. Vital signs
         a. If patient was seen prior to surgery, compare these measurements with preoperative visit
      4. Significant changes in health history since preoperative visit
      5. Upper respiratory infections
         a. Pulmonary congestion
         b. Fever
      6. Nausea/vomiting

7. Skin disruptions
   a. Specifically at surgical site
      i. Shave prep
      ii. Area of controversy
      iii. AORN recommendations is that hair that does not interfere with surgery should be left intact
         (a) Hair removal is often unnecessary
         (b) Possibly harmful
         (c) Relationship between shaving and increased wound infection
            (i) Depilatories and clippers are often used instead of razors
            (ii) Less incidence of skin nicks
               a) Lower postoperative skin infections
               b) Incidence of increased infection from earlier shave preps
               c) Microscopic nicks serve as good medium for bacterial growth
         (d) If shaving necessary, many surgeons now prefer it be done just prior to surgery

C. Intravenous access
   1. Policies regarding intravenous access vary greatly from facility to facility
   2. Insertion of venous access may be responsibility of admitting nurse
      a. CRNA
      b. IV team nurse
      c. Anesthesiologist
   3. Needle gauge
      a. Depends on patient needs
      b. Most ambulatory surgery patients will not require blood
         i. 20 gauge is adequate
         ii. 22 gauge may be needed for elderly patients with small, fragile veins
      c. A.M. admission patients, however, may be facing more complicated procedures
         i. Large-bore needle (18 gauge) for fluid and blood administration is recommended

D. Medication protocol
   1. Goals of preoperative medications
      a. Reduce anxiety
      b. Reduce incidence of nausea/vomiting
      c. Decrease oral secretions
      d. Decrease potential for laryngospasm
      e. Related potential for aspiration
         i. Decrease gastric acidity and volume
      f. Antibiotics
         i. Prophylaxis for subacute bacterial endocarditis (SBE)
            (a) Generally given prior to dental, gastrointestinal, genitourinary, oral, and respiratory procedures
   2. Anesthesia preparations
      a. General anesthesia
      b. Regional anesthesia
      c. Monitored Anesthesia Care (MAC) anesthesia
         i. Local sedation
   3. Provide emotional support during regional administration
      a. Positioned so patient can see nurse
      b. Maintain eye contact

      c. Hold hand if necessary

      d. Supportive conversation

   4. Physical support

   5. Emergency equipment readily available

      a. Oxygen

      b. Suction

      c. Potential for complications

         i.   Drug reactions

         ii.   Perforation of vessel or body cavity

         iii. Hemorrhage

         iv. Respiratory arrest

         v.   Cardiac arrest

E. Emotional support

   1. Provide emotional support while completing preparations

   2. Calm, unhurried demeanor can help calm patient and reduce anxiety

      a. Soft music

      b. Subdued lighting

      c. Warm colors

      d. Paintings on walls

         i.   Outdoor, nature settings

      e. Soothing voice

F. Documenting and reporting care

   1. Preoperative nursing care documented according to facility's policy

      a. Charting should be simple while complete

         i.   Checklist, fill-in, graphs

         ii.   Allow space for narrative documentation if needed

      b. Include:

         i.   Vital signs

            (a) Including height and weight

         ii.   Allergies

         iii. Emotional assessment

         iv. Medications

            (a) Patient's own

            (b) Any administered for surgery

         v.   Special preoperative preparations needed

         vi. Specific/unusual findings

            (a) Bruises

            (b) Unsuccessful IV attempts

            (c) Reactions to medications

            (d) Disposition of valuables

            (e) Responsible adult for home transport

            (f) Infectious diseases

            (g) Positioning requirements

            (h) Prostheses

            (i) Hemiparesis

            (j) Presence of dialysis catheter

                (i)   Use of nonaffected arm for blood pressure and venipuncture

            (k) Special requests of patient

                (i)   Wearing religious medal

                (ii)   Where family is waiting

Bibliography

1. Boike, L., Canala, L., Kozminski, K., Wynd, C. A. (1995). Development of an outpatient perioperative care record. *Journ Post Anes Nurs*, 10(3).
2. Brumfield, V.C., Kee, C.C., Johnson, J.Y. (1996). Preoperative patient teaching in ambulatory surgery settings. *AORN J*, 64(6).
3. Burden, N. (1993). *Ambulatory Surgical Nursing*. Philadelphia: Saunders.
4. Drain, C. (1994). *The Post Anesthesia Care Unit: A Critical Care Approach*, 3rd ed., Philadelphia: Saunders.
5. Kerridge, R., Lee, A., Latchford, E. (1996). The perioperative system: A new approach to managing elective surgery. *Anaesth Intensive Care*, 23(5).
6. Lancaster, K.A. (1997). Patient teaching in ambulatory surgery. *Nurs Clin North Am*, 32(2).
7. Lisko, S.A. (1995). Development and use of videotaped instruction for preoperative education of the ambulatory gynecological patient. *Jour Post Anes Nurs*, 10(6).
8. McGrory, A., Assmann, S. (1994). A study of investigating primary nursing, discharge teaching, and patient satisfaction of ambulatory cataract patients. *Insight*, 19(2).
9. Murphy, E.K. (1995). Evolving nursing care practices. *Surgical Services Management*, 1(4).
10. Oberle, K., Allen, M., Lynkowski, P. (1994). Follow-up of same day surgery patients: A study of patient concerns. *AORN J*, 59(5).
11. Pica-Furey, W. (1993). Ambulatory surgery—hospital based vs. freestanding: A comparative study of patient satisfaction. *AORN J*, 57(5).
12. Swan, B.A. (1996). Assessing symptom distress in ambulatory surgery patients. *Medsurg Nursing*, 5(5).
13. Williams, G.D. (1997). Ambulatory surgery: Preoperative assessment and health history interview. *Nurs Clin North Am*, 32(2).

REVIEW QUESTIONS

1. Patients who visit the ASC prior to the day of surgery

   A. Experience increased anxiety on the day of surgery
   B. Are no less anxious than those who did not visit
   C. Have decreased anxiety levels on the day of surgery
   D. Ask more questions than those who did not visit
   E. Require longer recovery periods overall

2. The primary goal of preoperative preparation for ambulatory surgical patients includes

   A. Assessment of the patient's physical status
   B. Promotion of the wellness concept
   C. Provision of emotional support
   D. Reduction of the patient's anxiety level
   E. All of the above

3. Physical examination of the skin includes observations of

   A. Color
   B. Turgor
   C. Lesions
   D. Bruising
   E. All of the above

4. Common fears related to surgery include
   (1) The possibility of not waking after anesthesia
   (2) Making a fool of oneself
   (3) Having an unplanned procedure performed
   (4) Waking up during the surgery

   A. 1, 4
   B. 3, 4, 5
   C. 1, 2, 5
   D. 1, 3, 4
   E. All of the above

5. According to AORN, hair that does not interfere with surgery should be left intact because
   (1) Microscopic nicks serve as good medium for bacterial growth
   (2) Hair removal is often considered unnecessary
   (3) Shaving the operative area is possibly harmful
   (4) Increased risk of skin and wound infections

   A. 1, 2
   B. 3, 4
   C. 2, 3, 4
   D. 1, 3, 4
   E. All of the above

6. Significant changes in health history since the preoperative visit should be reported, especially

   A. Fever
   B. Upper respiratory infections
   C. Nausea/vomiting
   D. Pulmonary congestion
   E. All of the above

7. Returning the patient's sensory aids as soon as possible after surgery

   A. Encourages adequate communication
   B. Fosters patient independence and dignity
   C. Promotes wellness philosophy
   D. None of the above
   E. All of the above

8. Providing information about the Patient Self-Determination Act requires that the patient
   (1) Receive information about advance directives
   (2) Have advance directives in place prior to surgery
   (3) Receive information about their rights under state law

   A. 1, 2, 3
   B. 2 only
   C. 1, 3
   D. 1 only

9. The nurses' role in obtaining patient consent for surgery is to
   (1) Ensure patient understands what is being done
   (2) Explain the entire scope of the procedure
   (3) Only be a witness to the patient's signature
   (4) Answer questions the patient may have

   A. 1, 3
   B. 2, 4
   C. 1, 2, 3
   D. 1, 3, 4
   E. 2, 3, 4

10. The ideal interpreter for a patient who does not speak English or who is sensory impaired is

   A. A family member
   B. A hospital employee
   C. Flash cards
   D. Video tapes

ANSWERS TO QUESTIONS

1. C
2. E
3. E
4. E
5. E

6. E
7. E
8. C
9. D
10. B

Postoperative Patient Assessment and Discharge Criteria—Phases I and II

Rose Ferrara-Love
Duquesne University
Mercy Providence Hospital
Pittsburgh, Pennsylvania

I. **Immediate Postanesthesia Care—Phase I**
   A. Focus of care
      1. Observe patient's physiologic status and intervene appropriately in a way that encourages uneventful recovery from anesthesia and surgery
      2. Provide safe environment for the patient experiencing limitations in physical, mental, and emotional function
      3. Avoid or immediately treat complications in the immediate postanesthetic period
      4. Uphold the patient's right to dignity, privacy, and confidentiality
      5. Encourage a sense of wellness and self-confidence needed for early discharge
   B. Patient outcome
      1. Return to consciousness
         a. Avoid heavy sedation
            i. Possible overnight admission
            ii. Prolongs recovery period
      2. Encourage self-care
         a. Promotes self-confidence
         b. Promotes sense of wellness, not illness
      3. Maintain patient dignity
         a. Use patient's name
         b. Maintain eye contact

Objectives

1. Plan the focus of nursing care for the ambulatory surgery patient.
2. Characterize ways to ensure patient satisfaction in the ambulatory surgery setting.
3. Explain staffing ratios for Phase I and Phase II PACU.
4. Identify key points of anesthesia report upon arrival to PACU.
5. Demonstrate initial patient assessment parameters.
6. Describe extubation criteria in the PACU.
7. Discuss causes of hemodynamic changes in the PACU.
8. Examine causes of alterations in level of consciousness after anesthesia.
9. Assess patient readiness for transfer from Phase I to Phase II following spinal or epidural anesthesia.
10. Compare PACU scoring systems.

      c. Use therapeutic touch

         i.   Includes voice, tone, facial expressions, etc.

    4. Resolution of effects of major regional anesthesia

    5. Patient satisfaction

      a. Provide privacy

      b. Early reunion with family/responsible others

II. Equipment and Environmental Concerns

  A. Suggested 1.5 beds available for each operating room

    1. 2 beds per OR suite may be needed for:

      a. Short procedures

      b. Pediatric cases

  B. Physical environment

    1. Well-lighted area

    2. Visibility of all patients in the PACU from any area

    3. Freestanding facility

      a. Access from PACU to lobby waiting area for family members

    4. Hospital-based facility

      a. Situated between OR suite and Phase II area

         i.   Separate rooms or sections are recommended for Phase I and Phase II areas

           (a) Provides ease in progression from OR to Phase II

    5. Amenities

      a. Bathrooms

      b. Changing/dressing areas

      c. Bedside chair

      d. Room for family member or responsible other to visit

      e. Diversionary materials

         i.   Current magazines, radio, television, videos, etc.

      f. Noninstitutional decor

         i.   Promotes sense of wellness

           (a) Wallpaper

           (b) Draperies

           (c) Greenery

           (d) Windows

           (e) Wall decorations

           (f) Supplies in modern cabinets

  C. Emergency preparation

    1. Emergency call system

    2. Emergency equipment/medications

III. Policies, Procedures, and Staffing

  A. Policy manual per institutional guidelines

    1. Address broad range of nursing duties and administrative practice specific to PACU

    2. Annual review of policies

    3. Staff participation in ongoing revision

  B. Outside certifying bodies

    1. Joint Commission for Accreditation of Healthcare Organizations

    2. American Hospital Association

    3. State Health Department

    4. Third–party payers

      a. Medicare

      b. Medicaid

      c. Insurance companies

C. Staffing ratios
  1. Table 8–1 highlights worksheet for determining full-time equivalent staffing (FTEs)
  2. ASPAN Standards of PeriAnesthesia Nursing Practice, 1998
     a. Phase I
        i. Class 1:2—one nurse to two patients who are
           (a) One unconscious, stable without artificial airway and over the age of 9 years; and one conscious, stable and free of complications
           (b) Two conscious, stable and free of complications
           (c) Two conscious, stable, 11 years of age and under; with family or competent support staff present
        ii. Class 1:1—one nurse to one patient
           (a) At the time of admission, until the critical elements are met
           (b) Requiring mechanical life support and/or artificial airway
           (c) Any unconscious patient 9 years of age and under
           (d) A second nurse must be available to assist as necessary
        iii. Class 2:1—two nurses to one patient
           (a) One critically ill, unstable, complicated patient
     b. Phase II
        i. Class 1:3—one nurse to three patients
           (a) Over 5 years of age within ½ hour of procedure/discharge from Phase I
           (b) 5 years of age and under within ½ hour of procedure/discharge from Phase I with family present
        ii. Class 1:2—one nurse to two patients
           (a) 5 years of age and under without family or support staff present
           (b) Initial admission of patient post procedure

Table 8–1 • FORMULA FOR DETERMINING DAILY STAFFING NEEDS

Number of patients scheduled in each class × Hours of care required for each class (average time in PACU for each class) × Nurse/patient ratio required for each class, with minimum of 2 nurses present for each classification

Example: Class III patients scheduled = 4 × 2 (nurse/patient ratio of 1:1, minimum 2 nurses)
     Average PACU stay for class III = 2 hours
     $4 \times 2 = 8$
     $8 \times 2 = 16$ hours, or 2 full-time equivalents (FTEs)

To schedule staff according to patient acuity, use the average hours of PACU care patients in each classification required.

Example: Class I patients require an average of 1 hour in PACU. Class II patients stay in PACU an average of 1½ hours. Class III patients may average 2 or more hours in PACU depending on the types of procedures (cardiovascular, organ transplant, etc.) most often performed that require transfer to the intensive care unit (ICU) after stabilization in PACU. Use the number of patients in each class × the hours of care required to obtain the nursing care hours required. Divide the nursing hours required by 6.5 to obtain the number of full-time equivalents (FTEs) needed. FTEs calculated at 6.5 hours represent 100% productivity based on an 8-hour shift, allocated as follows:

Breaks	2 @ 15 min = 30 min
Meal	1 @ 30 min = 30 min
Clothing change	2 @ 5 min = 10 min
Discharge, transport, or report	10 min
Maintenance of supplies/equipment	10 min

Total 1.5 hours per 8-hour shift per nurse

Litwack, K. (1995). *Core Curriculum for Post Anesthesia Nursing Practice*, 3rd ed. Philadelphia: Saunders.

  iii. Class 1:1—one nurse to one patient

   (a) Unstable patient of any age requiring transfer

 c. Phase III

  i. Class 1:5—one nurse to five patients

IV. **Transfer of the Patient to a PACU**

 A. Transporting teams responsible for patient until responsibility accepted by PACU nurse

  1. Anesthesia report

   a. History

   b. Medications

   c. Anesthetic agents/doses

    i. Untoward responses

     (a) Treatment

     (b) Result

   d. Vital signs

  2. Circulating nurse report

   a. Surgery performed

   b. Preoperative status

    i. Emotional

    ii. Psychosocial

   c. Laboratory results

  3. Medical record

   a. Provides information not included in verbal report

  4. Deferring verbal report

   a. Patient's condition is unstable

    i. Immediate safety assured by all participants before report provided

V. **Initial Patient Assessment and Care Planning**

 A. Systems assessment

  1. Usually rapid initial head-to-toe assessment

   a. Focus on vital functions

    i. Airway

    ii. Circulatory

  2. Comprehensive assessment

  3. Subjective assessment

   a. Patient's input

    i. Alertness

    ii. Lucidity

    iii. Orientation

    iv. Motor abilities

     (a) Sensory/motor control following regional anesthesia

    v. Comfort level

    vi. Presence of nausea

  4. Assessments are ongoing

   a. Concurrent with nursing interventions

VI. **Respiratory Adequacy**

 A. Assessment

  1. Auscultation of breath sounds

  2. Assessment of chest expansion

   a. Ease and depth of respirations

   b. Use of accessory muscles

   c. Skin and mucous membrane color

3. Administration of oxygen
    a. Considered standard following heavy sedation or general anesthesia
    b. Face mask
        i. Simple
        ii. Aerosol
    c. Nasal cannula
4. Body's oxygen demand increases with:
    a. Shivering
        i. By 400% or more
    b. Pain
    c. Anxiety
    d. Hypotension
    e. Hypertension
    f. Dysrhythmias
        i. Tachydysrhythmias
    g. Rapid fluctuations in intravascular volume
    h. Thromboembolic events
    i. Left ventricular failure
    j. Catecholamine release
B. Monitoring equipment
    1. Primary
        a. Eyes/ears
            i. Observation
            ii. Auscultation
            iii. Palpation
    2. Mechanical
        a. Respirometer
            i. Detect lung volumes
                (a) Tidal volume
                (b) Vital capacity
            ii. Negative Inspiratory Force (NIF) Meter
                (a) Least amount of negative force to initiate inhalation
        b. Arterial blood gas analysis (ABGs)
            i. Invasive, often painful arterial blood sample for analysis
        c. Pulse oximeter
            i. Measures ratio of oxygenated hemoglobin to the total amount of hemoglobin and expresses it as a percent of saturation
                (a) Analyzes color of blood with two light-emitting diodes and a photodetector
            ii. Noninvasive
                (a) Detects oxygen saturation of hemoglobin in circulating blood
                (b) Sensitive to changes in blood content oxygen
                    (i) Heralds hypoxic event before clinical signs
                (c) Considered "standard of care" monitoring in anesthesia and PACU settings
            iii. Advantages
                (a) Simplicity
                (b) Noninvasive
                (c) Continuous display
                (d) Sensitivity to changes in blood oxygen levels
                (e) Ability to be applied to all ages
                (f) Relatively low expense

      iv. Disadvantages
        (a) Motion at sensor site
        (b) Low perfusion of the arterial bed being monitored
           (i)   Hypothermia
           (ii)   Hypotension
           (iii)   Large doses of vasopressors
        (c) Significant dysrhythmias
        (d) Carbon monoxide or methemoglobin in the blood
        (e) Severe anemia
           (i)   Hemoglobin level less than 5g per dL
        (f) Venous pulsation
           (i)   Sensor is too tight
        (g) Electrical interference
        (h) Interference from ambient or extrinsic light sources
        (i) Circulation intravenous dyes
      v.   Complications
        (a) Burns/blisters
           (i)   Usually on infants/children
        (b) Pressure necrosis

   d. Capnography
      i.   Monitors exhaled carbon dioxide
        (a) End-tidal CO_2
      ii.   Intraoperative monitoring of patients under general anesthesia
        (a) Used in PACU for critically ill patients
           (i)   Often not applicable for ambulatory surgery

C. Airway obstruction
  1. Result of soft tissue displacement in upper airway and mouth
    a. Tongue most obvious and frequent cause
    b. Relieved by:
      i.   Turning patient to side
      ii.   Mandibular extension or jaw thrust
      iii. Insertion of artificial nasal or oral airway
      iv. Gentle backward tilt of head
      v.   Towel roll under shoulders
      vi. Persistent cases
        (a) Manual extension of tongue

  2. Laryngospasm
    a. Muscles of larynx contract causing reflex closing of the vocal cords
      i.   Protective mechanism against foreign material entering larynx and trachea
      ii.   Irritation of larynx
        (a) During initial or "twilight" period of emergence
        (b) Airway secretions
        (c) Artificial oral or nasal airways
        (d) Blood
        (e) Insult of instrumentation on airway
    b. Symptoms
      i.   Dyspnea
      ii.   Hypoxemia
      iii. Hypercarbia
      iv. Use of accessory muscles of respiration
      v.   Suprasternal retraction

vi.   Absent or crowing breath sounds
vii. In awake patients
    (a) Agitation
    (b) Anxiety
    (c) Panic
c. Prevention of laryngospasm
  i.   Extubate patient either while still deeply anesthetized or after completely awake
    (a) Protective reflexes have returned
  ii. Reduce environmental stimuli for patients who are coughing or exhibiting signs of laryngeal irritation while emerging from anesthesia
  iii. Administer humidified oxygen to moisten upper airway
  iv. Administer intravenous lidocaine before extubation
    (a) Controversial practice
d. Treatment of laryngospasm
  i.   Summon anesthesia help
  ii. Remove obvious irritant
  iii. Gently suction mouth and upper airway
  iv. Extend neck
    (a) Maintain anterior displacement of mandible
  v.   Avoid unnecessary movement of patient's head and neck
    (a) Reduces stimulation of already irritated airway
  vi. Administer humidified oxygen
  vii. Display a calm demeanor for the benefit of the semiconscious or awake patient
  viii. Persistent or total laryngospasm
    (a) 100% oxygen under pressure
      (i) Bag–valve–mask
    (b) IV sedation or paralysis
      (i) Succinylcholine 0.5 mg/kg IV
    (c) Atropine to reduce upper airway secretions
    (d) Reintubation
      (i) Cricothyrotomy/tracheotomy
        a) Rare occurrence

D. Aspiration
  1. Risk factors
    a. Larger gastric volumes compared with hospitalized patients
    b. Obesity
    c. Hiatal hernia
    d. Pregnancy
    e. Nasogastric tube
    f. Deflated or incompetent endotracheal cuff
    g. Recent alcohol ingestion
  2. Prevention
    a. Preferred
      i.   Instructions for NPO restrictions
        (a) Alcohol should be avoided day before surgery
          (i) New NPO studies for *healthy patients* with no increased risk of aspiration
            a) No solid food day of surgery
            b) Unrestricted clear liquids up to two hours before surgery

        c) Oral medications with 30 cc water up to one hour prior to surgery

        d) H$_2$ receptor antagonist with clear liquids

   ii.   Preventative measures on day of surgery

      (a) Histamine antagonists

      (b) Antacids

      (c) Antiemetic therapy

      (d) H$_2$ receptor blockers

         (i)   Cimetidine (Tagamet)

            a) Night before and morning of surgery most beneficial

         (ii)   Ranitidine (Zantac)

         (iii) Famotidine (Pepcid)

      (e) Lateral positioning for unconscious patients

3. Symptoms

   a. Mild

      i.   Dyspnea

      ii.   Cyanosis of varying degrees

      iii. Tachycardia

      iv. Abnormal lung sounds

   b. Severe

      i.   Immediate bronchospasm

      ii.   Hypoxemia

      iii. Respiratory arrest

        (a) Cardiac arrest

4. Treatment

   a. Depends on severity of symptoms

      i.   Amount and pH of aspirant

        (a) 25 cc can cause significant pulmonary involvement

        (b) pH 2.5 and volume of 0.4 ml/kg critical point

          (i)   Serious lung parenchymal damage

   b. Immediate oxygen administration

   c. Notify anesthesiologist

5. Aspiration of vomitus

   a. Oxygen administration

      i.   May need reintubation

   b. Lower head of bed

   c. Lateral position

   d. Suction airway

   e. Steroids

   f. Antibiotics

   g. Chest X-ray

      i.   Positive findings of aspiration absent in 10% patients

E. Pulmonary edema

  1. Predisposing factors

    a. Laryngospasm

    b. Narcotics

    c. Administration of naloxone

    d. Intravenous fluid overload

    e. Allergic reactions

    f. Pulmonary emboli

    g. Pre-existing congestive heart failure

2. Symptoms
    a. Tachycardia
    b. Dyspnea
    c. Tachypnea
    d. Confusion
    e. Wheezing
        i.   Rales
        ii.   Crackles
    f. Decreased blood pressure
    g. Paroxysmal nocturnal dyspnea
    h. Chest X-ray findings
        i.   Cardiomegaly
        ii.   Upper lobe pulmonary veins
    i. Increased jugular vein distension
3. Noncardiogenic pulmonary edema (negative pulmonary pressure edema)
    a. Uncommon
        i.   Caused by laryngospasm
        ii.   Naloxone
    b. Symptoms
        i.   Normal blood pressure readings
        ii.   Decreased lung compliance
        iii. Chest X-ray findings
            (a) Normal heart size
            (b) No congestive heart failure
4. Treatment
    a. Reduce cardiac workload
    b. Reduce hypoxemia
        i.   Upright position
        ii.   Oxygen administration
        iii. Suction airway as appropriate
    c. Reduce venous congestion
        i.   Diuretics
F. Hypoventilation
    1. Causes
        a. Residual effects of anesthetic agents
            i.   Muscle relaxants
            ii.   Analgesics
        b. Pain
            i.   Chest/abdominal surgery
                (a) Splinting prevents expansion of chest/abdominal muscles
    2. Treatment
        a. Administer oxygen
        b. Elevate head of bed
            i.   Encourages chest movement
                (a) Obese patients
                (b) Pre-existing respiratory compromise
        c. "Stir-up" regimen
            i.   Every 10–15 minutes
                (a) Encourage respiratory effort
                    (i)   Deep breathing
                    (ii) Coughing
                        a) If not contraindicated by surgery, such as cataract extraction with lens implant

      ii.   Increase circulation and alertness
          (a) Turning from side to side
          (b) Exercising extremities

3. Apnea
  a. Requires aggressive ventilatory support
      i.   Symptoms may be masked by general anesthesia
          (a) Lethargy
          (b) Confusion
          (c) Restlessness
          (d) Anxiety
          (e) Dysrhythmias
          (f) Cyanosis
          (g) Decreased $PaCO_2$
             (i)   May lead to respiratory acidosis
          (h) Hypertension followed by hypotension
          (i) Decreased urinary output

4. Treatment
  a. Pharmacologic cause
      i.   Narcotics
          (a) Intravenous narcotic antagonist—naloxone (Narcan)
             (i)   1 µg/kg (0.01 mg/kg)
                a) Repeated 5–10 minutes
             (ii)   Side effects
                a) Cessation of analgesia
                b) Agitation
                c) Hypertension
                d) Noncardiogenic pulmonary edema
                e) Atrial and ventricular dysrhythmias
                f) Cardiac arrest
      ii.   Muscle relaxants
          (a) Depolarizing muscle relaxant
             (i)   Succinylcholine (Anectine)
             (ii)   Short-acting
                a) Not pharmacologically reversed
                b) Action is self-limiting, effects usually dissipated before
                   admission to PACU
             (iii)   "Phase II block"
                a) Mimic characteristics of nondepolarizing blockade in *large*
                   doses >3 mg/kg
                b) Requires pharmacological reversal
          (b) Nondepolarizing muscle relaxants
             (i)   Reversed with anticholinesterase agents (neostigmine,
                 pyridostigmine, edrophonium)
                a) Can cause vagal reactions (specifically bradycardia)
                b) Usually administered in combination with a vagolytic agent
                   (atropine or glycopyrrolate)
          (c) Reparalysis (or recurarization)
             (i)   Major cause of respiratory depression
             (ii)   Inadequate pharmacologic reversal
                a) Effects of muscle relaxant extend beyond effects of reversal
                   agent

           (iii)   Other factors include
                a) General anesthetics
                b) Hypothermia
                c) Antidisrhythmics (quinidine, procainamide, and calcium channel blockers)
                d) Respiratory acidosis
                e) Metabolic alkalosis
                f) Hypokalemia
                g) Hypocalcemia
                h) Local anesthetic agents (including lidocaine given as antidisrhythmics by IV drip or bolus postoperatively)
                i) Furosemide IV in doses of 1 mg/kg
                j) Dehydration
                k) Hyponatremia
                l) Antibiotics, particularly mycins and aminoglycosides

G. The intubated patient
   1. Nursing care
      a. Constant nursing observation
      b. Administration humidified oxygen
         i.   Compensate for bypassed upper airway
         ii.   Provides moisture to artificially inspired air
      c. Protect patient from aspiration by maintaining cuff inflation
         i.   Position patient properly
         ii.   Suction as appropriate
      d. Ensure proper position of endotracheal tube by:
         i.   Auscultation of breath sounds
         ii.   Observation of symmetrical chest expansion
      e. Provide emotional support and explanations to awakening patient
      f. Evaluate for signs of sufficient recovery to allow for safe extubation
   2. Extubation criteria
      a. Return of muscle strength after muscle relaxants
         i.   Equal hand grasps
         ii.   Able to initiate head lift from bed and sustain at least 5 seconds
      b. Respiratory parameters
         i.   Tidal volume at least 5 ml/kg
         ii.   Vital capacity at least 15–20 ml/kg
         iii. Negative inspiratory force of 20–25 cm water pressure
      c. Patient should respond appropriately to questions
         i.   "Yes" or "no" head movements
         ii.   Other forms of communication
             (a) Sign/picture board
             (b) Writing
         iii. Protrude the tongue
         iv. Open eyes widely
      d. Swallow and cough reflexes present
      e. Regular respiratory pattern >10 breaths per minute
      f. After extubation close observation for hypoventilation
         i.   Presence of endotracheal tube may have stimulated patient to remain awake and breathing adequately

VII. Circulatory Adequacy
   A. Blood pressure
      1. Hypotension

    a. Reflection of several factors
        i.   Cardiac output
        ii. Arterial blood volume
        iii. Peripheral vascular resistance
        iv. Viscosity of the blood
        v.   Elasticity of arterial walls
    b. Affected by:
        i.   General anesthetic agents
           (a) Many cause cardiac depression and decreased peripheral vascular resistance
        ii. Regional anesthetic agents
           (a) Sympathetic nerve blockade
              (i)   Dilated vessels can result in drop in blood pressure
        iii. Changes in fluid status
           (a) Dehydration due to NPO status
           (b) Inadequate intravenous replacement
           (c) Blood loss
              (i)   May cause hypotension
        iv. Individual's preoperative health status
           (a) Anxiety levels
              (i)   Preoperative blood pressure may be artificially high
           (b) Preoperative sedation
           (c) Antihypertensive medications
        v.   Early postoperative ambulation
           (a) However, gradual change in position is recommended to prevent hypotension
    c. Treatment of hypotension
        i.   Continued oxygen therapy
        ii. Gentle movement of the patient
        iii. Supine positioning
        iv. Elevation of the legs
        v.   Infusion of intravenous fluids
        vi. Pharmacologic intervention in more persistent cases
           (a) Adrenergic agents
              (i)   Ephedrine
              (ii)   Phenylephrine (Neo-Synephrine)
              (iii) Metaraminol (Aramine)
              (iv) Isoproterenol (Isuprel)
           (b) Anticholinergic agents
              (i)   Atropine
              (ii)   Glycopyrrolate
2. Hypertension
    a. Causes
        i.   Often difficult to pinpoint
        ii. Sympathetic nervous system activity
        iii. Pain
        iv. Discomfort
        v.   Anxiety
        vi. Full bladder
        vii. Respiratory depression
           (a) Hypoxemia and hypercarbia effect aortic and carotid chemoreceptors
              (i)   Cause vasoconstriction resulting in hypertension

     viii. Fluid overload

     ix. Anesthetic agents/other drugs
  - (a) Ketamine
  - (b) Naloxone
  - (c) Pancuronium
  - (d) Oxytocin

     x. Hypothermia
  - (a) Shivering
    - (i) Increased metabolic activity increases oxygen consumption, carbon dioxide production, increases cardiac workload
  - (b) Peripheral vasoconstriction
    - (i) Conserve body warmth

     xi. Pre-existing state of health
  - (a) >37 million people in U.S. are hypertensive
    - (i) Essential hypertension
      - a) Cause unknown

b. Treatment

     i. Treat cause
  - (a) Pain
    - (i) Analgesics
  - (b) Fluid overload
    - (i) Have patient void
    - (ii) Straight catheterize
    - (iii) Diuretics
  - (c) Anxiety
    - (i) Anxiolytic agents
  - (d) Pre-existing state
    - (i) Antihypertensive agents
      - a) Own medications preoperatively
      - b) Nifedipine (Procardia) sublingual
      - c) Hydralazine (Apresoline) IV bolus
      - d) Propranolol (Inderal) IV bolus
      - e) Nitroglycerine sublingual
      - f) Calcium channel blockers
      - g) Alpha or beta blockers
      - h) Smooth muscle relaxants

c. Hypertension with tachycardia

     i. Particularly dangerous
  - (a) Treat tachycardia first
    - (i) Fluids
    - (ii) Beta blockers
  - (b) Hypertension
    - (i) Labetalol (Trandate, Normodyne)
    - (ii) Esmolol (Brevibloc)

d. Hypertensive crisis

     i. Diastolic pressure >120 mm Hg
  - (a) If untreated
    - (i) Damage to organs
    - (ii) Death

     ii. Perioperative causes include:
  - (a) Vasoconstriction due to catecholamine release
    - (i) Pain
    - (ii) Shivering

    (b) Hypothermia
    (c) Hypervolemia
    (d) Inadequate ventilation
    (e) Withholding patient's usual antihypertensive medications
    (f) Interactions with:
        (i)   Monoamine oxidase inhibitors (MAOIs)
        (ii) Antidepressants
B. Cardiac status
  1. Constant assessment of pulse for rate, rhythm, amplitude
    a. Weak, absent, or irregular pulses
      i.   Hypovolemia
      ii.   Decreased cardiac output
      iii. Myocardial ischemia
        (a) Prior cardiac compromise
            (i)   Increase risk of cardiac complications postanesthesia
        (b) Cannot measure myocardial oxygenation directly
            (i)   Clinical symptoms
            (ii) ECG changes
            (iii) Chest pain
            (iv) Change in skin color
            (v)   Diaphoresis
            (vi) GI sequelae
      iv.   Acute MI
        (a) Previous MI single most important risk factor for perioperative
            patient
            (i)   Nonurgent surgery should be delayed until at least 6 months
                  post MI to reduce perioperative morbidity
        (b) Early signs of perioperative acute infarction or ischemia
            (i)   ECG changes
                  a) T wave inversion and ST segment depression of 1 mm or
                     more below baseline indicative of ischemia
                  b) ST elevation indicates actual myocardial injury
                  c) Later presence of Q wave of 0.03 sec. is definitive for
                     infarction and tissue necrosis*
            (ii) Subjective changes described by patient
                  a) Anginal pain (often constant)
                  b) Nausea, vomiting
                  c) Diaphoresis
                  d) Feeling of impending doom or dying
            (iii) Silent MI
                  a) Only 25% patients who have MIs in the postoperative
                     period experience typical anginal pain
                  b) Most often seen in elderly, diabetic, and hypertensive
                     patients
      v.   Cardiac dysrhythmias
      vi.   Local pathology of the artery in extremity in question
    b. Bounding pulses
      i.   Excitement

---

*Note: ST segment and T wave changes are not absolutely diagnostic of an acute MI. They may be caused by digitalis therapy, hypothermia, electrolyte abnormalities, or dysrhythmias. These changes should be considered as one parameter of the diagnosis, which supports clinical evaluations and diagnostic enzyme tests.

    ii. Hypertension

    iii. Fluid overload

   2. Assess elderly especially for:

    a. Uncompensated congestive heart failure

    b. Pulmonary edema

   3. Cardiac monitoring

    a. Alarm parameters established

     i. Alarm system should be activated

    b. Lead II monitoring typically used in PACU

     i. Superiority in dysrhythmia detection

     ii. No information on inferior areas of heart

      (a) Right coronary artery supply

VIII. Fluid and Electrolyte Balance

 A. Most ambulatory surgery procedures not associated with significant alterations in fluid and electrolyte status

   1. Average adult requires 2,200 ml of fluid each day

    a. Most ambulatory surgery patients can compensate for fasting and intraoperative fluid status

    b. Those who cannot maintain homeostatic balance are:

     i. Small children

     ii. Debilitated adults with the following disease processes

      (a) Renal

      (b) GI

      (c) Endocrine

      (d) Cardiovascular

     iii. Elderly

     iv. Particularly thin or emaciated

   2. Other factors related to fluid/electrolyte disturbance

    a. Stress

     i. Fear

     ii. Anxiety

      (a) Retention of water and sodium

    b. GI disturbances

     i. Nausea/vomiting

     ii. Nasogastric suctioning

     iii. Bowel preparation

      (a) Loss of sodium and potassium

    c. Excessive bleeding

 B. Blood administration

   1. Usually not common in the ambulatory setting

    a. Used to treat unexpected hemorrhage

    b. Significant blood loss may be expected

     i. Lipolysis

     ii. Lipectomy

   2. Autologous blood donation

    a. More than 5% of blood donations are autologous

     i. Several units are donated weeks before surgery

      (a) Fresh, unfrozen blood can be stored up to 42 days

       (i) Depends on local blood bank policies

      (b) Last unit must be drawn 72 hours before surgery

       (i) Allow for regeneration of patient's blood volume

        (c) Other criteria for autologous donation
            (i)   Cardiovascular stability
                 a) No recent significant cardiac disease
            (ii)   Between 12 and 75 years of age
            (iii)   No history of seizures in adult life
            (iv)   Minimal hemoglobin level of 11 g/dL
                 a) 34% hematocrit
            (v)   No active infections
            (vi)   No bone marrow cancer
           (vii) Availability of adequate venous access for blood collection
        (d) Low body weight may prevent withdrawal of full unit
            (i)   Does not preclude autologous donation
        (e) Although self-donated, autologous units are crossmatched
            (i)   Increases chance of clerical error during processing
 3. Transfusion precautions
   a. No difference in policies for autologous or allogeneic transfusion
      i.   Secure blood from blood bank
      ii.   Identify patient
     iii.   Identify blood bag
        (a) Two nurses usually identify patient and blood
            (i)   One nurse and another professional is acceptable
                 a) CRNA
                 b) MD
      iv.   Initiate transfusion
        (a) Monitor patient throughout
            (i)   Include temperature in assessment
      v.   Respond to any untoward reactions
        (a) Volume overload
        (b) Bacterial contamination
        (c) Air emboli
        (d) Hypotension
            (i)   Bacterial contamination
            (ii)   Venous emboli
        (e) Hypocalcemia
            (i)   Citrate intoxication
        (f) Hypersensitivity to plastics or stabilizers in tubing and bag
        (g) Anaphylaxis and hemolytic reactions
            (i)   Urticaria (hives)
            (ii)   Chest tightness or pain
            (iii)   Dyspnea
            (iv)   Hyperthermia
            (v)   Wheezing
                 a) Discontinue infusion immediately
                 b) Maintain patent IV with new tubing and solution
                 c) Notify physician
                 d) Monitor vital signs
                 e) Administer oxygen
                 f) Diphenhydramine (Benadryl) IV is antihistamine of choice
                 g) Protocol may require urine and blood specimens sent to blood bank with tubing and remaining blood in bag for analysis

      b. Securing blood products may be more difficult in freestanding surgical center
         i.   Need contract with local blood bank
         ii. Procedure for rapid procurement when needed
             (a) Transfer of blood products must be efficient to address emergencies

  4. Other options for transfusion
      a. "Priming" bone marrow during autologous harvesting by adding erythropoietin
      b. Intraoperative blood salvage (IBS)
         i.   Blood lost by patient is processed by centrifugation and returned to patient
             (a) Often approved by Jehovah's Witness patients provided blood not processed outside of operating room
      c. Autotransfusion devices
         i.   Blood from patient drains into collecting bag and transfused directly to the patient
             (a) Collection of blood for 2–4 hours and transfused over two hours
             (b) Often used with total joint replacements and cardiac surgery

C. Artificial blood sources
  1. Basic property of blood is oxygen/carbon dioxide transport and hemodynamic stability
  2. Two types of substitutes under development
      a. Perfluorochemical emulsions (PFC)
         i.   Chemically inert liquids
         ii. High solubility for gases
         iii. Advantages
             (a) High O_2 solubility
             (b) Inert liquid
             (c) Adequate supply
         iv. Disadvantages
             (a) Long tissue half life
             (b) Short vascular half life
                (i)   Less than 19 hours
             (c) Higher than normal PO_2 level is needed
             (d) Little is known about toxic effects
      b. Hemoglobin solutions
         i.   Hemoglobin purified and reduced to a powder
             (a) Mixed with saline and infused
         ii. Advantages
             (a) Ability to carry oxygen at normal PO_2 levels
         iii. Disadvantages
             (a) Toxicities and impurities from residual red cell membrane (stroma)
                (i)   Effects predominately renal
             (b) Vasoconstriction
             (c) Short vascular half life
             (d) Uncertain supply

D. Non-blood volume substitutes
  1. Volume expanders
      a. Dextran
         i.   Synthetic plasma substitute
         ii. Advantages
             (a) Administered through standard IV tubing

(b) Relatively inexpensive
(c) Readily available
(d) No risk of disease
   iii. Disadvantages
     (a) Hypersensitivity reactions
      (i)   Usually in first 30 minutes of infusion
     (b) Interfere with platelet function
      (i)   Transient prolongation of bleeding time
     (c) Certain methods of typing and crossmatching have been affected by Dextran
  b. Hetastarch (Hespan)
   i.   Artificial colloid
   ii.   Inexpensive
   iii. Derived from corn starch
     (a) Closely resembles human glycogen
   iv. Available in 6%/0.9% sodium chloride solution
   v.   Minimal coagulation effects
   vi. Less likely to produce allergic reactions

E. Oral intake
  1. Preferred in ambulatory surgery patients
    a. Encouraged once patient is awake and sufficiently alert
      i.   All protective reflexes are present
      ii.   No nausea
    b. Raising patient's head promotes easy swallowing without choking
    c. Appropriate fluids
      i.   Water/ice
      ii.   Avoid citrus juice, coffee
        (a) May cause nausea/vomiting
  2. Continue IV fluids until oral intake is tolerated

F. Urinary status
  1. Average daily output of 600 ml is necessary to excrete waste products of metabolism
    a. Optimal amount to ensure kidney function and adequate hydration is 30 ml/hr
    b. Hypovolemia, hypothermia, and body's reaction to stress can decrease urine production
  2. Urinary retention
    a. Spinal/epidural anesthesia
    b. Surgical manipulation
    c. Use of local anesthetics surrounding structures
      i.   Assess bladder for distention particularly after:
        (a) Urinary procedures
        (b) Inguinal herniorrhaphy
        (c) Gynecologic procedures
          (i)   Palpable in lower pelvis
          (ii)   Firm, domed area above pubis
    d. Other symptoms of bladder distention
      i.   Restlessness
      ii.   Lower abdominal pain
      iii. Hypertension
      iv. Tachycardia
      v.   Anxiety

        vi. Tachypnea

       vii. Diaphoresis

          (a) May mimic hypoxic symptoms

    e. May require catheterization

  3. Urination may be required for home discharge

    a. Discharge from Phase I to Phase II may be done if not uncomfortable and not distended

    b. Allow patient to use bathroom if sufficiently recovered

IX. Temperature Regulation

  A. Normothermia

    1. Hypothalamus

      a. Regulatory center

        i. 98.6° and 99.5° F (36°–37.5° C)

    2. Major sites of heat production

      a. Byproduct of metabolism

        i. Muscles

          (a) 25% body heat production

        ii. Liver

          (a) 50% body heat production

        iii. Glands

          (a) 15% produced by brain

    3. Heat loss mechanisms in surgery

      a. Conduction of heat from body to cold surfaces it touches

      b. Convection—heat loss to air current

      c. Radiation—electromagnetic energy loss to colder objects in room

        i. Accounts for 65% heat loss

      d. Evaporation from skin during preps and through respiratory system and urine

  B. Hypothermia—core body temperature <95° F (35° C)

    1. Patient factors affecting body temperature in surgery

      a. Patient weight

        i. Thin patients loose more heat and generate less heat than heavier counterparts

      b. Length of surgical exposure of skin and internal structures

      c. Site of surgery

        i. Peritoneal exposure significantly increases heat loss

      d. Intravenous infusion of room-temperature fluids

      e. Cool irrigants and skin prep solutions

      f. Ambient room temperature

        i. Constant air circulation increases environmental effect of cool room temperature

          (a) Children—6 months to 2 years

            (i)   Greater degree of heat loss

               a) Larger body surface area compared to muscle mass

            (ii)   OR temperature 76° F

               a) Higher for newborns and premature babies

          (b) Elderly

            (i)   Shrinking muscle mass and decreasing subcutaneous fat layer

               a) Less able to conserve heat

    2. Anesthesia factors

      a. Depress thermoregulatory center

      b. Neuromuscular relaxants stop muscle activity

         i.   Also prevent shivering

      c. Inhalation agents

         i.   Respiratory heat loss from unwarmed oxygen and inhalation gas delivery

   3. Prevention of heat loss

      a. Increasing room temperature

      b. Heated blankets

      c. Warmed irrigation and prep fluids

      d. Foil blankets to prevent radiation of patient's body heat

      e. IV fluid warmers

      f. Respiratory circuits

         i.   Provide for heat conservation

      g. Head covering for patient

         i.   >50% body heat may be lost as radiation from scalp

   4. Benefits

      a. Decrease in oxygen requirements

         i.   Protect body tissues from hypoxemia

   5. Drawbacks

      a. Slows metabolic rate

         i.   Effects of medications greatly enhanced

            (a) Active drug remains in body longer

            (b) Less drug needed to produce desired effect

   6. Treatment in PACU

      a. Observation

         i.   Cyanosis of extremities

            (a) Vasoconstriction of distal vessels

               (i)   Physiologic response to conserve heat

               (ii)   May preclude accurate oxygen saturation measurements by pulse oximetry

        ii.   Dysrhythmias

            (a) Secondary to hypothermia

        iii. Reparalysis (or recurarization)

            (a) Dose of reversal agents effective in hypothermic patient is no longer effective when metabolic rate increases in response to warmer temperature

      b. Warming measures

         i.   Heated blankets

        ii.   Forced air heat

        iii. Radiant heat

        iv. Warmed IV fluids

        v.   Covering head and upper torso

C. Shivering

   1. Major mechanism of heat production

   2. Spontaneously without known cause in normothermic patient

   3. Uncomfortable and unpleasant for the awakening patient

   4. Untoward effects

      a. Hypertension

      b. Self-injury

         i.   Operative site

        ii.   Teeth

    c. Increase in oxygen demands

      i.   4–5 times normal

    d. Prolonged PACU time

      i.   Expense in additional PACU time, supplies, and medications

    e. Diffuse muscle aches for days after surgery

      i.   Intensity of muscle activity

        (a) Should be reported to Phase II nurse for postoperative instruction regarding analgesia unrelated to surgical site

  5. Treatment

    a. Oxygen therapy

      i.   Observe for signs of hypoxia

    b. Medications

      i.   Narcotics

        (a) Meperidine (Demerol)

          (i)   80% effectiveness with 12.5–25 mg IV doses

      ii.   Opiate agonist–antagonist analgesic

        (a) Butorphanol tartrate (Stadol)

          (i)   95% effective within 5 minutes

D. Hyperthermia

  1. Malignant hyperthermia (MH)

    a. Serious, hypermetabolic state

      i.   Genetic in origin

      ii.   Triggered by certain anesthetic agents and muscle relaxants

        (a) for more detailed information see Chapter 23

X. Level of Consciousness

A. Unconscious patients should never be left unattended

  1. Protective reflexes absent

  2. Cognitive abilities absent

    a. Patients totally dependent upon PACU nurse for protection from the environment

B. Accepted that hearing is first sense to return upon awakening

  1. Speaking to the patient in calm, low tones helps arouse and orient semiconscious patients

    a. Periodic, frequent attempts should continue until the patient responds **except in:**

      i.   Signs of upper airway irritation

        (a) Gagging, coughing

          (i)   Administer oxygen

          (ii)   Position to avoid aspiration

          (iii) Allow to awaken slowly without intervention to decrease risk of laryngospasm

      ii.   Use of ketamine

        (a) Severe hallucinations can follow administration

          (i)   If ketamine-induced delirium occurs:

            a) Diazepam (Valium) 5–10 mg IV

            b) Thiopental 50–75 mg IV

    b. Avoid extraneous noises (laughter, personal conversations, etc)

      i.   May be distorted and confuse or agitate awakening patient

C. Emergence delirium (emergence excitement)

  1. Signs/symptoms

    a. Restlessness

    b. Thrashing of extremities

      c. Combativeness

      d. Crying

      e. Moaning

      f. Screaming

      g. Irrational talking

      h. Disorientation

  2. Causes

      a. Preoperative medications

         i.   Scopolamine

      b. Pain

      c. Bladder distention

      d. Feelings of suffocation during awakening

      e. Possible cerebral hypoxia

      f. Psychological preoperative preparation

         i.   Fear of surgery

            (a) Body disfigurement

               (i)   Children and adolescents particularly

         ii.   Surgical diagnosis

  3. Untoward effects

      a. Self injury

         i.   Limbs

         ii.   Tongue

      b. Straining or opening suture lines

      c. Dislodging IV lines

      d. Self-extubation

  4. Treatment

      a. Gentle physical restraint

         i.   Total physical restraint may increase agitation

         ii.   May need several nurses or other personnel

      b. Pharmacologic treatment

         i.   Narcotics

            (a) Meperidine

            (b) Fentanyl with droperidol (Innovar)

            (c) Morphine

            (d) Methadone

         ii.   Physostigmine (Antilirium)

            (a) Use is controversial as reversal agent to end episode of emergence delirium

            (b) Useful in reversing effects of scopolamine or other anticholinergic drugs

               (i)   Dose in 1 mg increments IV slowly

                   a) Do not exceed 3 mg total

                   b) Can cause severe bradycardia

D. Delayed awakening

  1. Causes

      a. Impaired metabolism, ventilation, circulation due to:

         i.   Type and amount of preoperative medication

            (a) Benzodiazepines

            (b) Neuroleptic agents

            (c) Narcotics

            (d) Barbiturates

ii.   Intraoperative medications
    (a) Inhalation agents
    (b) Narcotics
    (c) Barbiturates
iii. Other drugs self-administered prior to anesthesia
    (a) Cimetidine
    (b) Lidocaine
    (c) Antihypertensives
    (d) MAOIs
    (e) Antidepressants
iv.   Hypothermia
v.   Malignant hyperthermia
vi.   Metabolic diseases
vii. Cardiovascular pathology
    (a) Hypertension
    (b) Hypovolemia
    (c) Myocardial ischemia
viii. Respiratory inadequacy
    (a) Narcotic induced
    (b) Pathologic in nature
ix.   Increased intracranial pressure
x.   CVA
xi.   Undiagnosed intraoperative seizure
xii. Embolism

XI. Positioning
  A. Ensure proper body alignment
    1. Provide comfort and safety
      a. Lateral positioning
        i.   Prevention of aspiration
        ii. Support patient's head and neck
        iii. Position extremities to avoid damage to nerves, tendons, and muscles
          (a) Avoid hyperextension of joints
            (i)   Can result in pain and damage to joint structure
        iv. Opposing skin surfaces should be separated with padding
        v.   Prolonged unconsciousness or immobility
          (a) Provide gentle passive range of motion
          (b) Frequent repositioning
    2. Promote cardiovascular and respiratory homeostasis
      a. Reposition slowly to avoid compromise
        i.   Reassess after repositioning
    3. Special surgical-specific positioning
      a. Extremities
        i.   Elevated above heart level
          (a) Prevent bleeding and edema
            (i)   Promotes healing
            (ii) Decreases pain
      b. Plastic surgery
        i.   Fowler's position
          (a) Head, face, neck, breast
            (i)   Promotes healing
            (ii) Prevents bleeding
      c. Eye and ear surgery
        i.   Usually surgeon specific

XII. Operative Site

   A. Assess wounds and/or dressings

      1. Bleeding

         a. Frank bloody drainage

         b. Rapid filling of collection systems

         c. Bruising

         d. Skin discolorations

         e. Swelling

            i.   Indicative of hematoma formation

         f. Excessive swallowing following ENT procedures

            i.   Subjective complaints of drainage in back of throat

         g. Heavy vaginal flow

         h. Excessive hematuria

      2. Intra-abdominal

         a. May not appear until blood loss is significant

         b. Signs and symptoms

            i.   Apprehension

            ii.   Hypotension

            iii.   Tachycardia

            iv.   Splinting

            v.   Abdominal pain

            vi.   Tenderness and rigidity

            vii.   Pallor

            viii.   Diaphoresis

      3. Laparoscopic procedures

         a. Particular risk for occult bleeding

            i.   Potential for laceration or inadvertent burning of abdominal vessels and organs

      4. Treatment

         a. While waiting for surgeon

         b. Reduce or stop any excessive bleeding

            i.   Manual pressure

            ii.   Elevation of site if possible

            iii.   Specific protocols

                (a) Ice or cool compresses to surrounding area

                (b) Increase IV infusion rate

                (c) Sedation

                (d) Pressor agents

                (e) Blood replacement

                   (i)   Colloids

                   (ii)   Blood products

                (f) Oxygen therapy

                (g) Resuturing incision or packing body cavity

                 (i)   Sterile supplies should be readily available

                (h) May return to OR

                 (i)   Consent must be obtained from family member

                     a) Sedated patients cannot sign legal document

         c. Airway involvement

            i.   Constant reassurance

            ii.   Position appropriately

            iii.   Gentle suction of mouth

                (a) Do not place suction catheter near site of hemorrhage

XIII. Peripheral Circulation
  A. Surgically involved extremity assessment
    1. Circulatory compromise
      a. Constriction
        i.   Encircling bandage
              (a) ACE wrap
              (b) Cast
        ii.   Thrombus
        iii. Embolus
        iv.   Internal pressure
              (a) Hemorrhage
    2. Peripheral pulses
      a. Palpated bilaterally for presence, strength, symmetry
        i.   Numerical description
              (a) Absent—0
              (b) Weak and thready—1+
              (c) Normal—2+
              (d) Full and bounding—3+
      b. If not palpable:
        i.   Reposition extremity and palpate pulse site again
        ii.   May need a doppler ultrasound stethoscope (DUS)
              (a) Noninvasive
              (b) Uses sound-wave frequency to detect movement of red blood cells
                  in underlying vessels
    3. Pulse oximeter
      a. Visual depiction of pulse strength on affected extremity
    4. Skin color and nailbed color
      a. Vasoconstriction in hypothermic patient may mimic cyanosis due to more
         severe causes
      b. Blanching or redness from an intraoperative tourniquet may persist
        i.   Evaluate for resolution of tourniquet-related symptoms
    5. Capillary refill
      a. Quick return of color to nailbed or distal area of skin blanched by pressure
        i.   Normally occurs in 3–5 seconds
        ii.   Helpful when dressing on extremity eliminates visual evaluation of all
              but tips of digits
XIV. Analgesia
  A. Pain
    1. Complex phenomenon
      a. Stimulation of nociceptors
        i.   Free nerve endings throughout body
              (a) Chemical
              (b) Thermal
              (c) Mechanical (surgical)
        ii.   Impulses transmitted via spinal cord
              (a) Afferent nerve fibers
        iii. Brain
              (a) Consciously perceived as pain
    2. Personal experience
      a. Variable between people
        i.   Variable within same people at different times
      b. Emotional impact of pain

       i.   Preoperative counseling
          (a) General description of what can be expected
          (b) Direct relationship between preoperative education and decreased analgesic needs
             (i)   Less fear
                 a) Decreases feelings of powerlessness
             (ii)   Earlier ambulation
                 a) Analgesia will be given
                 b) Discharge will not be attempted without adequate pain relief
   c. Pain-relieving techniques
       i.   Proper body mechanics
          (a) Body alignment
          (b) Positioning
       ii.   Encouragement of patient's efforts
   d. Soothing conversation
   e. Hand holding
       i.   Pain often exacerbated by fear and anxiety
   f. Massage
   g. Awake patients
       i.   Positive encouragement of relaxation
          (a) Distraction
             (i)   Imagine pleasant visions, sounds, and smells
             (ii)   Guided imagery
          (b) Counting
          (c) Rhythmic breathing
       ii.   Requires
          (a) Patient acceptance
          (b) Nursing skills
          (c) Preoperative discussion and practice
   h. Local infiltration
       i.   Explanations of local anesthesia if surgeon routinely does so
3. Transcutaneous electrical nerve stimulator (TENS)
   a. Stimulation of cutaneous afferent nerve pathways
       i.   Inhibit perception of pain
          (a) Possible release of endorphins attach to opiate receptors and block transmission of painful stimuli
          (b) Usually used for chronic pain
             (i)   Does have post surgical applications
4. Operative site affects pain levels
   a. More discomfort
       i.   Thoracic
       ii.   Abdominal
       iii. Rectal
   b. Less discomfort
       i.   Breast
       ii.   Scrotal
       iii. Chest wall
       iv. Extremity
5. Anesthesia technique
   a. Regional
       i.   Usually longer period of analgesia

    b. Local anesthetic infiltration

       i. Effective in reducing surgical site pain

    c. Intraoperative narcotics

6. Social issues

    a. Culture affects pain tolerance

       i. Nervous or anxious people

       ii. Those with particularly protective families

         (a) Difficulty in managing pain

7. Pain is subjective

    a. No one knows how much pain the patient is really having

    b. Objective observations are only clues

       i. Vital signs

         (a) Hypertension

         (b) Tachycardia

         (c) Tachypnea

       ii. Restlessness

       iii. Facial expression

       iv. Splinting

       v. Posturing

       vi. Mood

       vii. Voice

       viii. Refusal to be repositioned

    c. Nurses' role is not to judge patient's pain

       i. Assess thoroughly

         (a) Location

         (b) Intensity

            (i) Pain scale rates patient's perception of pain intensity

              a) Numerical (0–10)

              b) Faces (smiling–crying)

              c) Colors (blue–red)

         (c) Type

       ii. Provide appropriate interventions

         (a) Relive discomfort

8. Other sources of postoperative pain

    a. Bladder distention

    b. Uncomfortable positioning

    c. Joint pain

       i. Arthritis

       ii. Gout

    d. Decubitus ulcers

    e. Pre-existing diseases

    f. Placement of intravenous catheters

    g. Drainage tubes

       i. Chest tubes

       ii. Jackson-Pratt

       iii. Autotransfusion

    h. Gastric distention

    i. Postoperative complications

       i. Embolic events

       ii. Myocardial ischemia or infarction

       iii. Pulmonary ischemia

       iv. Hemorrhage

       v. Ruptured viscus

B. Ambulatory surgery expectations
   1. Analgesic needs will be met
   2. Discourage use of "pain"
      a. Focus on "discomfort"
         i.   Different connotation
         ii. Fits philosophy of wellness
              (a) Exception is patient in extreme pain
              (b) May seem unfeeling or trite to use "discomfort"
C. Untoward effects if inadequate analgesia
   1. Respiratory dysfunction
      a. Secondary to wound splinting
      b. Shallow respirations
         i.   Respiratory acidosis
   2. Tachycardia
   3. Hypertension
   4. Increased peripheral resistance
   5. Increased cardiac output
   6. Increased myocardial oxygen demand
   7. Gastric stasis
      a. Paralytic ileus
      b. Increased incidence of nausea/vomiting
         i.   Increased risk of aspiration
   8. Endocrine and metabolic changes
D. Analgesics
   1. Assessment prior to administration
      a. Often awakening from general anesthesia
         i.   Poorest inherent pain relief
         ii. Psychologically less able to handle pain
              (a) Compared with wakefulness and full control capacity
         iii. Magnified in half-awake state
         iv. Restless
              (a) Cause may be hypoxic
      b. Naloxone (Narcan)
         i.   Administered as reversal agent
         ii. Also reverses analgesia
              (a) Additional narcotics may produce additive effects once Narcan
                  wears off
   2. Challenge
      a. Provide adequate analgesia without oversedation
         i.   Smallest effective dose
         ii. Incremental administration favored
         iii. Narcotics
              (a) Most effective treatment in PACU
              (b) Following general anesthesia
                  (i) Close observation for potential:
                       a) Cumulative effects
                       b) Respiratory depression
                       c) Prolonged somnolence
                       d) Nausea/vomiting
      b. Dosage
         i.   Individual calculation essential

      (a) Patients vary significantly in:
         (i)   Weight
         (ii)   Age
         (iii) Sensitivity to drug actions
         (iv) Personal need or desire for certain level of comfort
      (b) Medication history
         (i)   Rarely takes any medications so usually require smaller doses
         (ii)   Heavy alcohol, tobacco, or drug use
             a) May decrease effectiveness of pharmacologic therapy through mechanism called enzyme induction
             b) Causes increased production of hepatic enzymes

c. Metabolism (biotransformation)

    i.   Converts lipid-soluble drugs into water-soluble usually inactive metabolites

      (a) Allows excretion through renal tubules

      (b) Hepatic microsomal enzymes responsible for most metabolic changes

         (i)   Chronic increase in hepatic enzymes increases rate of drug metabolism

             a) Increased doses are needed to produce therapeutic effect

3. Routes of administration

   a. Choice depends on patient's individual experience with pain and response to medication

   b. Transdermal and nasal agents

    i.   Still under clinical trials

    ii. May have widespread application in ambulatory surgery

   c. Intravenous agents

    i.   Rapid onset of action

    ii.   Rapid onset of side effects

      (a) Apparent in PACU

    iii. Fentanyl

      (a) 50 times more potent than morphine

      (b) Effective, rapid-acting

      (c) Produces minimal sedative hangover

         (i)   Give in small incremental doses

             a) Single 50 μg (one ml) usually appropriate for average-weight adult

             b) Potential for respiratory complications

      (d) Does not evoke histamine release

      (e) Minimal cardiovascular changes

         (i)   Can cause bradycardia

             a) Usually avoided with pulse rate <50

      (f) Action

         (i)   30–60 minutes with IV administration

         (ii)   Up to 3 hours with IM administration

    iv. Patient-controlled analgesia (PCAs)

      (a) Infusion pump method of intravenous postoperative narcotic pain control

      (b) Usually reserved for inpatient use

      (c) Manufacturers are developing miniaturized, battery-operated, or completely disposable systems for home and outpatient use

    d. IM administration

       i.   Usually ordered out of habit for hospitalized patients

      ii.   May be incompatible with goals of:

         (a) Rapid analgesia

            (i)   Studies have shown that ⅓ patients given IM narcotics usually continue with moderate to severe pain

         (b) Quick arousal

            (i)   IM administration accompanied by sedative effects

            (ii)   Increased hypotensive and respiratory depression

                a) Requires longer observation period

         (c) Rapid ambulation

         (d) Rapid discharge

     iii.   Other IM medications

         (a) Hydroxyzine (Vistaril, Atarax)

         (b) Phenothiazine derivatives

            (i)   Promethazine (Phenergan)

         (c) Potentiate narcotic effects

            (i)   Use cautiously in ambulatory surgery patients

                a) Significant sedation

            (ii)   Have antiemetic and anxiolytic properties

  e. Oral

       i.   Once believed only method for ambulatory surgery

         (a) Increasing complexity of ambulatory surgery procedures, oral analgesics not always sufficient

         (b) Providing immediate and effective pain relief important aspect

            (i)   Preventing severe pain easier than controlling it

         (c) Produces effective serum levels after administration of IV medication

         (d) Non-steroidal anti-inflammatory drugs (NSAIDs)

            (i)   Ibuprofen

            (ii)   Ketorolac

                a) May cause gastric irritation

                b) Can interfere with coagulation mechanism

4. Opioid agonist–antagonist

  a. Pentazocine (Talwin)

  b. Butorphanol tartrate (Stadol)

  c. Nalbuphine (Nubain)

       i.   Reduce pain when given without previous narcotics

      ii.   When given in presence of narcotics

         (a) Antagonistic characteristics reverse narcotic effect resulting in:

            (i)   Pain

            (ii)   Anxiety

            (iii)   Loss of sedation

     iii.   Contraindicated in chronically narcotic-dependent

         (a) Causes severe withdrawal symptoms

5. NSAIDs

  a. Ketorolac tromethamine (Toradol)

       i.   Parenteral agent

      ii.   IM route

         (a) 30–90 mg depending on weight

            (i)   Effective as 12 mg morphine or 100 mg meperidine

      iii. Few side effects
- (a) Nausea, dyspepsia, drowsiness, and GI pain
  - (i)   3–9%
- (b) Edema, diarrhea, dizziness, headache, tinnitus, peptic ulcer, sweating, and injection site pain
  - (i)   <3%
- (c) Respiratory function not altered
- (d) No significant cardiovascular effects

      iv. Often given with narcotic to obtain added analgesic benefits
- (a) Does not produce additive effects with narcotic administration

      v. No potential of addictive abuse
- (a) Ideal for narcotic-addicted patient

      vi. Liver metabolism

      vii. Renal excretion
- (a) 50% excreted unchanged
- (b) Use with caution in patients with kidney or liver dysfunction and the elderly

      viii. Onset of action
- (a) 10 minutes

      ix. Peak effect
- (a) 45–90 minutes
- (b) 6 hours' approximate duration
  - (i)   Administering ketorolac 45–60 minutes prior to the end of surgery in the operating room helps prevent pain of an injection

XV. Nausea and Vomiting
- A. Primary goal is to prevent rather than treat
  - 1. Obtain history of postoperative nausea and vomiting
  - 2. Prophylactic
    - a. Histamine blockers
    - b. Antiemetics
- B. Nausea subjective
  - 1. Often difficult to describe
  - 2. Unpleasant
  - 3. May or may not result in retching or vomiting
- C. Other predisposing factors
  - 1. Obesity
    - a. Usually increased gastric volumes
  - 2. Hiatal hernia
  - 3. Type of surgery
    - a. Laparoscopy
    - b. Ovum retrieval
    - c. Abdominal procedures
    - d. Pediatric strabismus
    - e. Orchipexy
    - f. ENT
      - i. Due to blood entering the stomach
  - 4. Anesthetic technique
    - a. Regional and local anesthetic approaches lower incidence
    - b. Nitrous oxide implicated as significant causative factor
      - i. Gravitates to any air-filled area of stomach and bowel
        - (a) Abdominal distention and pressure
      - ii. Collects in middle ear affecting vestibular system

    c. Propofol (Diprivan)
        i. Newer anesthetic agent for induction and maintenance
           (a) Low (1–3%) incidence of N/V
               (i) 10-mg dose may be beneficial as antiemetic agent

D. Vomiting
  1. Complex occurrence
    a. Involves skeletal muscles and autonomic nervous system
    b. Reflex
  2. Direct stimulation of vomiting center
    a. Located near the dorsal nucleus of the vagus nerve in the medulla
    b. Chemoreceptor trigger zone (CTZ)
        i. Three afferent nerve pathways
           (a) Cortical
               (i) Emotional
                   a) Stress, depression, and fear
               (ii) Organic
                   a) Hypoxia
                   b) Pain
                   c) Hypotension
                   d) Increased intracranial pressure
                   e) Hypovolemia
               (iii) Sensory
                   a) Sights and smells of OR or PACU
           (b) Visceral
               (i) Viscera and vagal nerve
                   a) Delayed gastric emptying
                   b) Abdominal distention
                   c) Handling abdominal contents during surgery
                   d) Pneumoperitoneum for laparoscopic procedures
                   e) Primary GI disorders
                   f) Cardiac disease
           (c) Vestibular
               (i) Tremors
               (ii) Motion
                   a) Patient with strong history of motion sickness may have vomiting due to vestibular afferent activity
               (iii) Otitis media
               (iv) ENT procedures
               (v) Anesthetics and narcotics
        ii. Response to stimulation via efferent nerve pathways
           (a) Respiratory center
               (i) Diaphragm
           (b) GI tract
               (i) Upper abdominal muscles
               (ii) Figure 8–1

E. "Central vomiting"
  1. Direct effect on CTZ
  2. Decreased cerebral blood flow
  3. Circulating drugs
    a. Narcotics
    b. Inhalation agents
    c. Intravenous anesthetic agents
    d. Amphetamines

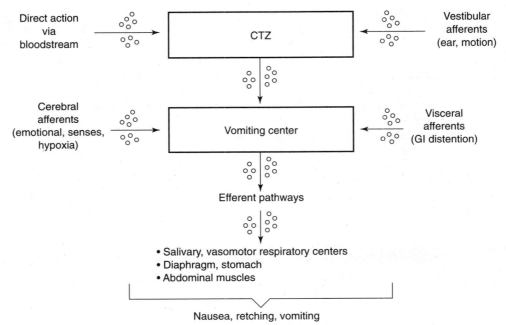

Figure 8–1.   Multiple pathways to and from the emetic center.

   e. Cardiac glycosides
   f. Ergot rates
   g. Chemotherapeutic agents
  F. Nursing interventions
   1. No single approach to prevention or treatment of nausea and vomiting effective due to diverse etiology
   2. In unconscious patient protection of airway
    a. Avoid aspiration of stomach contents
   3. Provide positive reinforcement to relieve anxiety
   4. Avoid sights, smells, or conversations near the patient that could stimulate nausea or vomiting
   5. Move and ambulate patient slowly
   6. Allow patient to awaken slowly without aggressive stimulation
   7. Maintain endotracheal tube cuff until extubation
   8. Provide adequate analgesia
   9. Use caution with oral intake
    a. Avoid coffee, citrus juices
   10. Limit irritation of upper airway
    a. Reduce gagging
    b. Limit secretions
    c. Remove artificial airways as soon as possible
    d. Gentle oral suction for blood and other secretions
   11. Provide privacy for the patient who is vomiting
    a. Reassure to avoid embarrassment
  G. Antiemetic agents
   1. Should reduce GI symptoms without oversedation
   2. Agents that block responsible receptors most effective
    a. Droperidol (Inapsine)
    b. Chlorpromazine (Thorazine)

    c. Trimethobenzamide (Tigan)

       i. Dopamine antagonists suppress CTZ activity

    d. Table 8–2 for additional antiemetic agents and their properties

XVI. **Progression of Care**

  A. Orientation

    1. Frequent orientation to surroundings

    2. Explanations

      a. Link with reality

      b. Aid in return of cognitive abilities

  B. Operative site

    1. Monitor for:

      a. Hemorrhage

      b. Swelling

      c. Compression of extremities

  C. Movement and ambulation

    1. Gradual

      a. Elevate head of bed slowly

      b. Exercise extremities

      c. Sitting on edge of bed or carrier

      d. Sitting in recliner

      e. Ambulation

        i. With each level assess

          (a) Vital signs

            (i) Specifically hypotension

          (b) Dizziness

          (c) Nausea

          (d) Faintness

        ii. If any symptoms occur, progress is slowed or reversed until symptoms subside

XVII. **Emotional and Psychological Support**

  A. Ideally begun with preoperative visit and assessment

  B. PACU nurse first line with normalcy after surgery/anesthesia

    1. Use of positive language promoting wellness and self-sufficiency

      a. Address fears patient expresses

        i. Pathology or surgical outcome

        ii. Family or friends waiting

        iii. Returning home with no nursing or medical attention

        iv. Ability to deal with pain at home

        v. Concern with family's ability to deal with postoperative needs

      b. Assure that anything said or done in the PACU is kept confidential

  C. Encourage family and friends in care discussions

    1. Family visitation in PACU fosters self-care model

      a. Reduces anxiety and stress level

      b. May reduce length of stay

    2. Prolonged PACU stay should be communicated to the family to reduce their anxiety

XVIII. **Special Needs of Patients After Local and Regional Anesthesia; Nursing Care After Epidural and Spinal Anesthesia**

  A. Many patients undergoing brachial plexus, intravenous, periorbital, or other regional blocks may bypass Phase I completely

  B. Patients undergoing central regional blocks (epidural and subarachnoid or spinal) are admitted to Phase I until major effects of the anesthesia have passed

    1. Complications following epidural or spinal

Table 8–2 • ANTIEMETICS

GROUP/DRUG	ACTION/USES	DOSAGE RANGES/ROUTES FOR ADULTS	SIDE EFFECTS/SPECIAL NOTES
Phenothiazines			
Prochlorperazine (Compazine)	Antiemetic, anxiolytic, tranquilizer	PO 5–10 mg IM 5–10 mg deep IM Rectal 25 mg IV 5–10 mg **slowly**—use great caution due to hypotension	orthostatic hypotension, ECG changes, tachycardia, extrapyramidal reactions, sedation, pseudoparkinsonism, EEG changes, dizziness, occular changes, blurred vision, dry mouth, constipation, urinary retention
Chorpromazine (Thorazine)	Antiemetic, anxiolytic	IM (deep) 12.5–25 mg	orthostatic hypotension, tachycardia, ECG changes, seizures, sedation, extrapyramidal reactions, urine retention, dry mouth, constipation, neuroleptic malignant syndrome
Promethazine (Phenergan)	Anti-motion sickness, anticholinergic	IM (deep) 12.5–25 mg (reduce with CNS depressants)	hypertension, hypotension, sedation, drowsiness, dry mouth; **NEVER** give epinephrine to treat hypotension caused by promethazine because it could further lower blood pressure
Others			
Trimethobenza-mide (Tigan)	Antiemetic— depresses CTZ, sedative, weak antihistamine	PO 250 mg IM 200 mg (deep IM) onset in 15 minutes, lasts 2–3 hours Rectal 200 mg	hypotension, seizures, drowsiness, coma, diarrhea
Benzquiamide (Emete-con)	Antiemetic	IM (preferred) 50 mg, onset in 15 minutes, peak 15 minutes, lasts 3–4 hours IV 25 mg **very slowly,** decrease dose if patient on pressor agent or on epinephrine-like drug or in cardiac patient	sudden rise in blood pressure and transient dysrhythmias (PVCs, PACs, and atrial fibrillation), hypotension, drowsiness, anorexia, dry mouth, urticaria, rash, diarrhea
Ondansetron (Zofran)	Depresses CTZ and $5HT_3$ receptor	PO 16 mg, 1 hour prior to anesthesia induction IV 4 mg undiluted over 2–5 minutes	diarrhea, constipation, musculoskeletal pain, urine retention, chest pain, injection site reaction, fever, hypoxia

(continued)

Table 8-2 • **ANTIEMETICS** *Continued*

GROUP/DRUG	ACTION/USES	DOSAGE RANGES/ROUTES FOR ADULTS	SIDE EFFECTS/SPECIAL NOTES
Droperidol (Inapsine)	Potent tranquilizer (neuroleptic agent), anxiolytic Potentiates narcotics and CNS depressants	IV 0.625-1.25 mg (reduce dose when given with narcotics or CNS depressants) onset 3–10 minutes, peak 30 minutes, lasts 3–6 hours	hypotension, tachycardia, laryngospasm, bronchospasm, extrapyramidal effects, drowsiness, hyperactivity
Dimenhydrinate (Dramamine)	Antiemetic, anti-motion sickness Depressant action on hyperstimulated labyrinthine function	IM 50 mg IV (dilute) 50 mg in 10 ml, slowly over at least 2 minutes IV infusion 50–100 mg in 500 ml solution	palpitations, drowsiness, headache, dizziness, confusion, nervousness, insomnia (especially in children), blurred vision, dry mouth
Metoclopramide (Reglan)	Increases gastric motility	IM 10 mg (5–20 mg range) onset	restlessness, anxiety, suicidal ideation, seizures, hallucinations, transient hypertension, hypotension
Hydroxyzine (Vistaril, Atarax)	Antiemetic, anxiolytic Potentiates narcotics	IM 25–10 mg (deep) decrease up to ½ when given with CNS depressants (12.5–50 mg IM) **Do not give IV or SQ**	drowsiness, dry mouth, marked discomfort at injection site
Diphenhydramine (Benadryl)	Competes for H1 receptor site	IM (deep) 10–50 mg IV 10–50 mg PO 25–50 mg	palpitations, hypotension, tachycardia, dry mouth, epigastric distress, drowsiness, vertigo, sedation, dizziness, restlessness, seizures, diplopia, blurred vision, urinary retention, thickening of bronchial secretions
Scopolamine (Transderm-Scop)	Anti-motion sickness Anti-muscarinic activity Acts on vestibular pathway and directly on vomiting center	1 patch behind the ear 4 hours before surgery delivers 0.5 mg over 72 hours	palpitations, tachycardia, paradoxical bradycardia, disorientation, restlessness, hallucinations, dry mouth, blurred vision, dilated pupils; **wash hands before and after application to avoid unintentional contact with the drug**

    a. Hypotension
       i.   Vasodilation of large portion of vasculature
          (a) Blood pools in lower extremities
          (b) Arteries and arterioles not able to constrict
             (i)   Compensatory mechanism lost
      ii. Maintain IV fluids
          (a) Until full motor and sensory functions return

          iii.   Aggressive therapy includes ephedrine 10–25 mg, diluted and given IV slowly
- b. Tachycardia
- c. Bradycardia
- d. Hypothermia
    - i.   Peripheral dilation
    - ii.   Warm carefully
        - (a) Can potentiate vasodilation
            - (i)   Result in hypotension
- e. Pressure injury
    - i.   Maintain proper body alignment
    - ii.   Elevate heels from mattress
- f. Unnoticed trauma to tissue
    - i.   Gentle passive range of motion
    - ii.   Repositioning
- g. Epidural hematoma
    - i.   Hemorrhage at injection site rare
        - (a) Internal pressure from hematoma can result in permanent neurologic damage
            - (i)   Rapid onset of neurologic deficit after the block has resolved
            - (ii)   Severe back pain
        - (b) Surgical intervention must occur within 12 hours to prevent permanent damage
- h. High or total spinal
- i. Post-dural puncture (spinal) headache

C. Spinal anesthesia
1. Technically easier and less time-consuming
2. Appropriate for ambulatory surgery patients

D. Epidural anesthesia
1. Ability to control titration of medication through a continuous catheter
2. Low incidence of foreign or infectious material into cerebrospinal fluid (CSF)

E. Resolution of anesthetic effects
1. Sensation generally returns first to areas most distal to the site of injection
    - a. Return of neurologic function is reverse to the sequence it was lost
        - i.   Autonomic control may return prior to movement and sensation, then usually in this order
            - (a) Proprioception (location of extremity in relation to the body) is usually first to return
            - (b) Pressure
            - (c) Movement
            - (d) Touch
            - (e) Pain
            - (f) Temperature
            - (g) Sympathetic functions
                - (i)   Vasomotor
                - (ii)   Bladder control
2. Figure 8–2 shows dermatome level to assess sensory and motor return
    - a. Major landmarks
        - i.   T4—sensation at nipple line
        - ii.   T10—sensation at umbilicus
        - iii.   L2 and L3—raising knee
        - iv.   L4 and L5—flexion of the knee
        - v.   S1 and S2—dorsiflexion of the foot

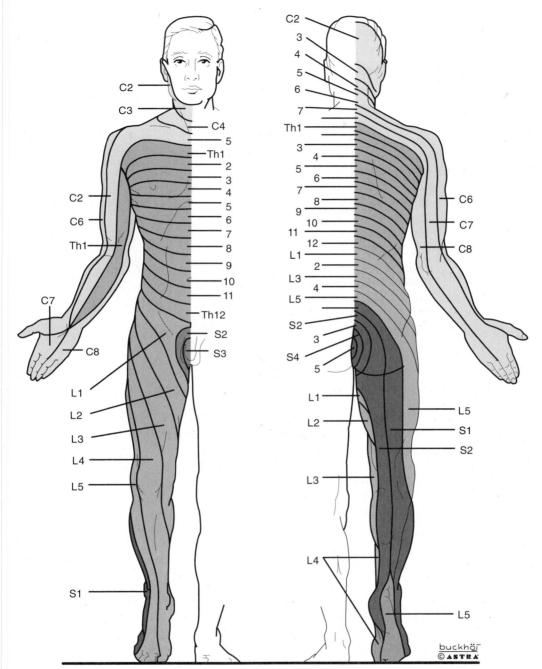

Figure 8–2. Dermatomes. (From ASTRA, "The House of Regional Anesthesia." Astra USA. Inc., 50 Otis Street, Westboro, MA 01581-4500. Reproduced with permission.)

F. High or total spinal anesthesia
1. Upper extremities and/or respiratory and cardiac functions are involved
   a. Incidence is rare
   b. May be caused by:
      i. Increased intrathecal pressure from coughing or straining
      ii. Too rapid injection or too large a volume injected
      iii. Positioning of the patient in head-down inclination before anesthetic agent has set at intended spinal level

2. Treatment
   a. Usually instituted in OR
   b. Mechanical ventilation
      i.   Oxygen therapy
   c. Intravenous fluids
   d. Vasopressors
   e. Atropine or glycopyrrolate
      i.   Treatment of bradycardia
   f. Emotional support
G. Autonomic innervation and urinary bladder tone
   1. Bladder distention may occur
      a. Decreased bladder muscle tone after sympathetic blockade
         i.   Restlessness
         ii.   Hypotension
         iii. Bradycardia
         iv.   May or may not feel suprapubic pain
               (a) Depends on level of sensory block
      b. Treatment simple
         i.   Have patient void if possible
         ii.   Insert urinary catheter to drain bladder
         iii. Provide specific instructions for bladder care
               (a) When to phone or return for follow-up care if not voided by specific time
                   (i)   Use patient's language
H. Post-dural puncture headache
   1. Cause
      a. Leakage of CSF through dural puncture site
         i.   Decrease in intrathecal pressure allows traction on pain-sensitive intracranial sensors
         ii.   Will usually appear within a few hours of the puncture
               (a) More likely becomes evident after 1 or 2 days
                   (i)   May take as long as 6 days to occur
               (b) Pain usually occipital
                   (i)   May also occur in frontal or vertex areas or behind the eyes
                         a) More intense when patient sits up or stands, moves head, flexes neck, or coughs
                         b) Relieved with abdominal pressure
   2. Other signs of CSF leakage
      a. Neck muscle aches
      b. Double vision
      c. Other types of visual disturbances
      d. Auditory difficulties
   3. Occurrence is rare
   4. Prevention may be accomplished with use of:
      a. Small-gauge needles
      b. Conical-tipped needles (*example:* Whitacre)
         i.   Spread or split rather than cut dural fibers
      c. "Wet tap"
         i.   Inadvertent dural puncture with a large-bore needle
               (a) Prevent flow of CSF into epidural space
                   (i)   Anesthesiologist injects saline into epidural space prior to removal of the needle to increase epidural pressure
                   (ii) Blood patch may also be performed

5. Treatment
   a. Several hours of recumbent position not effective in preventing post-spinal headaches
   b. Analgesics
   c. Subdued lighting
   d. Limited noise
   e. Aggressive hydration
      i.   Intravenous
      ii. Oral if tolerated
   f. Abdominal binder
      i.   Increases epidural venous plexus pressure
   g. IV caffeine may be effective treatment
   h. Severe or unrelenting headache
      i.   Epidural blood patch
           (a) Patient's own blood (10 cc) is injected into epidural space surrounding original dural puncture
               (i)   Clots around puncture site
               (ii) Stops CSF leak
           (b) Immediate relief of headache usually occurs

XIX. **Documentation of Care**
   A. Charting formats should provide ease of documentation and accommodate
      1. Typically short procedures
      2. Frequent admissions
      3. Rapid turnover
   B. Form should allow checkoff documentation and charting by exception
   C. Narrative notes should focus on individual patient responses
      1. Specific descriptions of operative site
      2. Associated information
   D. Vital signs easily documented and readable
   E. Scoring parameters easily understood

XX. **Discharge from a PACU—Phase I**
   A. Anesthesiologist usually responsible for discharge from Phase I
      1. Internal policy may require physician's attendance for discharge at time of readiness
      2. Predetermined criteria from the medical staff may allow the PACU nurse to discharge patients
   B. Discharge criteria
      1. Written criteria should address parameters of physical and cognitive recovery
      2. Appropriate to the unit or location patient is transferred
      3. Numeric scoring systems provide objective methods with which to evaluate and describe patient's condition
         a. Used upon admission, throughout the PACU stay, and at discharge
         b. Aldrete Scoring System
            i.   Measures five parameters with scoring ranges from 0–2
                 (a) Activity
                 (b) Respiration
                 (c) Circulation
                 (d) Consciousness
                 (e) Color
            ii. Score of 9 or 10 is generally required for PACU Phase I discharge
                 (a) May not reach this score for pre-existing conditions
                     (i)   Para- or quadriplegic

(ii)   Raynaud's disease
    a) Persistent peripheral cyanosis
(b) Criticism of inclusion of color and ignoring blood pressure
    (i)   Color is subjective finding affected by:
        a) Surrounding wall or curtain color
        b) Type of lighting
        c) Mucous membrane color not indicative of oxygenation
(c) Table 8–3 shows the Aldrete Modified Phase I PACU Scoring System

c. REACT (**R**espiration, **E**nergy [movement], **A**lertness, **C**irculation, and **T**emperature) Scoring System

4. Scoring systems are limited and do not address many important aspects of patient's condition
   a. Presence of nausea/vomiting
   b. Pain
   c. Emotional status
   d. Chills/shivering
   e. Condition of operative site
      i.   Hemorrhage
      ii. Edema
   f. Fluid status
   g. Urinary status
   h. Cognitive abilities
   i. Peripheral circulation
   j. Temperature
      i.   These parameters must also be considered in the decision for PACU discharge

Table 8–3 • ALDRETE'S MODIFIED PHASE I POSTANESTHESIA SCORING SYSTEM

PATIENT INDEX	STANDARD	SCORE
Activity	Patient is able to move . . .	
	4 extremities*	2
	2 extremities	1
	0 extremities	0
Respiration	Patient is . . .	
	able to deep-breathe and cough	2
	dyspnea or limited breathing	1
	apnic, obstructed airway	0
Circulation	Patient's BP ± . . .	
	20% of preanesthesia value	2
	10–49% of preanesthesia value	1
	50% of preanesthesia value	0
Consciousness	Patient is . . .	
	fully awake	2
	arousable (by name)	1
	nonresponsive	0
Oxygen Saturation	Patient's S_pO_2 . . .	
	>92% on room air	2
	>90% supplemental O_2	1
	<90% even with supplemental O_2	0

*Voluntarily or to command

5. After spinal or epidural anesthesia
   a. Return of strength and sympathetic innervation must be evaluated
      i.   Depending on facility policy patients may be transferred to Phase II with continued bedrest until spinal effects resolved
      ii. Most PACUs require patients to have return of movement and sensation prior to discharge
   b. Ensuring the absence of orthostatic hypotension may be main criterion
      i.   Safe discharge with a <10% drop in mean arterial pressure in response to two tests
           (a) Checking blood pressure in both sitting and supine positions

C. Transfer and report
   1. Comprehensive assessment prior to discharge
      a. Condition of operative site
      b. Vital signs
      c. Level of consciousness
      d. Comfort
   2. Skin care
      a. Remove any antiseptic solutions
         i.   Avoid skin irritation
         ii. Prevents staining of clothing
      b. Blood or surgical drainage should be removed
         i.   Aesthetic reasons
         ii. Safety of patients, family, and staff
         iii. Emotional reasons
   3. Surgical site
      a. Dressing dry and intact
      b. Wound drainage bags emptied
      c. Urinary drainage bags emptied
   4. Personal dignity
      a. Patient's sensory aids returned
         i.   Eyeglasses
         ii. Dentures
         iii. Hearing aid
   5. Complete report to Phase II nursing staff
      a. Operative course
         i.   Include medications for blood pressure, heart rate, etc.
      b. PACU course
         i.   Physician's orders completed in Phase I
         ii. Medications administered
              (a) Antibiotics
              (b) Analgesics

XXI. **Patient Assessment and Care Planning PACU—Phase II**
   A. Transporting and accepting nurses should cooperate in settling the patient safely
      1. Phase I nurse should have patient's current vital signs before relinquishing responsibility for the patient's care to Phase II nurse
   B. General nursing care
      1. Stability of vital signs
         a. Including cardiovascular and respiratory status
      2. Progression and encouragement of ambulation
      3. Nutrition and fluid status
      4. Prevention or aggressive treatment of nausea and vomiting
      5. Provision of adequate analgesia

  6. Observation of the operative site
   a. Associated symptoms of complications
  7. Psychosocial support
   a. Including speedy reunion with family or significant others
  8. Educational needs
 C. Initial assessment in Phase II
  1. Assess critical areas
   a. Airway
    i. Respiratory adequacy
   b. Circulation
  2. Complete assessment
   a. Vital signs
    i. Heart rate
     (a) Rhythm
    ii. Blood pressure
    iii. Temperature
    iv. Respiratory effort
   b. General appearance
   c. Level of consciousness
   d. Neurovascular and muscle strength
   e. Inspection of operative site
    i. Associated drainage devices
   f. Level of comfort
   g. GI status
   h. Urinary bladder status
    i. Patency of Foley catheter if applicable
   i. Intravenous fluids and site
   j. Skin condition
    i. Patient position
   k. Assignment of numeric score if applicable
XXII. Progression of Care in PACU—Phase II
 A. Ambulate slowly with gradual progression
  1. Dangle at side of bed before standing
  2. Sitting in recliner
  3. Ambulation
 B. Safety measures
  1. Wheels of stretcher locked
  2. Position stretcher close to floor
  3. Eliminate environmental hazards
   a. Wet floors
   b. Obstacles on floor
  4. Having sufficient number of assistants for ambulating patients
   a. Based on patient's size and ability to ambulate
  5. Using nonslip shoes or slippers
  6. Assess patient frequently
   a. Vital signs
    i. Hypotension
   b. Dizziness/faintness
 C. Fluids and nutrition
  1. Safety measures
   a. Presence of gag and swallow reflexes
   b. Allow patient to sit up prior to taking fluids

    c. Water or ice is usually first
      i.   Least likely to cause lung damage if aspirated
    d. Progress slowly to other fluids and food
      i.   Avoid nausea and vomiting
      ii. Usually prompt nausea and vomiting
         (a) Dairy products
         (b) Coffee
         (c) Citrus juices
      iii. Many believe room-temperature fluids cause less nausea than hot or cold
    e. After general anesthesia
      i.   Avoid nausea/vomiting with bland foods
         (a) Crackers or dry toast
  2. Nausea and vomiting
    a. Three predominant determinants of postoperative nausea
      i.   Predisposition to nausea and vomiting
         (a) History of motion sickness
         (b) Previous experience with postoperative nausea and vomiting
      ii. Appropriate prophylactic therapy
         (a) Use of histamine blockers
         (b) Antiemetics
         (c) Bland foods postoperatively
      iii. Psychological expectations
         (a) Self-fulfilling prophesy
            (i)   Encourage patient to expect nausea-free recovery period

XXIII. Discharge from a PACU—Phase II
  A. Begins with preadmission planning
    1. Acceptable transportation arrangements
    2. Telephone numbers that will be needed by the physician or nurse to contact family member or supporting adult on the day of surgery
    3. Acceptable plan for supporting adult to be with the patient
    4. Need for money, credit card, and/or insurance cards to obtain postoperative prescriptions
    5. Proper clothing to wear postoperatively
    6. Items to bring for postoperative use
      a. Crutches
      b. Braces
      c. Sunglasses
    7. Preparation of home environment
      a. Accessibility of necessary items if mobility is compromised
      b. Provision for meals
      c. Bathroom accessibility
      d. Securing postoperative medical supplies
      e. Removing obstacles
  B. Criteria for Phase II discharge
    1. Adequate recovery from anesthesia **not** from surgical procedure
      a. Parameters focus on standards such as:
        i.   Return of reflexes
        ii. Respiratory adequacy
        iii. Consciousness
        iv. Surgical site
        v.   Issues of transportation

      vi. Home support

     vii. Understanding of instructions

2. Time limitations
    a. Better measurements for determining discharge are patient's physical and psychological conditions
    b. Difficult to estimate
        i. Wide variation in patient response and procedures
    c. Facility protocols
        i. Patient load
        ii. Staffing
        iii. Age/health of population
        iv. Anesthesia used

3. Psychomotor tests
    a. Used during early development of ambulatory surgery programs
    b. Currently used occasionally to determine recovery after general anesthesia
        i. Most are too cumbersome and time-consuming to be useful
        ii. May reflect cognitive return while psychomotor impairment remains or vice versa
            (a) Simple tests like counting and adding the sum of a number of coins may be used
                (i) Provided patient could perform these tasks prior to anesthesia

4. Level of consciousness
    a. Consciousness is an obvious necessity prior to discharge
        i. Acceptable level of sedation at discharge is more elusive
            (a) Return to preoperative level of orientation
                (i) Surroundings
                (ii) Person
                (iii) Time
                (iv) Aware of and assistance with transfer from the surgical facility to home environment
        ii. Patients who remain sleepy
            (a) Should understand that sleepiness does not necessarily constitute a contraindication to being at home as long as the patient is not left alone
            (b) Need responsible adult who:
                (i) Understands responsibility as guardian
                (ii) Willing to fulfill this responsibility

5. Reflexes
    a. All protective airway reflexes must be present before discharge
        i. Swallow
        ii. Cough
        iii. Gag
    b. Pay particular attention to these parameters after procedures that have involved manipulation of or administration of topical anesthesia to the upper airway
        i. Usually patient must demonstrate adequate swallowing prior to discharge
            (a) If physician orders NPO status for several hours after discharge, instructions should include:
                (i) Specific time parameters to observe before drinking fluids
                    a) Water is suggested as the initial fluid
                (ii) Avoid talking while drinking and concentrate on swallowing

    c. Blinking
        i.   Following eye surgery
        ii.   Prevents drying of or injury to cornea
           (a) Bandage the eye with upper lid closed
               (i)   Until return of protective reflexes **or**
               (ii)   Seen by surgeon

6. Vital signs
    a. Stable vital signs for 30 minutes prior to discharge
        i.   Should be checked
           (a) On admission to Phase II
           (b) After ambulation
           (c) Prior to discharge
        ii.   Some facilities require vital signs be checked every 30 minutes or at other intervals during the Phase II stay
    b. Blood pressure
        i.   Should be similar to preoperative value ($\pm$ 20 mm Hg)
           (a) Often admission blood pressure may be elevated due to anxiety
               (i)   Better gauge is reading from preadmission visit or physician's office
    c. Pulse
        i.   Should be regular in rate and rhythm
        ii.   Reflect preoperative status of the patient
    d. Respirations
        i.   Return of preanesthesia respiratory status
           (a) No symptoms of upper airway compromise without:
               (i)   Wheezing
               (ii)   Snoring
               (iii) Stridor
               (iv) Labored breathing
               (v)   Crowing
        ii.   Pre-existing pulmonary disease
           (a) Specific physician's evaluation and discharge order
               (i)   Asthma/emphysema
                    a) Thorough assessment throughout postanesthesic period
           (b) No acute exacerbation of pre-existing disease should be present at time of discharge
           (c) Comparison of pre- and postoperative oxygen saturation levels helps assessment of discharge readiness
    e. Temperature
        i.   Typical criteria may state that patient's oral temperature:
           (a) Must be between 96° F and 100° F prior to discharge **or**
           (b) Variation of no more than 2° F from patient's preoperative admission temperature

7. Surgical site
    a. No active bleeding should be present
        i.   Signs of potential bleeding
           (a) Observation of dressing or surgical site for:
               (i)   Increased girth
               (ii)   Distention
               (iii) Swelling
               (iv) Vaginal flow/hematuria
               (v)   Frequent swallowing

        (b) Tachycardia

        (c) Hypotension

  8. Extremity circulation

    a. Use of pneumatic tourniquet may complicate postoperative assessment because of skin color changes in the immediate postoperative period

      i. Pale, flushed, or mottled

        (a) Until normal circulation has been established for a period of time

        (b) Patients should not be discharged until skin color and capillary refill have returned to normal limits

    b. Plaster or fiberglass casts or any encircling dressing

      i. Compromise circulation

        (a) Requires frequent extremity assessment

          (i) Skin color

          (ii) Pulses

          (iii) Capillary refill

          (iv) Motor and sensory integrity

          (v) Temperature not reliable

            a) Exposure to cool room temperatures

        (b) Comparison of operative and nonoperative extremity useful to determine surgically-induced deficits

  9. Gastrointestinal status

    a. Many facilities require patients tolerate oral fluids with limited or no nausea/vomiting

    b. Patients who are discharged without oral intake are usually well hydrated with intravenous fluids prior to discharge

    c. Instructions for prevention or decrease in postoperative nausea/vomiting at home should be reinforced with the patient and family

      i. Limit heavy or spicy foods

      ii. Remain recumbent until nausea subsides

      iii. Avoid rapid position changes

      iv. Base oral intake on desire to eat and drink

10. Comfort level

    a. Unrealistic to expect every patient will be totally pain-free at discharge

      i. Patient should not be discharged in acute distress

      ii. Pain should be controlled with oral analgesics

        (a) Addition of local anesthesia at the operative site results in greater comfort for a longer period

          (i) Patients should be cautioned against increased activity at home because of absent of minimal pain from the local anesthetic

    b. Parenteral analgesia may be necessary prior to discharge for the patient who is expected to have a higher level of discomfort at home

      i. Goal is to have patient comfortable, not too sedated

      ii. Must have responsible person in the home to care for her/him

11. Ambulation

    a. Ambulation without dizziness or faintness

      i. Consistent with preoperative status and procedure restrictions

    b. Romberg test is used in some facilities to identify longer recovery period

      i. Positive test characterized by loss of sense of position and balance when standing upright with feet together and eyes closed

    c. Spinal/epidural anesthesia

      i. Return of sensation and strength must be present along with proprioception (sense of position of the legs and feet)

12. Urinary status
    a. Difference of opinion and practice regarding the need for all patients to void prior to discharge
    b. Patients with potentially complicating conditions should void spontaneously prior to discharge
        i. To avoid complications at home
            (a) Males with diagnosed/undiagnosed prostatic hypertrophy
            (b) Inadequate hydration
            (c) Primary kidney disease
            (d) Surgical procedures
                (i) Inguinal herniorrhaphy
                (ii) Rectal/pelvic procedures
                (iii) Urinary procedures
                    a) May cause hematuria resulting in clots that may obstruct urinary flow
        ii. Spinal/epidural anesthesia
            (a) Sympathetic nervous system controls the bladder and urethra
                (i) Return of bladder function announces the end of the effects of sympathetic blockade
                    a) Also indicates vasomotor function is adequate for maintaining normotension when patient stands and ambulates
    c. Pain and anxiety may be increased when the staff and patient focus on the patient's need to void
    d. Abdominal examination to determine bladder distention should be done
13. Physical, emotional, and psychological factors
    a. The above criteria indicates physical aspects of care have been addressed for discharge
    b. Patient may express vague complaints, difficult to explain
        i. "Something is not quite right"
        ii. Better to slow discharge process and avoid potential complications from occurring in the home
    c. Avoid "rushing" the patient
        i. Even if care provided is of high quality the patient who feels pressured to leave after surgery will perceive the entire experience to be substandard
        ii. Provide clear explanations that highlight realistic expectations before sedation and surgery
            (a) Normal to:
                (i) Feel tired and sleepy for the remainder of the day following surgery
                    a) Due to sedation and analgesics
                (ii) Forget parts of the day
                    a) Amnesic effects of sedation and anesthesia
                (iii) Have some discomfort
                    a) Cannot render patient completely pain-free
                (iv) Mild nausea
                (v) Dizziness
                (vi) Headache
                (vii) Mild sore throat
                (viii) General muscle aches
                    a) Especially if the patient has arthritis

    iii. Emotional responses following surgery
      (a) May be individual reaction
      (b) May be response to surgical outcome
        (i)   Biopsy report
        (ii) Extensive alteration in body image
        (iii) Relief of receiving positive report
      (c) Individual behavioral responses
        (i)   Patients may question behavior during the immediate postanesthetic period
          a) Reassure that behavior was appropriate
          b) Confidentiality is maintained
        (ii) Pleasant/unpleasant dreams
          a) Reassure that dreaming is not unusual
          b) Allow patient to talk about these dreams
        (iii) Confusion
          a) Necessary to differentiate the cause of confusion
          b) Pharmacologic side effects on anesthesia
          c) Psychological response to stress
          d) Pre-existing psychiatric conditions

14. Discharge instructions

15. Verbal and written instructions
    a. Given to both patient and responsible adult
      i.   Home care
        (a) Incisional care
        (b) Medications
      ii. Emergency medical attention

16. Primary responsibility for instructions is physician
    a. Anesthesiologist provides instructions relating to potential side effects of anesthesia
    b. Surgeon provides parameters for general care and medication instructions
    c. Nurse acts as agent who relays and explains physician's instructions
      i.   Answers questions
      ii. Explains instructions so patient and responsible other can understand them

17. Instructional content
    a. General expectations
      i.   Reassure that minor symptoms may occur and are not serious
        (a) Headache
        (b) Fatigue
        (c) Muscle soreness/weakness
        (d) Sore throat
      ii. Symptoms not to be ignored
        (a) Bleeding at surgical site
        (b) Swelling of affected area
          (i)   Numbness and/or tingling of affected extremity
        (c) Emergency contact numbers
        (d) Go to nearest emergency department if unable to contact physician
      iii. Activity
        (a) General anesthetic and sedatives alter judgment and reflexes
          (i)   No driving for 24 hours
          (ii) Avoid signing legal documents
          (iii) No alcoholic beverages for 24 hours

      b. Medications
         i.   Review action and effect of prescribed medications
            (a) Include side effects
            (b) How to take medications
                (i)   Empty stomach or with food
                (ii)   What type of fluids to use
                (iii) Take with other medications or alone
        ii.   Indicate on discharge instruction sheet when next dose of prescribed medication is due
      c. Driving
         i.   Reinforce issue of no driving for at least 24 hours after anesthesia
        ii.   Surgeon may prohibit driving until seen postoperatively
      d. Diet
         i.   Caution against spicy or heavy foods day of surgery
            (a) Prevent gastric distress
        ii.   Increased oral fluids encouraged at home
            (a) Especially following urologic procedures
        iii. Patient experiencing nausea needs special instructions
            (a) Resting flat with head slightly elevated
            (b) Limit oral intake
            (c) Avoid foods and beverages that might potentiate nausea
            (d) Bland foods prior to taking oral medications might help
      e. Activity
         i.   Limitations and expectations should be explained
      f. Operative site
         i.   Instructions for appropriate operative site care
            (a) Dressing removal
                 (i)   When
                (ii)   Incision open to air or covered again
            (b) Incision care
            (c) Bathing/showering restrictions for wound care
            (d) Bleeding
                 (i)   Guidelines for acceptable amount of drainage
      g. Preventing infection
         i.   Care of incision and dressings emphasized
        ii.   Symptoms of infection explained to patient and family
      h. Sexual activity
         i.   Clarify physician's instructions
C. Discharge scoring systems
   1. One specific for ambulatory surgery patients
      a. Chung's Post Anesthesia Discharge Scoring System (PADSS)
         i.   Measures home readiness
        ii.   Five criteria
            (a) Vital signs
                 (i)   Similar to preoperative values
                (ii)   BP ± 20 mm Hg
            (b) Ambulation and mental status
            (c) Nausea and vomiting
            (d) Pain
            (e) Surgical bleeding and fluid intake/output
      b. See Table 8–4
      c. Final assessment prior to discharge from facility

Table 8–4 • PADSS

PATIENT INDEX	STANDARD	SCORE
Vital Signs	Patient's BP . . .	
	within 20% of preoperative value	2
	20–40% of preoperative value	1
	>40% of preoperative value	0
Ambulation	Patient is able to ambulate . . .	
	gait steady; no dizziness	2
	with assistance	1
	inadequately, dizziness present	0
Nausea/Vomiting	Patient's experience of nausea/ vomiting is . . .	
	minimal	2
	moderate	1
	severe	0
Pain	Patient's pain level is . . .	
	minimal	2
	moderate	1
	severe	0
Surgical Bleeding	Bleeding from operative site is . . .	
	minimal	2
	moderate	1
	severe	0

Note: Total possible score is 10; patients scoring ≥9 are considered fit for discharge from Phase II

    2. Level of recovery should meet discharge criteria
      a. Patient should express his/her readiness for discharge
    3. Describe instructions for home care
    4. Check for patient belongings
      a. Including medications
    5. Accompany patient to transportation
    6. Inform patient of follow-up phone call
      a. Usually within 24 hours
      b. Monday morning if surgery is on Friday

XXIV. Extension of Care
    A. Patients may not achieve adequate level of recovery to return home without professional assistance
    1. Home health care
      a. Arrangements should be made prior to day of surgery if possible
    2. Recovery care centers
      a. Separate facilities, not capable of performing surgical procedures
        i. Designed for nursing care of healthy postoperative patients
          (a) Require extensive nursing care and pain control after surgery
        ii. May provide around-the-clock care for patients at 25–30% lower cost than regular hospitalization
    3. 23-hour hospital admission
      a. For patients experiencing anesthetic- or surgical-related complications
        i. Prolonged nausea/vomiting
        ii. Pain
        iii. Bleeding

(a) Falls under umbrella of ambulatory surgery for most third-party payers

(b) May require preapproval from insurance companies

XXV. Focusing on "Success"

A. Often difficult to measure and define

  1. Four focus points in PACU nursing care

    a. Catalyst who helps the patient return as closely and rapidly as possible to preoperative condition and to their families

    b. Being totally attentive for potential complications and helping to avoid them whenever possible

    c. Discharging the patient as awake, pain-free, and nausea-free as possible

    d. Ensuring that each patient is treated with dignity and as a person who is important and special

XXVI. Special Considerations in PACU Care

A. Medical support

  1. Individual facilities differ in the chain of medical responsibility involved with the patient

    a. Anesthesiologist

      i. The ASA Standards for Postanesthesia Care provide definite statements in that regard

    b. Surgeon

B. Quality improvement practices

  1. Involvement in ongoing clinical studies and identify valuable trends affecting current and future patient care

  2. All members of the anesthesia team should be involved in quality improvement

  3. Evaluation of nursing care occurs both at discharge and during follow-up contact

C. The PACU as a treatment and anesthesia site

  1. Considered an excellent location because it is fully equipped

    a. ECG monitors

    b. Noninvasive blood pressure monitors

    c. Pulse oximetry

    d. Oxygen

    e. Suction

    f. Emergency equipment

  2. Often PACUs are used at sites for therapeutic procedures

    a. Pain clinic procedures

      i. Epidural steroid injections

      ii. Stellate ganglion blocks

      iii. Other sympathetic blocks

    b. Electroconvulsive shock therapy (ECTs)

    c. Blood transfusions

    d. Chemotherapy

  3. Administration of local or regional anesthesia prior to surgery

  4. PACU nurse's role

    a. May act as physician assistant

      i. Secure further supplies

      ii. Apply solutions or drapes

      iii. Adjust equipment

      iv. Reposition patient

   b. Patient supporter
      i.   Emotional support
   c. Monitor patient
      i.   Vital signs
      ii. Monitor pattern
      iii. Response to procedure

Bibliography

1. Aker, J. (1994). Immediate care in the postoperative period. *Curr Rev Post Anesth Care Nurses*, 16:146–156.
2. Aker, J. (1995). Neuromuscular relaxants: A primer. *Curr Rev Post Anesth Care Nurses*, 17:113–124.
3. Anderson, R., Crohg, K. (1976). Pain as a major cause of postoperative nausea. *Can Anaesth Soc J*, 23:336.
4. ASPAN Standards of PeriAnesthesia Nursing Practice. (1998). Thorofare, NJ: ASPAN.
5. Axelsson, K., Mollefors, K., Olsson, J., et al. (1985). Bladder function and spinal anesthesia. *Acta Anaesth Scand*, 29:315.
6. Bauer, J., (1996). Who is that new nurse? *J Peri Anesth Nurs*, 11:374.
7. Biddle, C. (1995). Should we really be "banking" on autologous blood? *Curr Rev Post Anesth Care Nurses*, 17:45–52.
8. Bodner, M. (1990). Presentation to the American Society of Anesthesiologists. Las Vegas.
9. Bosek, V. (1995). The role of non-steroidal anti-inflammatory agents in perioperative pain therapy. *Curr Rev Post Anesth Care Nurses*, 17:133–140.
10. Callahan, L. (1993). Anesthesia for electroconvulsive therapy. *Curr Rev Post Anesth Care Nurses*. 15:9–16.
11. Callahan, L. (1994). The effect of surgical stress on postoperative care of the patient. *Curr Reviews for Post Anesth Care Nurses*, 15:129–136.
12. Ciufo, D., Dice, S., Coles, C. (1995). Rewarming hypothermic postanesthesia patients: A comparison between a water coil warming blanket and a forced-air warming blanket. *J Post Anesth Nurs*, 10:155–158.
13. DeFazio-Quinn, D.M. (ed). (1997). Ambulatory surgery. *The Nursing Clinics of North America*. Philadelphia: Saunders.
14. Domino, K. (1996). Anesthetic management in the patient with chronic obstructive pulmonary disease. *Curr Rev Post Anesth Care Nurses*, 18:25–36.
15. Drain, C. (1994). *The Post Anesthesia Care Unit: A Critical Care Approach to Post Anesthesia Nursing*. Philadelphia: Saunders.
16. Einhorn, G., Chant, P. (1994). Postanesthesia care unit dilemmas: Prompt assessment and treatment. *J Post Anesth Nurs*, 9:28–33.
17. Feeley, T. (1993). The design and staffing of a modern post anesthesia care unit. *Curr Rev Post Anesth Care Nurses*, 15:129–136.
18. Fiorentini, S.E. (1993). Evaluation of a new program: Pediatric parental visitation in the postanesthesia care unit. *J Post Anesth Nurs*, 8:249–256.
19. Frost, E.A.M. (1990). *Post Anesthesia Care Unit: Current Practices*, 2nd ed. St. Louis: Mosby.
20. Grove, T.M. (1996). Management of problems in the post anesthesia care unit: Part I. *Curr Rev Post Anesth Care Nurses*, 18:1–8.
21. Grove, T. (1996). Management of problems in the PACU: Part II. *Curr Rev Post Anesth Care Nurses*, 18:9–16.
22. Heres, E., Gravlee, G. (1995). Approaches and techniques to minimize blood transfusions. *Curr Rev Post Anesth Care Nurses*, 17:69–76.
23. Ignatavicius, D., Workman, M., Mishler, M. (1995). *Medical Surgical Nursing—A Nursing Process Approach*, 2nd ed. Philadelphia: Saunders.
24. Jacobsen, W. (1992). *Manual of Post Anesthesia Care*. Philadelphia: Saunders.
25. The Joint Commission. (1994). *1994 Accreditation Manual for Hospitals*. Oakbrook Terrace, IL: JCAHO.
26. Kahn, R. (1996). Approaching common problems in the PACU. *Curr Rev Post Anesth Care Nurses*, 19:161–168.
27. Kang, S.B., Rudrud, L., Nelson, W., Baier, D. (1994). Postanesthesia nursing care for ambulatory surgery patients post-spinal anesthesia. *J Post Anesth Nurs*, 9:101–106.
28. Knowles, R. (1996). Standardization of pain management in the postanesthesia care unit. *J Peri Anesth Nurs*, 11:390–398.
29. Kotrilla, K., Hovorka, K., Erkola, O. (1987). Nitrous oxide does not increase the incidence of nausea and vomiting after isoflurane anesthesia. *Anesth Analg*, 66:761–765.
30. Kovac, A.L. (1997). The difficult postoperative patient with nausea and/or vomiting. *Curr Rev Peri Anesth Nurses*, 19:25–36.
31. Krenzischek, D.A., Frank, S.M., Kelly, S. (1995). Forced-air warming versus routine thermal care and core temperature measurement sites. *J Post Anesth Nurs*, 10:69–78.
32. Lau, W.C., Tremper, K.K. (1995). Blood substitutes: Today and tomorrow. *Curr Rev Post Anesth Care Nurses*, 17:69–76.
33. Litwack, K. (1991). *Post Anesthesia Care Nursing*. St. Louis: Mosby.
33a. Litwack, K. (1995). *Core Curriculum for Post Anesthesia Nursing Practice*, 3rd ed. Philadelphia: Saunders.
34. Lyon, L.J. (1997). *Basic Electrocardiography Handbook*. New York: Van Nostrand Reinhold.
35. Maree, S. (1994). Aspiration prophylaxis: An update. *Curr Rev Post Anesth Care Nurses*, 16:61–72.
36. Marley, R.A., Moline, B.M. (1996). Patient discharge from the ambulatory setting. *J Post Anesth Nurs*, 11:39–49.

38. Nachman, J.A. (1993). Postoperative nausea and vomiting. *Curr Rev Post Anesth Care Nurses*, 15:37–44.

39. Nachman, J. (1994). Pulse oximetry: History, technical aspects and clinical considerations. *Curr Rev Post Anesth Care Nurses*, 16:73–80.

40. NDH. (1997). *Nursing 97 Drug Handbook.* Springhouse, PA: Springhouse Corporation.

41. Omoigui, S. (1992). *The Anesthesia Drug Handbook.* St. Louis: Mosby.

42. Perry, K. (1996). Increasing patient satisfaction: Simple ways to increase the effectiveness of interpersonal communication in the PACU. *J Post Anesth Care Nurs*, (1995). 9:153–156.

43. Pflug, A., Aasheim, G., Foster, C. (1978). Sequence of return of neurological function and criteria for safe ambulation following subarachnoid block. *Can Anaesth Soc J*, 25:133.

44. Poole, E.L. (1993). The effects of postanesthesia care unit visits on anxiety in surgical patients. *J Post Anesth Nurs*, 8:386–394.

45. Reed, C. (1996). Care of postoperative patients with pulmonary edema. *J Peri Anesth Nurs*, 11:164–169.

46. Reiser, L.S. (1993). Regional anesthesia: PACU considerations. *Curr Rev Post Anesth Care Nurses*, 20:167–176.

47. Saga-Rumley, S.A. (1997). Intravenous regional anesthesia (IRA). *Curr Rev Peri Anesth Nurses*, 19:65–76.

48. Sullivan, L.M. (1994). Factors influencing pain management: A nursing perspective. *J Post Anesth Nurs*, 9:83–90.

49. Vogelsang, J., Hayes, S. (1989). Stadol attenuates postanesthesia shivering. *J Post Anesth Nurs*, 4:222–227.

50. Watcha, M.F., White, P.F. (1992). Postoperative nausea and vomiting: Its etiology, treatment, and prevention. *Anesthesiology*, 77:162–284.

51. Wetchler, B.V. (ed). (1985). *Anesthesia for Ambulatory Surgery*. Philadelphia: Lippincott.

REVIEW QUESTIONS

1. According to the American Society of PeriAnesthesia Nurses, the recommended nurse:patient ratio for a patient requiring mechanical ventilation is

   A. 1:4
   B. 1:1
   C. 1:2
   D. 1:3

2. In Phase II PACU, a staffing ratio of 1:4 is acceptable for which of the following?

   A. Over 5 years of age, awake, and stable
   B. Over 5 years of age within 30 minutes of procedure or discharge from Phase I
   C. Less than 5 years of age with family present
   D. There is no standard for a 1:4 staffing ratio

3. An *initial* assessment of the patient admitted to PACU Phase I should focus on

   A. Respiratory and circulatory parameters
   B. Motor function
   C. Anesthesia report
   D. Level of consciousness

4. All of the following regarding autologous blood donation are true except

   A. More than 5% of blood donations are autologous
   B. Fresh, unfrozen blood can be stored up to 42 days
   C. Only one nurse has to check autologous blood before transfusion
   D. The last unit of autologous blood must be drawn at least 72 hours before surgery
   E. The patient should be between 12 and 75 years of age

5. All of the following regarding discharge criteria are true except

   A. Written criteria should address parameters of physical and cognitive recovery
   B. Criteria should be appropriate to the unit or location to which the patient is being transferred
   C. Criteria can be based on a numeric scoring system that provides objective methods with which to evaluate and describe the patient's condition
   D. The Aldrete discharge scoring system requires a score of 7 or more for discharge from PACU Phase I
   E. When predetermined discharge criteria are established by the medical staff, the PACU nurse is allowed to discharge the patient

6. The REACT discharge scoring system

   A. Measures the same parameters as the Aldrete scoring system
   B. Is considered somewhat more reliable as it measures the patient's temperature and not color as a parameter
   C. Measures color in addition to the same parameters as the Aldrete scoring system
   D. Is considered less reliable than the Aldrete scoring system because it uses color as a parameter

7. Mr. S. received a spinal anesthesia for knee arthroscopy surgery. Which of the following is the best indicator that the sypathetic blockade is resolved?

   A. Is able to point toes toward head
   B. Is able to void spontaneously
   C. Is feeling pain in operative site
   D. Has sensation with proprioception to feet

8. Treatment for a post-dural puncture or spinal headache includes which of the following?

   A. Maintaining NPO status
   B. Applying an abdominal binder
   C. Allowing the patient to ambulate
   D. Infusing IVs at KVO rate

9. When does discharge planning begin?

   A. With the preadmission phone call
   B. On the day of surgery
   C. When the patient arrives in PACU Phase I
   D. When the patient is ready to leave the facility

10. Discharge instructions should contain the following information except

    A. Phone numbers for surgeon and emergency department
    B. Time next medication dose is to be taken at home
    C. Increase in acceptable amount of wound drainage
    D. Call the surgeon if feelings of weakness and fatigue last through the night

ANSWERS TO QUESTIONS

1. B	6. B
2. D	7. B
3. A	8. B
4. C	9. A
5. D	10. D

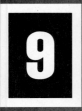

Patient and Family Education

Janet L. Ridder (late)
Hinsdale Hospital
Hinsdale, Illinois
Joyce C. Hadley
Inova Health Systems
Falls Church, Virginia

PATIENT EDUCATION:

The process of influencing human behavior.

I. **Who (Assessment)**
   A. Identify learning needs of the patient and family
      1. Methods of assessment
         a. Use of open-ended questions
            i. "Tell me what you already know about the day of surgery."
            ii. "Can you tell me more?"
            iii. "Go on."
         b. Direct observation of verbal and nonverbal cues
      2. Identify current knowledge level regarding impending procedure
         a. Previous experience
         b. Prior education (as in physician's office)
         c. Patient perception and expectation
         d. Potential misinformation from friends and other sources
      3. Assess patient/family/responsible adult's preferred method of learning
      4. Lack of questions from patient/family/responsible companion should not be interpreted as understanding of surgical/procedural intervention

Objectives

1. List learner characteristics to be assessed in the process of patient and family education.
2. State the three domains of learning behaviors.
3. Identify the domain of a sample learning objective.
4. Compare and contrast various methods of teaching.
5. List outcome standards related to assessment of patient and family education.
6. Describe an individualized teaching plan for a pediatric patient.

B. Learner characteristics
  1. Demographic and physical
    a. Primary language
      i. Provide interpreter when English is not spoken
      ii. Recognize limitations of vocabulary if family/significant other does interpretation
    b. Special learning considerations
      i. Reading level (current education level)
        (a) Use of vocabulary
        (b) Ability to communicate
      ii. Note any sensory impairments
        (a) Orientation and memory
        (b) Sight or hearing
          (i) Provide appropriate teaching materials, for instance:
            a) Prosthetics as necessary
            b) Braille materials
            c) Sign language interpreter (certified, when possible)
      iii. Physical condition
        (a) Level of comfort/discomfort
        (b) Energy level
        (c) Alertness
        (d) Overall appearance
      iv. Developmental level
        (a) Intellectual
        (b) Emotional
      v. Age
        (a) Pediatrics: plan teaching based on child's developmental age
          (i) Infant (birth–12 months): hallmarks—fear of separation and stranger anxiety
            a) Tell parent when/where he/she may be present with child
            b) Instruct parent to bring familiar object to stay with infant
            c) Discuss attendance of parents at induction when appropriate
        (b) Toddler (walking–2 years): hallmark—fear of separation, fear of bodily harm, limited time concept
          (i) Begin with very general concepts, using doll or stuffed animals
          (ii) Consider suggestions as above (infant)
        (c) Preschool (2–5 years): hallmark—separation anxiety persists, understands simple explanations
          (i) Demonstrate use of equipment on doll or stuffed animals
          (ii) Puppets are effective at this age
        (d) School-age (6–11 years): hallmark—fear of the unknown, loss of control, needs approval, companionship and successful performance
          (i) Explain procedures clearly and demonstrate when applicable
          (ii) Use simple drawings and correct equipment for demonstrations
          (iii) Allow child to make some choices
            a) "Flavor" of mask
            b) Ride or walk to the OR
        (e) Adolescent (12–18 years): hallmark—fears loss of control, isolation from peers—self esteem is fragile
          (i) Talk *to* the adolescent, not over his/her head
          (ii) Emphasize that privacy will be provided
          (iii) Tours are good for this age

(f) Adult (18–65): hallmark—concerned about survival; may deny fears; learning is goal directed and participative
- (i) Reflect patient's own words
  - a) May be misunderstood if he/she says "gaseous" and you say "flatulent"
  - b) Verbal and behavioral "messages" may differ—discover which is real

(g) Geriatric (65+): hallmarks—be sensitive to differences between chronological and physiological ages
- (i) Assess the individual; **do not assume** that all geriatric patients are hard-of-hearing or slow to learn
- (ii) Recognize that elders may be slower to learn new information or skills
- (iii) Consider mini-mental status exam for baseline function when indicated

2. Psychosocial
   a. Health beliefs
   b. Attitudes and motivation
      i. Patient perception of disease or condition and its seriousness is a critical factor in determining readiness to learn
   c. Stress and coping skills
   d. Obstacles to health learning
      i. Anxiety
         (a) Low levels enhance learning
         (b) Moderate and high levels inhibit learning
   e. Social support
      i. Include family/responsible adult in the teaching/learning considerations
C. Teaching characteristics
   1. Knowledge of teaching/learning principles
      a. Use common language (not complex medical terms or jargon)
      b. Anxiety and pain impede learning
      c. Learning needs to be reinforced
         i. Retention is enhanced when more senses are affected **and/or**
         ii. There are more repetitions of information
      d. Knowledge of teaching tools available
      e. Knowledge of content

II. Why (Objectives or Learning Goals)

A. Learning objectives or goals are really statements of the (realistic) hoped for outcome
   1. Must be *shared* objectives—your task: ensure that patient understands material
   2. Participants in the process may have different expectations of the outcome
      a. Patient, post-cataract extraction: "I just want to play golf again"
      b. Hospital/surgical center: "Make the patient happy with the experience and prevent post-discharge complications"
      c. Ambulatory surgery nurse: "Get the patient home with the necessary skills of self-care to prevent infection and support return to ADLs"
   3. Patient/family must be involved in setting the goals
   4. What a patient or family member is to learn should be stated in the form of an objective (e.g., "I will promote healing by changing my dressing correctly")
B. Benefits of learning that have been demonstrated/proposed in research and literature
   1. Diminish fear and anxiety
   2. Decrease incidence of postoperative complications
   3. Increase compliance with health-care regimens
   4. Increase ability to select coping strategies

        5. Decrease recovery time

        6. Decrease postoperative pain

        7. Improve patient preparation prior to procedure

        8. Increase family/responsible adult support

        9. Assist in return to normal activities of daily living (ADLs)

  C. Development of teaching plan

        1. Teaching plan parallels nursing process (see Figure 9–1)

        2. Consider verbal or written contract with patient and other learners, especially valuable with adolescents

  D. Classification of goals of learning (behaviors) are listed as **domains**

        1. Cognitive—includes intellectual abilities and knowledge; examples of preoperative teaching objective in this domain:

          a. To describe the reason for applying an ice collar after tonsillectomy

          b. To state which symptoms should be reported immediately to the physician

        2. Affective—includes attitudes, feelings and values; examples:

          a. To accept the feelings of loss after miscarriage

          b. To desire to change smoking habits

        3. Psychomotor—includes motor skills; examples:

          a. To demonstrate correct use of crutches

          b. To change catheter bag aseptically

  E. Formulate teaching plan

III. What (Content of Teaching Plan)

  A. Individualize teaching plan based on identified needs

  B. Generic content

        1. Provide overview of expected procedure and events

          a. Describe environments

          b. Sequence of events (where and when to arrive, what to bring, flow of events, when to expect to be discharged)

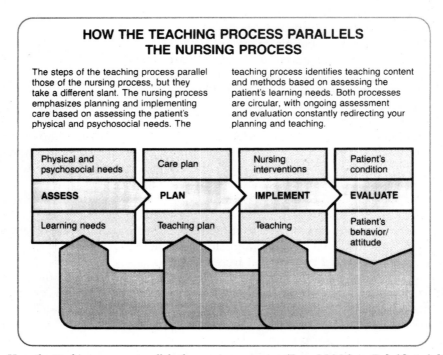

Figure 9–1. How the teaching process parallels the nursing process. (From McMahon, E. [ed.] et al. [1991]. *How to Teach Patients.* Springhouse, PA: Springhouse Publishing.)

2. Describe behaviors patient is expected to demonstrate
   a. Adherence to food- and drink-intake instructions
   b. Express understanding about taking medications before surgery—take them or "hold" them
   c. Preparing/wearing appropriate clothing
   d. Arranging responsible adult caretaker for discharge and for home recovery
3. Describe probable alterations in comfort level and strategies for reducing the pain and discomfort
   a. Wound/pain discomfort—what to expect
   b. Sore throat after general anesthesia with intubation
   c. Requesting pain medication
   d. Nonpharmacologic methods for reducing pain: ice chips or packs, guided imagery, distraction
4. Describe probable tactile, auditory, and verbal sensations that patient will experience in the operating room and PACU
5. Explain equipment patient will see or hear in the operating room
6. Describe postoperative behaviors patient is expected to demonstrate
   a. Passive exercises
   b. Ambulation
   c. Deep breathing and coughing
   d. Dressing care
   e. Resumption of diet, fluids, prescribed medications, and activities
   f. Signs and symptoms to report
   g. Provide contact in case of emergency before and after surgery/procedure
7. Patient/family/responsible adult should be able to:
   a. Cite reasons for each postoperative instruction provided
   b. Demonstrate coughing, deep breathing, incisional splinting, passive leg exercises (these and other tactics as appropriate to surgical procedure)
   c. Describe anticipated steps in postoperative activity resumption
C. General points to consider
   1. Sequence content of activities to facilitate learning
   2. Break instructions into manageable steps
   3. Instill confidence by reinforcing learning
   4. Anticipate potential problems
      a. Share tactics for reminding patient about medication timing
      b. Place a handwashing reminder with the dressing materials
   5. Include both preoperative and postoperative information
   6. Explain reasons for and benefits of behaviors
   7. Do not assume that a low educational level equates to low intelligence
   8. Keep it simple—avoid overloading the patient with information
D. Procedure-specific content
   1. Refer to procedure section of this book (see Chapters 26–38)
   2. Include education related to the types of anesthesia and how it impacts postoperative care
      a. General anesthesia
         i. Explain that patient will be asked to take frequent deep breaths and will probably receive oxygen in PACU to help eliminate anesthetic agents
         ii. Explain the monitoring, vital signs, and questioning that occur in PACU and their value in the recovery process
         iii. Explain that pain medication is available; encourage patient to request it if needed

    b. Local anesthesia
       i. Explain availability of adjunctive medications for relaxing patient (address fear of being awake and observing operation on self)
       ii. Explain positioning, draping, and tourniquet processes as expected in the OR
       iii. Instruct patient to alert nurse or physician to discomfort experienced during procedure
       iv. Explain postoperative routine (vital signs, getting up, preparing for discharge)

IV. How (Effective Learning Tools and Teaching Methods)
  A. Written
    1. Books, pamphlets, institution-specific handouts
    2. Materials should be presented at about sixth-grade level
    3. Criteria for use
      a. Analyze reading level
      b. Make adjustments for visually impaired, such as large print
      c. Provide written materials in patient's predominant language
    4. Review written information verbally with the patient; validate patient's comprehension by asking questions
  B. Audio
    1. Audio cassette; not so popular since advent of video cassette
    2. Criteria for use
      a. Consider for use with patients with low literacy skills or extensive visual impairment
  C. Visual
    1. Pictures, picture books, video cassette, computer-aided instruction
    2. Criteria for use
      a. If purchased material, ensure that content is consistent with practice and appropriate for patient
    3. Consider lending library for checkout from physician's office or preadmission testing site
    4. Interactive computer programs, especially with video
  D. Individual and group teaching
    1. 1:1 interviews, scheduled group discussions for specific types of surgery, facility tours
    2. Criteria for use
      a. Assess patient needs; always validate with the learner if the learning needs were met
  E. Common pediatric teaching methods
    1. Types
      a. Family preoperative interview (often in conjunction with pretesting)
        i. Demonstrate use of mask or equipment on a doll
        ii. Use of print materials specifically designed for pediatric populations (coloring books, videos); create pediatric materials at the fourth-grade level
      b. Facility tours
      c. Play therapy
      d. Filmed modeling

V. When and Where (. . . is the Best Time to Teach?)
  A. Timing of preoperative instructions
    1. Research results do not support a specific time frame; studies have been done, but none have had strong results that support a specific optimal time

2. Generally, teaching that is given immediately prior to a procedure is not well retained (learning principle: anxiety impedes learning)
3. Younger children **do** need explanations closer to the actual event (until their sense of time is well-developed)
    a. State the more fearsome information last
B. Environment for teaching should be:
    1. Conducive to learning
    2. Designed to reduce anxiety levels (color, decor)
    3. Undisturbed (reduce excess noise and distractions)
    4. Away from active surgical flow
    5. Private

VI. How (Do You Evaluate Teaching?)
A. Method—concurrent and retrospective
    1. Self report of patient/family/responsible adult
        a. Verify that objectives were met
            i.   After the teaching session
            ii. Also with a follow-up phone call
    2. Direct observation in skill-specific situations (psychomotor domain)
    3. Retain copy of signed teaching sheets to validate teaching efforts
B. Methods of measurement—use of outcome standards

NOTE: An example: 90% of patients stated on follow-up phone call that teaching met all their needs for self-care at home after surgery. The questions that the other 10% of patients expressed after discharge were recorded and tracked; the most frequent question was about dressing care for a specific surgery. The information for that surgery was revised to improve the quality of care.

1. Compile aggregate data for quality outcome indicators
2. Validate effectiveness of teaching effort by:
    a. Observation
    b. Written test
    c. Oral test
    d. Interview
    e. Checklist
3. Teaching effectiveness is measured by assuring that the patient (family or responsible adult) can demonstrate the knowledge; the patient/family/responsible companion should be able to:
    a. State time surgery is scheduled and time of arrival to hospital/surgicenter
    b. State where patient will be located after surgery
    c. List monitoring and therapeutic devices or materials most likely to be used during the postoperative period
    d. State location of family waiting area, telephones, rest rooms, and food service areas
    e. Ask questions regarding impending surgery
    f. Perform expected behaviors
        i.   Taking or holding medications as ordered
            (a) Encourage use of cues: timers, sticky notes, or clocks for reminders
        ii. Maintaining or omitting intake of fluids/foods as ordered
4. Demonstrate knowledge of potential physical and psychological effects of surgery
    a. The patient/family/responsible adult should be able to:
        i.   Describe the anticipated physical and psychological effects of surgical intervention
        ii. Express feelings regarding surgical intervention and its expected outcomes

5. Demonstrate knowledge of coping mechanisms that can be used in response to surgical intervention
   a. Medication
   b. Exercise
   c. Other nonpharmacologic pain relief
   d. Relaxation
   e. Family support
   f. Nursing support
   g. Counseling
   h. Community resource access

Bibliography

1. American Society of Post Anesthesia Nurses. (1989–1994). *J Post Anesth Nursing.*
2. American Society of PeriAnesthesia Nurses. (1994–present). *J Perianesth Nursing.*
3. Anderson, C. (1990). *Patient Teaching & Communication in an Information Age.* Albany: Delmar.
4. Burden, N. (1993). *Ambulatory Surgical Nursing.* Philadelphia: Saunders.
5. Cunningham, D. (1993). Improving your teaching skills. *Nursing, 93,* December.
6. Doak, C., et al. (1985). *Teaching Patients with Low Literacy Skills.* Philadelphia: Lippincott.
7. Eddy, M.E., Coslow, B.I. (1991). Preparation for ambulatory surgery: A patient education program. *J Post Anesth Nursing,* 6(1):5–12.
8. Ellerton, M., Merriam, C. (1994). Preparing children and families psychologically for day surgery: An evaluation. *J Adv Nursing,* 19(6):1057–62, June.
9. Haines, N. (1992). Same day surgery, coordinating the education process. *AORN J,* 55(2):573–580.
10. Kneedler, J. (ed.) (1990). *CNOR Study Guide.* Denver: National Certification Board, Perioperative Nursing, Inc.
11. Knowles, M. (1990). *The Adult Learner: A Neglected Species,* 4th ed. Houston: Gulf Publishing.
12. Kratz, A. (1993). Preoperative education: Preparing patients for a positive experience. *J Post Anesth Nursing,* 8(4):270–275.
13. Lancaster, K. (1997). Patient teaching in ambulatory surgery. In Greenfield, E., DeFazio-Quinn, D. (eds.) *The Nursing Clinics of North America.* Philadelphia: Saunders.
14. Lunow, K., Jung, L. (1993). Comprehensive perioperative care: Patient assessment, teaching, documentation. *AORN J,* 57(5):1167–1177.
15. McMahon, E., et al (eds.) (1991). *How to Teach Patients.* Springhouse, PA: Springhouse Corporation.
16. Meeker, B.J., Rodriquez, L.S., Johnson, J.M. (1992). A comprehensive analysis of preoperative patient education. *Today's OR Nurse,* 14(3):11–18.
17. Micheli, A. (1997). Advances and emerging topics in perioperative pediatric nursing. In *Nursing Clinics of North America.* Philadelphia: Saunders.
18. Murray, R.B., Zentner, J.P. (1997). *Health Assessment Promotion Strategies Through the Life Span,* 6th ed. Stamford, CT: Appleton and Lange.
19. Parnass, S.P. Ambulatory surgery patient priorities. In Brinsko, V., Litwack Saleh, K. (eds.) (1993). *Nursing Clinics of North America.* Philadelphia: Saunders.
20. Rankin, S., Duff, K. (1990). *Patient Education: Issues, Principles and Practices.* Philadelphia: Lippincott.
21. Redman, B. (1997). *The Process of Patient Education,* 8th ed. St. Louis: Mosby Yearbook.
22. Stewart, E.J., Algren, C., Arnold, S. (1994). Preparing children for a surgical experience. *Today's OR Nurse,* 16(2):9–14.
23. Yount, S., Schloesser, M. (1991). A description of patient and nurse perceptions of preoperative teaching. *J Post Anesth Nursing,* 6(1):17–25.

REVIEW QUESTIONS

1. When assessing a patient for learning readiness, the use of open-ended questions is encouraged. Which of the following represents an open-ended question?

   A. "Where do you live?"
   B. "What kind of surgery are you scheduled to have?"
   C. "Can you tell me more about what you know about the day of surgery?"
   D. "Do you expect to go home after your surgery?"

2. Mandy, a four-year-old, will be least helped by which of the following teaching strategies?

   A. A video about her proposed procedure
   B. A description in simple terms, using puppets, of the surgical events
   C. Touring the outpatient facility
   D. A discussion of the processes of the procedure

3. When providing patient education, the Ambulatory Surgery nurse is aware that:

   A. Elderly patients respond best to a higher pitched voice
   B. She must be sure patient can respond to information appropriately
   C. When several staff members participate in an education session, it is easier for the family to understand
   D. Information should be presented at eighth-grade level

4. Before beginning patient education, it is important for the nurse to:

   A. Indicate to patient/family/significant other how goals were chosen
   B. Make sure patient understands the goals
   C. Facilitate the patient in devising own goals
   D. Establish educational goals for patient and family

5. The literature indicates that learning:

   A. Diminishes fear/anxiety
   B. Reduces the need for surgery
   C. Reduces morale of family
   D. Inhibits patient satisfaction

6. Which statement best reflects a patient goal for the postoperative course of events?

   A. "Your family must be involved to help you get well."
   B. "I will help prevent infection in my wound by changing my dressing twice a day."
   C. "You will resume your usual activities by tomorrow."
   D. "Ask my son about that one."

7. The three domains of learning are:

   A. Cognitive, assertive, and psychomotor
   B. Psychomotor, environmental, and affective
   C. Deliberate, affective, and cognitive
   D. Cognitive, affective, and psychomotor

8. Printed materials for adults should be directed to which grade level?

   A. Third
   B. Fourth
   C. Fifth
   D. Sixth

9. Printed materials for children should be directed to which grade level?

   A. First
   B. Second
   C. Third
   D. Fourth

10. How can the ambulatory surgery nurse best validate the effectiveness of teaching efforts?

   A. Observe interaction of family members
   B. Assure patient can describe the surgical methods
   C. Assure that patient/family member is able to relate accurately the events of the operative day
   D. Observe that the patient is able to quickly recall his/her phone number

ANSWERS TO QUESTIONS

1. C
2. B
3. B
4. C
5. A

6. B
7. D
8. D
9. D
10. C

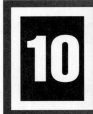

Environmental and Equipment Management

Cheryl Mullen
Bedford Ambulatory Surgical Center
Bedford, New Hampshire
Debby Niehaus
Bethesda North Ambulatory Surgery Center
Cincinnati, Ohio

I. **Facilities**
  A. Hospital-integrated
    1. Main operating suites used for ambulatory patients
    2. May have designated preoperative and postoperative areas
    3. Scheduling requires same protocols as inpatients
    4. Admitting process coordinated by ambulatory unit or hospital admitting
    5. Preoperative lab and diagnostic tests done outpatient prior to or on day of surgery
    6. Nursing staff may handle the processing of same day and A.M. admit patients
    7. Family members of both ambulatory and inpatients may share a waiting area
    8. Operating room scheduled specifically for ambulatory patients or interspersed with inpatients
    9. Advantages
      a. Allows sharing of personnel in different care areas
      b. Increased utilization of equipment and supplies
      c. Rapid admission to hospital if acute care is required
      d. Sharing of costs related to capital equipment expenditures

1. Identify the practice settings for ambulatory surgical nursing and physical structure of units.
2. Identify components of a safe environment in which to deliver competent care to all perianesthesia patients in the ambulatory surgical setting.
3. List the minimum required policies and procedures for safety, infection, latex allergy, and emergencies necessary for an ambulatory surgical unit.
4. Identify handling of issues of safety, infection control, and biohazards in the ambulatory setting.
5. List special consideration of caring for latex sensitive/allergy patients.

    10. Disadvantages
        a. Less control of scheduling and delays due to priority of inpatient surgical emergencies
B. Hospital-separated
    1. Physically separate ambulatory surgery department affiliated with the hospital
    2. Located within the hospital complex, adjacent to the hospital, or at an off-site location
    3. Designated preoperative, intraoperative, and postoperative areas
    4. Dedicated staff, equipment, policies and procedures, and separate care areas
    5. Organizationally separate structure from hospital-based operating rooms
    6. Exclusive facility for ambulatory surgery patient population
    7. Advantages
        a. Convenient scheduling
        b. Availability of hospital services and resources
        c. Easy admission of patient to hospital if acute care is required
        d. Sharing of unique equipment with hospital-based surgery unit
    8. Disadvantages
        a. Decreased opportunity for sharing of personnel
        b. Duplication of instruments and equipment
        c. Necessity for cross training of staff
C. Freestanding
    1. May be independently owned and operated, may or may not be hospital affiliated
    2. Operated as a for-profit enterprise or a not-for-profit
    3. May be owned by entrepreneurs, physicians, and nurses
    4. Types of ownership varies
        a. Corporate
        b. Joint venture
        c. Independent
    5. Frequently owned by health-care corporation chain
    6. Growing segment of health-care industry
    7. Advantages
        a. Cost effective
        b. Decreased bureaucracy
        c. User-friendly atmosphere
    8. Disadvantages
        a. Decreased reimbursement for some insurance carriers
        b. Decreased perception of patient safety
D. Office-based
    1. Similar to freestanding
    2. Safe and cost-effective surgery in physician's office
    3. May be operated as for-profit enterprise
    4. Advantages
        a. Schedule flexibility for patients and physicians
        b. Cost effectiveness of the procedure
        c. Staff expertise is specific to procedures performed
    5. Disadvantages
        a. Strict patient selection criteria
        b. Cannot provide many services offered by larger ambulatory facilities
E. Recovery center
    1. Facility with an internal or adjacent overnight recovery unit

2. Alternative for the patient and family when skilled nursing care is desirable, but acute care medically unnecessary
3. Generally equipped with private rooms in a hotel-like decor
4. Family members allowed to stay with patient if desired
5. Recovery center admission criteria
   a. Anticipated stay less than 72 hours
   b. Patient and/or family member staying, must be able to provide basic self-care needs
   c. Adequate pain management achieved within 72 hours
   d. Patient must have adequate psychomotor and cognitive skills to learn proper self-care techniques for discharge to home
6. Advantages
   a. Cost effective
   b. Nonthreatening, home-like atmosphere
   c. Family encouraged to participate in care
   d. Promotes early independence from health-care providers
7. Disadvantages
   a. Requires larger structural facility
   b. Separate staff required
   c. 24-hour nursing coverage necessary
   d. Increased need for ancillary services
   e. Provision for access to emergency care and hospital admission

II. **Physical Structure**
A. Lobby and reception area
   1. Exterior signs to direct to facility entrance or route to follow to department
   2. Area conveys sense of cleanliness, warmth, comfort, and professionalism
   3. Reception desk in sight of entrance door
   4. Knowledgeable receptionist/clerk to direct or answer questions
   5. Positive first impression by personnel
   6. Waiting area comfortable and relaxing
   7. Comfortable furniture, well-positioned lighting, nearby telephone, and rest rooms
   8. Handicapped accessible
   9. Diversion—television, music, reading materials, vending machines, nourishment (separate from waiting patients)
   10. Separate, enclosed play area for families with children, whenever space permits
B. Business and administrative area
   1. Office space for clerical, scheduling, and billing services
   2. Office space as needed for executive director, nurse manager, anesthesia personnel, doctor dictation/consult room, conference room/staff education area
   3. Promotion of health and emotional well-being of business staff
      a. Appropriate lighting, ventilation, and temperature control
      b. Windows that provide natural light
      c. Furnishings for comfort and good body mechanics
      d. Noise reduction measures
      e. Standard office equipment
      f. Telephone answering machine or voice mail
      g. Computerized management information system
C. Consultation and diagnostic area
   1. Located close to reception for easy accessibility
   2. Two-way communication system for summoning assistance

3. Consultation room
    a. Table and chairs for interviewing
    b. Supplies for documentation needs
    c. AV equipment for educational process
    d. Provision for privacy
    e. Lab area for obtaining patient specimens and appropriate supplies
    f. Bathroom handicapped accessible
    g. Stretcher for ECG or lab work
    h. Safety measures if radiology services provided, i.e., lead aprons, dose badges for staff
D. Preoperative Admitting
    1. Open floor plan allows constant visualization
    2. Minimal separation by curtains or glassed walls/doors
    3. Partial walls provide audio and visual separation
    4. Distinctly separate postoperative area
    5. Bathrooms
    6. Lockers for storage of personal belongings
    7. Scales, adult/infant
    8. Toys for children
    9. Recliners or stretchers (depends on anesthesia practice)
    10. IV poles
    11. Oxygen delivery and suction equipment accessible when sedation administered preoperatively or for special needs
    12. Monitoring devices, emergency equipment, and drugs readily available
    13. Access to nurse emergency call system
    14. Relaxing decor
        a. Calming colors
        b. Quiet surroundings with restricted traffic
        c. Soft music
    15. Resource 5—*Recommended equipment for preanesthesia phase, PACU phase I, phase II, phase III—ASPAN Standards of Perianesthesia Practice, 1998*
E. Operating room
    1. Follow recommended practice of the Association of Operating Room Nurses (AORN)
    2. Equipment and accessibility to emergency crash carts, medicines, and defibrillator
    3. Emergency power generator and lighting fixtures
    4. Back-up oxygen supply
    5. Anesthesia supplies and drugs
    6. Two-way communication for summoning help and contacting pre- and postoperative areas
    7. Considerations for storage, cleaning supplies, sterilizing of equipment, clerical needs, infection control, patient privacy
    8. Ensure safety, spill kits, and MSDS information available
        a. Routine inspection of electrical devices
        b. Grounding devices
        c. Restraining straps
        d. Pillows and padding for positioning
        e. Anesthesia waste gas scavenging
    9. Strict adherence to principles of asepsis
    10. Inclusion of windows provides emotional support to patients and staff
        a. Tinted, one-way glass

       b. Positioned in a restricted access area

       c. Vertical blinds for total darkness when necessitated by procedure

   11. Close proximity to Phase I PACU, ideal if OR corridors communicate directly with PACU

F. Phase I PACU

   1. Maintain adequate respect for patients' physical and psychological needs

   2. Adequate space to allow nursing care from either side, head, and foot of patient's stretcher

   3. Patient care supplies readily accessible

   4. Each station includes:

       a. Oxygen delivery system

       b. Vacuum station, suction

       c. Monitoring devices—cardiac monitor, pulse oximeter, noninvasive blood pressure monitor, and temperature

   5. Ice machine

   6. Patient warming device, thermal blanket warming device

   7. Easy accessibility to patient care supplies

   8. Close proximity to anesthesia administration

   9. Open room design for optimal visualization

   10. Distinct separation of postoperative patients and those patients having other procedures in the Phase I PACU, i.e., chronic pain procedures, preop administration of regional block

   11. Room that serves to provide patient isolation

   12. Provision for beverages/snacks

   13. One or more work desks within sight of patients

   14. Adjoins Phase II

   15. Hospital-based PACU

       a. Assign ambulatory patients to an area separated from sicker inpatients

   16. Freestanding center

       a. Favor liberal visiting policy, close proximity to waiting room

       b. Outside access to allow for ambulance transfer of patients to acute-care hospital if required

   17. Resource 5—*Recommended equipment for preanesthesia phase, PACU phase I, phase II, phase III—ASPAN Standards of Perianesthesia Practice, 1998*

G. Phase II PACU

   1. Casual, home-like atmosphere

   2. Provides continued nursing care and observation (emergency supplies available)

   3. Provides setting for education and instructions

   4. Allows reunion with family and friends

   5. Encourages self-care, ambulation, and a return to a level of function as close to the preoperative state as the procedure allows

   6. Room that serves to provide patient isolation

   7. Private rooms may be provided

   8. Open design less private, but allows for optimum visualization

       a. Opportunity for socialization with other patients/families

       b. Provision necessary for privacy related to care, i.e., partial walls, curtains, screens

   9. Stretchers/recliners depending on surgery and type and duration of anesthesia

   10. Discharge area large enough to accommodate at least one family member/significant other

   11. Separate area for pediatric patients if possible

12. Nourishment center for beverages/light foods
13. Television and VCR for diversion, teaching videos
    a. May choose not to have TV, can prolong discharge if patient/family too interested in program
14. Cabinets or furniture for storage of patient care items
15. Bathroom(s) in close proximity
16. Accessible to waiting area
17. Floor plan allows for efficient patient discharge
    a. Separate exit door for convenience/privacy
    b. Short route for those patients who are discharged ambulating
    c. Wheelchair ramp available and protected from weather
    d. Protective floor mats positioned inside doorways
18. Resource 5—*Recommended equipment for preanesthesia phase, PACU phase I, phase II, phase III—ASPAN Standards of Perianesthesia Practice, 1998*

III. Support Services

A. Supplies and equipment
   1. Storage for equipment and supplies available, efficiently positioned
   2. Outside shipments unboxed in receiving area, separate from sterile supplies to decrease the potential of introducing contaminants to restricted areas
   3. Inventory system in place for rapid location and retrieval of specific items
   4. Equipment stored adjacent to or near area of intended use
   5. Protected space for delicate instruments and equipment
   6. Resource 5—*Recommended equipment for preanesthesia phase, PACU phase I, phase II, phase III—ASPAN Standards of Perianesthesia Practice, 1998*
B. Housekeeping and linen
   1. Cleaning supplies and equipment stored out of sight of patients/visitors
   2. General housekeeping duties performed during downtimes
   3. Cleaning solutions and chemicals properly labeled and stored safely with adequate ventilation
   4. Provisions for supplies and personnel assigned to clean operating rooms between cases
   5. Separate mop sinks
   6. Maintain separation of soiled and clean linens
   7. Scrub clothing stored within confines of changing rooms
   8. Linen delivery carts outside of restricted areas to avoid contamination
C. Mechanical and electrical
   1. Preliminary evaluation and testing of all new equipment
   1. Inspected for safety, proper function before use
   2. Labeled with inspection sticker according to facility procedure
   3. Hospital-integrated facility
      a. Maintenance/clinical engineering responsible for servicing and safety of equipment
   4. Freestanding facility
      a. An individual(s) may be assigned or contracted for mechanical work
      b. Other staff members should have basic knowledge and written instructions of services
         i.   Electrical breaker switches
         ii. Water shut-off valves
         iii. Back-up oxygen sources
         iv. Piped-in gas shut-off valves
         v.   Emergency generator
         vi. Security system

        vii. Air conditioner

        viii. Humidifier controls

     c. Emergency service technician telephone number readily available

  D. Staff support services

    1. Comfort and safe working environment provided for staff members and physicians

    2. Separate or shared lounge for staff and physicians' use distant from clinical area

    3. Area for education, completion of projects, and staff meetings

    4. Reference library, reading material

    5. For physicians:

      a. Adequate parking near entrance, separate from patients' entrance

      b. Quiet area for dictation, telephoning, and completion of paperwork

      c. Easy access to medical records

IV. Safety Considerations

  A. General

    1. Dependent on physical conditions of facility

    2. Policies and procedures in place

    3. Safety-minded attitude and practice of staff members

    4. Practice habits of employees and physicians

    5. Administrative support reflective of compliance with safety standards

  B. Patients

    1. Care delivered by competent health providers

    2. Identification of patient—verbal and/or wrist band

    3. Special needs and/or allergies clearly communicated and noted

    4. Safeguard of valuables and personal possessions

    5. Safety practices in place to protect patient during dependence on staff

    6. Patient is appropriately attended and observed

      a. Side rails up

      b. Safety straps in place

      c. Nurse present, patient never left unattended

    7. Appropriate and safe equipment is available

      a. Faulty devices and equipment removed from service (lock out/tag out)

      b. Electrical equipment safely grounded/patient grounded

      c. Equipment used per manufacturer's recommendations

      d. Electrical, monitoring, and laser equipment pass biomedical inspection

    8. Medications stored and administered safely

    9. Health-care decisions made thoughtfully with regard to each individual patient

   10. Prevent spread of infectious disease

      a. Universal precautions

      b. Aseptic technique

      c. Employee, patient, and/or visitor health issues

      d. Notify anesthesiologist/physician of fever, cough, wheezing, or flu symptoms on admission

      e. Ask parents of pediatric patients regarding recent exposure to communicable diseases such as chicken pox

  C. Visitors

    1. Well-marked signage

    2. Dry, nonskid floors in waiting areas

    3. Uncluttered, well-lighted hallways

    4. Proper storage of toys

    5. Do not allow visitors to assist in patient transport/lifting

    6. Proper disposal of waste and needles

    7. Proper report and follow-up of noted/observed injuries

D. Employees
 1. Personal security provided
 2. Policies and practices in place to prevent spread of disease
  a. Universal precautions
  b. Aseptic technique
 3. Policies and practices in place to prevent exposure to or injury from radiation, laser equipment, and electrical and other equipment utilized
  a. Prevent skin injury
   i.   Electrical
   ii. Thermal
   iii. Chemical
   iv. Mechanical
 4. Individual health practices are encouraged
 5. Ongoing educational programs provided
 6. Storage of chemicals and dangerous materials considers safety of personnel
  a. Stored properly with adequate ventilation
  b. Labeled properly
  c. Spill kits, gloves, and eye protective gear available
  d. Material Safety Data Sheets (MSDS) readily available
  e. Policy and procedure for handling and care of hazardous materials
 7. Employees in high-risk areas are protected from anesthesia waste gases
 8. Policy in place regarding employee incidents, injury, or exposure to a biologic hazard
  a. Access to emergency care is readily available
  b. Incident or exposure reporting completed
  c. Investigation and follow-up include plan to prevent future incident or exposure
E. Safety management program
 1. Process to review, as frequently as necessary, but no less than every 2 years, all applicable service safety policies and procedures
 2. Promotion of an ongoing hazard surveillance program, including response to product safety recalls
 3. Reporting of all accidents involving patients, visitors, or staff, including evaluation, conclusion, recommendations, and action taken
 4. Use of safety-related information in the orientation of new employees and continuing education of all employees
 5. Annual evaluation of the effectiveness of the safety program
V. **Policies and Procedures**
A. Fire disaster
 1. Basic fire-prevention methods and codes per National Fire Protection Association
 2. A written plan for fire safety and evacuation adopted and posted
 3. Department heads/supervisors responsible for all employees under their supervision to be informed and trained in fire safety
 4. Information on types of fire extinguishers and appropriate use of each
 5. Techniques for patient evacuation demonstrated and practiced
 6. Telephones posted with fire alert number
 7. Fire drills/disaster drills are performed at least once per quarter
 8. Annual staff education updating fire safety by the department head/supervisor
B. Safety
 1. Establish standards for education and training, and establish credentials of caregivers
 2. Inspection and maintenance of equipment

      3. Body mechanics

      4. Hazard avoidance—chemical and biohazard; universal precaution; MSDS book

      5. Electrical safety/fire safety

      6. Annual review of safety policies/procedures by department head/supervisor

C. Infection control

      1. Hand washing to prevent spread of or acquiring nosocomial contaminates

         a. Hand washing necessary when gloves removed to prevent contamination if glove torn

         b. Hand washing between care of patients

         c. Hand washing and new gloves if contamination and to prevent cross contamination

         d. Universal precaution for patient and staff benefits handling all blood and body fluids

            i. Centers for Disease Control (CDC) guidelines

      2. Sterile technique (asepsis or aseptic) to maintain sterile field for surgery or treatments

         a. Surgical asepsis is the practice to provide area and objects as free of microbes as possible

         b. Medical asepsis is the practice that reduces and prevents transmission of microbes from one person or one area to another

      3. Patients requiring isolation will be cared for in a designated area in phases I and II postanesthesia areas (as detailed by institution's Infection Control Committee)

         a. Body substance isolation (precaution); protects against contact of:

            i. Blood, saliva, semen

            ii. Urine, feces, vaginal secretions, amniotic fluid

            iii. Wound drainage, cerebrospinal fluid, synovial fluid

         b. Protective barrier of:

            i. Gloves, mask

            ii. Goggles or safety glasses

            iii. Hair and shoe covers, waterproof gown

         c. Respiratory isolation for airborne disease (tuberculosis, childhood disease exposure)

            i. Measles, pertussis, chicken pox, colds

            ii. Recent cough, fever, congestion, croup

            iii. Staff highly susceptible or pregnant should not be exposed to these patients

         d. Patients with contact or acquired communicable disease should not be done in ambulatory setting, but if no diseases present but possible patient exposure

            i. Susceptible personnel should not care for these patients

            ii. Protective barrier for care workers immune to disease are not required

      4. If alternative care area utilized because of absence of an isolation room, postanesthetic care is delivered by a PACU nurse with isolation policy or special needs adhered to

      5. Terminal cleaning procedures

         a. Clean, sterilize, or disinfect equipment and supplies

         b. Environmental sanitation—careful disposal of sharps

      6. Handling and disposal of biohazardous waste and environmental sanitation

      7. Personal protective equipment readily available

      8. Annual review of infection-control policies and procedures

D. CPR

      1. Annual review of CPR by department head/supervisor

      2. Demonstration of competency of all staff in CPR every two years for renewal

E. Dress code
   1. Determined by proximity and frequency of access to ORs
      a. Unrestricted area—traffic not limited, street clothes may be worn
      b. Semi-restricted—processing and storage areas for instruments and supplies, corridors leading to the restricted areas of the surgical suite; staff to wear surgical attire, patients must wear gowns and hair coverings
      c. Restricted—operating rooms, clean core and scrub sink; surgical attire and masks required
F. Waste gas levels
   1. Monitor in Phase I per Occupational Safety Health Administration (OSHA)
G. Universal precautions
   1. In compliance with Centers for Disease Control (CDC), OSHA, Joint Commission for Accreditation of Healthcare Organizations (JCAHO), or American Association of Ambulatory Healthcare (AAAHC)
H. Unscheduled admissions/cancellations
   1. No patient should be scheduled for ambulatory surgery knowing that patient will require admission to an acute-care hospital setting
   2. Admissions due to unforeseen circumstances
      a. Uncontrolled pain management
      b. Prolonged nausea, vomiting
      c. Extensive surgery (incision or extended time for procedure beyond what was scheduled)
      d. Need for monitoring (rule out heart attack, stroke, or need for ventilator support)
      e. Unable to meet discharge criteria (VS, diabetes, hypertension, cardiac, respiratory status)
   3. Cancellations
      a. Patient not NPO per anesthesia requirements
      b. Uncontrolled diabetes, hypertension, cardiac condition, acute illness
      c. Lab work or pregnancy test in question
      d. Insurance/financial coverage, patient consent, or competency questionable
      e. Provision of required transportation and/or competent home-care support lacking

VI. Emergency Drugs and Equipment

   Resource 6—*Emergency Drugs and Equipment–ASPAN Standards of Perianesthesia Nursing Practice, 1998*

VII. Latex Allergy/Sensitivity
A. Identification of known patient sensitivity/allergy to latex when scheduled and prior to admission
   1. Identification of patient with possible latex allergy done preoperatively in physician's office
   2. Communication from office of patient latex allergy/sensitivity when surgery scheduled
   3. Patient scheduled as first case of day
   4. Nursing staff notified that patient scheduled with potential latex allergy
   5. Follow established surgical unit perioperative latex allergy policy and procedure guidelines
   6. Documentation and communication of latex allergy patient care needs to:
      a. Preadmission testing, radiology, laboratory, pharmacy
      b. Nursing unit

       c. Central distribution for latex free supplies

       d. Perioperative team members

   B. Preanesthesia care

     1. Obtain history including any latex allergy testing and results

     2. Identify patients not previously identified but high risk for being latex sensitive

       a. Rash, pruritis, edema, or burning after tape, Band-Aid, rubber gloves, blowing up a balloon, or latex condom use

       b. Skin eruption at exam site when gloves used in dental or obstetrical exams

       c. Patients with multiple drug and in particular food allergies

         i. Tropical fruits, kiwi, banana, tomatoes, potatoes, avocado, strawberries

       d. Multiple gastrointestinal or genitourinary procedures (i.e., spina bifida)

       e. Patients with occupational exposure to latex (i.e., health-care or food workers)

     3. Document and communicate patient information

     4. Follow unit policy and procedure

       a. Patient to be done as first case of the day

       b. Provide latex-free environment preop by separating by distance or separate room for preop preparation

       c. Provide latex-free areas in OR, PACU, and discharge units

       d. Allergy noted on bracelet, chart inside and out, and signs posted on doors or bed

     5. Have latex-free supply cart with all needed supplies, i.e., latex-free IV set with stopcocks

     6. Have crash cart available with drugs and supplies needed in case of anaphylaxis

     7. Support family and patient, and reassure that staff aware of latex allergy and needs

   C. Intraoperative care

     1. Communication and documentation to OR staff of latex allergy

     2. Latex-free surgery supplies and preparation of surgery suite

       a. Area should be isolated such as last suite at end of corridor

       b. Outside traffic and closed room maintained while patient in area

       c. Open packs and supplies in hall or sterile sub room adjoining suite

       d. OR table should be covered, and all monitoring equipment latex free or covered

     3. Notify anesthesiologist that latex-free anesthesia supplies needed in suite

     4. Have latex-free supplies and emergency drugs and equipment readily available

   D. Postanesthesia care

     1. Utilize latex-free care products and provide care in separate or distant location

     2. Follow policy and procedure guidelines to provide latex-free environment

     3. Give support to patient throughout; provide patient/family education

     4. Provide home care information and list of latex-containing and latex-free products

     5. Remind to carry wallet information and/or Medic-Alert band

     6. May need to carry epinephrine auto injectable or diphenhydramine

     7. Notify family care physician and may report to manufacturer on product reaction, or government agency if reaction to a medical device

     8. Careful documentation, communication, and following policies and procedure are mandatory

VIII. Orientation/Ongoing Training Programs

   A. Preparation of the orientee for the expected scope of practice in perianesthesia care

   B. Formulation of the skills and the knowledge required to function effectively

   C. General safety management issues, departmental safety plans, special hazards related to assigned duties, safety practices specific to the ages of the patients served

   D. *ASPAN Competency Based Orientation and Credentialing Program (1997 edition)*

IX. Hazard Identification
A. Policies for handling dangerous materials are available and communicated to all employees
B. Unit specific material safety data sheets (MSDS) for all toxic materials stored in the building or department and are easily accessible to all employees

X. Transportation
A. Perianesthesia nurse assures the availability of safe transport of patient on discharge
B. Perianesthesia nurse determines the mode, number, and competency level of accompanying personnel required based on patient needs
C. Policy in place for transport of a patient from a freestanding facility to a full-service acute-care hospital to be utilized in emergency situations

Bibliography

1. Allen, A., Culbertson, M. (1990). Environmental safety: An essential element of quality care. *J Post Anesth Nurs*, 5(4):291–294.
2. American Society of PeriAnesthesia Nurses. (1997). *ASPAN Competency Based Orientation and Credentialing Program*. Thorofare, NJ: ASPAN.
3. American Society of PeriAnesthesia Nurses. (1998). *ASPAN Standards of Nursing Practice*. Thorofare, NJ: ASPAN.
4. Burden, N. (1993). *Ambulatory Surgical Nursing*. Philadelphia: Saunders.
5. Burden, N. (1992). Telephone follow-up of ambulatory surgical patients following discharge is a nursing responsibility. *J Post Anesth Nurs*, 7(4):256–261.
6. Dechart, C. (1989). The joy of building a freestanding ambulatory surgical center. *J Post Anesth Nurs*. 4(2):106–108.
7. Drain, C.B. (1994). *The Post Anesthesia Care Unit*, 3rd ed. Philadelphia: Saunders.
8. Frost, E.A.M. (1990). *Post Anesthesia Care Unit*, 2nd ed. St . Louis: Mosby.
9. Howard, G. (1995). *Administrative Manual for Ambulatory Care Facilities*. Lakewood, CO: Medical Consultants Network.
10. Joint Commission for Accreditation of Healthcare Organizations. (1994). *Accreditation Manual for Ambulatory Health Care*, Vol. 2. Oakbrook Terrace, IL: JCAHO.
11. Litwack, K. (1995). *Core Curriculum for Post Anesthesia Nursing Practice*, 3rd ed. Philadelphia: Saunders.
12. Luckmann, J. (1991). *Saunders Manual of Nursing Care*. Philadelphia: Saunders.
13. Marshall Erdman and Assoc. Inc. (1994). *Organizing, Designing, and Building Medical Office/Ambulatory Healthcare Facilities*. Madison, WI.
14. Meeker, M.H., Rothrock, J.C. (1995). *Alexander's Care of the Patient in Surgery*, 10th ed. St. Louis: Mosby.
15. Michel, L.L., Myrick, C. (1990). Current and future trends in ambulatory surgery and their impact on nursing practice. *J Post Anes Nurs*, 3(3):347–349.
16. Redmond, M. (1993). Infection control monitoring in the ambulatory surgical unit. *J Post Anes Nurs*, 8(1):28–34.
17. (1996). Latex allergy: Recognition and perioperative management. *JOPAN*, 11(1)/February: 6–12.
18. Trihealth, Inc. (1997). *Corporate Policy, Latex Sensitivity and Allergy Precautions*. Cincinnati: Trihealth.
19. Wood, P. (1994). Essential reading for ambulatory surgical nurses. *J Post Anes Nurs*, 9(1):26–27.

REVIEW QUESTIONS

1. Criteria for admission to a Recovery Center includes

   A. Anticipated length of stay greater than 72 hours
   B. Necessity for acute care
   C. Adequate pain management achieved within 72 hours
   D. Patient unable to provide basic self care needs

2. An important consideration in the design of the preoperative admitting area is to provide

   A. Total patient privacy
   B. Constant patient visualization
   C. Minimal stimulation
   D. Socialization with other patients

3. An alternative location is utilized for providing postanesthesia care to a patient requiring isolation. The care will be provided by the

   A. OR nurse
   B. Med-surg nurse
   C. Nurse Manager
   D. PACU nurse

4. A disadvantage of a hospital-integrated ambulatory surgery setting is

   A. Decreased scheduling control and delays
   B. Cost
   C. Unavailability of staff
   D. Management obstacles

5. Patient goals in the Phase II PACU include all but which of the following:

   A. Provide acute care until discharge
   B. Encourage self-care
   C. Encourage ambulation
   D. Assist return to preoperative state

6. Safety considerations are dependent on

   A. Physical conditions of facility
   B. Policies and procedures
   C. Staff attitude
   D. All of the above

7. Employee expectations of a safe environment include

   A. Provision of personal security
   B. Policies and practices in place to prevent spread of disease
   C. Provision of ongoing educational programs
   D. All of the above

8. Foods that cause reaction or sensitivity by patients who may be at risk for latex allergy include

   A. Cheese, milk, dairy products
   B. Tropical fruits, bananas, strawberries
   C. Walnuts, peanuts, pecans
   D. Shellfish and seafood

9. Handwashing should be done

   A. After gloves are removed to prevent contamination if glove is torn
   B. Between patient care
   C. To prevent spread of or acquiring nosocomial contaminates
   D. After handling blood and body fluids
   E. All of the above

10. Policies and procedures for Fire/ Disaster include all of the following except

   A. Basic fire-prevention methods and codes per the National Fire Protection Association
   B. Policies and procedures to prevent injury from radiation exposure
   C. Information on types of fire extinguishers and appropriate use of each
   D. Techniques for patient evacuation

ANSWERS TO QUESTIONS

1. C
2. B
3. D
4. A
5. A

6. D
7. D
8. B
9. E
10. B

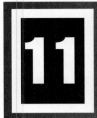

Cardiopulmonary Care and Emergency Support

Melody Heffline
Southern Surgical Group, LLC
West Columbia, South Carolina

I. **Cardiovascular and Pulmonary Assessment**
   A. Cardiovascular
      1. Management goals
         a. Cardiac output increases 25–50% to meet increased tissue oxygen demands without myocardial oxygen debt—debt reflected in chest pain, ECG changes, cardiac failure
         b. Promote myocardial oxygen delivery to exceed myocardial oxygen demand
      2. Assessment parameters
         a. Blood pressure
            i. Maintain adequate diastolic pressure
            ii. Cuff size ⅓–½ circumference of extremity
            iii. Too narrow—false high; too wide—false low
            iv. Evaluates—heart as a pump, blood volume, systemic vascular resistance
         b. Heart rate
            i. Establish baseline for patient
            ii. Rate 60–100 beats/minute
            iii. Rhythm regular, S1 and S2 sounds
            iv. Assess for rubs, murmurs
            v. Identify cardiac medications—especially beta blockers (decrease HR, increase contractility); know cardioselective (affects B_1 receptors) vs. noncardioselective (affects B_1 and B_2 receptors) (See Table 11–1)
         c. Urine output
            i. 30 cc/hr.—ideal adult output

1. Describe the components of a detailed cardiopulmonary assessment, including normal and abnormal findings.
2. Identify possible cardiopulmonary complications occurring in the postanesthetic period in the ambulatory surgery patient.
3. Identify assessment findings and treatments for various cardiopulmonary complications.
4. Describe the use of supportive cardiopulmonary therapy for the postanesthesia patient in ambulatory surgery.

      ii.   Usually don't have Foley catheter for constant assessment—assess over time

      iii. Balance intake and output

   d. Color and temperature of extremities

      i.   Establish baseline for patient

      ii.   Warm, pink extremities indicate adequate circulation

      iii. Cool, pale extremities indicative of lack of blood flow; assess for cause (volume vs. thrombus)

      iv. Cyanosis is a late sign of decompensation

   e. Skin turgor

      i.   Establish baseline for patient

      ii.   Skin should return to normal position when pinched

      iii. Poor turgor indicative of fluid imbalance

      iv. Skin loses elasticity with aging

   f. Mental status

      i.   Establish baseline for patient

      ii.   Alert, oriented, or return to baseline indicative of adequate cardiac output to brain

      iii. Most sensitive indicator of brain function is level of consciousness; may indicate lack of perfusion if altered

3. Complications

   a. Hypotension

      i.   Definition: systolic blood pressure >20% below baseline

      ii.   Assessment findings

         (a) Low blood pressure

         (b) Decreased urine output (oliguria to anuria)

         (c) Tachycardia, tachypnea

         (d) Pale, cool, clammy extremities

         (e) Disorientation to unconsciousness

         (f) Nausea

         (g) Chest pain

      iii. Potential causes

         (a) Decreased intravascular volume

         (b) Left ventricular failure

         (c) Decreased vascular tone

         (d) Exhaustion of catecholamines (e.g., prolonged pain)

      iv. Treatment

         (a) Oxygen therapy

         (b) Assess and replace intravascular volume

         (c) For ventricular failure—coronary vasodilators, decrease afterload, inotropic support

         (d) Maximize vascular tone—discontinue vasodilators, administer vasoconstrictive agents

         (e) Pain management

Table 11–1 • CARDIOSELECTIVE BETA BLOCKERS

Atenolol (Tenormin)
Betaxolol (Kerlone)
Bisoprolol (Zebeta)
Metoprolol (Lopressor)
Metoprolol (Toprol XL)

       v.   Prevention through monitoring of preoperative, intraoperative, and postoperative volume status and titration of vasoactive/cardiac medications

b. Hypertension

    i.   Definition: >20–30% above baseline blood pressure

    ii.   Assessment findings

        (a) Elevated blood pressure

        (b) Signs of sympathetic stimulation

        (c) Headache with extreme elevations

        (d) Decreased level of consciousness (LOC) with disruption of cerebral autoregulation and cerebral hemorrhage

        (e) Signs of ventricular failure and pulmonary edema with longstanding elevations (>190/100 for 3 hours or more)

    iii.   Potential causes

        (a) Pre-existing disease

        (b) Central nervous system damage

        (c) Cardiovascular impairment

        (d) Excess catecholamine production (e.g., pain, emotional stress)

        (e) Hypoxemia/hypercarbia

        (f) Endocrinopathies

        (g) Hypothermia

        (h) Excess intravascular volume

        (i) Sudden withdrawal or overdose of medications

        (j) Visceral distention

        (k) Pre-eclampsia

    iv.   Treatment

        (a) Alleviate cause

           (i)   Restart antihypertensives

           (ii)   Maximize cardiac function

           (iii)   Pain/stress management

           (iv)   Maximize respiratory function

           (v)   Rewarming

           (vi)   Correct fluid overload (fluid restriction and diuretics)

           (vii) Decrease visceral distention (Foley catheter, nasogastric tube)

    v.   Prevention

        (a) Assess for potential causes early

        (b) Patients to take antihypertensives on day of surgery

c. Cardiac dysrhythmias (See Advanced Cardiac Life Support overview starting on page 181.)

d. Hemorrhage

    i.   Definition: loss of intravascular volume

    ii.   Assessment findings

        (a) Visible blood on dressings, in drains, emesis

        (b) Restlessness

        (c) Swelling at surgical site

        (d) Hypotension and signs of hypovolemia

        (e) ENT—frequent swallowing, hemoptysis, vomiting blood

        (f) Abdominal—increased girth, abdominal pain and hardness

    iii.   Potential causes

        (a) Loss of vascular integrity

        (b) Coagulation disorders

    iv.   Treatment

        (a) Stop active bleeding

          (b) Support circulation—transfusion usually not indicated unless hemoglobin <7 or hematocrit <21, unless autologous blood available or patient is symptomatic

          (c) Patient comfort measures—decrease anxiety, keep warm, pain management

      v.   Prevention

          (a) Assess for bleeding disorders preop

          (b) Assess for medications that interfere with coagulation and discontinue prior to surgery

          (c) Monitor closely postoperatively

   e. Peripheral circulatory compromise

      i.   Definition: decreased/absent blood flow to an extremity

      ii. Assessment findings

          (a) Color changes of extremity (pale, flushed to blue)

          (b) Swelling if obstructed venous return

          (c) Diminished/absent pulses

          (d) Delayed/absent capillary refill

          (e) Pain, paresthesia

     iii. Potential causes

          (a) Bandage, splint, cast too tight

          (b) Occurrence of thrombus/embolus

      iv. Treatment

          (a) Relieve restriction to blood flow by loosening constricting bandages

          (b) Possible return to surgery for thrombectomy/embolectomy

      v.   Prevention

          (a) Use caution when applying bandages

          (b) Frequent evaluation of extremities

B. Pulmonary

  1. Management goal—provide adequate gas exchange necessary to maintain normal tissue metabolism

  2. Assessment parameters

   a. Skin color

      i.   Establish baseline for patient

      ii. Indicative of gas exchange

     iii. Cyanosis indicative of inadequate oxygenation

      iv. Absence of cyanosis not indicative of adequate oxygen delivery (See other assessment parameters)

   b. Pattern of breathing

      i.   Assess adequacy of ventilation

      ii. Adult rate 12–30, tidal volume of 5–7 ml/kg

     iii. Examine rate, rhythm, and patency of airway

          (a) Rapid with shallow volume and jerky movements

             (i)   Residual neuromuscular blockade

             (ii) Decreased pulmonary compliance (pulmonary edema, atelectasis, pneumonia, pneumothorax, splinting from pain)

          (b) Slow, deep

             (i)   Narcotics

             (ii) Central nervous system conditions (e.g., stroke)

          (c) Stridor

             (i)   Upper airway obstruction

             (ii) Hypocalcemia

             (iii) Hydrocephalus

(d) Kussmaul—rapid and deep
  (i)   Severe acidosis (e.g., diabetic ketoacidosis)
  (ii) Lactic acidosis
  (iii) Malignant hyperthermia
(e) Prolonged expiratory phase—obstructive airway disease
c. Auscultation of breath sounds
  i.   Normal—vesicular, bronchial, bronchovesicular
  ii. Abnormal—wheezes, rales (crackles), rhonchi (gurgles)
d. Pulse oximetry
  i.   Requires pulsating vascular bed
  ii. SpO_2 >90% = paO_2 >60 mm Hg (with normal oxyhemoglobin curve)
  iii. SpO_2 <90% indicative of hypoxemia, proceed to arterial blood gas if need to validate full oxygenation status
  iv.   Assess for anemia: affects oxygen delivery which may lead to ischemia; hemoglobin >9–10 usually sufficient
e. End-tidal CO_2 (assess prior to extubation if available)
  i.   Normal 35–45 mm Hg
  ii. Elevations indicative of obstruction of pulmonary blood flow
f. Lung volumes (assess prior to extubation)
  i.   Tidal volume (vT): 5–7 ml/kg
  ii.   Vital capacity (VC): 10–15 ml/kg
  iii. Increased with obstructive diseases (COPD, emphysema, bronchitis)
  iv.   Decreased with restrictive conditions (kyphoscoliosis, effusion, pneumothorax, atelectasis, fibrosis, pulmonary edema)
3. Complications
  a. Hypoventilation
    i.   Definition: inadequate ventilation to maintain oxygenation
    ii. Assessment findings
      (a) Rate <10–12
      (b) SpO_2 <90% and/or retention of CO_2
      (c) Shallow respirations (vT <5–7 cc/kg if intubated)
    iii. Potential causes
      (a) Poor respiratory drive (e.g., residual anesthetics, loss of stimulation, somnolence)
      (b) Poor muscle function (e.g., abdominal surgery, obesity, neuromuscular disorders, residual anesthetics)
      (c) High production of carbon dioxide
      (d) Acute or chronic lung disease
    iv. Treatment
      (a) Treat cause
      (b) Stimulation to arouse
      (c) Reverse residual anesthetics
      (d) Intubation and mechanical ventilation
  b. Hypoxemia/hypercapnia
    i.   Definition: low oxygen content in arterial blood, elevated pCO_2 in arterial blood
    ii. Assessment findings
      (a) SpO_2 <90%
      (b) pCO_2 >45 mm Hg (blood gas); patient with COPD may have elevated PCO_2 at baseline
      (c) Shallow respirations, decreased breath sounds
      (d) Agitation to somnolence

        (e) Hypotension to hypertension

        (f) Bradycardia to tachycardia and/or ventricular ectopy

  iii. Potential causes

        (a) Low inspired concentration of oxygen

        (b) Hypoventilation

        (c) Dead space ventilation (pulmonary embolus)

        (d) Intrapulmonary shunt (pulmonary edema, atelectasis—most common)

  iv. Treatment

        (a) Oxygen therapy

        (b) Stimulation to arouse and/or reversal of residual anesthetic if hypoventilation

        (c) Increased mobility

        (d) Incentive spirometry

        (e) Correction of pulmonary edema

c. Airway obstruction

  i. Definition: blockage of air flow into the lungs

  ii. Assessment findings

        (a) Partial—snoring, stridor, decreased vT, retraction of chest, use of accessory muscles, abdominal breathing movements, decreased SpO_2, cyanosis (late sign)

        (b) Complete—inspiratory effort silent, exaggerated; cyanosis leading to respiratory/cardiac arrest if not corrected

  iii. Potential causes

        (a) Relaxation of soft tissues due to anesthetics, neuromuscular disease (tongue most common)

        (b) Excessive secretions

        (c) Improperly placed artificial airway

        (d) Anatomy—obesity, large/short neck, no jaw

        (e) Swelling—surgical procedure, anaphylaxis, edema

  iv. Treatment

        (a) Stimulation

        (b) Reposition airway (jaw thrust/chin lift)

        (c) Correct placement of artificial airway

        (d) Suctioning of secretions

        (e) Possible reintubation and mechanical ventilation

        (f) Reversal of anesthetics

  v. Prevention

        (a) Proper positioning—lateral, head down if patient not awake

        (b) Constant assessment until able to maintain own airway

        (c) Careful administration of narcotics

d. Pneumothorax

  i. Definition: penetration of pleural cavity creating loss of negative intrapleural pressure or air in pleural space

  ii. Assessment findings (depend on degree of pneumothorax)

        (a) Tracheal deviation toward unaffected (contralateral) side

        (b) Asymmetrical chest excursion

        (c) Diminished/absent breath sounds on affected side

        (d) Hyperresonance on percussion of affected side

        (e) Cyanosis

        (f) Dyspnea

        (g) Severe apprehension

        (h) Chest pain

    iii. Potential causes
- (a) Central line placement
- (b) Positive-pressure ventilation
- (c) Intercostal/paravertebral block
- (d) Emphysema bleb rupture
- (e) Surgical chest procedures

    iv. Treatment
- (a) Small (<20%)—oxygen, bed rest, observation
- (b) Larger/patient symptomatic—chest tube placement

e. Laryngospasm
    i. Definition: obstruction secondary to tonic contraction of laryngeal and pharyngeal muscles
    ii. Assessment findings
- (a) Complete—absent breath sounds
- (b) Incomplete—stridor
- (c) Agitation
- (d) Decreased SpO_2

    iii. Potential causes
- (a) Blood/vomitus/mucous on vocal cords
- (b) Nasal/oral airway
- (c) Mechanical irritation after intubation, laryngoscopy, or suctioning
- (d) Irritation due to inhalation agents
- (e) Coughing
- (f) History of smoking

    iv. Treatment
- (a) Incomplete—oxygen therapy; slow, deep breath and cough; calming measures
- (b) Complete/progression of incomplete—positive pressure ventilation with 100% oxygen; small doses of succinylcholine (may be necessary to assist with ventilation and/or reintubate after administration)
- (c) Decrease airway irritation and/or swelling with intravenous administration of steroids and/or lidocaine
- (d) Reassurance of patient and family

    v. Prevention
- (a) Extubate when deeply anesthetized or awake
- (b) Suction prior to extubation; gentle suction if needed after extubation
- (c) Remove artificial airways promptly upon return of reflexes
- (d) Intravenous administration of lidocaine/steroids prior to extubation

f. Bronchospasm
    i. Definition: reflex bronchiolar constriction resulting in airway closure
    ii. Assessment findings
- (a) Wheezing
- (b) Tachypnea, dyspnea
- (c) Decreased lung compliance
- (d) Decreased SpO_2
- (e) Use of accessory muscles
- (f) Restlessness
- (g) Tightness in chest

    iii. Potential causes
- (a) Pre-existing bronchospastic disease
- (b) Airway irritation (e.g., secretions, aspiration, intubation, suctioning)
- (c) Histamine release

        (d) Allergic reaction

        (e) Pulmonary edema

        (f) Environmental factors (e.g., odors, perfumes)

        (g) History of smoking

    iv. Treatment

        (a) Decrease irritation of airway

        (b) Administer bronchodilators—may use inhaled or parenteral; beta-agonists primary treatment

        (c) Humidified oxygen

    v. Prevention

        (a) Identify predisposed preoperatively

        (b) Consider pretreatment of patient

        (c) No smoking 24 hours prior to surgery

        (d) Reduce anxiety and stress

g. Pulmonary edema

    i. Definition: accumulation of fluid in the alveoli

        (a) Cardiogenic—usually occurs as a result of underlying cardiac disease or fluid overload

        (b) Negative-pressure (NP)—follows airway obstruction and attempts to breathe against closed glottis

    ii. Assessment findings

        (a) Dyspnea, orthopnea

        (b) Cough with white to pink, frothy sputum

        (c) Restlessness and anxiety

        (d) Wheezes and rales

        (e) Tachycardia with weak thready pulse

        (f) Decreased compliance

        (g) Hypoxemia

        (h) Infiltrates on chest X-ray

    iii. Potential causes

        (a) Underlying cardiopulmonary disease

        (b) Intravenous fluid overload

        (c) Aspiration

        (d) Administration of narcotic antagonist (NP and cardiogenic)

        (e) Allergic reactions/anaphylaxis

        (f) Sepsis

        (g) Dissiminated intravascular coagulation (DIC)

        (h) Airway obstruction (NP)

    iv. Treatment

        (a) Oxygen therapy

        (b) Remove/treat cause

        (c) Elevate head of bed

        (d) Measures to decrease venous return—legs dependent, administer diuretics, fluid restriction, vasodilating agents

        (e) Consider afterload reduction

        (f) Monitor for hypotension with diuretic therapy

        (g) Cardiogenic patient may need digoxin to improve contractility

    v. Prevention

        (a) Identify predisposed preoperatively

        (b) Careful fluid administration

h. Aspiration

    i. Definition: entry of foreign body, blood, or gastric contents into the tracheobronchial tree

    ii.   Assessment findings (depend on type/degree of aspiration)
       (a) Foreign body—cough, atelectasis, obstruction
       (b) Blood—minor to complete airway obstruction, hypoxemia, hypercarbia
       (c) Gastric contents—bronchospasm, hypoxemia, atelectasis, pulmonary edema, hypotension
    iii. Potential causes
       (a) Obesity
       (b) Hiatal hernia
       (c) Pregnancy
       (d) Peptic ulcer
       (e) Loose teeth
       (f) Diminished pharyngeal reflexes
       (g) Full stomach
       (h) Insufflation of abdomen during laparoscopy
       (i) Trendelenburg position
    iv. Treatment
       (a) Depends on severity/cause
       (b) Remove foreign body
       (c) Suctioning for blood, gastric contents
       (d) Correct hypoxemia
       (e) Intubation and ventilation if severe
       (f) Antibiotic therapy and theophylline if severe
       (g) Steroids may be considered
    v.   Prevention
       (a) Maintenance of NPO status
       (b) Constant monitoring of unconscious or heavily sedated patient
       (c) Position patient side-lying, head down
       (d) Prompt removal of artificial airways to prevent gagging
       (e) If topical anesthesia, demonstrate return of protective reflexes prior to taking oral fluids
       (f) Medications may be used to decrease secretions (anticholinergics), neutralize gastric secretions (nonparticulate antacids), decrease acidity and volume of gastric contents (histamine H_2-receptor antagonist), foster gastric emptying (metaclopramide), reduce incidence of nausea and vomiting (antiemetics)

II. Supportive Cardiopulmonary Therapy
A. Oxygen administration and airway adjuncts
  1. Airway control
    a. Most common obstruction from the tongue
    b. Head-tilt/chin-lift maneuver opens airway
    c. If neck injury, use jaw thrust without head tilt
    d. Place fingers under anterior mandible to lift; never place hands behind neck—use caution at ramus of jaw due to potential to damage facial nerve (Figure 11–1)
  2. Adjuncts
    a. Oropharyngeal airways
      i.   Semicircular hard plastic device
      ii. Holds tongue away from posterior pharynx
      iii. Prevents biting endotracheal tube
      iv. Insert backward and rotate into position (Figure 11–2)
      v.   Must still maintain proper head position
      vi. Measure teeth to ramus of jaw for proper fit

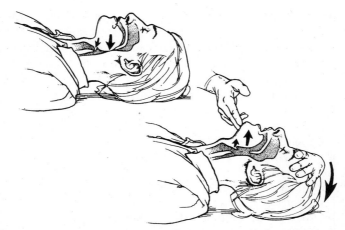

Figure 11–1. Opening the airway. Top: Airway obstruction produced by tongue and epiglottis. Bottom: Relief by head tilt–chin lift. (From *Textbook of Advanced Cardiac Life Support*, 1994. Copyright American Heart Association. Reproduced with permission.)

        vii. May stimulate nausea and vomiting or precipitate laryngospasm in the conscious/semiconscious patient

        viii. May cause worsening of obstruction if not properly placed or if too large

        ix. Assess for proper placement—bilateral breath sounds

    b. Nasopharyngeal airways

        i.   Soft plastic or rubber device

        ii. Used when oropharyngeal airway cannot be used

        iii. More tolerated by semi-conscious, but may still cause stimulation of gag reflex producing laryngospasm

        iv. Measure nares to ramus of jaw for proper fit (Figure 11–3)

        v.   Larger internal diameter, longer tube

        vi. Insert with water-soluble lubricant or anesthetic jelly close to midline on floor of nostril—rotate slightly if resistance is met

        vii. Tube too long may enter the esophagus

        viii. May cause bleeding of nasal mucosa

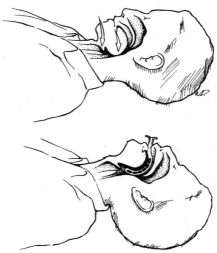

Figure 11–2. Placement of correctly inserted oropharyngeal airway. Top: Before insertion, incorrect head position. Bottom: After insertion, showing head tilted and oropharyngeal airway in place. (From *Textbook of Advanced Cardiac Life Support*, 1994. Copyright American Heart Association. Reproduced with permission.)

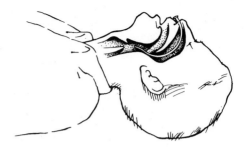

Figure 11–3. Nasopharyngeal airway in place. Note head tilted back for proper insertion. (From *Textbook of Advanced Cardiac Life Support, 1994.* Copyright American Heart Association. Reproduced with permission.)

    ix. Must still maintain proper head position
    x. Assess for proper placement—bilateral breath sounds
  c. Endotracheal intubation
    i. Isolates the airway, maintains patency, reduces risk of aspiration, allows suctioning, allows for delivery of high oxygen concentrations, provides route for drug administration, enables delivery of high tidal volumes
    ii. Maximum interruption of ventilation 30 seconds
    iii. In adults, may provide cricoid pressure to facilitate intubation and prevent vomiting—apply with thumb and index finger at anterolateral aspect of cricoid cartilage
    iv. Indications: cardiac arrest, inability of conscious patient to ventilate adequately, inability of patient to protect airway, inability to ventilate patient by conventional means
    v. Once in place no longer necessary to synchronize ventilation with chest compressions—perform asynchronously at 12 to 15 ventilations per minute with tidal volume of 12–15 ml/kg
    vi. Equipment needed: laryngoscope, proper size endotracheal tube, stylet, 10 cc syringe, water-soluble lubricant, suction equipment, tape
    vii. Proper placement: usually at 20–22 cm mark at front teeth in adult, bilateral breath sounds and symmetrical chest expansion, 2–3 cm above carina by chest x-ray
    viii. Placement in right mainstem: no breath sounds left lung—reposition tube
    ix. Other complications: lips or tongue compressed between blade and teeth, teeth chipped, pharyngeal trauma, vomiting, aspiration, esophageal intubation
 3. Oxygen administration
  a. Components of oxygen delivery system
    i. Oxygen supply
    ii. Flowmeter or valve handles for cylinder
    iii. Tubing connecting supply to administration device
    iv. Humidifier
  b. Nasal cannula
    i. Low-flow system—inspired concentration depends on flow of oxygen and tidal volume of patient
    ii. Each liter of flow increase provides O_2 concentration increase of approximately 4% up to six liters per minute
    iii. Used for minimal or no respiratory distress or inability to tolerate mask
  c. Face mask
    i. Usually well-tolerated
    ii. Need oxygen flow greater than five l/min—recommended eight to ten l/min
    iii. System provides 40–60% oxygen concentrations

    d. Face mask with oxygen reservoir
       i. Requires flow of six l/min to provide 60%; ten l/min will provide almost 100%
       ii. Provides constant flow of oxygen into attached reservoir
       iii. Used for patients requiring high concentrations of oxygen who are spontaneously breathing
    e. Venturi mask
       i. Provides high gas flow with fixed oxygen concentration
       ii. Used with patients who require oxygen in lower concentrations, e.g., COPD
       iii. Provides concentrations of 24%, 28%, 35%, 40%

B. Mechanical ventilation for emergency use
  1. Mechanical means to provide ventilatory support to maintain adequate alveolar ventilation
  2. Indication for use
    a. Acute ventilatory failure
    b. Used with caution in COPD patient to avoid complications related to chronic ventilatory insufficiency
    c. Hypoxemia—paO_2 less than 50 mm Hg
    d. Cardiac arrest
  3. Types of ventilators
    a. Negative pressure—uses negatively applied pressure to the thorax (e.g., iron lung)
    b. Positive pressure—gases driven into lungs
       i. Pressure-cycled—delivers preset pressure of gas to lungs (e.g., Bennett PR-2 and Bird-Mark-7)
       ii. Volume-cycled—deliver preset volume of gas to lungs; will deliver volume of gas regardless of pressure required; preset pressure limits provide safety (e.g., MA-1, MA-2, Bear-2)
       iii. Time-cycled—length of time allowed for inspiration is controlled and volume and pressure vary (e.g., Babybird, Sechrist IV, Engstrom, Servo 900)
  4. Commonly monitored ventilator settings
    a. Tidal volume (vT)
       i. Air in and out of lungs one breath
       ii. Normal 5–7 cc/kg, ventilator set at higher levels of 10–15 cc/kg to decrease risk of atelectasis and stimulate production of surfactant
       iii. Too low results in hypoventilation
       iv. Too high may place patient at risk for pneumothorax and cardiovascular system depression
    b. Fraction of inspired oxygen (FiO_2)
       i. Expressed as decimal—$1.0 = 100\%$
       ii. In emergency situations set at 50–100%
       iii. Increase or decrease based on PaO_2
       iv. Prolonged use of greater than 60% may result in oxygen toxicity
       v. Set at lowest levels possible for COPD patient to avoid obliteration of hypoxic drive
    c. Ventilation mode
       i. Assist/control (A/C)
          (a) Assist mode—ventilator sensitive to patient inspiratory effort; patient breath triggers ventilator to give mechanical breath
          (b) Control mode—ventilator delivers the breath at preset rate based on time; very uncommon

        (c) Assist/control mode—assist sensitive to patient allowing some control, but control functions as backup in event patient does not trigger ventilator; every breath is ventilator breath; may be used initially because takes over work of breathing; not a long-term mode of ventilation

    ii.   Intermittent mandatory ventilation (IMV)

        (a) Patient breathes spontaneously through ventilator circuit

        (b) Ventilator provides breath at preset rate

        (c) Patient breathes between ventilator breaths at own rate

        (d) Synchronous IMV synchronizes ventilator to follow patient expiration; more comfortable to patient

        (e) Decreases risk of hyperventilation and provides better ventilation—perfusion distribution, facilitates weaning process

d. Rate (f)

    i.   Critical to establish adequate minute ventilation

    ii.   Minute ventilation (VE)—amount of air moving in and out of lungs in one minute $VE = vT \times f$

    iii.   Too low results in hypoventilation and respiratory acidosis

    iv.   Too high results in hyperventilation and respiratory alkalosis

e. Positive end-expiratory pressure (PEEP)

    i.   Provides alveoli with constant amount of positive pressure at the end of each expiration

    ii.   Can be used with A/C or IMV

    iii.   Opens previously collapsed alveoli, prevents atelectasis, improves gas exchange

    iv.   Monitored by airway pressure manometer—should fall back to 0 if no PEEP

    v.   Complications increase as PEEP increases—barotrauma and decreased cardiac output due to decreased venous return to right side of heart

f. Continuous positive airway pressure (CPAP)

    i.   Uses same principle as PEEP but does not require ventilator

    ii.   Continuous flow of positive pressure so airway pressure never drops to zero

    iii.   Allows patient to breathe spontaneously through ventilator circuit

    iv.   Can be delivered by mask or T-piece

g. Pressure support (PS)

    i.   Provides positive pressure to alveoli but supports inspiratory phase, augmenting tidal volume

    ii.   Purpose is to decrease work of breathing through supporting inspiratory efforts

    iii.   Primarily used as tool for weaning

h. Peak airway/inspiratory pressure (PAP, PIP)

    i.   Pressure required to deliver volume varies depending primarily on airway resistance and lung compliance; amount of pressure required is PIP

    ii.   PIP <40 cm H_2O desirable

    iii.   High PIP increases risk of barotrauma

    iv.   Increasing indicative of increased airway resistance or decreased lung compliance

    v.   Decreasing indicative of improvement in airway resistance or lung compliance

i. Alarms

    i.   Low exhaled volume—loss of tidal volume or leak in system; disconnect, leak in cuff

      ii.   High pressure—increased airway resistance; coughing, biting tube, mucous plug/secretions, water in tubing

  5. Effects on body systems

    a. Cardiovascular effects

      i.   Relative increase in intrathoracic pressure causes increase in central venous pressure; reduces blood return to right heart

      ii.   Decreases preload and stroke volume reducing cardiac output; also causes squeezing of heart by lungs during inspiratory phase

      iii. Manifests as reduction in blood pressure, especially if patient is hypovolemic

    b. Pulmonary effects

      i.   Alters relationship of ventilation to perfusion in lungs

      ii.   Causes gases to flow through the path of least resistance; increased ventilation to healthy lung with decreased ventilation to diseased lung

      iii. Pushes blood to peripheral lung and dependent areas; perfusion greatest in periphery and ventilation greatest in larger airways

    c. Neurovascular effects

      i.   Increases intracranial pressure (ICP) initially; with settings designed to decrease pCO_2 will decrease ICP

      ii.   Decreases cerebral perfusion pressure (CPP)

      iii. CPP = Mean Arterial Blood Pressure − ICP

      iv. Assess for decrease in cardiac output sufficient to decrease blood pressure

    d. Renal effects—decreases urinary output through decreased cardiac output and redistribution of renal blood flow

    e. Gastrointestinal effects—decreases blood flow into intestinal viscera causing visceral ischemia

C. Basic life-support overview

  1. Recognize need for immediate action

  2. Perform steps promptly and effectively

    a. Airway—determine unresponsiveness

      i.   Shake victim, call out

      ii.   Get help if no response (Code, 911)

      iii. Place in position to provide effective resuscitation measures—supine, firm flat surface

      iv. Open airway—head-tilt/chin-lift or jaw thrust

    b. Breathing—determine breathlessness

      i.   Look for chest to rise and fall

      ii.   Listen for air leaving lungs

      iii. Feel for air flowing out of lungs

      iv. Create airtight seal for effective breathing

      v.   Provide appropriate airway opening for ventilation

      vi. Administer two initial breaths

    c. Circulation—determine pulselessness

      i.   Assess carotid pulse (adult/child), brachial (infant)—at least 5 to 10 seconds

      ii.   If present, perform rescue breathing

        (a) One breath every 3 seconds infant/child

        (b) One breath every 5 seconds adult

      iii. If pulseless, begin compressions

        (a) 5 compressions:1 breath infant/child

        (b) 15 compressions:2 breaths adult one rescuer

        (c) 5 compressions:1 breath adult/child two rescuers

        (d) Rate: 80–100 adult/child, at least 100 infant

    d. Complications

        i. Gastric distention due to excess ventilation volume—maintain open airway and limit ventilation to point that chest rises, use slow inflation time during ventilation

        ii. Rib/sternal fractures, pneumothorax, hemothorax, lung contusions, liver/spleen lacerations, fat emboli—use proper hand position, apply pressure lower ½ of sternum, do not press on ribs with fingertips, use steady rhythm rather than jabbing motion for compressions

D. Advanced cardiac life-support overview

  1. Primary survey—focus on basic CPR and defibrillation

    a. Airway—open

    b. Breathing—ventilation

    c. Circulation—chest compressions

    d. Defibrillation

  2. Secondary survey—return to ABC's but at advanced level

    a. Airway—advanced airway control, intubation

    b. Breathing—positive-pressure ventilation

    c. Circulation—IV access, CPR, pharmacology

    d. Differential diagnosis—possible reasons for arrest

  3. Dysrhythmia identification

    a. Causes

        i. Disturbances in automaticity—speeding/slowing

        ii. Disturbances in conduction—too slow/fast

        iii. Combinations of altered automaticity and conduction

    b. Normal ECG (Figures 11–4 and 11–5)

        i. P wave—represents origination of impulse in sinus node; abnormality indicates impulse origination in some other area of heart; atrial depolarization

        ii. PR interval—represents conduction through atria and AV node and into Bundle of His

        iii. QRS complex—represents conduction through bundle branches; ventricular depolarization

        iv. T wave—ventricular repolarization

    c. Identification of dysrhythmias

        i. Evaluate QRS complex

           (a) Ventricular fibrillation (VF)—no organized depolarization, therefore no normal-looking QRS complexes, no cardiac output; may be coarse (Figure 11–6) or fine (Figure 11–7), irregular rhythm

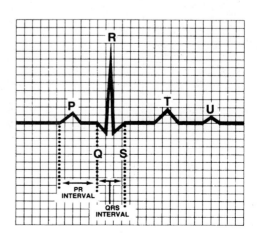

Figure 11–4. The electrocardiogram. (From *Textbook of Advanced Cardiac Life Support, 1994.* Copyright American Heart Association. Reproduced with permission.)

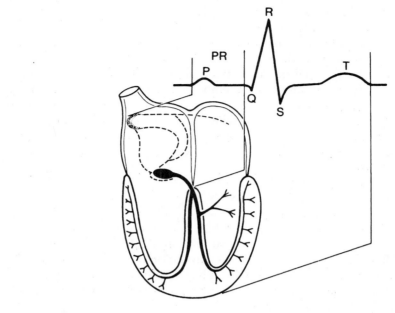

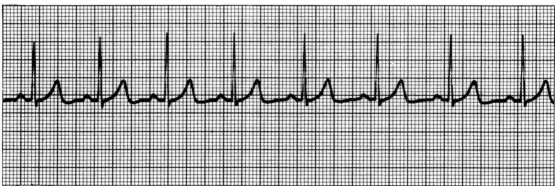

Figure 11–5.   Relation of an electrocardiogram to the anatomy of the cardiac conduction system.   (From *Textbook of Advanced Cardiac Life Support, 1994.* Copyright American Heart Association. Reproduced with permission.)

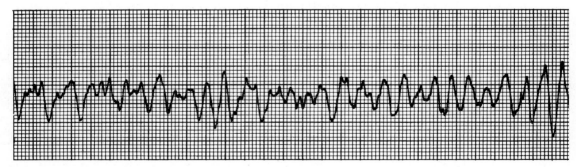

Figure 11–6.   Coarse ventricular fibrillation. Note high amplitude waveforms, which vary in size, shape, and rhythm, representing chaotic ventricular electrical activity. There are no normal-looking QRS complexes. (From *Textbook of Advanced Cardiac Life Support, 1994.* Copyright American Heart Association. Reproduced with permission.)

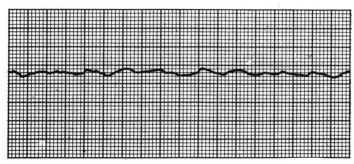

Figure 11–7. Fine ventricular fibrillation ("coarse" asystole). In comparison with Fig. 11–6 amplitude of electrical activity is much reduced. Note complete absence of QRS complexes. Slow undulations like this are virtually indistinguishable from asystole.   (From *Textbook of Advanced Cardiac Life Support, 1994.* Copyright American Heart Association. Reproduced with permission.)

(b) Ventricular asystole—total absence of ventricular electrical activity, no cardiac output, verify in two leads, may have P waves due to atrial activity (Figure 11–8)

(c) Ventricular tachycardia (VT)—three or more ventricular beats together at rate greater than 100, no normal-looking QRS complexes, usually regular rhythm, may be well tolerated or life-threatening, hemodynamic consequences depend on presence/absence of myocardial dysfunction and rate of VT (Figure 11–9)

(d) Premature ventricular complex (PVC) abnormal QRS usually wider than 0.12 seconds, fully compensatory pause (Figure 11–10); indicative of ventricles firing prematurely (Figure 11–11); may occur isolated or in pairs (couplets) (Figure 11–12); may also occur from different foci in ventricles (multifocal/multiformed) (Figure 11–13); may occur every other beat (bigeminy) (Figure 11–14); every third beat (trigeminy), or every fourth beat (quadrigeminy); occurring too close to T wave may result in VT or VF (Figure 11–15)

ii. Evaluate P wave

(a) Atrial fibrillation—atrial rate too rapid to be counted; no organized atrial activity, therefore no P waves; irregular ventricular rhythm; normal QRS unless aberrant conduction present (Figures 11–16 and 11–17)

(b) Atrial flutter—atrial rate usually 300 but may range from 220 to 350, atrial rhythm regular, ventricular rhythm usually regular but may be irregular, P waves resemble flutter/sawtooth waves (Figures 11–18, 11–19, and 11–20)

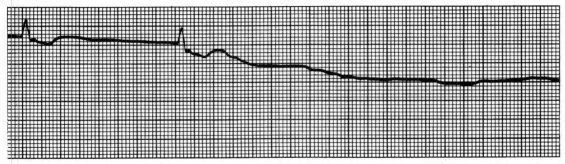

Figure 11–8. Ventricular asystole. Only two QRS complexes are seen, probably representing ventricular escape beats. They are followed by an absence of electrical activity. These are not normal looking.   (From *Textbook of Advanced Cardiac Life Support, 1994.* Copyright American Heart Association. Reproduced with permission.)

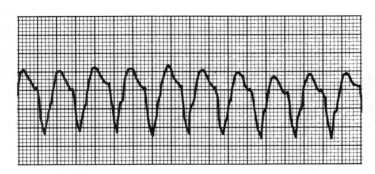

Figure 11–9. Ventricular tachycardia. The rhythm is regular at a rate of 158 beats per minute. The QRS is wide. No evidence of atrial depolarization is seen. (From *Textbook of Advanced Cardiac Life Support, 1994.* Copyright American Heart Association. Reproduced with permission.)

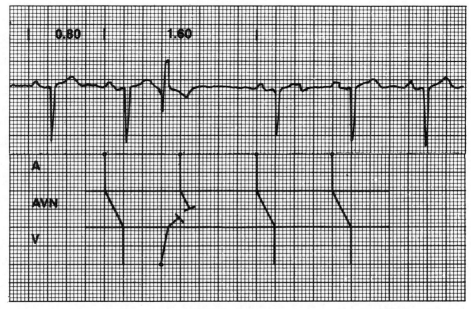

Figure 11–10. Premature ventricular complex with fully compensatory pause. Two normal sinus beats are followed by premature, wide QRS that is not preceded by P wave. As illustrated in accompanying ladder diagram, firing of sinus node was not disturbed, so next sinus beat comes at expected time. Hence interval between normal beat preceding and following PVC is twice normal sinus interval. This is a fully compensatory pause. Sinus impulse that occurs coincident with PVC depolarizes atria but cannot reach ventricles because it is blocked in AV node by refractory period of impulse that arose in ventricle and is attempting to reach atria retrogradely. Neither impulse can be conducted through AV node because it is blocked by refractory period of the other. A, atrium; AVN, AV node; V, ventricle. (From *Textbook of Advanced Cardiac Life Support, 1994.* Copyright American Heart Association. Reproduced with permission.)

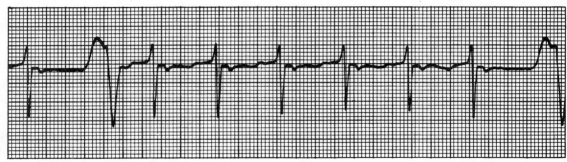

Figure 11–11. Premature ventricular complex. (From *Textbook of Advanced Cardiac Life Support, 1994.* Copyright American Heart Association. Reproduced with permission.)

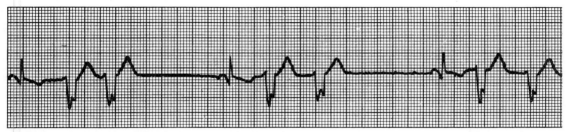

Figure 11–12.   Pairs of premature ventricular complexes.   (From *Textbook of Advanced Cardiac Life Support, 1994.* Copyright American Heart Association. Reproduced with permission.)

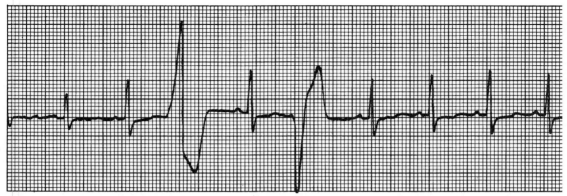

Figure 11–13.   Multiformed premature ventricular complexes. Note variation in morphology and in coupling interval of PVCs.   (From *Textbook of Advanced Cardiac Life Support, 1994.* Copyright American Heart Association. Reproduced with permission.)

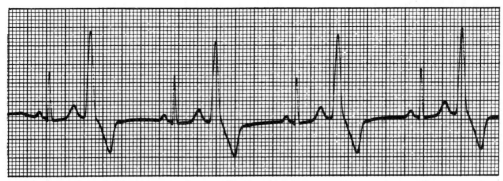

Figure 11–14.   Ventricular bigeminy. Note that every other beat is PVC. Both coupling interval and morphology remain constant; hence they are unifocal.   (From *Textbook of Advanced Cardiac Life Support, 1994.* Copyright American Heart Association. Reproduced with permission.)

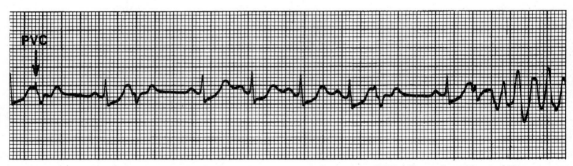

Figure 11–15. R-on-T phenomenon. Multiple PVCs are present. On right, a PVC falls on downslope of T wave, precipitating ventricular fibrillation. (From *Textbook of Advanced Cardiac Life Support, 1994.* Copyright American Heart Association. Reproduced with permission.)

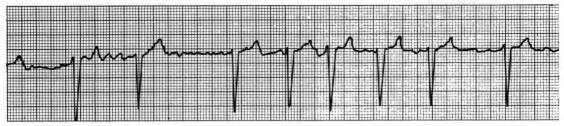

Figure 11–16. Atrial fibrillation with controlled ventricular response. Note irregular undulations of baseline representing atrial electrical activity (fibrillatory waves). The fibrillatory waves vary in size and shape and are irregular in rhythm. Conduction through the AV node occurs at random; hence ventricular rhythm is irregular. (From *Textbook of Advanced Cardiac Life Support, 1994.* Copyright American Heart Association. Reproduced with permission.)

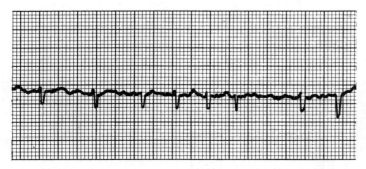

Figure 11–17. Atrial fibrillation with rapid ventricular response. (From *Textbook of Advanced Cardiac Life Support, 1994.* Copyright American Heart Association. Reproduced with permission.)

Figure 11–18. Atrial flutter. The atrial rate is 250 beats per minute, and the rhythm is regular. Every other flutter wave is conducted to ventricles (2:1 block), resulting in regular ventricular rhythm at a rate of 125 beats per minute. (From *Textbook of Advanced Cardiac Life Support, 1994.* Copyright American Heart Association. Reproduced with permission.)

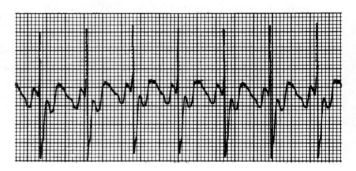

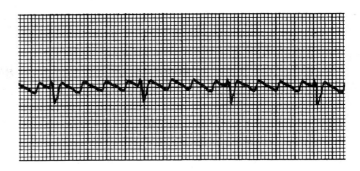

Figure 11–19. Atrial flutter with high-grade AV block. Atrial rhythm is regular (260 beats per minute), but only every fourth flutter wave is followed by a QRS (4:1 conduction). (From *Textbook of Advanced Cardiac Life Support, 1994.* Copyright American Heart Association. Reproduced with permission.)

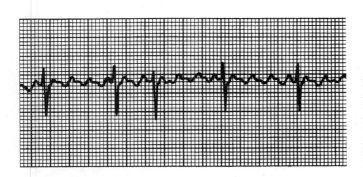

Figure 11–20. Atrial flutter with variable AV block. Atrial rhythm is regular, but variable AV block is present (2:1, 4:1 conduction ratios), resulting in irregular ventricular rhythm. (From *Textbook of Advanced Cardiac Life Support, 1994.* Copyright American Heart Association. Reproduced with permission.)

iii. Evaluate relationship between P waves and QRS
  (a) First-degree block—delay in impulse passage from atria to ventricles, results in prolonged PR interval beyond 0.20 seconds, P waves and QRS normal (Figure 11–21)
  (b) Second-degree block, type I (Wenckebach) block at level of AV node results in progressively longer PR interval until a beat is blocked, atrial rhythm regular, normal P wave and QRS (Figure 11–22)
  (c) Second-degree block, type II—below level of AV node, associated with poorer prognosis, PR interval remains constant and may be normal or prolonged (Figure 11–23)
  (d) Third-degree block—complete absence of conduction between atria and ventricles, P waves normal, atrial and ventricular rhythms regular but independent of each other, ventricular rate 40–60 (Figure 11–24)

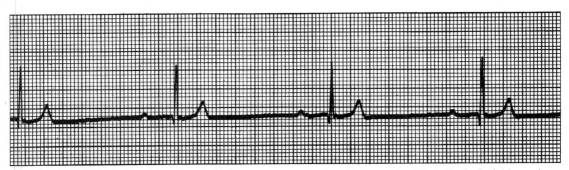

Figure 11–21. First-degree AV block. The PR interval is prolonged to 0.31 second. (From *Textbook of Advanced Cardiac Life Support, 1994.* Copyright American Heart Association. Reproduced with permission.)

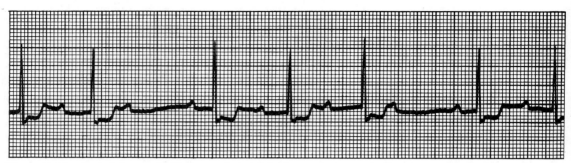

Figure 11–22.   Second-degree AV block type I. Atrial rhythm is nearly regular, but there are pauses in ventricular rhythm because every fourth P wave does not conduct into ventricles. Note progressive prolongation of PR interval, indicating increasing conduction delay in AV node before nonconducted beat. There are four P waves and three QRS complexes in this example, respresenting a 4:3 cycle. The QRS complexes are normal.   (From *Textbook of Advanced Cardiac Life Support, 1994.* Copyright American Heart Association. Reproduced with permission.)

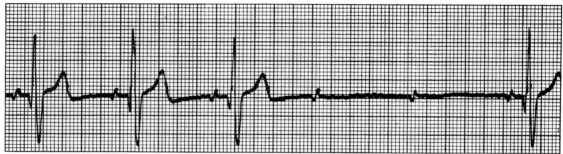

Figure 11–23.   Second-degree AV block type II. In this example three conducted sinus beats are followed by two nonconducted P waves. The PR interval of conducted beats remains constant, and QRS is wide.   (From *Textbook of Advanced Cardiac Life Support, 1994.* Copyright American Heart Association. Reproduced with permission.)

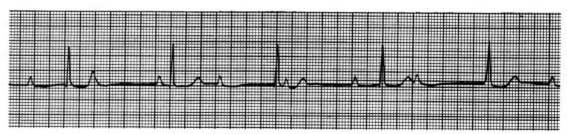

Figure 11–24.   Third-degree AV block occurring at level of AV node. Atrial rhythm is slightly irregular owing to presence of sinus arrhythmia. Ventricular rhythm is regular at slower rate (44 beats per minute). There is no constant PR interval. The QRS complexes are narrow, indicating they are of supraventricular origin but below level of block.   (From *Textbook of Advanced Cardiac Life Support, 1994.* Copyright American Heart Association. Reproduced with permission.)

    (e) Sinus tachycardia—characterized by normal-looking QRS, rate greater than 100, regular rhythm, upright P waves in leads I, II, and AVF; evaluation and treatment of causes usually sufficient to resolve (pain, hypoxemia, hypovolemia) (Figure 11–25)

    (f) Sinus bradycardia—characterized by normal-looking QRS, rate less than 60, regular rhythm, upright P waves in leads I, II, and AVF; evaluate and treat causes (hypothermia, hypothyroidism, MI, vagal response); treat rhythm only if symptomatic (Figure 11–26)

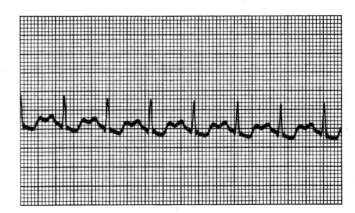

Figure 11–25. Sinus tachycardia. Note regular rhythm at the rate of 121 beats per minute. Each QRS is preceded by upright P wave in lead II. (From *Textbook of Advanced Cardiac Life Support, 1994.* Copyright American Heart Association. Reproduced with permission.)

4. Select appropriate algorithm (Refer to *Textbook for Advanced Cardiac Life Support* by Cummins for algorithms)
   a. Universal algorithm
   b. Ventricular fibrillation (VF)/pulseless ventricular tachycardia (VT) algorithm
   c. Pulseless electrical activity (PEA) algorithm
   d. Asystole algorithm
   e. Bradycardia algorithm
   f. Tachycardia algorithm
   g. Acute pulmonary edema/hypotension/shock algorithm
   h. Acute myocardial infarction algorithm
5. Pharmacology
   a. Epinephrine
      i.   Natural catecholamine with alpha and beta adrenergic effects
      ii. Cardiovascular responses
           (a) Increased systemic vascular resistance
           (b) Increased systolic and diastolic BP
           (c) Increased electrical activity in myocardium
           (d) Increased coronary and cerebral blood flow
           (e) Increased strength of myocardial contraction
           (f) Increased myocardial oxygen requirements
           (g) Increased automaticity
      iii. Indications
           (a) VF/pulseless VT
           (b) Asystole
           (c) PEA
           (d) Infusion for profoundly symptomatic bradycardia

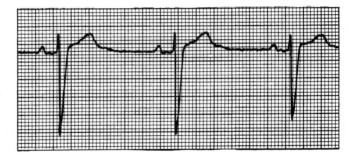

Figure 11–26. Sinus bradycardia. Sinus rate is 46 beats per minute and rhythm is regular. (From *Textbook of Advanced Cardiac Life Support, 1994.* Copyright American Heart Association. Reproduced with permission.)

iv. Dose
  (a) Routine: 1 mg IV every 3–5 minutes
  (b) Intermediate: 2–5 mg IV every 3–5 minutes
  (c) Escalating: 1–3–5 mg IV 3 minutes apart
  (d) High: 0.1 mg/kg IV every 3–5 minutes
  (e) Can be given via endotracheal tube: 2–2.5 mg diluted in 10 ml normal saline

b. Atropine
  i. Parasympatholytic; enhances sinus node automaticity and atrioventricular conduction; direct vagolytic action
  ii. Indications
    (a) Symptomatic bradycardia
    (b) Relative bradycardia (patient where tachycardia would be more beneficial)
    (c) First-degree AV block
    (d) Mobitz type I AV block
    (e) Bradyasystolic cardiac arrest
    (f) Use with caution in Mobitz II AV block and third-degree block—watch for paradoxical slowing
  iii. Dose
    (a) Without cardiac arrest—0.5–1 mg, repeated at 5-minute intervals
    (b) With asystolic cardiac arrest—1 mg repeated every 3–5 minutes if asystole persists, 3 mg (0.4 mg/kg) = fully vagolytic dose
    (c) Administration of doses less than 0.5 mg may precipitate paradoxical bradycardia
    (d) Can be given via endotracheal tube: 1–2 mg diluted in 10 ml normal saline
  iv. Precautions
    (a) Tachycardia
    (b) Use caution in presence of myocardial ischemia
    (c) Excessive doses may precipitate anticholinergic syndrome: delirium, tachycardia, coma, flushed/hot skin, ataxia, blurred vision

c. Lidocaine
  i. Antiarrhythmic: decreases automaticity
  ii. Indications
    (a) VT and VF
    (b) Ventricular ectopy
    (c) Wide-complex tachycardias of unknown origin
  iii. Dose
    (a) Refractory VF/pulseless VT: 1.0–1.5 mg/kg initial dose, total dose 3 mg/kg
    (b) After restoration of spontaneous circulation: 2–4 mg/minute drip (2 Gms. in 500 D5W)
    (c) Noncardiac arrest: 1.0–1.5 mg/kg bolus followed by infusion of 2–4 mg/minute, may repeat bolus of 0.5–0.75 mg/kg up to 3 mg/kg
    (d) Can be given via endotracheal tube 2–2.5 times dose with 10 mg normal saline
  iv. Precautions
    (a) Neurological changes, myocardial and circulatory depression with excessive doses
    (b) Neurological changes: drowsiness, disorientation, decreased hearing ability, paresthesia, muscle twitching
    (c) Myocardial depression: heart block

d. Procainamide
  i.   Antiarrhythmic: suppresses automaticity, useful in some cases where lidocaine fails
  ii. Indications
       (a) Persistent cardiac arrest due to VF
       (b) Rarely used to treat VT due to prolonged time to administer effective doses
       (c) Recurrent VT and PVCs not suppressed with lidocaine
       (d) Supraventricular arrhythmias
  iii. Dose
       (a) PVC's: 20–30 mg/minute until suppressed, hypotension develops, QRS widens by 50% of original width or 17 mg/kg is reached
       (b) Maintenance IV infusion: 1–4 mg/minute (2 Gms. in 500 D5W)
  iv. Precautions
       (a) Hypotension most pronounced after rapid injection
       (b) ECG and blood pressure monitoring essential
       (c) Tendency to produce arrhythmias greater in presence of hypokalemia and hypomagnesemia
e. Bretylium
  i.   Adrenergic neuronal blocking agent with direct myocardial effects
  ii. Indications
       (a) VF and VT refractory to other therapy
       (b) Not first-line drug
  iii. Dose
       (a) VF: 5 mg/kg by rapid injection, 10 mg/kg in 5 minutes, 10 mg/kg at 5- to 30-minute intervals up to 35 mg/kg
       (b) Refractory VT without pulse: 500 mg in 50 mg D5W, inject 5–10 mg/kg over 8–10 minutes, repeat dose in 10–30 minutes
       (c) Infusion of 2 mg/minute (2 Gms in 500 D5W)
  iv. Precautions
       (a) Postural hypotension: treat with IV fluids and supine position
       (b) Hypertension and tachycardia
       (c) Nausea and vomiting
       (d) Use with caution in presence of digitalis toxicity
f. Verapamil
  i.   Calcium channel blocker: exerts direct negative chronotropic and inotropic effects
  ii. Indication—paroxysmal supraventricular tachycardia (PSVT); avoid in patients with wide-QRS tachycardia unless known with certainty to be supraventricular in origin
  iii. Dose
       (a) Single dose: 2.5–5.0 mg IV over 1–2 minutes
       (b) Repeat dose: 5–10 mg in 15–30 minutes, 5 mg every 15 minutes up to 30 mg or desired response is reached
       (c) Administer over 3 minutes in older patients
       (d) Ages 8–15, 0.1–0.3 mg/kg over 1 minute; repeat dose is 0.1–0.2 mg/kg 15–30 minutes after first dose
g. Adenosine
  i.   Endogenous purine nucleoside
       (a) Slows conduction through AV node
       (b) Interrupts AV-nodal reentry pathways
       (c) Can restore normal sinus rhythm in PSVT
       (d) Half-life less than 5 seconds

      ii. Indications
        (a) PSVT termination
        (b) Diagnosis of supraventricular arrhythmias
     iii. Dose
        (a) Initial: 6 mg rapid bolus (1–3 seconds)
        (b) Repeat in 1–2 minutes 12 mg rapidly
     iv. Precautions
        (a) Administration may be followed by brief period of asystole
        (b) Flushing, dyspnea, chest pain usually resolve within 1–2 minutes

h. Magnesium
       i. Cofactor in enzymatic reactions
        (a) Essential to function of sodium-potassium ATPase pump
        (b) Physiological calcium channel blocker
        (c) Blocks neuromuscular transmission
      ii. Indications
        (a) Reduction in incidence of postinfarction ventricular arrhythmias
        (b) Torsades de pointes: a special form of VT with a gradual alteration and in amplitude and direction of electrical activity
     iii. Dose
        (a) VT: 1–2 Gms diluted in 10 ml D5W, give over 1–2 minutes
        (b) VF: administer IV push
        (c) Torsades de pointes: may use up to 5–10 Gms
     iv. Precautions
        (a) Hypotension or asystole on administration
        (b) Hypermagnesemia: depressed reflexes, flaccid paralysis, circulatory collapse, respiratory paralysis, diarrhea

i. Sodium bicarbonate
       i. Buffer agent
      ii. Indications
        (a) Pre-existing metabolic acidosis
        (b) Hyperkalemia
        (c) Tricyclic or phenobarbital overdose
        (d) Considered only after confirmed interventions (defibrillation, compressions, intubation, epinephrine)
     iii. Dose
        (a) Initial dose: 1 mEq/kg IV
        (b) Repeat half dose every 10 minutes using blood gases to measure acid-base status
     iv. Precautions
        (a) Intracellular acidosis may occur
        (b) Hypernatremia and hyperosmolality

6. Principles of defibrillation
  a. Must be early in arrest period
  b. Chance of successful recovery decreases quickly over time
  c. Only means of termination of VF, most common rhythm associated with cardiac arrest
  d. Overcoming transthoracic impedance
       i. Sufficient energy level to overcome
      ii. Appropriate electrode size—standard paddle
     iii. Appropriate electrode/skin contact—gel pads
     iv. Number and time interval of previous shocks
        (a) Initial shock 200 joules
        (b) Follow immediately after verifying rhythm with 200–300 joules

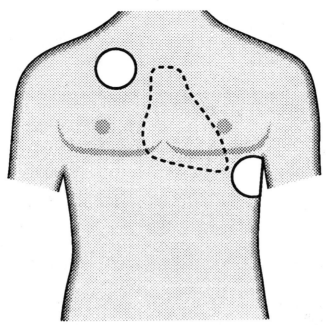

Figure 11–27. Recommended anterior-apex position for defibrillation. The anterior electrode should be to the right of the upper sternum below the clavicle. The apex electrode should be placed to the left of the nipple with the center of the electrode in the midaxillary line.   (From *Textbook of Advanced Cardiac Life Support, 1994.* Copyright American Heart Association. Reproduced with permission.)

   (c) Repeat verification of rhythm and immediately follow with 360 joules
   (d) Pediatric energy levels: 1 joule/lb or 2 joules/kg, double energy level for successive shocks
  v. Appropriate phase of ventilation: shock at end expiration
  vi. Distance between electrodes: proper chest placement of electrodes (anterior electrode to the right of the upper sternum and apex electrode to the left of the nipple with center of electrode at mid-axillary line) (Figure 11–27)
 e. Defibrillation safety
  i. Perform away from wet areas (e.g., water on floor from spilled IV fluids or humidifier bottles)
  ii. Use appropriate conductive materials to prevent burning of patient skin
  iii. Remove transdermal medication patches to prevent arcing of electricity
  iv. Clear prior to shock to prevent injury to rescue team members

Bibliography

1. Burden, N. (1993). *Ambulatory Surgical Nursing.* Philadelphia: Saunders.
2. Cummins, R.O. (1994). *Textbook of Advanced Cardiac Life Support.* Dallas: American Heart Association.
3. Drain, C.B. (1994). *The Post Anesthesia Care Unit: A Critical Approach to Post Anesthesia Nursing.* Philadelphia: Saunders.
4. Einhorn, G.W., Chant, P. (1994). Postanesthesia care unit dilemmas: Prompt assessment and treatment. *J Post Anesth Nurs,* 9:28–33.
5. Hogenson, K.D. (1992). Acute Postoperative Hypertension in the Hypertensive Patient. *J Post Anesth Nurs,* 7:38–44.
6. Jacobsen, W. (1992). *Manual of Post Anesthesia Care.* Philadelphia: Saunders.
7. Litwack, K. (1995). *Post Anesthesia Care Nursing.* St. Louis: Mosby.
8. Seibel, H.M. (1995). *Mosby's Guide to Physical Examination,* 3rd ed. St. Louis: Mosby-Yearbook.
9. Wagner, K.D. (1992). Mechanical ventilation. In Kidd, P.S., Wagner, K.D., *High Acuity Nursing.* Norwalk, CT: Appleton & Lange.

REVIEW QUESTIONS

1. Oxygen debt in the postoperative period may manifest as any of the following except

   A. Cardiac dysrhythmias
   B. Chest pain
   C. Hypertension
   D. ST changes

2. Hypotension in the postoperative period may be caused by which of the following?

   A. Decreased intravascular volume, left ventricular failure, decreased vascular tone
   B. Decreased intravascular volume, right ventricular failure, increased vascular tone
   C. Increased intravascular volume, excess catecholamines, increased vascular tone
   D. Increased intravascular volume, decreased vascular tone, immobility

3. Which of the following is a false statement regarding the assessment of skin color?

   A. Absence of cyanosis is indicative of adequate oxygenation
   B. Color should be assessed preoperatively to determine normal for each individual
   C. Cyanosis is indicative of inadequate oxygenation
   D. Skin color may reflect the adequacy of gas exchange

4. Rapid, shallow, jerky movements may be indicative of which of the following?

   A. Central nervous system problems
   B. Lactic acidosis
   C. Narcotics
   D. Residual neuromuscular blockade

5. Proper endotracheal tube placement may be confirmed by all of the following except

   A. Confirming equality of bilateral breath sounds
   B. Confirming the presence of bubbling over the epigastrium
   C. Direct visualization of the tube passing through the vocal cords
   D. Observing the chest wall for equal thoracic expansion

6. All of the following are indications for use of mechanical ventilation except

   A. Acute ventilatory failure
   B. Cardiac arrest
   C. Hypoxemia
   D. Pneumonia

7. The ventilator low-exhaled volume alarm will trigger when

   A. The patient bites the ET tube
   B. The patient coughs
   C. There is a leak in the system
   D. There is water in the tubing

8. Systemic effects of mechanical ventilation include all of the following except

   A. Altered ventilation-perfusion relationships
   B. Decreased preload
   C. Increased intracranial pressure
   D. Increased mesenteric blood flow

9. The primary survey for advanced cardiac life support consists of all of the following except

   A. Airway
   B. Breathing
   C. Circulation
   D. Differential diagnosis

10. All of the following may be useful in overcoming transthoracic impedance during defibrillation except

    A. Appropriate electrode/skin contact
    B. Appropriate electrode size
    C. Appropriate phase of ventilation
    D. Interruption of shocks for reassessment

ANSWERS TO QUESTIONS

1. C
2. A
3. A
4. D
5. B

6. D
7. C
8. D
9. D
10. D

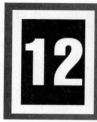

Pre-Existing Medical Conditions

Kim Litwack
University of New Mexico
College of Nursing
Albuquerque, New Mexico

Objectives

1. Identify patients at an increased perioperative risk.
2. Recognize the reasons for the increased risk.
3. State the specific perioperative nursing care priorities for the high-risk patient.
4. Be proactive in reducing perioperative morbidity and mortality.

I. **Pre-existing Medical Conditions**
   A. Increase ASA classification
   B. Increase perioperative risk, morbidity, and mortality
   C. May require multiple medications
      1. Increased potential for drug interactions
      2. Increased potential for laboratory test alterations
      3. Increased potential for noncompliance
   D. Level of disease control may jeopardize ambulatory status
II. **Cardiovascular Diseases**
   A. Hypertension
      1. Definition: systolic >140 mm Hg and/or diastolic >90 mm Hg
      2. Incidence: 20–25% of U.S. population; males >females
      3. Significance: risk factor for coronary artery disease, cerebrovascular accidents, congestive heart failure, renal failure
      4. Etiology/findings
         a. Medical evaluation/clearance
            i. Mild hypertension: within 2 months of surgery
            ii. Moderate hypertension: within 2 weeks of surgery
            iii. Severe hypertension (diastolic >115 mm Hg): immediate evaluation with surgery canceled

      b. Advise patient to take routine prescription antihypertensive medication on day of surgery with a sip of water

      c. Ask about presence of heart disease during preoperative interview

B. Coronary artery disease (CAD)

  1. Definition: accumulation of plaque within the coronary arteries

  2. Incidence: extremely common, males >females, age >35

  3. Significance: increased risk for myocardial infarction (MI), hypertension, renal disease, arrhythmias, congestive heart failure, sudden death

  4. Etiology: physiologic, environmental, aging, diet, biochemical

  5. Treatment: coronary vasodilators (nitrates), activity, diet, education

  6. Perioperative significance

      a. If history of MI, elective surgery should wait minimum of 6 months to decrease risk of reinfarction with very high mortality

      b. Requires evaluation and clearance from a cardiologist

      c. May increase intraoperative monitoring requirements

      d. Assess for signs of congestive heart failure (CHF); if present, surgery is canceled

      e. Signs of CHF include:

        i. Shortness of breath

        ii. Dyspnea on exertion or nocturnal

        iii. Jugular venous distension

        iv. Crackles

        v. Edema

      f. Assess incidence and triggers of chest pain

        i. If new onset (<2 months) or unstable, postpone surgery pending cardiologist evaluation

        ii. All prescription medications to be taken on morning of surgery with sip of water

C. Congestive heart failure (CHF)

  1. Definition

      a. Left- and/or right-sided heart dysfunction producing decreased systolic emptying and decreased ventricular compliance

      b. Heart is unable to meet demands of peripheral tissues

  2. Incidence

      a. Most common inpatient diagnosis for patients >65 years of age

      b. Males >females for age 40–75

      c. Males = females for over age 75

  3. Significance: increased risk for pulmonary edema, dyspnea, peripheral edema

  4. Etiology: CAD, myocardial infarction, rheumatic heart disease, volume overload

  5. Treatment: diuretics, inotropic therapy, oxygen, low-sodium diet

  6. Perioperative significance

      a. If symptomatic (see CAD), surgery is canceled

      b. Auscultate breath sounds on arrival, on admission to PACU Phase I, and prior to discharge

      c. Strict intake and output records

      d. Increased perioperative mortality (10–50%)

      e. Obtain cardiologist clearance prior to surgery

D. Mitral valve prolapse (MVP)

  1. Definition: prolapse or stenosis of mitral heart valve that results in resistance to left ventricular emptying (increased afterload)

  2. Incidence: age <30 congenital; age >70 degenerative

3. Significance: increased risk of angina, syncope, fatigue, dyspnea, click or heart murmur on auscultation, pulmonary embolism, arrhythmias
4. Etiology: congenital, rheumatic heart disease, aging
5. Treatment: prolapse often requires no treatment; stenosis requires valve replacement, digoxin or other anti-arrhythmic (including beta blocker or calcium channel blocker), low-sodium diet, education
6. Perioperative significance
   a. Patients require antibiotic endocarditis prophylaxis prior to dental work or other invasive procedures regardless of age, etiology, disease severity
   b. May be anticoagulated on warfarin; if so, check PT/INR (International Normalized Ratio)
      i. Patient may be asked to stop warfarin 3 days prior to surgery
   c. Risk of pulmonary edema is significant

E. Arrhythmias
   1. Definition: alteration in conduction system requiring pharmacologic or surgical (automatic implantable cardiac-defibrillator [AICD], pacemaker) intervention
   2. Incidence: very common (arrythmias)
      a. Use of pacemakers and AICDs increases with age
      b. Common outcome of coronary artery disease
   3. Significance: increased risk of myocardial infarction and progression to lethal arrhythmias
   4. Etiology: CAD, CHF, valve disease, myocardial infarction, hypoxia, hypercarbia, electrolyte imbalance, acid-base alterations
   5. Treatment: pharmacologic, education, pacemaker (heart block, asystole), AICD (ventricular fibrillation)
   6. Perioperative significance
      a. Patient to take anti-arrhythmic medications on day of surgery
      b. Inquire about type of pacemaker and setting (patient may have pacer ID card); document in chart (may need to call cardiologist)
      c. Have external pacemaker readily available
      d. Have cardiologist available, although not necessarily in the OR
      e. If patient has an AICD, cautery should not be used during surgery
         i. If cautery must be used, AICD is turned off
         ii. External defibrillator must be available in OR suite for immediate use if needed

III. **Pulmonary Diseases**
   A. Chronic obstructive pulmonary disease (COPD)
      1. Definition: term includes chronic bronchitis and emphysema
         a. Bronchitis presents with cough, increase sputum production, dyspnea, wheezing
         b. Emphysema presents with barrel chest, pursed lip breathing, decreased breath sounds
      2. Incidence: 20–30% of adults >40 years of age; male >female
      3. Significance: hypoxia, hypercapnia
      4. Etiology: cigarette smoking, air pollution, occupational exposure to smoke
      5. Treatment: bronchodilators, possibly anticholinergics and corticosteroids, patient education to stop smoking
      6. Perioperative significance
         a. Encourage patient to stop smoking 8 weeks prior to surgery; be aware that most patients will not comply
         b. General anesthesia may exacerbate symptoms/disease; regional anesthesia avoids intubation and use of controlled ventilation

      c. Patient's respirations controlled by hypoxic drive
         i. High flow, high concentration oxygen may produce apnea
         ii. Nasal cannula <3L oxygen preferred delivery system unless unable to maintain saturation
      d. Encourage deep breathing and coughing after general anesthesia; postoperative pulmonary infections common
      e. Ask patient to bring inhalers used to the facility on day of surgery
      f. Pulmonary function tests may be ordered preoperatively (rare)

B. Asthma
  1. Definition: tracheobronchial disorder characterized by obstruction to airflow secondary to narrowing of airways, edema, and inflammation
  2. Incidence: 10 million new cases each year; 50% patients <age 10; 7–19% of all children
  3. Significance: increased risk of laryngospasm/bronchospasm on induction, hypoxemia, decreased peak flow rates
  4. Etiology: allergic factors, smoke, infection, cold air, exercise
  5. Treatment: bronchodilators (beta-2 agonists), corticosteroids (acute asthma), mast cell stabilizers, education
  6. Perioperative significance
      a. Encourage patient to avoid known irritants to minimize perioperative wheezing
      b. Auscultate breath sounds pre- and postoperatively
      c. Increased risk of bronchospasm on intubation and emergence
      d. Ask patient to bring any inhalers used to the facility on the day of surgery
      e. If on steroids, determine last use/dose; may need steroid preoperatively
      f. Question patient on the frequency, severity, and management of attacks
      g. Cancel surgery if patient presents with upper respiratory infection

C. Smoking
  1. Definition: use of inhaled tobacco
  2. Incidence: extremely common; teenagers, adults, and elderly
  3. Significance: increased risk of COPD, heart disease, hypoxia, poor tissue healing
  4. Etiology: access to/use of product
  5. Treatment: cessation
  6. Perioperative significance:
      a. Patient has elevated carboxyhemoglobin levels
      b. Carbon monoxide has greater affinity for hemoglobin than does oxygen
      c. Increased risk of bronchospasm/laryngospasm on induction, intubation, emergence
      d. Encourage patient to stop smoking 8 weeks prior to surgery; be aware that most will not comply

IV. **Renal Diseases**
A. Acute renal failure (ARF)
  1. Definition: rapid, increasing azotemia with or without oliguria
  2. Significance: patient will experience urinary changes, fluid volume excess, metabolic acidosis, sodium alterations, potassium excess, calcium deficit and phosphate excess, nitrogenous waste accumulation
  3. Patient inappropriate for ambulatory surgery

B. Chronic renal failure (CRF)
  1. Definition: progressive, irreversible disruption of the excretory and regulatory function of the nephron
  2. Incidence: common—160,000 new cases/year; more common in African-Americans; rare in children; males = females

3. Significance: patients commonly diabetic with multiple laboratory alterations, hypertension, and anemia
4. Etiology: pyelonephritis, polycystic kidneys, autoimmune, diabetes, drug-induced nephropathy (antibiotics, NSAIDs), hypertension, congenital
5. Treatment: renal replacement therapy, hemodialysis, peritoneal dialysis, ultrafiltration, renal transplantation, diet, patient education
6. Perioperative significance
   a. Avoid nephrotoxic drugs
   b. Consider decreased doses of medications eliminated through kidneys
   c. Anemia may compromise oxygenation, especially with hematocrit <18%
   d. Monitor electrolytes and renal function preoperatively, especially potassium, BUN, and creatine
   e. Obtain preoperative glucose level in diabetic patients
   f. Avoid same-arm venipunctures/blood pressures if patient has A-V fistula for hemodialysis
   g. Increased risk for infection
   h. Determine date of last dialysis; if off schedule, anticipate fluid/electrolyte imbalance
   i. Avoid potassium-containing solutions
   j. Obtain preoperative weight
   k. Careful intake and output; may be on fluid restriction
   l. Poor tolerance for physiologic stress
   m. Instruct patient to take antihypertensive medications on day of surgery
   n. Use of Lactated Ringers or D_5LR may lead to acidosis; use ½ NS or D_5 ½ NS

V. Liver Diseases

A. Cirrhosis–liver failure
1. Definition: hepatic fibrosis producing portal hypertension including ascites, variceal bleeding, hepatic encephalopathy
2. Incidence: 30,000 deaths/year; males >females
3. Significance: inappropriate for ambulatory surgery
B. Hepatitis
1. Definition
   a. Acute hepatitis is an inflammatory disease of hepatocytes
   b. Chronic hepatitis (active): widespread destruction of hepatocytes causing cirrhosis and hepatic failure
   c. Chronic hepatitis (persistent): nonprogressive inflammatory disease confined to portal areas
2. Incidence (varies with etiology)
   a. Hepatitis A: 25% of cases
   b. Hepatitis B: 200,000 young adults/year
   c. Hepatitis C: most common cause of acute viral hepatitis; males >females
3. Significance: hepatitis in presence of alcoholism increases risk of cirrhosis
   a. Depending on extent of disease, may have alterations in coagulation, fluid and electrolytes, and wound healing
4. Etiology: viral
   a. Hepatitis A: transmitted enterically (fecal–oral via food)
   b. Hepatitis B: transmitted sexually, via contaminated blood (needle sticks) and body fluids
   c. Hepatitis C: transmitted via blood transfusions and body fluids, although in 50% of cases route of transmission unknown
5. Treatment: supportive as disease is viral
6. Prevention: vaccine Hepatitis B, Havrix (Hepatitis A) vaccine for high risk patients

    7. Perioperative significance

        a. Patients with acute hepatitis are inappropriate for ambulatory surgery

        b. Patients with chronic persistent hepatitis should be evaluated prior to surgery by a gastroenterologist

        c. Vigilance to universal precautions

        d. Consider obtaining preoperative liver enzymes to compare with previous levels

            i. Increases reflect worsening of disease

            ii. Requires medical evaluation prior to surgery

C. Alcohol abuse

    1. Definition: illness characterized by significant impairment associated with persistent and excessive use of alcohol

        a. Impairment may be physiologic, psychologic, or social

    2. Incidence: 10% of men; 3.5% of women; 11–15% of all adults; highest incidence is between 18–39 years of age

    3. Significance: associated with malnutrition, poor compliance, hypertension, pulmonary disease with concomitant cigarette use

    4. Etiology: biologic, psychologic, and sociocultural factors

    5. Treatment: detoxification and withdrawal of use

    6. Perioperative significance

        a. Compliance with pre- and postoperative instructions may be poor

        b. Determine usual consumption, time, and amount of last drink

        c. Malnutrition may compromise wound healing

        d. Aberrant responses to narcotics and benzodiazepines

        e. At risk for cirrhosis, alterations in coagulation, and bleeding

        f. Delirium tremens may require heavy sedation/restraints to prevent patient self-injury

            i. First sign of delirium tremens in patient still sedated following general anesthesia may be tachycardia

        g. Occurrence of delirium tremens in perioperative period associated with high incidence of morbidity and mortality

        h. Increased incidence of aspiration pneumonitis

        i. Concomitant pulmonary disease will require aggressive postoperative pulmonary hygiene

        j. Patients arriving intoxicated for ambulatory procedures should have surgery canceled

VI. Neuromuscular, Skeletal, Connective Tissue Diseases

A. Scoliosis

    1. Definition: C- or S-shaped lateral curvature of the vertebral spine

    2. Incidence: women >men (80% women)

    3. Significance: most commonly diagnosed and treated in childhood during maximal growth period

    4. Etiology: congenital, fracture, osteomalacia

    5. Treatment

        a. In childhood and adolescence: exercises, weight reduction, bracing, casting, surgery (spinal fusion with rod placement)

        b. In adults: spinal fusion

    6. Perioperative significance

        a. Severe deviations (>50 degrees) can compromise cardiopulmonary function; obtain preoperative pulmonary function tests

        b. Curvature can cause lower back pain

        c. Deformity may compromise intraoperative positioning

      d. Mitral valve prolapse present in 25% of patients; will require antibiotic prophylaxis

      e. Patients with concomitant myopathies likely to require postoperative ventilation; inappropriate as outpatients

      f. Pulmonary function may be decreased after general anesthesia requiring aggressive pulmonary care

B. Arthritis: rheumatoid and osteoarthritis

  1. Definitions

      a. Rheumatoid: chronic inflammatory disease of multiple joints producing disability and disfigurement

      b. Osteoarthritis: degenerative disease of articular cartilage with minimal inflammation

  2. Incidence

      a. Rheumatoid: 1/1000 children; females >males; most common between ages 30–50

      b. Osteoarthritis: 33–90% of all adults >65 years of age; 20 million patients

  3. Significance

      a. Rheumatoid: increased incidence of cardiopulmonary involvement

      b. Osteoarthritis: is the most common form of joint disease

  4. Etiology

      a. Rheumatoid: unknown, includes genetics, altered immune response, trauma

      b. Osteoarthritis: aging, genetics

  5. Treatment: goal is to maintain joint function and to minimize disability

      a. Rheumatoid: symptomatic, NSAIDs, gold, methotrexate, corticosteroids

      b. Osteoarthritis: NSAIDs and heat

  6. Perioperative significance

      a. Rheumatoid arthritis

         i. Joint stiffness worse in morning; consider afternoon scheduling

         ii. Pericardial effusion/thickening present in ⅓ of adults

         iii. Pleural effusion is the most common pulmonary alteration

      b. Osteoarthritis

         i. Corticosteroids not recommended; increased risk of degenerative joint changes

      c. Arthritis (both types)

         i. Cervical spine and temporomandibular joint (TMJ) involvement may restrict neck mobility for intubation; may require use of fiberoptic bronchoscopy

         ii. Limited joint mobility may compromise intraoperative positioning

         iii. NSAIDs can alter platelet function/coagulation, and cause mild anemia

         iv. Obtain preoperative coagulation studies, hemoglobin, and hematocrit

C. Neuromuscular diseases

  1. Muscular dystrophy

      a. Definition

         i. Progressive disease of muscle resulting in painless degeneration and atrophy of skeletal muscles

         ii. Due to increased permeability of skeletal muscle membranes and decreased cardiopulmonary reserve

      b. Inappropriate for ambulatory surgery

  2. Myasthenia gravis

      a. Definition: chronic autoimmune disease of the neuromuscular junction resulting in rapid exhaustion/weakness of voluntary skeletal muscles

      b. Incidence: 1/20,000 adults; females >males; females ages 20–30, males >60 years of age

    c. Significance: disease classified as Type I to IV based on skeletal muscle involvement and severity of symptoms
- i. Type I: involvement of only extraocular eye muscles
- ii. Type IIA: slow, progressive mild skeletal muscle weakness with respiratory muscle involvement
- iii. Type IIB: severe, rapidly progressive form of skeletal muscle weakness with or without respiratory muscle weakness
- iv. Type III: acute onset, rapid deterioration of skeletal muscle strength with high mortality
- v. Type IV: severe skeletal muscle weakness that results from progression of Type I or Type II

    d. Etiology: unknown; thymus gland abnormality

    e. Treatment: anticholinesterase drugs, corticosteroid, immunosuppressants

    f. Perioperative significance
- i. Not appropriate for ambulatory surgery if Type IIB, III, or IV
- ii. Will likely require prolonged postoperative ventilatory support
- iii. Anticholinesterase drugs alter effects of nondepolarizing muscle relaxants with variable responses
- iv. Very susceptible to respiratory depression

3. Parkinson's disease (Paralysis Agitans)

    a. Definition: slow adult-onset, progressive disease of central nervous system degeneration characterized by the classic triad of resting tremor, rigidity, and bradykinesia

    b. Incidence: 50,000 new cases/year; males >females; onset >60 years of age

    c. Significance: do not assume presence of mental status changes

    d. Etiology: possible genetic predisposition

    e. Treatment: no cure
- i. Goal is to control symptoms and to slow disease course
- ii. May include anticholinergics, beta blockers, amantadine, levodopa

    f. Perioperative significance
- i. Physical limitations may increase need for assistive devices
- ii. Continue levodopa on day of surgery—interruption of drug for 6–12 hours can result in loss of drug's therapeutic effect, including difficulty in maintaining ventilation
- iii. Levodopa may produce orthostatic hypotension, dysrhythmias, hypertension
- iv. Use of phenothiazines (Compazine) and butyrophenones (Droperidol) contraindicated—may produce extrapyramidal effects
- v. Depression common in advanced stages of disease (if MAO inhibitors are being used, notify anesthesiologist)

VII. Endocrine Diseases

    A. Diabetes mellitus (DM)

      1. Definition

        a. Chronic, systemic disease producing altered glucose metabolism and hyperglycemia

        b. Insulin dependent diabetes mellitus (IDDM, type I, ketosis-prone) commonly develops in childhood and adolescents
- i. Patient produces no insulin
- ii. Requires insulin to sustain life

        c. Non-insulin dependent diabetes mellitus (NIDDM, type II, non-ketosis prone) develops after age 35
- i. Commonly managed with diet and oral hypoglycemic agents
- ii. May require insulin

      d. Incidence: 2.4% of U.S. population (5.5 million people)

      e. Significance: increased risk of macroangiopathy (coronary artery disease, cerebrovascular disease, peripheral vascular disease), microangiopathy (retinopathy, nephropathy), and central nervous system disorder (autonomic nervous system neuropathy, peripheral neuropathy)

      f. Etiology

        i. IDDM: autoimmune, viral, genetic

        ii. NIDDM: genetic, obesity

      g. Treatment: diet, oral hypoglycemic agents, (not with IDDM) insulin, exercise

      h. Perioperative significance

        i. Ultimate goal is to mimic normal metabolism, avoid hypoglycemia, excessive hyperglycemia, ketoacidosis, and electrolyte disturbances

        ii. Patients will require glucose containing IV solutions to prevent hypoglycemia and insulin to prevent ketosis and hyperglycemia

          (a) Goal: blood glucose level of 120–180 mg/dL

        iii. Diabetic patients ideally scheduled early in the day to avoid prolonged NPO

        iv. Continue insulin on the day of surgery (some physicians request half normal dose—check facility policy); alternative is to hold insulin on day of surgery and to monitor blood glucose levels during surgery

        v. Oral hypoglycemic agents commonly held as hypoglycemia common without caloric intake

        vi. Obtain preoperative ECG, electrolytes, glucose (may vary with facility policy)

          (a) Most common cause of perioperative morbidity in diabetic patients is ischemic heart disease

        vii. Presence of autonomic nervous system dysfunction may increase risk of aspiration and cardiovascular instability

        viii. Peripheral neuropathy may influence selection of regional anesthesia

        ix. Limited joint mobility and obesity may make intubation difficult

        x. IV solutions commonly contain potassium

        xi. All supplemental insulin to be given IV to prevent unpredictable subcutaneous absorption

  B. Adrenocortical insufficiency (Addison's disease)

    1. Definition: inadequate secretion of aldosterone and testosterone caused by partial or complete destruction of the adrenal glands

    2. Incidence: 4/100,000; all ages; females >males

    3. Significance: endocrine and metabolic alterations

    4. Etiology: autoimmune, tuberculosis, AIDS, adrenal hemorrhage in anticoagulated patient

    5. Treatment: corticosteroid replacement

    6. Perioperative significance:

      a. Steroid dose may be increased for patients undergoing surgical procedure as patients are unable to increase release of endogenous cortisol to meet physiologic stress; can lead to cardiovascular collapse

      b. Most minor ambulatory procedures require no change of steroid dose

      c. Instruct patient to take steroid medication on morning of surgery

VIII. Hematologic Diseases

  A. Anemia

    1. Definition: deficiency of erythrocytes (red blood cells)

      a. Females: hemoglobin <11.5 g/dL (hematocrit 36%)

      b. Males: hemoglobin <12.5 g/dL (hematocrit 40%)

2. Incidence: common
3. Significance: will compromise oxygen delivery to cells
4. Etiology: iron deficiency (infants and small children only); chronic disease (GI bleed, menstrual loss); thalassemia (decreased synthesis of normal hemoglobin)
5. Treatment: ferrous sulfate; address source if chronic loss
6. Perioperative significance
   a. No minimally accepted standard of hemoglobin concentration required for surgery
   b. Low hemoglobin does not require transfusion
   c. Low hemoglobin does not compromise wound healing
   d. Low hemoglobin does not increase the risk of infection
   e. Decision to transfuse intended only to increase the oxygen-carrying capacity
      i. Patients with compromised oxygenation are not candidates for ambulatory surgery
B. Sickle cell anemia
   1. Definition: chronic hemoglobinopathy with varying quantities of hemoglobin-S (normal is hemoglobin A), resulting in vascular occlusion and compromised tissue oxygenation
   2. Incidence: sickle cell trait 8–10% of all African-Americans (defined as Hgb-S concentration <50%), 0.2% of all African-Americans with sickle cell disease (Hgb-S 70–98%), 1/500 African-Americans
      a. Also present in persons from India and Saudi Arabia
   3. Significance: characterized by chronic hemolysis (anemia) and acute vaso-occlusive crisis that causes organ failure and can be life-threatening
   4. Etiology: inherited, autosomal recessive
   5. Treatment: minimize factors that cause sickling, including hypoxia, acidosis, hypothermia, Hgb concentration <8.5 g/dL, dehydration, pain, infection
   6. Perioperative significance
      a. Patients in sickle cell crisis inappropriate for ambulatory surgery
      b. Patients with sickle cell trait not at increased risk during perioperative period
      c. Patient with sickle cell disease must be free of infection, hydrated, and hemodynamically stable preoperatively
      d. Obtain sickle cell lab test in all African-Americans under age 15
         i. If by age 15 patient has never been tested nor diagnosed, can omit
         ii. Most commonly diagnosed in childhood
      e. Anesthetic goal: avoid acidosis secondary to hypoventilation, maintain oxygenation, prevent circulatory stasis, maintain body temperature
      f. Postoperative goal: maintain oxygenation, maintain intravascular fluid volume, maintain body temperature, utilize analgesics
C. The anticoagulated patient
   1. Definition: administration of oral anticoagulant to induce alterations in coagulation to prevent thrombus formation
   2. Incidence: used in patients with synthetic heart valves, history of atrial fibrillation, sinus arrhythmia with enlarged left atrium, left ventricular dysfunction, CHF, history of thrombolic events
   3. Significance: concomitant valve disease/replacement
   4. Etiology: Coumadin therapy alone or with aspirin or dipyridamole
   5. Treatment: discontinue drug, vitamin K
   6. Perioperative significance
      a. Increased risk of surgical bleeding
      b. Coumadin ideally stopped 3 days before elective procedure
         i. May not be possible for patients with prosthetic valves

     c. Obtain day of surgery prothrombin time (PT)

     d. Consider bleeding time/platelet count

     e. Inquire about the use of aspirin and NSAIDs in addition to Coumadin use

     f. Increased risk of CVA with atrial fibrillation patients off Coumadin

IX. Infectious Diseases

A. HIV Infection/AIDS

1. Definition: destruction of lymphocytes with decline in immune function
2. Incidence: >250,000 infectious persons; young adults 25–44; males >females
3. Significance: increased risk of opportunistic infections in CNS, GI tract, lungs (TB)
4. Etiology: human immunodeficiency virus spread via sexual activity, blood transfusions, IV drug use, fetal transmission, needle stick
5. Treatment: none known; supportive, some disease-slowing with investigational drug therapy
6. Perioperative significance
   a. Meticulous attention to universal precautions
   b. Chest X-ray to rule out interstitial pneumonitis
   c. Must consider extent of organ system involvement when approving ambulatory status (pneumonia, dementia, cardiomyopathy, renal dysfunction)
   d. Asymptomatic patient who is HIV positive will respond in normal manner to anesthetic agents

B. Tuberculosis (TB)

1. Definition: bacterial pulmonary infection characterized by asymptomatic conversion of a TB skin test or presence of fever and nonproductive cough in an "at-risk" patient
2. Incidence: 100/100,000 population; males >females; increased risk with HIV positive patients, homeless, prisoners, Asian immigrants
3. Significance: can affect bones, joints, meninges, kidney, and skin
4. Etiology: mycobacterium tuberculosis via aerosol transmission
5. Treatment: isoniazid, rifampin, pyrazinamide, streptomycin in combination varying with severity of disease
6. Perioperative significance
   a. Highest risk of disease is within 8–12 weeks of exposure
   b. Rifampin colors urine, tears, and secretions orange
   c. Isoniazid can cause peripheral neuritis/hypersensitivity—can prevent with pyridoxine
   d. Compliance issues predominate with number of drugs/length of treatment
   e. Not infectious after 2 weeks of therapy and negative AFB culture
   f. Chest X-ray will show infiltrate with or without effusion
   g. Homeless patients will have significant discharge limitations
   h. Patients with active TB require respiratory isolation

X. Substance Abuse

A. Illicit Drug Use

1. Definition: self-administration of drug(s) that deviate(s) from accepted medical or social use, which, if sustained, can lead to physical and psychologic dependence
2. Incidence: varies with drug; includes cocaine, opioids, barbiturates, benzodiazepines, amphetamines, marijuana, hallucinogens
3. Significance: physical withdrawal requires inpatient hospitalization—should not be attempted in perioperative period
4. Etiology: biologic, social, environmental, psychologic factors

5. Treatment: medical management of withdrawal, behavioral, and supportive counseling
6. Perioperative significance
   a. Can manifest cross tolerance to drugs making it difficult to predict anesthetic and/or analgesic requirements; usually increased
   b. May have concomitant problems of HIV, hepatitis, TB, malnutrition
   c. Frequently has associated personality disorders
   d. Patients acutely affected by substances are not candidates for ambulatory surgery

XI. **Obesity**
   A. Definition: weight >20% of ideal body weight
      1. Morbidly obese: double normal body weight
   B. Incidence: 20–30% of adult men, 30–40% of adult women; females >males; all ages
   C. Significance: may have concomitant heart disease, diabetes, pulmonary insufficiency
   D. Etiology: food intake >energy expenditure; genetic, endocrine
   E. Treatment: medically supervised weight loss with nutritional counseling, increase exercise/activity
   F. Perioperative significance
      1. Increased risk of aspiration; administer metoclopramide, H-2 antagonist
      2. Decreased use of positive pressure ventilation to pre-oxygenate to prevent distention and vomiting
      3. Increased difficulty in intubation
      4. May be chronically hypoxemic and hypercarbic; sleep apnea common
      5. Increased duration of action of lipid-soluble drugs
      6. Increased morbidity due to cardiovascular disease
      7. Increased risk of deep venous thrombosis—consider anti-embolism precautions
      8. Increased risk of wound infection

Bibliography

1. Aker, J. (1993). Assessment and care planning for the cardiac patient undergoing non-cardiac surgery. *Anesthesia Today*, 5(1):8–11.
2. Burden, N. (1994). *Ambulatory Surgical Nursing*. Philadelphia: Saunders.
3. Brooks-Brunn, J. (1995). Minimizing pulmonary complications. *Heart and Lung*, 24(2):94–115.
4. Dambro, M. (1995). *Griffith's 5 Minute Clinical Consult*. Philadelphia: Lee and Fiberger.
5. Litwack, K. (1995). *Post Anesthesia Care Nursing*, 2nd ed. St. Louis: Mosby-Yearbook.
6. Litwack, K. (1995). *Postoperative Pulmonary Complications*. Sacramento: CME Resource.
7. McGoldrick, K. (1995). *Ambulatory Anesthesiology*. Baltimore: Williams and Wilkins.
8. Passannante, A. (1993). Anesthesia for the morbidly obese. *Welcome Trends in Anesthesiology*, 11(2):3–10.
9. Reilly, M. (1993). Anesthesia assessment and considerations for the patient with chronic pulmonary disease. *Anesthesia Today*, 4(4):12–16.
10. Stoelting, R., Dierdorf, S. (1993). *Anesthesia and Coexisting Disease*, 3rd ed. New York: Churchill-Lingstone.
11. Vender, J., Spiess, B. (1992). *Post Anesthesia Care*. Philadelphia: Saunders.

REVIEW QUESTIONS

1. Triggers for sickling for a patient with sickle cell anemia in the postoperative period include

   A. Incisional pain, hypoxemia, pulmonary infection

   B. Oxygen therapy, hypothermia, alkalosis

   C. Acidosis, vasodilation, infection

   D. Malignant hyperthermia, sepsis, aspiration

2. Which signs of congestive heart failure seen in the preoperative patient warrant cancellation of the case with referral to a cardiologist?

   A. Profound diuresis, low serum osmolality, polydipsia
   B. Syncope, orthostatic hypotension, fatigue
   C. Shortness of breath, jugular venous distension, rales
   D. Headache, polyuria, hyperglycemia

3. The drug class of choice for a patient with an acute asthma attack are

   A. Corticosteroids
   B. Beta agonists
   C. H-2 antagonists
   D. Antibiotics

4. Patients with which of the following pre-existing medical conditions are at an increased risk for congestive heart failure?

   A. Chronic persistent hepatitis
   B. Valvular heart disease
   C. Asthma
   D. Tuberculosis

5. The major predisposing factor for chronic obstructive pulmonary disease is

   A. Asthma
   B. Environmental exposure to pollutants
   C. Asbestos exposure
   D. Cigarette smoking

6. Preoperative management of a patient with chronic renal failure includes all of the following except

   A. Estimates of blood volume status
   B. Consideration of concomitant drug therapy
   C. Administration of supplemental insulin
   D. Continuation of antihypertensive therapy

7. The principle goal in the management of anesthesia for the diabetic patient includes avoiding all of the following except

   A. Hypoglycemia
   B. Excessive hyperglycemia
   C. Ketoacidosis
   D. A blood glucose level of 140 mg/dL

8. Which of the following statements is true concerning the obese patient?

   A. The risk of wound infection is increased
   B. The increased functional residual capacity of the obese patient suggests spontaneous ventilation intraoperatively
   C. The use of positive end expiratory pressure will increase cardiac output, thereby improving peripheral perfusion
   D. The supine position optimizes ventilation

9. The classic triad characterizing Parkinson's disease includes

   A. Bradykinesia, resting tremor, rigidity
   B. Polyuria, polydipsia, fatigue
   C. Epistaxis, nocturia, dysphagia
   D. Weakness, pseudohypertrophy of muscles, kyphosis

10. Which of the following statements about anemia is true?

   A. No patient should be admitted for surgery without a hemoglobin level of at least 12 g/dL
   B. Anesthetic drugs that reduce cardiac output will improve peripheral tissue oxygenation
   C. Shivering and hypothermia will increase the body's total requirements for oxygen
   D. Wound healing will be particularly problematic in the presence of moderate anemia

ANSWERS TO QUESTIONS

1.	A	6.	C
2.	C	7.	D
3.	B	8.	A
4.	B	9.	A
5.	D	10.	C

13

Fluid and Electrolyte Balance and Hematologic Considerations

Kathy Carlson
Abbott Northwestern Hospital
Minneapolis, Minnesota

I. **Fluid and Electrolyte Balance: Outpatient Issues**
   A. Assess clinical status with laboratory tests before ambulatory surgery
      1. Necessary only when warranted by a patient's health needs, medications, coexisting disease, and medical history, age, or physical examination
      2. Currently, there is no consensus that *any* lab measures are truly required for healthy, asymptomatic patients
      3. Presurgical assessment for ambulatory surgery parallels requirements for inpatient surgery to assure a given patient can safely withstand the stress of anesthesia and surgery
   B. Fluid, chemical, and hematologic considerations when determining a patient's acceptability for ambulatory surgery
      1. Surgical procedure will not induce extensive physiologic fluid or electrolyte shifts
      2. No large blood loss or infusion of fluid volume is anticipated
         a. Large blood loss is often associated with unplanned hospital admission
         b. Anticipated need for blood transfusion is a debatable issue

      i. Some surgeons transfuse autologous blood after liposuction, for example

      ii. For preterm infants less than 60 weeks of age, a hematocrit less than 30% increases risk of apnea

  3. *Before* the day of surgery, the patient's preoperative biochemical condition and organ function status are determined to be *stable*

    a. No increased risk of perianesthetic crisis is foreseen

    b. Increasingly, even aged and ASA classification III and IV patients are accepted for ambulatory surgery

    c. Clinically relevant laboratory tests—determined by clinical, surgical, or anesthetic need—are within normal limits (see Table 13–1)

    d. If no new clinical events occur, baseline assessment and lab results are considered acceptable for 3–6 weeks

    e. Verify stable fluid status and update specific tests, particularly potassium and glucose, on the day of surgery to detect any suspected new abnormalities

Table 13–1 • CLINICAL INDICATORS FOR PREANESTHETIC LABORATORY ASSESSMENT

OBTAIN PREOPERATIVE TEST	TO ASSESS
Potassium* if	
potassium-depleting diuretics	**hypokalemia:** lethal cardiac dysrhythmia
digoxin, especially with toxicity	
corticosteroids	
preoperative colon preparation or laxative	
chronic renal failure	**acidosis, hyperkalemia:** muscle weakness, including respiratory; metabolic dysfunction
Electrolyte panel and chemistries if	
renal failure	hyperkalemia, acidosis, BUN, and creatinine increases potential for renal failure
diabetes	
cardiopulmonary disease	renal function, acidosis
chemotherapy	
Glucose*	
diabetes mellitus	baseline preoperative status when insulin dependent, recheck preop
chronic corticosteroid use	possible hyperglycemia, need for insulin
Hemoglobin, Hematocrit	
infants less than one year old	normal physiologic anemia
renal disease	chronic anemia, suppressed RBC manufacture
anticoagulants	unrecognized bleeding potential and determine baseline status
malignancy, radiation/chemotherapy	suppressed bone marrow function, RBCs
use of nonsteroidal antiinflammatories	mild anemia
Coagulation: PT/PTT/INR/Platelets	
chronic anticoagulation	great risk of excessive or prolonged bleeding
warfarin stopped at least 3–7 days preop	risk of **intraspinal bleed** if spinal anesthetic *verify return to normal parameters*
chronic aspirin or nonsteroidal	altered platelet function
antiinflammatory drugs (NSAIDs)	potential for prolonged postsurgical bleeding —unresearched, but risk presumed less likely if risk of intraoperative bleeding is low

*Some recommend potassium and glucose values be updated on day of surgery.

■ BOX 13–1.   Perianesthetic Consideration: Fluids and Postoperative Nausea

Administering oral fluid too soon actually precipitates nausea; ability to tolerate oral fluids is no longer a discharge criterion in many facilities. The incidence of nausea, thirst, and vertigo has been reduced by liberal administration of IV fluid to build intravascular volume.

    C. "Routine" laboratory tests: questioning need vs. cost
       1. Today, a battery of "routine" laboratory tests for every surgical candidate is judged costly and medically unnecessary
       2. Studies have demonstrated that even new abnormal lab findings in asymptomatic patients *rarely* cause surgery to be canceled
         a. False-positive abnormal results in healthy, asymptomatic patients create undue concern, increase costs, and/or surgical delays
       3. Medical staff of individual facility establishes protocols for laboratory testing; appropriate preoperative labs remain a controversial, highly scrutinized issue
    D. Postanesthetic hydration and chemical concerns
       1. Infusing moderate volumes of isotonic IV fluid maintains fluid balance intraoperatively and postoperatively
       2. Postoperative nausea and vomiting (PONV) increases potential for hypovolemia, significantly delays discharge to home, and increases cost of care
         a. Infants, children, and elderly patients dehydrate easily
         b. Unrelenting, protracted vomiting can result in clinically significant chemical imbalances and result in hospital readmission
         c. Laparoscopy, strabismus correction, and surgery in the ear are highly associated with PONV

II. Physiologic Fluid Balance
    A. Body fluid compartments
       1. Extracellular Fluid (ECF)
         a. Location: fluid circulating *outside* of cells
           i. Intravascular fluid: blood and plasma equal about ⅓ of ECF volume
           ii. Interstitial fluid: fluid between cells equal about ⅔ of ECF volume
           iii. Transcellular fluid: present in cerebrospinal, intraocular, and gastric fluids
       2. Intracellular Fluid (ICF)
         a. Location: fluid *within* cells
         b. Contains nearly ⅔ of body's total water, or about 25 liters
       3. Factors influencing water distribution, which is regulated by osmosis
         a. Obesity and aging decrease total body water
         b. ECF comprises proportionately greater volume of child's body weight
         c. Water comprises nearly 75% of newborn's weight
         d. A woman's body contains a higher proportion of fat than a man's and so, less water
    B. Components distributed within body water
       1. Electrolytes: electrically active ions with either a positive or negative charge when dissolved in solution (See Table 13–2)
         a. Primary electrolytes in ECF
           i. Cation: positively charged ion
              (a) Sodium (Na^+)
           ii. Anion: negatively charged ion
              (a) Chloride (Cl^-)
              (b) Bicarbonate: (HCO_3^-)

Table 13–2 • PRIMARY ELECTROLYTES OF THE ECF AND ICF*

ECF ION	NORMAL SERUM VALUE	INDICATORS	
		DEFICIT (HYPO-)	EXCESS (HYPER-)
Sodium (Na^+) *regulates ECF osmolality and vascular fluid volume *active transport via sodium pump—to sustain high intracellular K^+	135–145 mEq/L	*Hyponatremia* *<130 mEq/L ↓ serum osmolality *salt diluted by excess retained water —bladder irrigations —electrolyte-free IVs —ADH oversecretion *Outcomes:* *weak muscles *confusion *nausea/vomiting *hypotension, seizure *coma if <115 mEq/L	*Hypernatremia* *>145mEq/L ↑ serum osmolality *excess salt from —water loss —inadequate osmotic diuresis —poor fluid intake *Outcomes:* *thirst *flushed skin *hypotension *oliguria *seizures, coma if extreme
Chloride (Cl^-) *preserve acid-base balance *reciprocal: if Cl^- depleted, HCO_3^- rises *combines w/ sodium to maintain osmolality	96–106 mEq/L	*Hypochloremia* *<98mEq/L *prolonged Cl^- loss gastric suction, diuresis *Metabolic Alkalosis* *patient hypoventilates	*Hyperchloremia* *>108 mEq/L *Cl^- gain *Metabolic Acidosis* *patient hyperventilates
Bicarbonate (HCO_3^-)	24–28 mEq/L	*Metabolic Alkalosis* *pH >7.45* *patient hypoventilates	*Metabolic Acidosis* *pH <7.35 *patient hyperventilates *hyperkalemia occurs
Osmolality (mOsm)	280–300/Osm/Kg	*Dehydration* *ECF concentrated	*Overhydration* *ECF dilute
Potassium (K^+) *ECF content small *potent effect on cell neuromuscular irritability *acidosis, catabolism move K^+ to serum *insulin, glucose shift K^+ back to cell	3.5–5.0 mEq/L	*Hypokalemia* *<3.5 mEq/L *reflects ECF loss* —diuretics —diarrhea, vomit —digitalis —bowel preps *if ECF depleted, ICF is also *muscle weakness *hypoventilation *flaccid paralysis *cardiac arrhythmias —more PVCs —U wave classic —conduction blocks *slow KCl doses*	*Hyperkalemia* *>5.0 mEq/L *gain in serum* —tissue lysis —acidosis from: —renal —diabetes —MH **CAN BE LETHAL** *muscle weakness *hypoventilates *paralysis *arryhthmias —peaked T wave —wide QRS —asystole *stat *insulin* carries K^+ back to ICF *dialyze renal patients *stop any K^+ intake

(Table continued on following page)

Table 13–2 • PRIMARY ELECTROLYTES OF THE ECF AND ICF* *Continued*

ECF ION	NORMAL SERUM VALUE	INDICATORS	
		DEFICIT (HYPO-)	EXCESS (HYPER-)
Magnesium (Mg^+) *promotes Ach release at neuromuscular junction *regulates K^+ *opposes Ca^{++}	1.5–2.5 mEq/L	*Hypomagnesemia* *<1.5 mEq/L **Causes:* —diarrhea, malabsorption —long-term vomiting —excess aldosterone **Signs:* *neuromuscular irritability *Cardiac: long PR wide QRS, flat T *K^+, Ca^{++}, and PO_4^-	*Hypermagnesemia* *>2.5 mEq/L **Causes:* —$MgSO_4$ infusion —ketoacidosis —chronic renal failure **Signs:* *CNS depression —sedation —muscle weakness *hypotension, bradycardia *if Mg^+ >12, hypoventilation
Phosphate (PO_4^-) *most stored in bone *essential for energy & acid-base balance *inverse relationship w/calcium: if $PO_4^-\uparrow$, $Ca^{++}\downarrow$ *need parathyroid hormone (PTH) to excrete	1–2 mEq/L (3–4.5 mg/dL)	*Hypophosphatemia* *<1.5 mg/dL **Causes:* —aspirin overdose —ketoacidosis —malabsorption —steroids —hypercalcemia *Outcome *energy depletion: —weak muscle —seizures —cardio-resp failure	*Hyperphosphatemia* *>4.5 mg/dL **Causes:* *laxative excess *supplement in diet *trauma *Outcome *cell death —renal failure —PTH decreases
Calcium (Ca^{++}) *Critical for —impulse conduction —cardiac contraction —coagulation *is stored in bone *present in blood (ECF): —ionized (50%) —protein bound *reciprocal relationship with phosphorus: when $Ca^{++}\uparrow$, $PO_4^-\downarrow$	4.5–5.3 mEq/L (8.5–10.5 mg/dL)	*Hypocalcemia* *<4.5 mEq/L **Causes:* —low albumin —renal failure (chronic) —hypoparathyroidism *Symptoms —tingling/weakness —twitching/tetany —low BP/EKG change —**postop laryngospasm**	*Hypercalcemia* *>4.5 mEq/L *Causes:* —immobility —malignancy —low PO_4^- —hyperparathyroidism *Symptoms —lethargy —short QT

*Electrolytes found in high concentration in ECF are in low concentration in ICF; similarly, the primary electrolytes of the ICF are present, but in low concentrations, in the ECF.

   b. Primary electrolytes in ICF
      i. Cations:
         (a) Potassium (K^+)
         (b) Magnesium (Mg^+)
      ii. Anions
         (a) Phosphorus (P), present in body fluid as Phosphate (PO_4)
         (b) A measure of the serum concentration of an electrolyte does not
             necessarily reflect the electrolyte content of intracellular electrolytes
 2. Undissolved particles: sugar, urea and protein are examples
   a. Large, osmotically active molecules
   b. Influence movement of water across permeable cell membranes
 3. Buffers: physiologic controls to regulate acids and bases
   a. Bicarbonate: immediate chemical buffer, present in ECF
      i. Regulate (buffer) pH by accepting or releasing acidic hydrogen ions (H^+)
      ii. Maintain serum's chemical neutrality, specifically pH = 7.4
      iii. Maintain a bicarbonate∶carbonic acid ratio of 20∶1 (See Table 13–3)
   b. Chemical buffers are present in all body fluids and include phosphate,
      hemoglobin, and protein
 4. Salts: potassium chloride (KCl) is one example
C. Forces of water distribution in the body
 1. Principles of water movement
   a. Water seeks to establish equilibrium between ECF and ICF
   b. Osmosis controls fluid movement between ECF and ICF
   c. Normal fluid balance requires both normal volume of water and normal
      concentrations of particles in solution
 2. Mechanisms of fluid distribution (See Table 13–4)
   a. Diffusion: movement of *particles* in solution across a semipermeable cell
      membrane from a concentrated solution toward a more dilute one
      i. Purpose: to equalize concentration of particles between compartments
      ii. Electrolytes are small and pass easily across cell walls
      iii. Though individual ions move randomly between ECF and ICF, net
           migration of ions is toward the dilute solution
      iv. Particle concentration and movement in solution affects water balance
   b. Osmosis: movement of *water* from a dilute space with few particles to a more
      densely concentrated space
      i. Purpose: to equalize compartment concentrations
      ii. Numbers and size of particles in ECF and ICF water often are unequal
         (a) Glucose, urea, and protein are large molecules that normally cannot pass
             from blood (ECF) through selectively permeable walls into cells (ICF)
         (b) Due to these large particles in the blood, ECF contains more particles
             (is more concentrated) than cells (ICF)
         (c) Net movement of water is toward the ECF, preventing cells from
             becoming waterlogged, edematous, and bursting
   c. Osmotic pressure: pressure exerted within a compartment by osmotically active
      particles in solution
      i. Differences in particle concentration between two compartments creates a
         concentration gradient
      ii. Pressure across this gradient moves (redirects) water across the gradient to
          equalize water between cells or fluid compartments
      iii. After water equilibrates, the concentrations of particles in solution become
           equal, but the volume of water in the compartments may not be equal

Table 13–3 • CARBONIC ACID REGULATION OF ACID-BASE BALANCE

Immediate response as directed by **Henderson-Hasselbach equation:**

Hydrogen + Bicarbonate $\rightleftarrows$ Carbonic Acid $\rightleftarrows$ Water + Carbon Dioxide

$$H^+ \quad + \quad HCO_3^- \quad \rightleftarrows \quad H_2CO_3 \quad \rightleftarrows H_2O + \quad CO_2$$

Acidic conditions (pH <7.35):	**Alkalotic** conditions (pH >7.45):
Bicarbonate ion is reabsorbed	Bicarbonate ion excreted
Recombines with hydrogen ion	Relative excess of hydrogen ion
Forms more carbonic acid	Less carbonic acid is formed

$H_2CO_3^-$ dissociates to water and CO_2

Respiratory rate & depth increase	Respiratory rate & depth decrease
CO_2 is exhaled (pCO$_2$ ↓)	CO_2 acccumulates (p$_a$CO$_2$ ↑)
pH restored (↑) toward 7.4	**pH restored (↓) toward 7.4**

    d. Osmolality: concentration of particles in serum, per kilogram
- i. Total number of "osmotically active" particles in a solution
  - (a) Reflected by concentration of serum sodium
  - (b) Water "follows" sodium to equalize concentration and establish equilibrium
- ii. Osmolality is primarily regulated by antidiuretic hormone (ADH)
  - (a) Released by the posterior pituitary
  - (b) Changes in osmolality sensed by baroreceptors at right atrium
  - (c) Stimulates aldosterone release which acts at the kidney to regulate sodium excretion or retention, and therefore water excretion or retention
  - (d) Secretion stimulated by stress such as pain, anesthetics, and surgery
- iii. Osmolality reflects body's hydration status (See Tables 13–5 and 13–6)
  - (a) Dehydration indicates ECF is concentrated; osmolality is high
    - (i) When serum sodium concentration is high, water shifts toward the area with high osmolality to dilute sodium and decrease the osmolality
    - (ii) Clinicians increasingly recognize that the significance of preoperative dehydration has been undervalued

Table 13–4 • REGULATORS OF FLUID & ELECTROLYTE EQUILIBRIUM

Diffusion:	Movement of *particles* like potassium or calcium through a cell's permeable wall from an area of high concentration to a lower concentration
Osmosis:	Movement of *water* from a dilute solution toward a more concentrated fluid
Concentration gradient:	Difference in concentration (**osmolality**) between two solutions that promotes fluid or, electrolyte movement
Osmotic pressure:	A physical force, determined by the number of particles in a solution (or its concentration), that causes water to move toward the concentrated solution
Oncotic pressure:	Osmotic force produced in vascular spaces by molecules like plasma proteins
Antidiuretic hormone (ADH):	Hypothalamic hormone released by the posterior pituitary gland in response to increased serum osmolality; ADH regulates **sodium** concentration and thereby the passive movement of water toward sodium

Table 13–5 • SYMPTOMS ASSOCIATED WITH CHEMICAL AND FLUID IMBALANCES

SYMPTOM	POSSIBLE CLINICAL SIGNIFICANCE
Cardiovascular	
Bounding pulse CVP, neck vein distention	Fluid overload, increased ECF
Weak or thready pulse	Dehydration, decreased ECF volume
Increased heart rate	May reflect fever, acidosis or ECF volume deficit
Irregular pulse	Cardiac arrhythmia—may signal $\downarrow K^+$
Hypotension, orthostatic	ECF volume deficit
Respiratory	
Increased rate and depth	Anxiety with hyperventilation can prompt respiratory alkalosis Perhaps compensation for retained carbon dioxide (acidosis)
Decreased rate and depth	Perhaps compensation for alkalosis and insufficient carbon dioxide Possible muscle weakness from $\uparrow Mg^+$ or $\downarrow K^+$ With somnolence, may signal oversedation
"Crackles" and rales at lung bases	Overhydration or cardiac congestion and failure
Neurologic	
Level of consciousness	Low or elevated sodium, dehydration, acid-base imbalance
Vertigo	ECF volume deficit
Muscle weakness	Severely elevated or low potassium, hypercalcemia, hypermagnesemia May reflect volume losses
Altered reflexes	Magnesium or calcium imbalance
Tingling	Hyperventilation with respiratory alkalosis Suspect calcium elevation
Excitability	Decreased calcium or magnesium
Skin	
Turgor at sternum	Dehydration if remains "tented" when pinched *Not reflective* of fluid status in elderly patients
Mucous membranes	Dryness may indicate ECF deficit

(iii) NPO status causes even the relatively healthy ambulatory surgery patient to be mildly dehydrated, perhaps about 5%
   a) Children can become significantly hypovolemic and hypoglycemic
   b) Preoperative deficit and surgical blood loss is replaced intraoperatively with an isotonic crystalloid solution (see Table 13–7)
(b) Overhydration indicates the ECF is dilute; osmolality decreases
   (i) When serum sodium concentration (osmolality) is low, water enters cells; serum sodium concentrates and osmolality increases
   (ii) Anesthetic medications ease the strain of fluid overload by dilating vasculature; ECF expands and diastolic filling in the heart improves

III. Physiologic Electrolyte Balance
   A. Principles of ion balance
      1. Balance is critical for normal cellular function, particularly for the anesthetic period (Refer to Table 13–2)
      2. Expect physiologic balance in the ambulatory surgery setting
      3. Selective presurgical assessment only (Refer to Table 13–1)
         a. Identify anesthetic and surgical risk related to individual patient's history and examination
         b. Some clinicians believe renal assessment with BUN and creatinine is indicated when a patient is elderly, has a systemic disease, or uses medications with potential for renal damage
      4. Noncritical illness and brief, elective procedures mean significant electrolyte imbalance is uncommon
      5. Potential imbalances may result from:
         a. Transient, mild respiratory acidemia related to anesthetic-induced hypoventilation and sedation
         b. Preoperative hypokalemia related to potassium-depleting pre-endoscopic bowel preparations or chronic medications such as diuretics or digoxin
         c. Physiologic stress related to surgery and a patient's anxiety alters homeostasis by increasing sodium and fluid retention

---

Table 13–6 • ISSUES OF FLUID IMBALANCE IN THE AMBULATORY SURGERY SETTING

POTENTIAL FOR DEHYDRATION	POTENTIAL FOR OVERHYDRATION

Extended preoperative NPO status
insufficient water intake relative to need
particular concern for infants, young children
clinical research reports:
   clear liquids safe until 2–4 hours preop
   —gastric volume and acidity normal
   —aspiration risk NOT increased
	Excessive fluid volume intake
	consumption greater than body's physiologic
	   capacity to circulate
	   —drinking or IV fluids
	   —inability to excrete water
	suspect renal failure
	insufficient ADH secretion
	break in cell wall integrity so proteins move freely
	   from ECF
	potential outcomes:
	   —tissue edema: pulmonary/peripheral
	   —dilutional serum hyponatremia
	   —congestive heart failure: increases perioperative
	    mortality risk by up to 50%

Fluid and electrolyte loss
postoperative nausea and vomiting (PONV)
   nearly ⅓ of surgical patients develop PONV
   effects are usually self-limiting within 24 hours
   children and elderly at particular risk for imbalance
   raises cost of care and patient dissatisfaction
diarrhea, enemas, and preoperative bowel cleansing
   preps
Increased serum osmolality
   extreme hyperglycemia in diabetics
   elevated BUN and creatinine with renal failure
   mannitol, hypertonic solutions or colloid
Inappropriate oversecretion of ADH
   endocrine disease, ventilators, cranial trauma	

Table 13–7 • CONSIDERATIONS FOR VOLUME REPLACEMENT

Purposes
- Replace insensible losses and restore volume from NPO deficit
- Infused volumes often are minimal in ambulatory surgery setting and primarily provide access for administering medications

Options

Isotonic solutions: reflect normal serum (ECF) osmolality
- Relatively little fluid moves between ECF and ICF
- 0.9% normal saline or lactated ringers are isotonic
  —approximately ⅔ redistributes into the ICF
  —⅓ remains in ECF
- Typically used for healthy patients undergoing elective surgery
  —Practitioners differ in preference for balanced electrolyte solution (lactated ringers) or physiologic saline (0.9 NS)

Hypotonic solutions: contains fewer particles than ECF
- More dilute so osmolality is lower than body fluid
- Water moves into ICF by osmosis, expanding water available to cells
- 0.45% normal saline or D_5W are hypotonic
- Glucose-containing solutions
  —Provide small amount of glucose for metabolic energy
  —May add to rise in serum glucose already elevated by physiologic stress response

Hypertonic solutions: contain more particles than ECF
- More concentrated than body fluids, so osmolality is higher
- Water is drawn by osmosis into the more concentrated compartment
  —ECF expands; water available in ICF shrinks
  —mannitol, 10% dextrose and water, blood, or plasma expanders like albumin, dextran and hetastarch are hypertonic
- Colloid seldom necessary and is controversial in ambulatory setting
  —boluses of isotonic crystalloid are usually adequate to treat hypotension

Volume Replacement
- Purpose: sufficient to support blood pressure, circulation, and urine volume
- During elective, outpatient surgery, significant fluid and electrolyte imbalance are rare
  —Replacement of volume deficits is calculated at 2–4 ml/Kg per hour

---

BOX 13–2.   Perianesthetic Consideration: Dehydration

Anesthesia decreases circulation and blunts compensatory sympathetic reflexes. Giving spinal, epidural, or general anesthesia to a dehydrated patient obliterates the vasoconstriction and slight heart rate increase that sustains blood pressure. **Profound hypotension** can occur if volume deficit is not replaced before anesthesia.

BOX 13–3.   Perianesthetic Consideration: Overhydration

History of congestive heart failure, or the heart's inability to effectively circulate the fluid volume in the vascular space (ECF), increases a patient's anesthetic mortality risk to an estimated 6%. Fulminant cardiogenic pulmonary edema during the postoperative period increases to over 15% in patients whose heart failure is uncorrected, compared with only 2% of patients with no cardiovascular disease.

> **BOX 13-4.   Perianesthetic Consideration: Electrolyte Balance**
>
> Administering anesthesia to a patient with electrolyte abnormalities seriously increases the risk of complication. Cardiac rhythm and contractility, neurologic conduction, and muscle strength all depend on electrolyte balance. Correct serum imbalances prior to induction, even though such intervention often delays or even cancels surgery.

      6. Most ambulatory surgery facilities have capability to monitor hemoglobin, hematocrit, and glucose

  B. Mechanics of electrolyte distribution

    1. Principles of ion movement

      a. Ions in solution passively move to achieve equilibrium between ECF and ICF

      b. Diffusion: movement of ions through the selectively permeable cell wall due to a difference in concentration between two areas; this difference is defined as a concentration gradient

        i. Ion (particle) movement occurs from the more concentrated solution to the less concentrated solution until the particle concentrations are equal

        ii. Physiologic factors within the body prevent major electrolytes in ECF and ICF from ever equalizing

          (a) Sodium pump

          (b) Large concentration gradients

IV. Hematology and Coagulation: Outpatient Issues

  A. Preoperative clinical assessment with laboratory tests

    1. Alterations can affect surgical outcomes, particularly related to tissue oxygenation and hemostasis

      a. Critically assess a patient's potential for anemia and coagulopathy

      b. Determine by reviewing clinical indications and medical history

      c. An absolute minimum value for presurgical hemoglobin has not been established

      d. Routine hemoglobin screening, though low cost, is neither required nor recommended for all preoperative patients (See Table 13–8)

      e. Preoperative hemoglobin is selectively recommended for:

        i.   Neonates to detect physiologic anemia

        ii. Elderly patients and menstruating women

        iii. Patients with bone marrow suppression, malignancy, or genetically determined anemic conditions

      f. A patient with a documented coagulation disorder is seldom an appropriate candidate for surgery in the nonacute ambulatory setting, although preanesthetic screening may uncover a patient's previously unrecognized coagulopathy

    2. When preoperative hemoglobin is low, continuing with surgery-as-planned is often decided by the acuity of anemia, patient's cardiopulmonary response, and any surgical urgency

  B. Hemoglobin

    1. Definition: transports oxygen to tissues via red blood cells (RBCs)

    2. Physiology

      a. RBC production is stimulated by erythropoetin which is produced by the kidney

      b. RBCs are actually produced in bone marrow and removed by the spleen

      c. Life span is approximately 120 days

    3. Perianesthetic concerns

      a. Sufficient RBC numbers to bind oxygen for delivery to tissues

Table 13–8 • PREANESTHETIC LABS: HEMATOLOGY AND COAGULATION

ASSESSMENT	NORMAL VALUES	CLINICAL SIGNIFICANCE
Hemoglobin (Hgb) *Essential carrier to transport oxygen to cells	14–18 gm/dL (men) 12–16 gm/dL (women)	Determine **anemia** **polycythemia**
Leukocyte (WBC) *immune response *indicate infection *significant increase *or* decrease may affect whether surgery proceeds	5,000–10,000	**leukocytosis:** reactive increase in number: response to infection, inflammation, or foreign body **leukopenia:** reduced number of circulating WBCs; indicate bone marrow suppression, chemotherapy, irradiation **Immunity altered:** increased infection risk
Prothrombin Time (PT) *monitor response to coumadin *often reflected as **International Normalized Ratio (INR)** —standardized calculation to adjust for lab inconsistency	12–16 seconds 1.0	Perioperative bleeding if INR prolonged; treatment with **Vitamin K** occurs over hours
Partial Thromboplastin Time (PTT) *monitor **heparin** therapy	30–45 seconds	Reverses spontaneously when heparin doses cease
Thrombin Time (TT) *assess thrombin activity and conversion of fibrinogen to fibrin	9–11 seconds	Indicates ability to form fibrin clot
Platelets *bleeding protection *both function and number important	150–400,000 mm^3	Required to support fibrin clot for lasting hemostasis —minimum: 50,000 mm^3 —medications affect function —life expectancy: 2 weeks

> b. A safe minimum hemoglobin measure is not absolutely established
> > i. Hemoglobin of 9–10 gm/dL is desired
> > ii. Anesthesia safely administered to patients with hemoglobin of 6–7 gm/dL
> > > (a) Patients with chronic renal failure whose erythropoetin is suppressed
> > > (b) Acutely ill Jehovah Witnesses who refuse blood on religious principles
> > > (c) Acute anemia is unlikely to occur in ambulatory surgery setting
> 4. Anemia: Hemoglobin or RBC deficit
> > a. Cardiovascular symptoms: vary with hemoglobin level and acuity of cell loss
> > > i. Acute loss produces more symptoms than chronic, possibly compensated loss
> > > ii. Decreasing oxygen saturation (SpO$_2$) during perianesthesia period
> > > iii. Hypotension, perhaps indicated by orthostatic changes
> > > iv. Tachycardia likely as compensatory way to sustain cardiac output
> > > > (a) Consider hypovolemia when perianesthetic patient's heart rate increases
> > > > > (i) A multipurpose indicator representing a response by sympathetic nerves of the autonomic system
> > > > > (ii) Also increases with stress, anxiety, fever

             (b) Patients with transplanted hearts cannot respond with tachycardia
                (i)   Denervated transplanted hearts lack autonomic responses
                (ii) Resting heart rate is approximately 100–110 beats/minute
                (iii) Fluid volume used to support preload and cardiac output

  b. Causes of hemoglobin loss
     i.   Hemorrhagic: trauma, surgical loss, gastrointestinal, uterine, nasal, vascular
     ii. Inadequate RBC production
        (a) Insufficient vitamin B_{12} for erythropoesis: pernicious anemia
        (b) Endocrine factors
           (i)   Insufficient erythropoetin production in chronic renal failure
           (ii) Inadequate intake of folic acid or iron: malnutrition
               a) Malignancy
               b) Malabsorption
               c) Dietary lack
           (iii) Hemodilution from fluid volume expansion: pregnancy
        (c) Bone marrow suppression
           (i)   Irradiation or chemical exposure: aplasia
           (ii) Chronic disease
               a) Infection, lupus erythematosis, steroids
               b) About 15% of asymptomatic HIV positive patients are anemic
        (d) Genetic predisposition: recessive traits alter a link in the chain of hemoglobin formation
           (i)   Mutation produces hemolytic anemias such as:
               a) Sickle cell anemia (See Table 13–9)
               b) Thalassemia: severe beta (Coley's) form predisposes to early death
    iii. Increased RBC destruction: impaired RBC function or jaundice-causing hemolysis
        (a) Pharmaceuticals, infections, burns, excessive physical stress
        (b) Cell trauma or consumption: prosthetic heart valves, blood pumps
  c. Perianesthesia nursing considerations and interventions related to anemia
     i.   Assure adequate oxygenation
        (a) Position the patient for lung expansion
        (b) Deliver supplemental oxygen
        (c) Support cardiac output
           (i)   Hydration with crystalloid, colloid if necessary
           (ii) Measure hemoglobin, particularly if oxygen saturation decreases
     ii. Limit oxygen demand
        (a) Reduce stress
        (b) Manage pain
    iii. Prevent hypotension
        (a) Support cardiac output
        (b) Identify orthostatic effects
           (i)   Gradually change position toward upright
           (ii) Note hypotension and mild tachycardia with position change

5. Polycythemia: exaggerated RBC, hemoglobin, hematocrit production
  a. Increased RBC production unrelated to erythropoetin level
     i.   One form (p. vera) occurs primarily in adults over 60 years
     ii. Significantly increases blood volume and viscosity, engorges veins
    iii. Hypertension, cardiac arrhythmia, thrombosis, tissue hypoxia can result
  b. Physiologic response by bone marrow to increased erythropoetin release
     i.   Adaptive response to altitude: normal compensation to environment

Table 13–9 • SICKLE CELL ANEMIA: PREDISPOSED BY HEREDITY

Genetic Characteristics:
  *Specific stimuli cause RBCs to alter shape and function
  *Formation of abnormal HbS rather than normal HbA
  *Trait carried by 10% of African-Americans (HbAS)
  *Disease affects fewer than 1% of African-Americans (HbSS)
Clinical Concern: HbS has decreased affinity for oxygen
  *Oxygen deficit causes cells to change shape and sickle (become concave)
  *Hemolytic anemia: hemolysis reduces RBC life to 10–15 days
  *Sickled cells rupture or clog small vessels
  *A sickling crisis can be stimulated during the perianesthesia period by:
    —Altered temperature (fever or cold)
    —Acidosis and hypoventilation
    —Dehydration (sluggish circulation, peripheral thrombosis, and infarction)
Clinical Outcomes
  *Ischemic pain, especially in limbs, joints, bones, and abdomen
  *Increased susceptibility to infection, limb ulcerations, and necrosis
  *Cerebral changes, altered renal function, and cardiopulmonary compromise related to infarction
Nursing Responses Focus on Prevention
  *Assure oxygenation: prevent hypoventilation and acidosis
    —Monitor respiratory quality, rate, and depth
    —Supplemental oxygen to maintain oxygen saturation and pO_2
    —Determine adequate reversal of muscle relaxants
    —Position patient for effective lung expansion
    —Early postoperative mobility
  *Promote peripheral circulation: minimize vasoconstriction
    —Maintain normothermia
    —Assure adequate hydration for blood flow and reduce blood viscosity
    —Regularly assess ischemia: limit peripheral blood stagnation
  *Reduce stress
    —Adequate analgesia
    —Prevent or control infection
    —Create a calming environment
  *Interview patients about family history and clinical symptoms
    —Preoperative exchange transfusions may precede some surgeries to build hematocrit to 40% and increase capacity for oxygenation

---

      ii. Pharmaceutically induced with parenteral erythropoetin in patients with chronic renal failure
      iii. To compensate perceived hypoxemia associated with chronic cardiopulmonary conditions
         (a) Valvular or structural cardiac anomalies impede cardiac outflow and therefore oxygen delivery to tissue
         (b) Pulmonary obstructive diseases like asthma, emphysema
   C. Leukocytes
     1. Definition: white blood cells (WBCs)
     2. Physiology: mediate immune response with assorted WBC types
     3. Leukocytosis: production *increases* to more than 10,000/mm^2 of blood
       a. Appropriate inflammatory response to "invasion" by foreign substances or infection
       b. Bone marrow proliferation (leukemias, lymphoma or myeloma, Hodgkins)
     4. Leukopenia: production *reduced* to fewer than 5,000/mm^2 of blood
       a. Bone marrow suppression by immunosuppression, radiation, toxins, or drugs

5. Perianesthesia nursing considerations and interventions related to altered WBC
   a. Report deviation from normal parameters
      i.   Preadmission tests might be first recognition of infection or leukemia
      ii. Leukopenia and unusual bruising may coexist with anemias and platelet dysfunction
   b. Obtain accurate history: ask pointed preanesthetic questions
      i.   Fevers, with or without chills?
      ii. Easy bruising or bleeding?
      iii. Increased fatigue?
      iv. Pain, especially in joints?
   c. Think "protection"
      i.   Avoid pressure to skin and joints, and provide soft surfaces against skin
      ii. Prevent hematoma during venipuncture and suctioning
      iii. Isolate as required: infectious vs. protective

D. Coagulation
   1. A chain of events to assure hemostasis
   2. Physiology: an intricate balance that requires:
      a. Adequate liver function to produce a cascade of interrelated clotting factors
      b. Functional platelets, normal calcium, and specific enzymes
      c. *Vascular integrity* assures "healthy" endothelial wall for
         i. Adherence of a platelet plug bound by a fibrin clot
         ii. Appropriate local constriction to limit local blood flow
      d. Synergy among a host of clotting factors (proteins) along the coagulation pathway
         i. Clotting pathways:
            (a) Extrinsic pathway: tissue injury triggers thromboplastin release and a sequence of events leading to fibrin clot formation
            (b) Intrinsic pathway: activation of proenzyme spurs a sequence of clotting factors
   3. Laboratory assessments of coagulation
      a. Prothrombin time (PT): assesses conversion of prothrombin to thrombin
         i.   Specific monitor for Coumadin, which affects the external coagulation pathway
         ii. If prolonged: significant bleeding risk during surgery, trauma, or soft tissue injury
            (a) Liver disease, vitamin K deficiency
            (b) Deficient fibrinogen, prothrombin, and clotting factors V, VII, X
         iii. Correct clinically with:
            (a) Vitamin K injections
            (b) Fresh frozen plasma
      b. Partial Thromboplastin Time (PTT): assesses intrinsic coagulation pathway
         i. Monitor if administering heparin
         ii. Detects alteration in clotting factors I, II, V, VIII, IX-XI
      c. Thrombin Time (TT): assesses thrombin activity to stimulate fibrin creation at coagulation's final stage
         i. Prolonged by fibrinogen (Factor I) deficiency
      d. Platelet count: number, shape, and size of circulating platelets
         i.   Surgical bleeding is rare if numbers are 100,000 or greater
         ii. Anticipate spontaneous bleeding if platelet numbers drop to 20,000 or fewer
         iii. Aspirin alters function for the life of the platelet, approximately 7 days
         iv. NSAID use alters platelet function, though recovery within 2 days

---

BOX 13–5.   Perianesthetic Consideration: von Willebrand's Disease

This usually mild-mannered inherited coagulopathy may not manifest until a surgical procedure prompts unstoppable bleeding. Aspirin or nonsteroidal antiinflammatory drugs (NSAIDs) can stimulate a similar response in patients with von Willebrand's disease. Inquiring during the preanesthesia interview about extended or easy bleeding can alert the clinician to identify a latent, unrecognized bleeding disorder.

---

   4. Coagulopathies: disorders of clotting sequence
     a. Idiopathic immune thrombocytopenic purpura (ITP): spontaneous bleeding
       i.   Autoimmune disorder: active antiplatelet antibodies and profoundly reduced platelet numbers
       ii. Acutely affects young children after immunization or viral infection with chicken pox, mumps, or measles
       iii. Chronic ITP affects adults, primarily women, under age 50
     b. Disseminated intravascular coagulopathy (DIC): clotting factor consumption
       i.   Simultaneous active bleeding and intravascular clotting capillaries
       ii. Reflects severe, overwhelming response to organ system crisis
       iii. Occurrence in ambulatory surgery setting is highly unlikely
     c. Hereditary coagulopathies
       i.   Hemophilia: sex-linked clotting factor deficiency affecting men
         (a) Hemophilia A: clotting factor VIII lacking
           (i) Significant bleeding into tissues and joints if active factor VIII is <5%
           (ii) PTT prolonged and PT normal
         (b) Hemophilia B (Christmas disease): clotting factor IX lacking
           (i) Intraoperative fresh frozen plasma (FFP) needed to support Factor IX
           (ii) PTT, PT, and TT all within normal limits
         (c) Disease prevents formation of stable clots
           (i) May require regular infusions of cryoprecipitate or FFP
       ii. von Willebrand's disease: common disorder affecting 1:800 men and women
         (a) Coagulopathy and effect
           (i)   Defective von Willebrand factor (vWF), the "carrier" Factor VIII
           (ii) Activity of Factor VIII in coagulation chain is therefore reduced
           (iii) Adequate numbers of platelets, though "stickiness" is impaired
         (b) Preoperative administrations
           (i) Desmopressin (DDAVP) can increase vWF
           (ii) Cryoprecipitate in scheduled twice-daily doses
   5. Perianesthesia nursing considerations and interventions related to coagulation
     a. Preanesthesia nursing assessment
       i.   A patient with a significant bleeding disorder is an unlikely candidate for outpatient surgery with discharge home
       ii. Identify at-risk patients: assess coagulation risk and bleeding history
         (a) Document date and time of most recent anticoagulant medication
           (i)   Coumarins and heparin
           (ii) Drugs that alter platelet function: aspirin, nonsteroidal antiinflammatories (NSAIDs)
           (iii) Chemotherapy agents that suppress bone marrow function
         (b) Assessment is critical
           (i) Risk of intraspinal or epidural hematoma increases if anticoagulated patient receives regional anesthesia
           (ii) Undetected coagulopathy can underlie persistent postsurgical bleeding

  b. Postanesthesia nursing assessment
    i. Observe often for insidious bleeding
      (a) Always look *under* the patient as well as at the wound itself
      (b) Increasing abdominal girth after laparoscopic procedures
        (i) An obese patient can accumulate a lot of blood in the abdomen before distention or tenderness is evident
      (c) Oozing and bruising from incisions or venipuncture sites
    ii. Link vital signs and oxygenation changes with bleeding potential
      (a) Continuously monitor oxygen saturation
        (i) Anemia often associated with coagulopathy: obtain a hemoglobin measure
        (ii) Persistent reductions may indicate undetected hemoglobin loss
      (b) Watch for respiratory compromise
      (c) Support blood pressure with adequate fluid volume

Bibliography

1. Burden, N. (1993). *Ambulatory Surgical Nursing.* Philadelphia: Saunders.
2. Carlson, K. (1995). *Certification Review for Perianesthesia Nursing.* Philadelphia: Saunders.
3. Cassidy, J., Marley, R.A. (1996). Preoperative assessment of the ambulatory patient. *J Perianesth Nurs*, 11(5):334–343.
4. Cote, C.J. (1995). NPO guidelines: Children and adults. In McGoldrich, K.E., ed, *Ambulatory Anesthesia: A Problem Oriented Approach.* Baltimore: Williams & Wilkins, pp. 20–32.
5. deFranco, M. (1994). Fluid and electrolyte balance. In Litwack, K., ed, *ASPAN's Core Curriculum for Post Anesthesia Nursing Practice*, 3rd ed. Philadelphia: Saunders, pp. 156–175.
6. Fleisher, L.A. (1997). Preoperative evaluation. In Barasch, P.B., Cullen, B.F., Stoelting, R.K., eds, *Clinical Anesthesia*, 3rd ed. Philadelphia: Lippincott, pp. 443–459.
7. Green, C.R., Pandit, S.K., Schork, M.A. (1996). Preoperative fasting time: Is the traditional policy changing? Results of a national survey. *Anesth Analg*, 83:123–8.
8. Lammers, P.K., Palmer, P.H. (1991). Surgeons discuss ambulatory surgery, legislative concerns, dangers of transfusions, surgical advances. *AORN J*, 53:16.
9. Lancaster, K.A. (1997). Care of the pediatric patient in ambulatory surgery. *Nurs Clin of North Amer*, 32(2): 441–455.
10. Lichtor, J.L., Wetchler, B.V. (1997). Anesthesia for ambulatory surgery. In Barasch, P.B., Cullen, B.F., Stoelting, R.K., eds, *Clinical Anesthesia*, 3rd ed. Philadelphia: Lippincott, pp. 1137–1155.
11. Litwack, K. (1997). Care of the special needs patient. *Nurs Clin of North Amer*, 32(2): 457–467.
12. Litwack, K. (1995). *Post Anesthesia Care Nursing*, 2nd ed. St. Louis: Mosby.
13. McGaffigan, P.A., Christoph, S.B. (1994). Assessment and monitoring of the post anesthesia patient. In Drain, C., ed., *The Post Anesthesia Care Unit: A Critical Care Approach to Post Anesthesia Nursing*, 2nd ed. Philadelphia: Saunders, pp. 284-S.
14. Marley, R.A. (1996). Postoperative nausea and vomiting: The outpatient enigma. *J Perianesth Nurs*, 11(3): 147–61.
15. Mecca, R.S., Sharnic, S.V. (1995). Common postanesthesia care unit problems. In McGoldrich, K.E., ed., *Ambulatory Anesthesia: A Problem Oriented Approach.* Baltimore: Williams & Wilkins, pp. 582–618.
16. Meeks, G.R., Waller, G.A., Meydrech, E.F., et al. (1992). Unscheduled hospital admission following ambulatory gynecologic surgery. *Obstet Gynecol*, 80:446.
17. Oertel, L. (1995). *Nurse Pract*, 20(9):15–22.
18. Pandit, U.A., Pandit, K.S. (1997). Fasting before and after ambulatory surgery. *J Perianesth Nurs*, 12(3): 181–187.
19. Pasternak, I.R. (1995). Screening patients; Strategies and studies. In McGoldrich, K.E., ed., *Ambulatory Anesthesia: A Problem Oriented Approach.* Baltimore: Williams & Wilkins, pp. 219.
20. Silinsky, J. (1994). The hematologic system. In Litwack, K., ed., *ASPAN's Core Curriculum for Post Anesthesia Nursing Practice*, 3rd ed. Philadelphia: Saunders, pp. 176–201.
21. Tibmar, K.J. (1993). Fluid and electrolyte abnormalities and management. In Vender, J.S., Speiss, B.D., eds., *Post Anesthesia Care.* Philadelphia: Saunders, pp. 157–177.
22. Welborn, L.G., Hannallah, R.S., Luban, N.L.C., et al. (1991). Anemia and postoperative apnea in former preterm infants. *Anesthesiology*, 74:1003.
23. Wetchler, B.V. (1990). *Anesthesia for Ambulatory Surgery*, 2nd ed. Philadelphia: Lippincott.

REVIEW QUESTIONS

1. Mr. S, age 75 years, complains of feeling weak when he arrives at 6:00 A.M. in the preanesthesia area. He is scheduled for an intraoperative colonoscopy and examination under anesthesia. He states he has been NPO since midnight, used his bowel prep with great results, and misses his morning coffee. The nurse considers that Mr. S's weakness *most likely* results from

   A. Caffeine deprivation and hypoglycemia related to preoperative stress
   B. Hypernatremia related to dehydration from fasting
   C. Hypokalemia related to electrolyte loss from bowel prep
   D. Lack of sleep and hypercalcemia related to age-induced hypovolemia

2. Ms. P's serum osmolarity measure of 350 mOsm affects her fluid and electrolyte status by

   A. Increasing diffusion of urea, glucose, and protein into the ICF
   B. Establishing an isotonic fluid balance
   C. Decreasing the osmotic shift of electrolytes from cells
   D. Causing fluid movement across a concentration gradient into the ECF

3. The preanesthesia nurse notes that 34-year-old Ms. D, who has end-stage renal disease, has an admission potassium of 6.9 mEq/L. The nurse *most expects* to see

   A. Fingertip tingling and muscle twitches
   B. Respiratory muscle weakness and a stat insulin and glucose infusion
   C. Inverted T waves, a stat injection of hypertonic potassium and bronchospasm
   D. Vasodilation and diaphoresis

4. A physiologic response to *raise* the serum pH is

   A. Increase respiratory rate to exhale carbon dioxide
   B. Conserve carbon dioxide by hypoventilation
   C. Renal retention of water, bicarbonate, and hydrogen ion
   D. Release of hydrogen ion into the serum by buffer systems

5. For the postsurgical patient whose pulse oximeter reading is 90%, the ambulatory surgery nurse considers the *most likely* potential of concurrent

   A. Hematocrit of 52% and a pCO_2 of 23mm Hg
   B. Hypothermia and pO_2 of 93mm Hg
   C. pO_2 of 60mm Hg and a hemoglobin of 8.2 gm%
   D. pCO_2 of 55 and hyperventilation

6. Stress and pain influence antidiuretic hormone secretion (ADH) by prompting

   A. Diuresis and renal excretion of sodium
   B. Potassium wasting and angiotensin formation
   C. Vasoconstriction and bicarbonate conservation
   D. Fluid and sodium reabsorption by renal tubules

7. Laboratory tests on the day of surgery are indicated in the preoperative ambulatory surgery setting

   A. Routinely to provide a basis for postoperative comparison
   B. Selectively when the patient uses diuretics or aspirin
   C. Consistently as a necessary basis for the anesthetic plan
   D. Only when suspecting a genetic condition will alter anesthetic choices

8. Biochemically, magnesium is

   A. More heavily concentrated in the blood than cells
   B. A depressant to muscle strength at serum levels of 2.0 mEq/L
   C. Required at the neuromuscular junction for acetylcholine release
   D. Reduced in patients with chronic renal failure and immobility

9. Mr. B's preanesthetic interview and record reveals he has sickle cell anemia. After anesthesia, the nurse observes him specifically for signs of sickling, including

   A. Tall, peaked T waves on EKG and slow awakening
   B. Hyperventilation, stridor, and wheezing
   C. Bleeding tendency and headache
   D. Abdominal or knee pain and hypoxemia

10. Unanticipated blood loss of 450 ml and more extensive repair complicated Mr. D's planned outpatient knee arthroscopy and anterior cruciate repair. Pending a hemoglobin result, he may still be discharged through the ambulatory surgery center. The Phase I postanesthesia nurse plans care that emphasizes

   A. Adequate fluid volume, gradual activity, and head elevation
   B. Trendelenberg position, platelet infusion, and ice on his knee
   C. Hypothermia, frequent neurovascular assessment, and immobility
   D. Prompt crutch instruction, cautious IV fluid rate, and 32 ventilations per minute

ANSWERS TO QUESTIONS

1. C
2. D
3. B
4. A
5. C

6. D
7. B
8. C
9. D
10. A

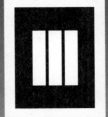

Lifespan
Considerations

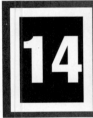

Human Growth and Development

Donna M. DeFazio Quinn
Elliot 1-Day Surgery Center
Manchester, New Hampshire

I. **Overview of Growth and Development**
   A. Definition
      1. Growth and development
         a. Often used interchangeably
         b. Each has distinct definition
      2. Growth
         a. Implies a change in quantity (quantitative change)
            i. An increase in physical size of a whole or any of its parts
            ii. Can be measured in:
               (a) Inches (height)
               (b) Kilograms or pounds (increased organ mass, weight)
               (c) Numbers (increased vocabulary, increased number of relationships with others, increased number of physical skills that can be performed)
         b. Increase in number and size of cells
            i. Reflected in an increase in the size and weight of the whole or any of its parts
      3. Development
         a. Complex concept not easily measured or studied
         b. Gradual growth and expansion; viewed as a qualitative change
            i. Increased function (skill) and complexity (capacity)
            ii. Occurs through growth, maturation, and learning

1. Define growth and development.
2. Identify the stages of growth and development.
3. Explain Freud's theory and Erikson's theory of psychosocial development.
4. List the four stages of cognitive development.
5. Discuss the five stages of language development.
6. Discuss the effects of positive influence on the development of self-esteem.
7. Identify eight factors that could influence growth and development.

     c. Move from lower case to a more advanced stage of complexity
       i.   Continuous orderly series of conditions
         (a) Leads to activities, new motives for activities, and eventual patterns of behavior
         (b) Expansion of capabilities to provide greater facility in functioning
     d. Development process is:
       i.   Continuous, complex, and irreversible
       ii. Involves aging
         (a) Most rapid during fetal stage
         (b) Is a lifelong process
     e. Progression of development
       i.   Simple to complex
         (a) Infant's vocalizations before speech refinement
       ii. General to specific
         (a) Infant's palmar grasp prior to acquiring finer control of pincer grasp
       iii. From head to toe (cepalocaudally)
         (a) Infant gains head and neck control prior to gaining control of trunk and limbs
       iv. From inner to outer (proximodistally)
         (a) Control of near structures before control of structures farther away from the body center
         (b) Infant coordinates arms to reach before gaining hand and finger coordination
     f. Predictability of development
       i.   Sequence of development is invariable
       ii. Precise age will vary
       iii. Wide norm range allows for individual variances
     g. Uniqueness of development
       i.   Each child has own genetic potential for growth and development
       ii. May be deterred or modified at any stage

II. Stages of Growth and Development

  A. Prenatal
    1. Period of life from conception to birth
      a. Crucial period in developmental process
      b. Health and well being of the infant directly related to adequate prenatal care
      c. Direct relationship between maternal health and certain manifestations in the newborn
  B. Newborn or neonatal
    1. From birth through the first month of life
    2. Major physical adjustment to extrauterine existence
  C. Infancy
    1. Begins at end of first month of life and ends at one year of age
    2. Period of rapid motor, cognitive, and social development
    3. Establishes basic trust
      a. Foundation for future relationships
  D. Early childhood (see Table 14–1)
    1. Toddler
      a. From 1 to 3 years
    2. Preschool
      a. From 3 to 6 years

Table 14–1 • EMERGING PATTERNS OF BEHAVIOR FROM 1 TO 5 YEARS OF AGE*

15 Months

Motor: Walks alone; crawls up stairs
Adaptive: Makes a tower of 3 cubes; makes a line with crayon; inserts pellet in bottle
Language: Jargon; follows simple commands; may name a familiar object (ball)
Social: Indicates some desires or needs by pointing; hugs parents

18 Months

Motor: Runs stiffly; sits on small chair; walks up stairs with one hand held; explores drawers and waste baskets
Adaptive: Makes a tower of 4 cubes; imitates scribbling; imitates vertical stroke; dumps pellet from bottle
Language: 10 words (average); names pictures; identifies one or more parts of body
Social: Feeds self, seeks help when in trouble; may complain when wet or soiled; kisses parent with pucker

24 Months

Motor: Runs well; walks up and down stairs, one step at a time; opens doors; climbs on furniture; jumps
Adaptive: Tower of 7 cubes (6 at 21 months); circular scribbling; imitates horizontal stroke; folds paper once imitatively
Language: Puts 3 words together (subject, verb, object)
Social: Handles spoon well; often tells immediate experiences; helps to undress; listens to stories with pictures

30 Months

Motor: Goes up stairs alternating feet
Adaptive: Tower of 9 cubes; makes vertical and horizontal strokes, but generally will not join them to make a cross; imitates circular stroke, forming closed figure
Language: Refers to self by pronoun "I"; knows full name
Social: Helps put things away; pretends in play

36 Months

Motor: Rides tricycle; stands momentarily on one foot
Adaptive: Tower of 10 cubes; imitates construction of "bridge" of 3 cubes; copies a circle; imitates a cross
Language: Knows age and sex; counts 3 objects correctly; repeats 3 numbers or a sentence of 6 syllables
Social: Plays simple games (in "parallel" with other children); helps in dressing (unbuttons clothing and puts on shoes); washes hands

48 Months

Motor: Hops on one foot; throws ball overhand; uses scissors to cut out pictures; climbs well
Adaptive: Copies bridge from model; imitates construction of "gate" of 5 cubes; copies cross and square; draws a man with 2 to 5 parts besides head; names longer of 2 lines
Language: Counts 4 pennies accurately; tells a story
Social: Plays with several children with beginning of social interaction and role-playing; goes to toilet alone

60 Months

Motor: Skips
Adaptive: Draws triangle from copy; names heavier of 2 weights
Language: Names 4 colors; repeats sentence of 10 syllables; counts 10 pennies correctly
Social: Dresses and undresses; asks questions about meaning of words; domestic role-playing

*Data are derived from those of Gesell (as revised by Knobloch), Shirley, Provence, Wolf, Bailey, and others. After five years the Stanford-Binet, Wechsler-Bellevue, and other scales offer the most precise estimates of developmental levels. In order to have their greatest value, they should be administered only by an experienced and qualified person. (From Behrman, R.E., Kliegman, R.M., Arvin, A.M. [1996]. *Nelson Textbook of Pediatrics*, 15th ed. Philadelphia: Saunders.)

    3. Characteristics
        a. Characterized by intense activity and discovery
        b. Marked physical and personality development
        c. Motor development advances steadily
        d. Acquire language skills
        e. Expand social relationships
        f. Learn role standards
        g. Gain self control and mastery
        h. Develop increasing awareness of dependence and independence
        i. Begin to develop a self-concept
    E. Middle childhood or school-age years
        1. From age 6 to 11 or 12 years
        2. Child is directed away from family group and centered around peer relationships
        3. Steady advancement in physical, mental, and social development
        4. Emphasis is on developing skill competencies
        5. Social cooperation and moral development take on importance
            a. Relevant for later life stages
        6. Critical period in the development of self-concept
    F. Later childhood or adolescence and young adulthood
        1. From the beginning of the twelfth year to the end of the twenty-first year
        2. Period of rapid maturation and change
        3. Considered to be a transition that begins with the onset of puberty and extends to the point of entry into the adult world
        4. Biologic and personality maturation are accompanied by physical and emotional turmoil
        5. Self-concept is redefined
        6. In late adolescence the child begins to internalize all previously learned values and focus on an individual rather than a group identity
III. **Theories of Development—Overview** (see Table 14–2)
    A. Freudian
        1. Psychosocial
        2. Emphasis on development of personality
    B. Erikson
        1. Psychosocial development

Table 14–2 • CLASSIC STAGE THEORIES

THEORY	0–1 INFANCY	2–3 TODDLERHOOD	3–6 PRESCHOOL	6–12 SCHOOL AGE	12–20 ADOLESCENCE
Freud: psychosexual	Oral	Anal	Oedipal	Latency	Adolescence
Erikson: psychosocial	Basic trust	Autonomy versus shame and doubt	Initiative versus guilt	Industry versus inferiority	Identity versus identity diffusion
Piaget: cognitive	Sensorimotor (stages I–IV)	Sensorimotor (stages V, VI)	Preoperational	Concrete operations	Formal operations

(From Behrman, R.E., Kliegman, R.M., Arvin, A.M. [1996]. *Nelson Textbook of Pediatrics*, 15th ed. Philadelphia: Saunders.)

C. Sullivan
  1. Interpersonal development
D. Piaget
  1. Cognitive development
E. Kohlberg
  1. Moral development
F. Skinner, Watson
  1. Learning theory; behaviorism
  2. Focus entirely on behavior
  3. Internalize processes such as thoughts and feelings
G. Maslow
  1. Humanistic
  2. Focus on characteristics that contribute to healthy personality development

IV. Freudian
A. Three components of personality
  1. Id
    a. Develops during birth
    b. The unconscious mind
    c. Inborn component that drives instincts
    d. Obeys pleasure principle of immediate gratification of needs
      i.   Raw libido seeking pleasure
  2. Ego
    a. Develops during toddler years
    b. Represents the conscious mind
      i.   Reality component
      ii. Mediates conflict
    c. Functions as conscious or controlling self
    d. Finds realistic means of gratifying instincts
    e. Blocks irrational thinking of the Id
  3. Superego
    a. Develops during preschool years
    b. Conscience
    c. Functions as moral arbitrator
      i.   Puts good or bad labels on behavior
    d. Represents the ideal
    e. Prevents individual from expressing undesirable instincts that could threaten social order
B. Psychosexual development (see Table 14–3)
  1. Stages of development
    a. Oral
    b. Anal
    c. Phallic
    d. Latency
    e. Genital
  2. Sexual instincts significant in development of personality
  3. Psychosexual used to describe any sensual pleasure
  4. Theory focuses on desire to satisfy biological needs
    a. Theory difficult to verify
    b. Of little value when attempting to predict future behaviors
    c. Psychosexual development usually complete by 6 years of age
C. Oral stage
  1. Birth to 1 year of age

Table 14–3 • PERSONALITY TRAITS ASSOCIATED WITH FREUD'S FIRST THREE STAGES OF PSYCHOSEXUAL DEVELOPMENT

STAGE	AGE	SOURCE OF PLEASURE	PERSONALITY TRAITS
Oral	Birth to 1 year	Oral activities —sucking —biting —chewing —vocalizing	Pessimism or optimism Determination or submission Gullibility or suspiciousness Admiration or envy Cockiness or self-belittlement
Anal	1 to 3 years	Anal region —withhold or expel feces	Stinginess or overgenerosity Constrictedness or expansiveness Rigid punctuality or tardiness Stubbornness or acquiescence Orderliness or messiness
Phallic	3 to 6 years	Genitals	Brashness or bashfulness Stylishness or plainness Gaiety or sadness Blind courage or timidness Gregariousness or isolationism

      2. Sources of pleasure
        a. Sucking
        b. Biting
        c. Chewing
        d. Vocalizing
      3. Oral personality traits
        a. Pessimism or optimism
        b. Determination or submission
        c. Gullibility or suspiciousness
        d. Admiration or envy
        e. Cockiness or self-belittlement
    D. Anal stage
      1. One to 3 years of age
      2. Focus on anal region
      3. Child develops ability to withhold or expel feces at will
      4. Toilet training can have lasting effects on personality development
      5. Anal personality traits
        a. Stinginess or over-generosity
        b. Constrictedness or expansiveness
        c. Rigid punctuality or tardiness
        d. Stubbornness or acquiescence
        e. Orderliness or messiness
   E. Phallic stage
      1. Three to 6 years of age
      2. Focus on genitals
      3. Recognition of difference between sexes
      4. Phallic personality traits
        a. Brashness or bashfulness
        b. Stylishness or plainness
        c. Gaiety or sadness
        d. Blind courage or timidness
        e. Gregariousness or isolationism

F. Latency period
   1. Six to 12 years of age
   2. Elaboration of previous learned traits and skills
   3. Physical and psychic energies funneled into acquiring knowledge and vigorous play
G. Genital stage
   1. Twelve years and over
   2. Begins at puberty
   3. Genital organs become major source of sexual tensions and pleasures
   4. Energy used to form friendships and prepare for marriage

V. **Erikson**
A. Theory of psychosocial development most widely used
B. Emphasis on health personality
   1. Stresses rational and adaptive natures of individual
   2. Explains child's behaviors in mastering developmental tasks
C. Eight stages of development
   1. Each stage has two components—favorable and unfavorable aspect of conflict
   2. Progression to next stage depends on resolution of conflict
   3. Conflict never mastered completely—remains a recurrent problem throughout life
D. Trust versus mistrust stage (Stage I)
   1. Birth to 1 year of age
   2. "Getting" and "taking in" from all the senses
   3. Exists only in relation to something or someone
   4. Consistent, loving care by mother essential to development of trust
   5. Mistrust develops when:
      a. Trust-promoting activities absent
      b. Basic needs inconsistently or inadequately met
   6. Individual develops quality of hope and belief that one can attain deep and essential wishes
      a. Results in faith and optimism
E. Autonomy versus shame and doubt stage (Stage II)
   1. One to 3 years of age
   2. Development centered on child's ability to control his/her body, him-/herself, and the environment
   3. Uses his/her power to do things independently
      a. Walking
      b. Climbing
      c. Selection and decision making
   4. Learns to conform to social rules
   5. Doubt and shame arise when:
      a. Child made to feel unimportant or self-conscious
      b. Choices are disastrous
      c. Shamed by others
      d. Forced to be dependent when he/she is capable of assuming control
   6. Achieves autonomy through imitation
      a. Parents are key socializing intermediaries
      b. Results in self-control and willpower
F. Initiative versus guilt stage (Stage III)
   1. Three to 6 years of age
   2. Characterized by vigorous, intrusive behavior and a strong imagination
   3. Explores physical world with all senses

       4. Develops a conscience
       5. Responds to an inner voice that warns and threats
       6. Guilt arises when:
         a. Child undertakes goals or activities that are in conflict with those of parent
         b. Made to feel activities are bad
       7. Achieves initiative through identification
         a. Family is key socializing agent
         b. Results in direction and purpose; ability to imagine and pursue
  G. Industry versus inferiority stage (Stage IV)
       1. Six to 12 years of age
       2. Carries tasks and activities through to completion
       3. Learns to compete and cooperate with others
       4. Learns rules
       5. Successful child develops a sense of mastery and self-assurance
       6. Inferiority develops when:
         a. Too much is expected of child
         b. Child believes he/she cannot meet standards set for him/her by others
       7. Achieves industry through education
         a. Teachers and peers are socializing agents
         b. Develops competence, skill, and intelligence to complete task
  H. Identity versus role confusion stage (Stage V)
       1. Twelve to 18 years of age
       2. Characterized by marked physical changes
       3. Engrossed in how he/she appears to others as compared with his/her own self-concept
       4. Struggle with:
         a. Ability to maintain current role and future role as defined by peers
         b. Integrating concepts and values with those of society
         c. Decision for an occupation
       5. Role confusion develops when unable to resolve core conflicts
       6. Mastering identity results in devotion and fidelity
       7. Achieves identity through peer pressure and role experimentation
 I. Intimacy versus isolation (Stage VI)
       1. Occurs in early adulthood
       2. Intimacy established on a sense of identity
       3. Capacity to develop:
         a. An intimate love relationship
         b. Intimate interpersonal relationships with friends, partners, and significant others
       4. Isolation develops when intimacy not present
       5. Intimacy develops when there is mutuality among peers
       6. Key socializing agents
         a. Lovers
         b. Spouses
         c. Close friends
       7. Develops affiliation and love
 J. Generativity versus stagnation stage (Stage VII)
       1. Young and middle adulthood
       2. Creation and care of next generation
       3. Essential element is to nourish and nurture
       4. Failure results in self-absorption and stagnation

      5. Key socializing agents are spouse, children, and cultural norms
        a. Results in production and care; commitment and concern for what has been generated
   K. Ego integrity versus despair stage (Stage VIII)
      1. Old age
      2. Results from satisfaction with life and acceptance of what has been
      3. Despair is a result of remorse for what might have been
      4. Ego integrity results in renunciation and wisdom and concern with life in the face of death
      5. Process achieved through introspection

VI. Sullivan
   A. Interpersonal development
      1. Recognizes importance of environment in development
      2. Has some predictive value
      3. Does not recognize biologic maturation process
   B. Emphasis on interpersonal relationships and importance of social approval or disapproval in developing a self-concept
      1. Unfavorable reactions result in tension and anxiety
      2. Favorable reactions result in comfort and security
   C. Infants
      1. Mother gratifies and comforts child
      2. Relationship gradually extends to other family members
   D. Toddler
      1. Becomes more outgoing
      2. Directs social gestures to wider audience
        a. Relatives
        b. Neighborhood children
      3. Engages in aspects of social learning
        a. Peer play
        b. Family events
   E. School age
      1. Wider range of relationships
        a. Authority figures at school and in community
      2. Develops peer relationships
      3. Shares intimacy and common interests with peers
   F. Adolescent
      1. Personal identity
        a. Friends of same sex
        b. Friends of opposite sex

VII. Piaget: Cognitive Development
   A. Cognition
      1. Process by which developing individuals become acquainted with the world and the objects it contains
      2. Cognitive development allows child ability to:
        a. Reason abstractly
        b. Think in a logical manner
        c. Organize intellectual functions into higher structures
   B. Sequence of four stages (Sensorimotor, Preoperational, Concrete Operational, Formal Operational)
      1. Prior practice or teaching has little effect on development of new cognitive skills
      2. Suitable cognitive maturity or readiness necessary to progress to next stage
   C. Sensorimotor stage of intellectual development
      1. Birth to 2 years of age

    2. Consists of substages that are governed by sensations through which simple learning takes place

    3. Progresses from simple reflex activities to simple repetitive behaviors that imitate behaviors

    4. Develops sense of cause and effect

      a. Directs behavior towards object

      b. Solves problems through trial and error

      c. High level of curiosity

      d. Develops sense of self through interactions with environment

        i. Able to differentiate self from environment

    5. Awareness that object has permanence

      a. Important prerequisite for all other mental activity

  D. Preoperational period of intellectual development

    1. Two to 7 years of age

    2. Egocentricity is predominant characteristic

      a. Defined as inability to put oneself in place of another

    3. Interprets objects and events in terms of their relationship or use of them

    4. Sees only his/her perspective

      a. Cannot see another's point of view

    5. Preoperational thinking is concrete and tangible

    6. Lacks ability to make deductions or generalizations

    7. Thoughts dominated by what he/she sees, hears, and experiences

    8. Increasing ability to use language to represent objects in his/her environment

    9. Increasing ability to elaborate on concepts and make simple associations between ideas

   10. Cannot understand that for every action or operation, there is an action or operation that cancels it

   11. Develops intuitive reasoning later in stage

   12. Begins to understand weight, length, size, and time

  E. Concrete operational stage

    1. Seven to 11 years of age

    2. Thoughts become more logical and coherent

    3. Able to problem solve

      a. Classifies, sorts, orders, and organizes facts

    4. Develops concept of permanence

    5. Able to deal with a number of different aspects of a situation simultaneously

    6. Unable to deal with the abstract

    7. Problem solves in concrete, systematic fashion, based on what he/she can perceive

    8. Thoughts become less self-centered

    9. Can consider points of view other than his/her own

   10. Develops socialized thinking

  F. Formal operational stage

    1. Twelve to 15 years of age

    2. Characterized by adaptability and flexibility

    3. Can think in terms of the abstract

    4. Able to draw logical conclusions from a set of observations

    5. Can make and test hypotheses

    6. May confuse the ideal with the practice

VIII. Kohlberg: Moral Development (see Table 14–4)

  A. Based on cognitive development theory

  B. Proceeds in an invariant sequence of stages

Table 14-4 • COMPARISON OF THEORIES OF GROWTH AND DEVELOPMENT

	PIAGET'S PERIODS OF COGNITIVE DEVELOPMENT	FREUD'S STAGES OF PSYCHOSEXUAL DEVELOPMENT	ERIKSON'S STAGES OF PSYCHOLOGICAL DEVELOPMENT	KOHLBERG'S STAGES OF MORAL DEVELOPMENT
Infancy	**Period 1 (Birth–2 Years): Sensorimotor Period** Reflective behavior is used to adapt to the environment; egocentric view of the world; development of object permanence.	**Oral Stage** Mouth is a sensory organ; infant takes in and explores during oral passive substage (first half of infancy); infant strikes out with teeth during oral aggressive substage (latter half of infancy).	**Trust versus Mistrust** Development of a sense that the self is good and the world is good when consistent, predictable, reliable care is received; characterized by hope.	**Stage 0 (0–2 Years): Naivete and Egocentrism** No moral sensitivity; decisions are made on the basis of what pleases the child; infants like or love what helps them and dislike what hurts them; no awareness of the effect of his/her actions on others. "Good is what I like and want."
Toddlerhood	**Period 2 (2–7 Years): Preoperational Thought** Thinking remains egocentric, becomes magical, and is dominated by perception.	**Anal Stage** Major focus of sexual interest is anus; control of bodily functions is major feature.	**Autonomy versus Shame and Doubt** Development of a sense of control over the self and bodily functions; exerts self; characterized by will.	**Stage 1 (2–3 Years): Punishment-Obedience Orientation** Right or wrong is determined by physical consequences: "If I get caught and punished for doing it, it is wrong. If I am not caught or punished, then it must be right."
Preschool Age		**Phallic or Oedipal/Electra Stage** Genitals become focus of sexual curiosity; superego (conscience) develops; feelings of guilt emerge.	**Initiative versus Guilt** Development of a can-do attitude about the self; behavior becomes goal-directed, competitive, and imaginative; initiation into sex role; characterized by purpose.	**Premorality or Preconventional Morality Stage 2 (4–7 Years): Instrumental Hedonism and Concrete Reciprocity** Child conforms to rules out of self-interest: "I'll do this for you if you do this for me"; behavior is guided by an "eye for an eye" orientation. "If you do something bad to me, then it's OK if I do something bad to you."

Table continued on following page

Table 14-4 • COMPARISON OF THEORIES OF GROWTH AND DEVELOPMENT *Continued*

	PIAGET'S PERIODS OF COGNITIVE DEVELOPMENT	FREUD'S STAGES OF PSYCHO-SEXUAL DEVELOPMENT	ERIKSON'S STAGES OF PSYCHO-LOGICAL DEVELOPMENT	KOHLBERG'S STAGES OF MORAL DE-VELOPMENT
School Age	**Period 3 (7–11 Years): Concrete Operations** Thinking becomes more systematic and logical, but concrete objects and activities are needed.	**Latency Stage** Sexual feelings are firmly repressed by the superego; period of relative calm.	**Industry versus Inferiority** Mastering of useful skills and tools of the culture; learning how to play and work with peers; characterized by competence.	**Morality of Conventional Role Conformity Stage 3 (7–10 Years): Good-Boy/Girl Orientation** Morality is based on avoiding disapproval or disturbing the conscience; child is becoming socially sensitive. **Stage 4 (Begins about 10–12 Years): Law and Order Orientation** Right takes on a religious or metaphysical quality. Child wants to do his/her duty, show respect for authority, and maintain social order; obeys rules for their own sake.
Adolescence	**Period 4 (11 Years–Adulthood): Formal Operations** New ideas can be created; situations can be analyzed; use of abstract thinking.	**Puberty or Genital Stage** Stimulated by increasing hormone levels; sexual energy wells up in full force, resulting in personal and family turmoil.	**Identity versus Role Confusion** Begins to develop a sense of "I"; this process is lifelong; peers become of paramount importance; child gains independence from parents; characterized by faith in self.	**Morality of Self-Accepted Moral Principles Stage 5: Social Contract Orientation** Right is determined by what is best for the majority; exceptions to rules can be made if a person's welfare is violated; the end no longer justifies the means; laws are for mutual good and mutual cooperation.
Adulthood			**Intimacy versus Isolation** Development of the ability to lose the self in genuine mutuality with another; characterized by love.	

Generativity versus Stagnation

Production of ideas and materials through work; creation of children; characterized by care.

Ego Integrity versus Despair

Realization that there is order and purpose to life; characterized by wisdom.

Stage 6. Personal Principle Orientation

Achieved only by the morally mature individual; few people reach this level; this person does what he/she thinks is right, regardless of others' opinions, legal sanctions, or personal sacrifice; actions are guided by internal standards; integrity is of utmost importance; may be willing to die for his/her beliefs.

Stage 7: Universal Principle Orientation

This stage is achieved by only a rare few; Mother Teresa, Ghandi, Socrates are examples; the individual transcends the teachings or organized religion and perceives him/herself as part the cosmic order; understands the reason for his/her existence and lives for his/her beliefs.

(From Ashwill, J.W., Droske, S.C. [1997]. *Nursing Care of Children Principles and Practice.* Philadelphia: Saunders.)

243

C. Cannot acquire higher levels of moral reasoning until appropriate cognitive development has occurred

D. Preconventional level of morality
1. Morality is external
    a. Children conform to rules imposed by adults
2. Stage 1—The punishment and obedience orientation
    a. Child determines if action is good or bad based on consequences
    b. Obeys those in power
    c. Avoids punishment
    d. Possesses no concept of the underlying moral order
3. Stage 2—The instrumental relativist orientation
    a. The right behavior is that which satisfies the child's own needs
    b. Possesses elements of fairness, reciprocity, and equal sharing
    c. Do not possess elements of loyalty, gratitude, or justice

E. Conventional level
1. Child concerned with:
    a. Conformity and loyalty
    b. Maintaining, supporting, and justifying the social order
    c. Personal expectations of those significant to him/her
2. Child values maintenance of family regardless of consequences
3. Stage 3—The interpersonal concordance or "good boy–nice girl" orientation
    a. Behavior that meets approval of others is viewed as good
    b. Conformity to the norm is the "natural" behavior
    c. Earn approval by being "nice"
4. Stage 4—The "law and order" orientation
    a. Correct behavior is:
        i.   Obeying rules
        ii. Doing one's duty
        iii. Showing respect for authority
        iv. Maintaining social order
    b. Rules and authority can be social or religious

F. Postconventional, autonomous, or principled level
1. Child reaches cognitive formal operational stage
2. Attempts to define moral values and principles
3. Stage 5—The social contract, legalistic orientation
    a. Correct behavior defined in terms of general individual rights and standards agreed to by society
    b. Emphasis on:
        i.   Legal point of view
        ii. Possibility of changing law in terms of societal needs and rational considerations

IX. Skinner, Watson: Learning Theory
A. Learning occurs when behavior changes as a result of experience
B. Child
1. Acquires new behaviors
2. Produces alterations in existing behavior through:
    a. Forming associations through conditioning
    b. Observing models
3. Behavior is determined (conditioned) by:
    a. Environmental events
    b. Experiences
    c. Consequences

4. Rewarded behaviors are repeated
5. Punished behaviors are not repeated
C. Conditioning
1. Learning through association
a. Establishing a connection between a stimulus and a response
2. Operant or instrumental conditioning
a. Involves rewards or reinforcements to encourage specific behaviors
b. Applicable to toddler and preschooler learning
3. Avoidance conditioning
a. Discourages undesirable behaviors through punishment
b. Success depends on child's subjective assessment of reward or punishment
X. **Maslow: Humanistic Theory**
A. Focuses on attributes or characteristics that contribute to healthy personality development
B. Concerned with uniqueness and potential of individuals
1. Humans motivated by two need systems
a. Basic
i.   Food, water, and shelter
b. Growth needs—internally motivated and reinforced
i.   Beauty
ii.   Self-fulfillment
2. Needs arranged in a hierarchy
a. Lower-level needs assume dominance
b. When one level need is satisfied, the next becomes predominant
C. Theory does not address developmental stages or shaping of human behaviors
XI. **Biologic Growth**
A. During childhood, variations in growth of tissues and organs produces changes in body proportions
B. First year
1. Period of rapid growth
2. Lengthening of trunk
3. Accumulation of subcutaneous fat
C. First year to puberty
1. Legs grow more rapidly
2. Body becomes slender and elongated
D. Puberty
1. Feet and hand sizes increase
a. Appear large in relation to rest of body
b. Source of embarrassment
2. Trunk growth increases
3. Onset of puberty approximately 2½ years earlier for girls than boys
4. Rapid linear growth followed by lateral growth
5. Child "fills out" during later stages of adolescent growth
E. Height
1. Occurs as a result of skeletal growth
2. Considered a stable measurement of general growth
3. When maturation of skeleton is complete, linear growth ceases
F. Weight
1. Weight gain considered indication of satisfactory growth progress in child
2. Variable
3. Subject to numerous intrinsic and extrinsic factors

G. Neurologic growth
   1. Rapid brain cell growth from 30 weeks to 1 year of age
   2. Growth consists of:
      a. Increase in cytoplasm around nuclei of existing cells
      b. Increase in number and intricacy of communication with other cells
      c. Advancing peripheral axions in relation to expanding body dimensions
   3. Brain growth
      a. Measured by head circumference
      b. Increases six times during first year
   4. Lymph tissue
      a. Lymph nodes, thymus, spleen, tonsils, adenoids, blood lymphocytes
         i.   Increase rapidly
         ii. Reach adult dimensions by age 6
         iii. Tissue reaches size approximately twice that of adult by age 12
            (a) Rapid decline to stable adult dimension by adolescence

XII. Language Development
A. Child born with mechanism and capacity to develop speech and language skills
   1. Requires intact physiologic function of:
      a. Respiratory system
      b. Speech control center in cerebral cortex
      c. Articulation and resonance structures of the mouth and nasal cavity
   2. Child also requires:
      a. Intact and discriminating auditory apparatus
      b. Intelligence
      c. A need to communicate
      d. Stimulation
B. Components of language
   1. Phenology—learned first
      a. Basic units of sound that are combined to produce words
   2. Semantics of language—learned next
      a. Words and sentences convey an expressed meaning
   3. Gain knowledge of syntax
      a. The form or structure of language (rules)
   4. Pragmatics
      a. Principles specifying how language is used in different contexts and situations
C. Stages of language development
   1. Prelinguistic stage
      a. Period before child speaks first meaningful word
      b. Develops systematically over first 10 to 12 months
      c. Involves crying, cooing, and babbling
   2. Holophrastic stage
      a. Speech consists of one- or two-word statements
      b. Includes holophrases
         i.   Single words with meaning of entire sentence
   3. Telegraphic stage
      a. Speech includes content words only
      b. From 18 to 24 months
   4. Preschool period
      a. Produce lengthy sentences
      b. Speech increases in complexity
      c. From 30 months to 5 years

5. Middle childhood period
   a. Refines language skill
   b. Increases linguistic competence
   c. From 6 to 14 years
   d. Uses bigger words
   e. Understands complex syntactic structures of language
D. Theories of language development
   1. Learning theory
      a. Language is acquired as child hears and responds to speech
      b. How child learns to speak (two theories)
         i. Operant conditioning—adults reinforce child's attempt to produce grammatical speech
         ii. Acquires language by listening to and imitating speech of adults
   2. Nativists theory
      a. Inborn linguistic processor specialized for language learning
      b. Critical period for language development exists
      c. Most proficient at learning language between 2 years of age and puberty
   3. Interactional proponents
      a. Child is biologically prepared to acquire language
      b. Recognizes crucial role of environment in language learning
E. Factors affecting language development
   1. Delayed, lack of, or impaired speech can result from:
      a. Congenital structural defects of mouth and nasopharynx
      b. Hearing deficit
      c. Neurological dysfunction
      d. Maternal deprivation
      e. Emotional factors

XIII. **Self-Concept and Self-Esteem**
   A. Self-concept
      1. Perception of whole self
      2. Not present at birth
         a. Develops gradually as a result of unique experiences
         b. Learned during childhood
         c. Is a product of socialization
      3. Is subjective; may not reflect reality
      4. Answers the question "Who am I?" and "What am I?"
      5. Formed by:
         a. Self-selected mental images
         b. Attitudes
         c. How he/she thinks others see him/her
   B. Self-esteem
      1. Personal, subjective judgment of one's worthiness
         a. Derived from and influenced by social groups
         b. Individual's perception of how he/she is valued by others
      2. Factors affecting child's development of self-esteem (Sieving and Zirbel-Donish, 1990)
         a. Temperament
         b. Personality
         c. Ability and opportunity to accomplish age-appropriate developmental tasks
         d. Significant others
         e. Social roles undertaken
         f. Expectations of social roles

Early Childhood Experiences

Trust
+
Success in early motor/verbal experiences

↓

Positive self-concept
High self-esteem

↓

Encouragement, plentiful and positive
recognition from significant others
•
Role models of appropriate emotional expression
•
Permitted to experience disappointment, fear,
frustration; given empathetic support
•
Encouraged and permitted to finish tasks and reach goals

↓

Sturdy identity
Self-actualizing behavior

Figure 14–1. Requisites of childhood self-system development to support self-actualization. (Adapted from Betz, C.L., Hunsberger, M., Wright, S. [1994]. *Family-Centered Nursing Care of Children*, 2nd ed. Philadelphia: Saunders.)

3. Methods to develop and preserve self-esteem
   a. Needs to feel worthwhile
   b. Needs recognition for achievements
   c. Needs approval of parents and peers
   d. For inappropriate behavior, stress "behavior" is unacceptable, not the child
   e. Needs constructive communication
      i.   Use of "I" messages
      ii. Conveys feelings and needs
      iii. Does not destroy child's self-esteem
4. Positive experiences during developmental phases (see Figure 14–1)
   a. Individual with sturdy identity
   b. High level of self-actualization during adulthood
5. Negative experiences during developmental phases (see Figure 14–2)
   a. Individual with frail identity
   b. Self-destructive behavior

XIV. **Factors Influencing Growth and Development**
   A. Heredity
      1. Inherent characteristics influence development
         a. Sex of child directs pattern of growth and behavior of others toward child
         b. Physical characteristics are inherited
            i. Can influence how child grows and interacts with environment
   B. Gender
      1. Sex differences that influence behaviors in childhood
         a. Boys
            i.   More aggressive physically
            ii. Engage in rough and tumble play
            iii. Aggressive fantasies
            iv. Competitive behavior more common
            v.   Difficulty sitting still

   vi.   Engage in more exploratory behavior
   vii.   High activity level in presence of other boys
   viii. Greater impulsiveness
   ix.   Subject to distraction
   x.   More extensive sphere of relationships
   xi.   Highly oriented toward peer groups
   xii.   Congregate in large groups
   xiii. View themselves as more powerful and with more control over events
   xiv. Respond to a challenge, especially when it appeals to their ego or
         competitive feelings
  b. Girls
   i.   More aggressive verbally
   ii.   More likely to associate in pairs or small groups
   iii.   Involved in more intense relationships with a few close friends
   iv.   More concerned with the welfare of the group
   v.   More apt to compromise in situations involving conflict
   vi.   May be superior regarding motivation to achieve
   vii.   More likely to comply to adult commands
   viii. More nurturant or helping behavior
C. Culture
  1. Ethnicity, demographic setting, socioeconomic class, parental occupation, and
     family structure
  2. Attitude and expectations differ with respect to the sex of the child
D. Lifestyle
  1. Different family structures
   a. Two-parent
   b. One-parent
   c. Extended family
   d. Other variations

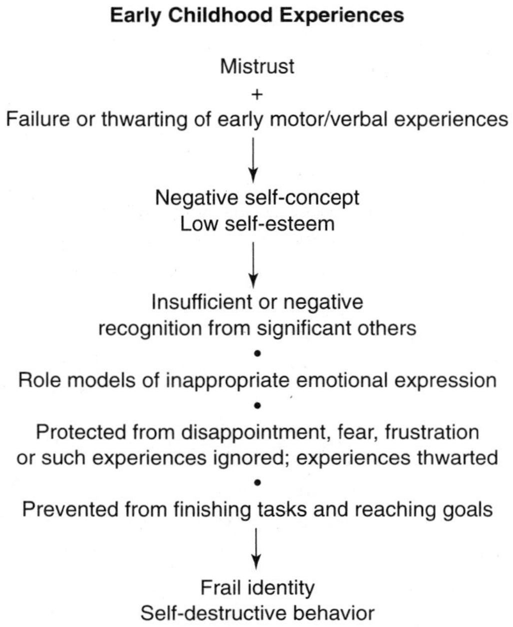

Early Childhood Experiences

Mistrust
+
Failure or thwarting of early motor/verbal experiences

↓

Negative self-concept
Low self-esteem

↓

Insufficient or negative
recognition from significant others
•
Role models of inappropriate emotional expression
•
Protected from disappointment, fear, frustration
or such experiences ignored; experiences thwarted
•
Prevented from finishing tasks and reaching goals

↓

Frail identity
Self-destructive behavior

Figure 14–2.   Requisites of childhood self-system development to support self-actualization.   (Adapted from Betz, C.L., Hunsberger, M., Wright, S. [1994]. *Family-Centered Nursing Care of Children,* 2nd ed. Philadelphia: Saunders.)

E. Play
   1. Activity with meaning and purpose
   2. May be directly related to expanding
      a. Social development
      b. Intellectual development
      c. Motor development
      d. Language development
   3. Play used to accomplish developmental tasks and master the environment
F. School
   1. Contributes to development in the form of:
      a. Skill training
      b. Cultural transmission
      c. Self-actualization
G. Neighborhood
   1. Offers child opportunity to experience world outside the home
      a. Accepting
      b. Supportive of child's physical and psychosocial needs
      c. Reinforcing of child's self-confidence and safety
H. Disease
   1. Disorders
      a. Skeletal (dwarfism)
      b. Chromosome anomalies (Turner syndrome)
      c. Disorders of metabolism
         i.   Vitamin D-resistant rickets
         ii. Mucopolysaccharidoses
         iii. Endocrine disorders
      d. Klinefelter syndrome and Marfan syndrome
      e. Chronic illness
      f. Congenital cardiac anomalies
      g. Respiratory disorders
         i.   Cystic fibrosis
      h. Malabsorption syndromes
      i. Defects in digestive enzyme systems
I. Neuroendocrine
   1. Possible relationship exists between hypothalamus and endocrine system that influences growth
   2. Peripheral nervous system may influence growth
      a. Muscles deprived of nerve supply degenerate
   3. All hormones affect growth in some manner
      a. Growth hormone, thyroid hormone, and androgens given to a person deficient in these hormones
         i.   Stimulates protein anabolism
         ii. Produces retention of elements essential for building protoplasm and bony tissue
J. Prenatal factors
   1. Smoking may produce smaller infant
   2. Fetal alcohol syndrome infants
      a. Exhibit prenatal and postnatal growth deficiencies in height and weight
      b. May produce significant central nervous system alterations that may not be evident until the child is older
   3. Fetal exposure to drugs such as marijuana, cocaine, and heroin
      a. Associated with intrauterine growth retardation and prematurity

4. Nutritional needs
   a. Poor nutrition may have negative influence on development from time of implantation of ovum until birth
   b. Severe maternal malnutrition associated with permanent reduction in total number of fetal brain cells
      i.   Has critical effect on child's intellectual functioning
K. Season, climate, and oxygen concentration
   1. Some evidence that:
      a. Growth in height faster in spring and summer months
      b. Growth in weight more rapid in autumn and winter
   2. Effects of hypoxia on growth
      a. Children with disorders that produce chronic hypoxia characteristically smaller than children of same chronological age
      b. Children native to high altitudes smaller than children of lower altitudes
L. Nutrition
   1. Single most important influence on growth
   2. Satisfactory nutrition closely related to good health throughout lifetime
   3. Malnutrition
      a. Defined as under-nutrition, primarily resulting from insufficient calorie intake
      b. May result from:
         i.   Inadequate dietary intake
            (a) Quality
            (b) Quantity
         ii.   Disease that interferes with:
            (a) Appetite
            (b) Digestion
            (c) Absorption
         iii. Excessive physical activity
         iv.   Inadequate rest
         v.   Disturbed interpersonal relationships
         vi.   Other environmental or psychological factors
M. Stress
   1. Abnormal conditions that tend to disrupt normal functions of the body or mind (Melloni and others, 1994)
   2. Some children more vulnerable than others
      a. Affected by age, temperament, life situation, and state of health
      b. Response can be behavioral, physiologic, or psychologic
   3. Methods of coping
      a. Respond by trying to change the circumstance (primary control coping)
         i.   Tantrums
         ii.   Aggressive behavior
      b. Trying to adjust to circumstances (secondary control coping) (Band and Weisz, 1988)
         i.   Withdrawal
         ii.   Submission
   4. Fear
      a. Emotional reaction to a specific real or unreal threat or danger
         i.   Child perceives threat
            (a) Person
            (b) Animal
            (c) Situation
         ii.   Perceives threat to be stronger than him-/herself and capable of harm

b. Alleviate fear by:
    i.   Presence of adult who will offer protection
    ii.   Becoming familiar with source of threat (animal)
N. Media
  1. Television
    a. Pervasive force
    b. Primary source of socialization in children
    c. Major source of information
       i.   Unhealthy messages regarding sex and violence
       ii.   Alcohol consumption synonymous with having a good time
       iii. Food products promoting unhealthy nutritional practices
  2. Reading materials
    a. Books, newspapers, magazines
       i.   Provide enjoyment
       ii.   Increase child's knowledge
  3. Movies
    a. Not closely associated with reality
    b. Usually provide opportunity for desirable social learning
    c. Child may be unable to distinguish between reality and fantasy
       i.   Results in fears

Bibliography

1. Ashwill, J.W., Droske, S.C. (1997). *Nursing Care of Children Principles and Practice.* Philadelphia: Saunders.
2. Band, E.B., Weisz, J.R. (1988). How to feel better when it feels bad: Children's perspectives on coping with everyday stress. *Dev Psychol*, 24:247–253.
3. Behrman, R.E., Kliegman, R.M., Arvin, A.M. (1996). *Nelson Textbook of Pediatrics*, 15th ed. Philadelphia: Saunders.
4. Betz, C.L., Hunsberger, M., Wright, S. (1994). *Family-Centered Nursing Care of Children*, 2nd ed. Philadelphia: Saunders.
5. Broyles, B.E. (1997). *Clinical Companion for Ashwill and Droske Nursing Care of Children Principles and Practice.* Philadelphia: Saunders.
6. Dox, I.G., Melloni, B.J., Eisner, G.M. (1994). *Melloni's Illustrated Medical Dictionary*, 3rd ed. Pearl River, NY: Parthenon.
7. Frederick, C., Reining, K. (1995). Essential components of growth and development. *J Post Anesth Nurs*, 10(1):12–17.
8. Sieving, R., Zirbel-Donisch, S. (1990). Development and enhancement of self-esteem in children. *J Pediatric Health Care*, 4(6):290–296.
9. Wong, D. (1995). *Nursing Care of Infants and Children*, 5th ed. St Louis, MO: Mosby.

REVIEW QUESTIONS

1. Growth

  A. Is a qualitative change
  B. Is a quantitative change
  C. Is the sum of select changes that take place during childhood
  D. Encompasses unrelated dimensions

2. Development

  A. Is a quantitative change
  B. Is a qualitative change
  C. Results in a decreased skill level
  D. Proceeds from an advanced stage of complexity to a simple stage of complexity

3. Characteristics of the toddler include all of the following except

  A. Marked physical and personality development
  B. Expanded social relationships
  C. Increasing awareness of dependence and independence
  D. Social cooperation and moral development

4. The adolescent period includes
   (1) Physical and emotional turmoil
   (2) Biologic and personality maturation
   (3) Redefinement of the self-concept
   (4) A focus on the individual self rather than group identity
   (5) Internalization of all previously learned values

   A. 1, 2
   B. 1, 2, 3, 5
   C. 1, 3, 4, 5
   D. All of the above

5. Piaget's theory of development focuses on

   A. Development of personality
   B. Psychosocial development
   C. Cognitive development
   D. Moral development

6. According to Freud, the Id
   (1) Develops at birth
   (2) Deals with the unconscious mind
   (3) Drives instinct
   (4) Seeks immediate gratification of needs
   (5) Functions as a moral arbitrator

   A. 1, 3, 5
   B. 3, 4, 5
   C. 1, 2, 3, 4
   D. 1, 2, 4, 5
   E. All of the above

7. The following personality traits are associated with Freud's oral stage of psychosexual development
   (1) Admiration or envy
   (2) Cockiness or self-belittlement
   (3) Orderliness or messiness
   (4) Stylishness or plainness
   (5) Pessimism or optimism

   A. 1, 3, 4
   B. 2, 4, 5
   C. 1, 2, 5
   D. 3, 4, 5
   E. All of the above

8. Kohlberg's theory of Moral Development

   A. Is based on the cognitive development theory
   B. Proceeds in no specific order
   C. States higher levels of moral reasoning can be acquired without appropriate cognitive development
   D. States morality is internal

9. In order for the child to develop speech and language skills
   (1) There must be intact physiologic function of the respiratory system
   (2) There must be a need to communicate
   (3) The auditory apparatus needs to be intact
   (4) The child must be intelligent
   (5) The child needs to be stimulated

   A. 1, 3
   B. 1, 2, 3
   C. 1, 3, 5
   D. All of the above

10. Factors influencing growth and development include all but

    A. Heredity
    B. Gender
    C. Culture
    D. Birth order
    E. Lifestyle
    F. Disease
    G. Nutrition
    H. Stress

ANSWERS TO QUESTIONS

1. B
2. B
3. D
4. D
5. C

6. C
7. C
8. A
9. D
10. D

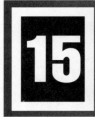

The Pediatric Patient

Donna M. DeFazio Quinn
Elliot 1-Day Surgery Center
Manchester, New Hampshire

I. **The Hospitalized Child**
   A. Outpatient approach
      1. Child arrives at facility morning of procedure
      2. Undergoes procedure
      3. Recovers from procedure
      4. Is discharged home same day
   B. Advantages
      1. Minimal separation from parents
      2. Decreased risk of infection due to decreased exposure to hospital environment
      3. Reduced psychological trauma to child and parents
      4. Decreased cost
   C. Disadvantages
      1. Outpatient facility may be freestanding
         a. Not connected to hospital
         b. May require transport to hospital if child requires overnight admission
      2. Does not allow for follow-up care and continued observation
      3. Can be a burden to family
      4. Less continuity of care
      5. Increased difficulty in managing pain
   D. Response to hospitalization
      1. Response varies according to:
         a. Developmental age
         b. Presence of support system
         c. Consistency of care providers
         d. Past exposure to hospital
   E. Factors affecting response (see Table 15–1)
      1. Age
         a. Preparation for hospitalization varies by age
         b. Based on child's growth and development

1. Discuss the stressors associated with hospitalization in the infant, toddler, preschooler, and school-age child.
2. Identify four nursing goals for performing the preoperative assessment.
3. Discuss the three degrees of dehydration in the pediatric patient.
4. Discuss the causes, signs and symptoms, and treatment of respiratory acidosis, respiratory alkalosis, metabolic acidosis, and metabolic alkalosis.
5. Identify four potential causes of hypothermia in the pediatric patient and discuss four precautionary measures for prevention.
6. Discuss the causes, signs and symptoms, and nursing interventions for stridor, croup, laryngospasm, bronchospasm, and airway obstruction in the pediatric patient.

Table 15–1 • DEVELOPMENTAL APPROACHES TO THE HOSPITALIZED CHILD

Infant

Anticipate needs and fulfill in a timely manner.

Provide opportunities for sucking and oral stimulation, use a pacifier if NPO.

Provide swaddling and soft talking to soothe.

Follow painful procedures with holding and cuddling.

Model appropriate behaviors to family members regarding stimulation, touch, verbalization and feeding (if appropriate).

Provide consistency in caregivers if possible (preoperatively and postoperatively).

Involve parents in the care of their infant as much as possible.

Older infant will anticipate painful procedures and fight.

Expect and inform parents about regression.

Limit the number of caregivers to whom the infant is exposed.

Request that parents bring the infant's security object (e.g., blanket, stuffed animal).

Encourage parents to be present during procedures (induction and PACU recovery—if facility policy permits).

Toddler

Expect regression, inform parents about behaviors.

Follow home routines and rituals (e.g., medicine taking, toileting).

Involve parents in the care of the toddler.

Employ all possible methods of pain control when the child must have a painful procedure done (e.g., IV insertion prior to anesthesia).

Anticipate temper tantrums when the child's frustration level is high.

Maintain a safe environment for physical acting out and temper tantrums.

Encourage the child to be independent (e.g., undressing self).

Provide support when the toddler needs to be dependent (e.g., hold after procedure, comfort during periods of parental separation).

Approach with positive attitude ("I am going to give you your medicine").

Preschooler

Take time for communication. Answer questions with simple, concrete explanations.

Explain all procedures honestly.

Expect egocentric behavior.

Provide for a safe and secure environment (e.g., object from home, underwear left on if not contraindicated).

Be consistent.

Ask the parents how the child usually copes in new situations.

Reassure the child that he/she did not cause the illness.

Involve parents in care and follow home routines and rituals.

Place the child with other children of the same age if possible.

Accept regression if it occurs; explain it to parents.

Encourage the child to be independent (e.g., medicine taking, dressing).

School Age

Inform the child of limits.

Involve the child in planning and implementing care (e.g., chose which arm for IV insertion if appropriate; hold gauze on venipuncture site).

Explain all procedures, and allow child time for questions and answers. Use medical and scientific terminology and diagrams or body outlines to explain the procedure.

Accept regression, but encourage independence.

Provide privacy.

Adapted from Ashwill, J.W., Droske, S.C. (1997). *Nursing Care of Children*. Philadelphia: Saunders, pp. 356–357.

    2. Cognitive development

    3. Family member's response

      a. Child knows when parent is upset

        i.   Anxiety transferred to child

        ii.   Child's anxiety level increases

          (a) Parent does not answer child's questions

          (b) Parent talks in whispers so child does not hear

      b. Reaction of family members dependent on:

        i.   Coping strategies

        ii.   Sociocultural environment

        iii. Availability of support systems

        iv. Prior experiences with hospitalization

      c. Nursing interventions to assist family members

        i.   See Table 15–2

II. Stressors Associated with Hospitalization

  A. Infant and toddler

    1. Separation anxiety (major stressor)

      a. Stages

        i.   Protest: child is agitated, resists caregivers, screams, cries, actively searches for parent, clings to parent, is inconsolable

        ii.   Despair: child becomes quiet, withdrawn, sad and apathetic, experiences hopelessness, refuses to play, acts disinterested

        iii. Detachment: child becomes interested in environment, appears content, plays quietly, does not search for parent, seems to form relationship with caregivers, may ignore parents if they return

    2. Fear of injury and pain

      a. Child may perceive reaction from parents

      b. Reaction affected by previous experiences

      c. Child reacts by crying, avoiding painful stimuli, pushing painful stimuli away

      d. Reaction may be result of intrusion on self, whether painful or not

    3. Loss of control

      a. Disruption of normal daily routines and rituals

      b. Offer choices to return some control to child

      c. May regress in behaviors associated with feeding, toileting, etc.

  B. Preschooler (early childhood)

    1. Separation anxiety

      a. Reaction less intense than infant and toddler

      b. Reactions include tantrums, regression, anger, uncooperativeness

      c. May repeatedly ask when parents will return or why they can't be there

    2. Fear of injury and pain

      a. Fear of mutilation

      b. Lack of understanding causes child to imagine that things are worse than they actually are

      c. Reacts to strangers, loud noises, machines, and equipment

      d. Reacts to intrusive procedures that cause bleeding

      e. Reaction based on previous experiences

      f. Child may cling to parent

      g. May fear illness caused by something they did wrong

      h. Pain

        i.   Reaction to pain includes

          (a) Crying

          (b) Restlessness

          (c) Whimpering

Table 15–2 • NURSING INTERVENTIONS RELATING TO FAMILY MEMBERS' RESPONSE TO HOSPITALIZATION OF CHILD

NURSING INTERVENTIONS	RATIONALE
1. Assess the physical and emotional needs of the family.	Identify factors that may interfere with appropriate adjustment to child's illness.
2. Orient the parents to the hospital/facility and provide information related to their physical needs (food, restrooms).	The physical needs of the parents must be met for them to meet the child's and their own emotional needs. Meeting these needs indicates support for the parents from the health-care giver.
3. Encourage the family to express their feelings and to ask questions about the child's illness/procedure.	Decreases anxiety and clarifies misconceptions.
4. Provide the family with information about the child's condition, treatment, and support systems.	Gives the parents a sense of control and decreases their anxiety.
5. Identify with the family the ways in which they are coping.	Individuals are not always aware of their coping mechanisms, and the nurse should evaluate the effectiveness of the family's coping mechanisms.
6. Refer the family to other professionals (social worker, clinical specialist, clergy) when their problems are not within the scope of nursing.	Early identification of family problems can decrease the possibility of escalation of the problems. Collaboration with other professionals can bring a holistic approach to the care of the child and family.
7. Assess the family's knowledge regarding ability to care for child at home.	A systematic approach should be used to assist the family in its readjustment to the home environment.
8. Provide information about the procedure and the expected outcomes. Tell the parents when they should consult the surgeon or nurse.	
9. Explain medications to be given at home, and provide written information about times, routes, side effects, and any special care to be taken when giving the medication.	
10. Explain any nutritional needs.	
11. Identify specific activities in which the child may or may not participate.	
12. Explain, demonstrate, and request a return demonstration of any treatments or procedures that will be done at home. This teaching should be an ongoing process that begins at the time of admission.	
13. Provide parent with a date for follow-up appointment with the surgeon.	
14. Provide parents with information about any referral agency needed for the child or family.	

Adapted from Ashwill, J.W., Droske, S.C. (1997). *Nursing Care of Children*. Philadelphia: Saunders, pp. 365–366.

         (d) Active resistance to caregiver

         (e) Screaming

      ii.   May be able to verbally express pain

      iii.   Can respond to pain-assessment tools

      iv.   Nursing assessment may not be truly accurate

   3. Loss of control

     a. Reacts to loss of control and disruption of routine

     b. May regress

       i.   Temper tantrums, toileting, etc.

       ii.   Exhibits negative behavior

 C. School age

   1. Separation anxiety

     a. Less affected because child is accustomed to periods of separation

     b. Reacts with inappropriate behavior

   2. Fear of injury and pain

     a. Fears

       i.   Death

       ii.   Disfigurement

       iii. Mutilation

       iv.   Procedures involving the genitals

     b. Child understands cause and effect

     c. May express guilt about illness

     d. Pain

       i.   Able to express concern regarding pain

       ii.   Methods to control reaction to pain

         (a) May want to watch procedure being performed

         (b) May request nurse to talk to them during procedure

   3. Loss of control

     a. Illness causes child to feel helpless and dependent

     b. Expresses anger at loss of independence

     c. Reactions include boredom, frustration, anger at caregivers, disinterest, refusing to cooperate

     d. Offer opportunities to promote independence

       i.   Assist in own care

       ii.   Assist with treatments

       iii. Make choices regarding fluid/food intake

III. Communicating with the Pediatric Patient

See Table 15–3.

 A. Types of communication

   1. Verbal

     a. Uses the spoken word

     b. May be hampered by language barriers

     c. May be misunderstood

   2. Nonverbal

     a. Most reliable

     b. Not so easily controlled

     c. Child's natural method of expression

 B. Communication skills

   1. Listening

     a. Nurse needs to understand level of language development and cognitive level of child

b. Need to provide child with explanations
  i.   Assists in establishing trust between child and nurse
2. Observation
  a. Provides cues about child
  b. Observe
    i.   Eyes
      (a) Happy
      (b) Sad
    ii. Quality of voice
    iii. Facial expression
      (a) Smiling/crying
      (b) Relaxed/tense
      (c) Makes eye contact/avoids eye contact
    iv. Body posture
      (a) Relaxed/stiff
      (b) Open or closed body posture (arms crossed in front of body versus arms loosely at sides)
      (c) Facing nurse/turned away from nurse
    v.   Movement
      (a) Holds still/resists touch by nurse
      (b) Moving around room/staying still near parent
      (c) Cooperative versus kicking and flailing
      (d) Nodding head with understanding
      (e) Biting, shaking, twitching, banging fist
    vi. Vocal clues
      (a) Crying
      (b) Whining
      (c) Silence
      (d) Tone of voice (shaky versus loud and confident)
    vii. Interaction between parent and child
      (a) How parent responds to child overall
      (b) How parent responds to child's behavior
        (i) Good behavior rewarded
        (ii) Unacceptable behavior receives attention
      (c) How parent physically handles child
      (d) How parent answers child's questions
      (e) How parent enlists the cooperation of the child
3. Silence
  a. Child may be quiet because he/she is:
    i.   Afraid
    ii. Shy
    iii. Angry
    iv. Busy
  b. Need to assess environment to determine cause of silence
  c. May be used by child to block communication
  d. May be used to promote positive communication
    i.   Allows child to process thoughts and feelings
    ii. Seeks to understand what has been communicated
C. Communicating at the child's level of understanding
  1. See Table 15–4

Table 15–3 • DEVELOPMENTAL MILESTONES AND THEIR RELATIONSHIP TO COMMUNICATION APPROACHES

DEVELOPMENT	LANGUAGE DEVELOPMENT	EMOTIONAL DEVELOPMENT	COGNITIVE DEVELOPMENT	SUGGESTED COMMUNICATION APPROACH
Infancy (0–12 months) The infant experiences the world through senses of hearing, seeing, smelling, tasting and touching.	Crying. Babbling. Cooing. Single-word production. Able to name some simple objects.	Dependent on others. High need for cuddling and security. Responsive to environment (sounds, visual stimuli, etc.). Distinguishes between happy and angry voices as well as familiar and strange voices. Beginning to experience separation anxiety.	Interactions are largely reflective. Begins to see repetition of activities and movements. Begins to intentionally imitate interactions. Short attention span (1–2 minutes).	Use calm, soft, soothing voice. Be responsive to cries. Engage in turn-taking vocalizations (adult imitates baby sounds). Talk and read regularly to babies. Prepare infant as you are about to perform care. Talk to infant about what you are about to do to him or her. Use slow approach and allow child time to get to know you.
Toddler (1–2 years) The toddler experiences the world through senses of hearing, seeing, smelling, tasting, and touching.	Two-word combinations emerge. Participates in turn talking in communication (speaker/ listener). "No" becomes a favorite word. Able to use gestures and verbalize simple wants and needs.	Strong need for security objects. Separation/stranger anxiety heightened. Participates in parallel play. Thrives on routines. Beginning development of independence; "Want to do by self." Still very dependent on significant adults.	Experiments with objects. Participates in active exploration. Begins to experiment with variations in activities. Begins to identify cause-and-effect relationships. Short attention span (3–5 minutes).	Learn the toddler's word for common items and use them in conversations. Describe activities and procedures as they are about to be done. Use picture books. Use play for demonstration. Be responsive to child's receptivity toward you and approach cautiously. Preparation should occur immediately prior to the event.

Preschool (3–5 years)			
Many words used are not fully understood by child. Further development and expansion of word combination (able to speak in full sentences). Upward growth in correct grammatical usage. Uses pronouns. Clearer articulation of sounds. Vocabulary rapidly expanding. May know words without understanding meaning.	Likes to initiate activities and make choices. Strives for independence but needs adult support and encouragement. Demonstrates purposeful attention-seeking behaviors. Learns cooperation and turn taking in game playing. Needs clearly-set limits and boundaries.	Begins developing the concepts of time, space, and quantity. Magical thinking becomes prominent. World view seen only from child's perspective. Short attention span (5–10 minutes).	Seek opportunities to offer choices. Use play to explain procedures and activities. Speak in simple sentences and explore relative concepts. Use picture and storybooks, puppets. Describe activities and procedures as they are about to be done. Be concise; limit length of explanations (less than 5 minutes). Engage in preparatory activities 1–3 hours prior to the event.
School Age (6–11 years)			
Communicates thoughts and appreciates viewpoints of others; words with multiple meanings and words describing things they have not yet experienced are not thoroughly understood. Expanding vocabulary enabling child to describe concepts, thoughts, and feelings. Development of conversational skills.	Interacts well with others. Understands rules to games. Very interested in learning. Builds close friendships. Beginning to accept responsibility for own actions. Competition emerges. Still dependent on adults to meet needs.	Able to grasp concepts of classification, conversation. Concrete thinking emerges. Becomes very oriented to "rules." Able to process information in serial format. Lengthened attention span (10–30 minutes).	Use photographs, books, diagrams, charts, videos to explain. Make explanations sequential. Engage in conversations that encourage critical thinking. Establish limits and set consequences. Use medical play techniques. Introduce preparatory materials 1–5 days in advance of the event.

From Ashwill, J.W., Droske, S.C. (1997). *Nursing Care of Children*. Philadelphia: Saunders, pp. 194–195, Table 10–3.

261

Table 15–4 • COMMUNICATING WITH THE CHILD IN THE PERIOPERATIVE SETTING

DON'T SAY	DO SAY	CHILD'S PERSPECTIVE
We are going to put you on a stretcher.	A special bed with wheels	Child may interpret as "stretch her"—"Why are they going to stretch me?"
The doctor will give you some gas.	The doctor will give you a special medicine that you will breathe through a mask like this (show mask)	"Why are they going to give me gasoline?"
The doctor will put you to sleep for your operation.	We will give you some medicine that will put you in a very deep sleep so the doctor can do the operation and you won't feel anything. When it's all over, you will wake up.	"They put my kitty to sleep and he never woke up."
The doctor will cut you open—make an incision	Make a tiny opening	"He's going to cut me with a knife?"
Take your vital signs	Check your temperature to see how warm you are and how fast your heart is beating.	Taking can be misinterpreted; Do not "take" anything from the child.
Put some electrodes on your chest	Put some sticky Band-Aids (stickers) on you so we can get a picture of your heart.	Involve child in process; supply child with printout of ECG that he/she will be able to take home and show his/her friends (great for show and tell)
Put a dressing on	You will have a bandage on	"Why will they dress me?"
Give you a shot—a little stick—just like a bee sting	Give you a little medicine under your skin	"When you get shot, you get hurt real bad." "Are you going to shoot me with a gun?"
Hook you up to a monitor	Attach some wires so you can see your heart beat on a TV screen	"Are you going to hook me like I hook the fish when I go fishing?"
Hurt	Boo-boo, owee, uncomfortable, discomfort	Communicate at child's developmental level with words he/she is familiar with.

D. Preoperative education
1. Include child in preparation
2. Communicate with child in language appropriate for age and developmental level
3. See Table 15–5

IV. **Preoperative Assessment**
A. Goals
1. Decrease anxiety level for child and parents
2. Establish a trusting relationship with child
3. Assist parents/family to:
   a. Design and implement a plan of care
      i.   Process (what's going to happen)
      ii. Expectations (time frames for preoperative, intraoperative, and postoperative)
      iii. Potential complications associated with procedure (pain, bleeding, nausea and vomiting, etc.)
   b. Plan preoperative preparation of child based on developmental level

Table 15–5 • EDUCATIONAL STRATEGIES ACCORDING TO AGE OF CHILD

DEVELOPMENTAL CHARACTERISTICS OF CHILD	EDUCATIONAL STRATEGIES
Infant (0–12 months) Unable to understand explanations but is sensitive to gentleness of voice, touch, and movement; infant can anticipate what will occur by physical signs (e.g., preparation of equipment, certain sounds associated with activity) Familiarity is a source of comfort Stranger anxiety occurs at 6–8 months of age	Main focus is to teach parents and caregiver Tone of voice and gentle handling communicate support to infant; prepare equipment and proceed with the activity as quickly as possible to reduce the amount of anticipated distress Talk to and touch infant before beginning a procedure Provide infant with favorite toy as soon as preparation begins Spend time with child before beginning a procedure or new activity; involve parent in activity
Toddler (1–3 years) Separation from parents is a primary threat Egocentric thinking View of world is that events are related to self Has developed limited coping skills, and ability to express emotions and feelings is limited Fantasizes about what will happen and why things are as they are Attention span short but can be increased with inclusion of sensory experiences Language skills limited Concept of time is limited	Encourage presence of parents for stressful events Careful explanations of reasons for events should be provided Machines and equipment should be described according to what they do and the sounds they make Use play as a method of expression; tell child it is OK to cry Use simple words child can understand; encourage expression of thoughts through doll and puppet play and verbal expression (e.g., "How does your puppet feel about . . . ?") Teaching sessions must be short (5–10 minutes) and should include equipment to touch and explore or a visual aid such as a book May interpret words literally; therefore, careful choice of simple words and short sentences is necessary Explanations should be given just before a procedure of short duration, such as an injection; if the procedure or event is more involved, the child should be told 2–3 hours before it occurs
Preschooler (3–6 yrs) Egocentric thinking continues Magical thinking continues Coping behaviors continue to be limited Fears of body mutilation peak at this age Ability to understand how body works increases Attention span is increasing	Explain why things are as they are; repeat such explanations to reduce potential for child feeling she or he has *caused* the situation Children should be asked to "repeat back" their perception and understanding of what has been told to them Reduce misconceptions by avoiding threatening words, such as "cut"; instead, say "make an opening" Encourage presence of parents for stressful events Give clear explanations about which body parts will and will not be affected (be clear about *how* it will be affected); feelings can be expressed through doll play, with demonstration of the procedure (i.e., where is the tube, the bandage, or the opening) Use visual aids of body models or picture outlines to enhance teaching; use correct anatomic terms Continue to provide information in short sessions (10–15 minutes) Involve child in the teaching sessions by doing something (e.g., handling equipment, drawing, or demonstrating on a doll)

(Table continued on following page)

Table 15-5 • EDUCATIONAL STRATEGIES ACCORDING TO AGE OF CHILD *Continued*

DEVELOPMENTAL CHARACTERISTICS OF CHILD	EDUCATIONAL STRATEGIES
Has increased verbal skills and questions "why" (questioning is child's way to learn about the events and people in the environment)	Provide opportunity for child to phrase questions; take the time to encourage further expression of questions, then provide information in a simple, clear response; questions at this age do not require long, complicated answers
Understands concrete explanations—only what he or she sees and touches	Actual equipment or miniature forms of equipment give child an understanding of environment
Interprets words literally	Some words used in health care are confusing (e.g., "take your vital signs" and "take your pulse"); it is better to explain what you will do (e.g., "listen to your heart")
Inability to conceptualize effect of event	Explain about the sensations that will be experienced
School-Age Child (6–12 years)	
Mastery becomes important at this age; is eager to learn and accomplish new skills and increase understanding of environment; has also acquired more skills, such as reading and verbal expression of ideas	Can use more books that teach the information through drawings, coloring books, and a variety of pencil-and-paper activities; encourage child to use language ability now to verbalize fears
Is beginning to have better understanding of causation but still cannot apply logic to abstract problems	Teaching should continue to focus on concrete aspects of the event; clarify misconceptions about causation
Concept of time has improved	Procedural information can be provided a day or two in advance
Attention span	Can pay attention for 30–45 minutes if actively involved
Peers are important support	Can hold educational sessions with groups of children who have similar problems
Increased neuromuscular development	Child can now perform skills that involve manipulation of equipment
Now more interested in self-management	Parents are still requested for support but child can be given more responsibility and in many instances can be given information separate from parents; children at this age may express some fears more freely to the health professional than to parents
Continues to view hospitalization as punishment	Continue to reassure and give explanations that reduce child's feelings of being the cause for the situation
Competitive behavior	Devise games that contain content to be learned

Adapted from Betz, C.L., Hunsberger, M., Wright, S. (1994). *Family-Centered Nursing Care of Children*. Philadelphia: Saunders, pp. 810–811.

4. Prevent postoperative complications
    a. Awareness of preoperative health status
        i. Cardiac
            (a) Congenital problems
        ii. Respiratory
            (a) Recent colds, congestion, asthma
        iii. Report any abnormal findings to anesthesiologist
B. Decision to perform procedure on an outpatient basis based on:
    1. Type of procedure to be performed
    2. Parental readiness and acceptance of procedure

3. Patient status
   a. Child in good health
   b. Generally ASA class I or II, occasionally class III
   c. If chronic illness, should be optimally prepared
C. Laboratory requirements
   1. Vary according to hospital/facility policy
   2. Current trend is towards no requirements for healthy children
   3. Generally only hematocrit for child less than 1 year of age
D. NPO guidelines
   1. Vary according to hospital/facility policy
   2. Stomach should be free of solids prior to anesthesia
   3. Clear liquids up to 2–4 hours preoperatively
E. Physical exam
   1. Use play therapy
      a. Perform procedure on teddy bear or doll first
      b. Have child hold stethoscope
      c. Have parent hold infant and approach from behind
   2. Listen to what the child has to say
   3. Give simple, easy-to-understand instructions; give one at a time
   4. Be honest with child
   5. Do painful procedures last
   6. Note birthmarks, bruises, loose teeth (document on record)

V. Preanesthesia Evaluation

See Table 15–6.

A. Performed by anesthesia provider and/or RN
   1. Evaluate for conditions requiring special treatment (e.g., anemia, asthma)
   2. Evaluate for recent exposure to communicable and infectious diseases (e.g., chicken pox, HIV, hepatitis)
   3. Counsel patient and parents regarding anesthesia and surgery
B. Physical exam
   1. General observation of the patient
   2. Vital signs
   3. Assess airway for potential difficulty with mask induction or intubation
   4. Assess respiratory status (presence of wheezing, coughing, etc.)
   5. Assess ability to perform venous access after induction
   6. Assess behavior to determine need for premedication
C. Implications of anesthesia to preexisting diseases (see Table 15–7)
   1. Chronically ill child may present for outpatient surgery
      a. Diagnostic or therapeutic procedure (e.g., insertion of venous access device)
D. Premedication
   1. Decrease fear and anxiety
   2. Allow easier transition of child from parents to anesthesia provider
   3. Techniques to assist in preparation of the child preoperatively (based on child's cognitive development)
      a. Explain purpose of procedure
         i.   Use pictures, diagrams, dolls, video, etc.
         ii. Use words child can understand
      b. Describe sequence of events
      c. Describe potential discomfort
      d. Allow time for ample discussion

Table 15–6 • THE PREANESTHETIC HISTORY

Child's Previous Anesthetic and Surgical Procedures
  Review anesthetic record for information about mask and endotracheal tube size, type and size of laryngoscope used, difficulties with mask ventilation or intubation

Perinatal Problems (especially for infants)
  Need for prolonged hospitalization
  Need for supplemental oxygen or intubation
  History of apnea and bradycardia

Other Major Illnesses and Hospitalizations

Family History of Anesthetic Complications, Malignant Hyperthermia (MH), or Pseudocholine-sterase Deficiency

Respiratory Problems
  Obstructive apnea, breathing irregularities, or cyanosis (especially in infants under age 6 months)
  History of snoring or obstructive breathing pattern
  Recent upper respiratory tract infection
  Recurrent respiratory infections
  Previous laryngotracheitis (croup)
  Asthma or wheezing during respiratory infections

Cardiac Problems
  Murmurs
  Dysrhythmias
  Exercise intolerance
  Syncope
  Cyanosis

Gastrointestinal Problems
  Reflux and vomiting
  Feeding difficulties
  Failure to thrive
  Liver disease

Exposure to Exanthems or Potentially Infectious Pathogens

Neurologic Problems
  Seizures
  Developmental delay
  Neuromuscular diseases
  Increased intracranial pressure

(Table continued on following page)

  4. Premedication should not be substituted for lack of preprocedure education
  5. Options for premedication
     a. Oral
        i.   Midazolam (not FDA approved)
             (a) 0.5 mg/kg PO
             (b) Nursing considerations
                 (i) May cause respiratory depression
        ii. Diazepam
             (a) 0.1–0.5 mg/kg PO
             (b) Nursing considerations
                 (i)   Slow onset
                 (ii) Prolonged action
                 (iii) Insufficient dose may cause disinhibition and decreased patient cooperation
        iii. Oral transmucosal fentanyl
             (a) Lollipop may be viewed by child as candy
             (b) 10 to 15 µg/kg oral transmucosal

Table 15–6 • THE PREANESTHETIC HISTORY *Continued*

Hematologic Problems
   Anemia
   Bleeding diathesis
   Tumor
   Immunocompromise
   Prior blood transfusions and reactions
Renal
   Renal insufficiency, oliguria, anuria
   Fluid and electrolyte abnormalities
Psychosocial
   Post-traumatic stress
   Drug abuse, cigarettes, alcohol
   Physical or sexual abuse
   Family dysfunction
   Previous traumatic medical and surgical experiences
   Psychosis, anxiety, depression
Gynecologic
   Sexual history
   Possible pregnancy
Current Medications
   Prior administration of corticosteriods
Allergies
   Drugs
   Iodine
   Latex products
   Surgical tapes
   Food allergies (especially soya and egg albumin)
Dental Condition (loose or cracked teeth)
When and What the Child Last Ate (especially in emergency procedures)

From Behrman, R.E., Kliegman, R.M., Arvin, A.M. (1996). *Nelson Textbook of Pediatrics*. Philadelphia: Saunders, p. 280.

        (c) Nursing considerations
            (i)   High incidence of itchy nose
            (ii) May cause respiratory depression, nausea, vomiting
    b. Nasal
       i.   Midazolam (not FDA approved)
          (a) 0.2 to 0.3 mg/kg intranasal
       ii. Ketamine
          (a) 3 mg/kg intranasal
    c. Intramuscular
       i.   Midazolam, ketamine
          (a) Painful
          (b) Reserved for sedation of highly distressed or uncooperative child
            (i)   Midazolam: 0.08 to 0.5 mg/kg IM
            (ii) Ketamine: 2 to 5 mg/kg IM
               a) Nursing considerations
                   Increases heart rate and blood pressure
               b) Accumulation of pharyngeal secretions may cause laryngospasm
               c) Contraindicated with increased intracranial pressure

Table 15–7 • SPECIFIC PEDIATRIC DISEASES AND THEIR ANESTHETIC IMPLICATIONS

DISEASE	IMPLICATION
Respiratory System	
Asthma	Intraoperative bronchospasm that may be severe
	Pneumothorax
	Optimal preoperative medical management essential; may require preoperative steroids
Difficult airway	May require special equipment and personnel
	Should be anticipated in children with dysmorphic features or acute airway obstruction as seen in epiglottitis, laryngotracheobronchitis, or airway foreign bodies
	Down syndrome patients may require evaluation of atlanto-occipital joint
	Patients with storage diseases may be at high risk
Bronchopulmonary dysplasia	Barotrauma with positive pressure ventilation
	Oxygen toxicity, pneumothorax a risk
Cystic fibrosis	Airway reactivity
	Risk of pneumothorax, pulmonary hemorrhage
	Atelectasis
	Assess for cor pulmonale
Sleep apnea	Must rule out pulmonary hypertension and cor pulmonale
	Requires careful postoperative observation for obstruction
Cardiac	
	Need for antibiotic prophylaxis for subacute bacterial endocarditis
	Use of air filters; careful purging of air from intravenous equipment
	Need to understand effects of various anesthetics on the hemodynamics of specific lesions
	Preload optimization and avoidance of hyperviscous states in cyanotic patients
	Possible need for preoperative evaluation of myocardial function and pulmonary vascular resistance
	Provide information concerning pacemaker function
Hematologic	
Sickle cell	Possible needs for simple or exchange transfusion based upon preoperative Hgb and percent Hgb S
	Importance of avoiding acidosis, hypoxemia, hyperviscosity states
Oncology	Pulmonary evaluation of patients who have received bleomycin, BCNU, CCNU, MTX, or chest radiation
	Avoidance of high oxygen concentration
	Cardiac evaluation of patients who have received anthracyclines; risk of severe myocardial depression with volatile agents
	Potential for coagulopathy

(Table continued on following page)

    d. Rectal
       i. Barbiturates
         (a) Methohexital
            (i) 1%–10% solution to 20–30 mg/kg per rectum
            (ii) Nursing considerations
               a) Unpredictable systemic bioavailability
               b) May cause rectal irritation or defecation
               c) Contraindicated in temporal lobe epilepsy or porphyria
         (b) Pentobarbital or secobarbital: 2–4 mg/kg per rectum
            (i) Nursing considerations

Table 15–7 • **SPECIFIC PEDIATRIC DISEASES AND THEIR ANESTHETIC IMPLICATIONS** *Continued*

DISEASE	IMPLICATION
Rheumatology	Limited mobility of TMJ, C-spine, arytenoid cartilages
	Requires careful preoperative evaluation
	May be difficult airway
Gastrointestinal	
Esophageal, gastric	Potential for reflux and aspiration
Liver	High overall morbidity and mortality in patients with hepatic dysfunction
	Altered metabolism of some drugs
	Potential for coagulopathy
Renal	Altered electrolyte and acid-base status
	Altered clearance of some drugs
	Need for preoperative dialysis in selected cases
	Succinylcholine to be used with extreme caution and only when serum potassium is shown recently to be normal
Neurologic	
Seizure disorder	Avoid anesthetics that may lower threshold
	Ensure optimal control preoperatively
	Preoperative anticonvulsant levels
Increased ICP	Avoid agents that increase cerebral blood flow
	Avoid hypercarbia
Neuromuscular disease	Avoid depolarizing relaxants; at risk of hyperkalemia
	May be at risk of malignant hyperthermia
Developmental delay	May be uncooperative at induction
Endocrine	
Diabetes	Greatest risk is unrecognized intraoperative hypoglycemia; if insulin is administered, monitor blood glucose intraoperatively; must provide glucose and insulin with adjustment for fasting condition and surgical stress
Skin	
Burns	Difficult airway
	Risk of rhabdomyolis and hyperkalemia from succinylcholine
	Fluid shifts
	Bleeding
	Coagulopathy

From Behrman, R.E., Kliegman, R.M., Arvin, A.M. (1996). *Nelson Textbook of Pediatrics.* Philadelphia: Saunders, p. 283.

        a) May cause paradoxical reaction
        b) Contraindicated in porphyria
    ii.   Benzodiazepines
        (a) Midazolam: 0.4–1 mg/kg per rectum
        (b) Diazepam: 0.1–0.5 mg/kg per rectum
    iii.   Ketamine: 8 to 10 mg/kg per rectum
  e. Anticholinergics
    i.   Current trend to limit use
        (a) Drying of secretions is unpleasant in awake child
        (b) Need for drying secretions diminished due to current available anesthetics
    ii.   Used when:
        (a) Prolonged surgery in prone position
        (b) Airway surgery

(c) Ophthalmic surgery to block the oculocardiac reflex
    iii. Nursing considerations
        (a) Atropine: can cause fever, extremely dry mouth, flushing, tachycardia
        (b) Glycopyrrolate
            (i) No CNS effects
            (ii) Long duration
        (c) Scopolamine
            (i) May cause confusion
            (ii) Long duration
6. Nursing interventions
    a. If premedication is administered
        i. Continuous observation of child necessary
            (a) Prevent from falling or becoming injured
            (b) Resuscitation equipment immediately available
        ii. Nursing staff skilled in airway management

VI. Intraoperative Anesthetic Considerations

Although the nurse is not involved in the administration of anesthetic agents, an understanding of anesthetic agents and techniques will assist the nurse in providing answers to both patient and parents questions as well as ensuring a safe postoperative recovery from the anesthetic agents.

A. Placement of intravenous catheter
    1. May be inserted prior to induction with older or cooperative child
        a. May use eutectic mixture of local anesthetics (EMLA)
        b. Requires application to site one to two hours in advance of venipuncture
    2. Usually inserted after mask induction on young child
B. Emotional responses to anesthetic induction (see Table 15–8)
    1. Decrease by allowing parent in operating room
    2. Hospital/facility policy dictates acceptance of this practice
C. Induction of anesthesia
    1. Induction technique dependent on:
        a. Specific patient risks

Table 15–8 • EMOTIONAL RESPONSES TO ANESTHETIC INDUCTION

AGE	TYPICAL RESPONSES AND IMPLICATIONS
0–8 months	Fewer anticipatory responses Generally calm with strangers Mask induction well tolerated
8 months to 2 years	Separation anxiety is high Most difficult mask induction Premedication, preinduction useful
3–7 years	Separation anxiety still present Mask induction aided by parental presence
7–11 years	Generally calm with mask induction Fear of needles Fear of loss of control
12–18 years	Generally prefers IV to mask induction

From Behrman, R.E., Kliegman, R.M., Arvin, A.M. (1996). *Nelson Textbook of Pediatrics.* Philadelphia: Saunders, p. 284.

   b. Disease status
   c. Preoperative medical condition
   d. Presence or absence of intravenous line
   e. Child's or parent's choice
2. Selected technique discussed with parents and child during preoperative interview
3. Allowing child to practice beforehand with selected equipment (inhalation mask) helpful
   a. Use play therapy
   b. Assist in decreasing child's anxiety level of new and unfamiliar procedure
   c. Involve parents as appropriate
4. Ideal method is one that causes the child the least distress
5. Intravenous induction
   a. Medically indicated if child is coming in for emergency surgery
      i.   Child is at increased risk for aspiration of gastric contents
6. Rapid sequence induction
   a. Patient inhales 100% oxygen prior to induction
      i.   Prolongs the time to arterial desaturation with apnea
   b. Anesthesia induced with rapid acting hypnotic and a muscle relaxant
   c. Cricoid pressure is applied to occlude the esophagus
      i.   Prevents reflux of gastric contents into the pharynx
7. Risks associated with rapid sequence induction
   a. Unknown if muscle paralysis will cause inability to intubate the trachea or ability to ventilate by mask
   b. The fixed dose of hypnotic may cause hypertension or hypotension
   c. The younger the infant, the shorter the time before child becomes hypoxic after pre-oxygenation induction
   d. Cricoid pressure does not protect against aspiration
D. Inhalation induction technique
1. Medically indicated in situations where spontaneous breathing needs to be preserved
   a. Foreign body in the airway
2. Most widely accepted technique of induction in the United States
3. Well accepted for children 4 to 10 years of age
4. Technique
   a. Proceed in quiet surroundings
   b. Avoid delays once in operating room
   c. Use flavored aromas on mask
   d. Administer nitrous oxide (odorless) in conjunction with oxygen first
   e. Introduce more aromatic vapor anesthetics

VII. Anesthetic Agents

For complete information regarding anesthetic agents, see Chapter 22.

VIII. Perianesthesia Considerations
   A. Metabolism
   1. Infants have greater nutritional requirements to minimize loss of body protein
      a. Develop disturbances more rapidly than adults
      b. Complications increase proportionately with increase in time of fluid restriction
   2. Infants and small children should have priority on surgery schedule in order to limit food and fluid deprivation to as short a time as possible

    3. Intake (may vary according to hospital/facility policy)
      a. Infants
        i.   Regular formula or diet up to six hours before anesthesia
        ii. Clear liquids up to 2 to 4 hours before
        iii. Should not miss more than two feedings
        iv. Oral intake resumes promptly after recovery from anesthesia
      b. Toddler/preschool children
        i.   Usually permitted clear liquids up to six hours preoperatively
      c. Children over 5 years of age
        i.   NPO after midnight or 8 hours prior to induction of anesthesia
        ii. Exceptions necessary for children with diabetes or other special problems
        iii. Postoperative oral intake resumed as tolerated
  B. Fluid and electrolyte balance
    1. Infants and young children more vulnerable to changes (see Table 15–9)
    2. Dehydration
      a. Dehydration causes disturbances in acid-base balance
        i.   Caused by decrease in fluid intake or fluid loss
        ii. Causes rapid extracellular fluid loss
        iii. Results in electrolyte imbalance
        iv. Results in intracellular fluid loss
        v.   Causes cellular dysfunction
        vi. Can result in hypovolemic shock and death
      b. Degrees of dehydration (Ashwill, 1997)
        i.   Mild
           (a) 3–5% loss of body weight
           (b) Fluid volume loss less than 50 ml/kg

Table 15–9 • **PEDIATRIC DIFFERENCES RELATED TO FLUID AND ELECTROLYTE BALANCE**

Infants

Can lose fluids equal to their extracellular fluid (ECF) within 2–3 days due to the higher percentage of water in the ECF

Have a decreased ability to concentrate urine, due to immature renal function

Have a higher peristalsis

Have an immature lower esophageal sphincter, which makes them more prone to gastroesophageal reflux, which can lead to dehydration and electrolyte disturbances

Have a harder time compensating for acidosis due to decreased ability to acidify urine

Infants and Young Children

Have a higher metabolic turnover of water due to a higher metabolic rate (if losses are not replaced rapidly, imbalance occurs)

Are unable to verbalize or communicate thirst

Infants and Children

Have a proportionately greater body surface area in relation to body mass, resulting in greater potential for fluid loss via the skin and GI tract

Have a higher proportionate water content (premature infants have 90%, full-term infants, 75%–80%, preschool-age children 60%–65%, and adolescents and adults approximately 55%), with a larger proportion of fluid in the extracellular space

Have a lower functioning immune system, with more tendencies to infectious diseases, fever, food intolerances and allergies, gastroenteritis, and respiratory infections, all of which can result in fluid and electrolyte disturbances and fluid volume deficit

---

From Ashwill, J.W., Droske, S.C. (1997). *Nursing Care of Children.* Philadelphia: Saunders, p. 673.

Table 15–10 • **MAINTENANCE FLUID REQUIREMENTS AND MINIMUM URINE OUTPUT**

Fluid Requirements by Body Weight

Up to 10 kg:	100 ml/kg/day
10–20 kg:	100 ml/kg/day + 50 ml/kg/day for each additional kg between 10 and 20 kg
20+ kg:	150 ml/kg/day + 20 ml/kg/day for each additional kg over 20 kg

Hourly Infusion Rates
To obtain hourly infusion rate, divide total amount required by 24.

Minimum Urine Output by Age Group

Infants and toddlers:	>2–3 ml/kg/hr
Preschoolers and young school-age:	>1–2 ml/kg/hr
School-age and adolescents:	0.5–1 ml/kg/hr

Adapted from Ashwill, J.W., Droske, S.C. (1997). *Nursing Care of Children.* Philadelphia: Saunders, p. 681.

      ii.   Moderate
         (a) 6–9% loss of body weight
         (b) Fluid volume loss less than 50–90 ml/kg
      iii. Severe
         (a) 10% or more loss of body weight
         (b) Fluid volume loss 100 ml/kg or greater
   c. Nursing assessment
      i.   Measure intake and output
      ii. Assess skin color, temperature, and turgor
      iii. Assess perfusion
         (a) Vital signs
            (i)   Rapid, weak thready pulse
            (ii) Increased respiratory rate
            (iii) Decreased blood pressure
      iv. May be irritable, lethargic, confused; infant cry may be high pitched and weak
   d. Treatment (see Table 15–10)
      i.   Correct imbalance
      ii. Treat underlying cause
 C. Hypervolemia
  1. Infants and toddlers at increased risk
   a. Excessive IV fluid administration
   b. Increase in antidiuretic hormone and aldosterone being produced in response to stress of surgery
  2. Signs and symptoms
   a. Restlessness
   b. Increased activity
   c. Periorbital edema
      i.   Presents before alterations in vital signs
      ii. May be more prominent on dependent side (side child is lying on)
   d. Tachycardia
   e. Dyspnea
      i.   Accompanied with grunting respirations **and**
      ii. Adventitious lung sounds

3. Interventions
   a. Administer IV fluids using graduated fluid chamber (soluset) or infusion pump
   b. Monitor intake and output
   c. If periorbital edema noted, decrease IV fluid rate
   d. Notify physician
D. Disturbances in acid-base balance
   1. Need to maintain pH between 7.35 to 7.45 (see Chapter 13)
      a. Crucial in order to maintain:
         i. Cellular function
         ii. Enzyme activity
         iii. Neuromuscular membrane potentials
      b. Respiratory system and kidney work to maintain pH within normal limits
      c. Respiratory system works rapidly
      d. Renal system works slower; 1 to 2 days
   2. Acidosis (pH below normal)
      a. Lungs
         i. Respiratory rate and depth increase
         ii. Removes CO_2
         iii. Increases pH
      b. Kidneys
         i. Excrete hydrogen ions
         ii. Conserve bicarbonate
         iii. Increase pH
   3. Alkalosis
      a. Lungs
         i. Respiratory rate and depth decrease
         ii. Decrease pH
      b. Kidneys
         i. Conserve hydrogen ions
         ii. Decrease pH
   4. Imbalance involving respiratory or metabolic mechanism
      a. Types of imbalances
         i. Respiratory acidosis
            (a) Causes
               (i) Pulmonary disease
               (ii) Airway obstruction
               (iii) Respiratory failure
               (iv) CNS depression from sedation or anesthesia
            (b) Signs and symptoms
               (i) Increased heart rate
               (ii) Dysrhythmias
               (iii) Increased respiratory rate and depth
            (c) Treatment
               (i) Aimed at correcting ventilation defect
                  a) Oxygen
                  b) Intubation
                  c) Mechanical ventilation
                  d) Administration of sodium bicarbonate
         ii. Respiratory alkalosis
            (a) Causes
               (i) Hyperventilation

          (ii) Hypoxia
          (iii) Compensation from metabolic acidosis
          (iv) Sepsis
      (b) Signs and symptoms
          (i)   Increased respiratory rate and depth
          (ii) Dysrhythmias
      (c) Treatment
          (i)   Oxygen
          (ii) Rebreathing mask
          (iii) Mechanical ventilation
          (iv) Sedatives
   iii.   Metabolic acidosis
      (a) Causes
          (i)   Increased metabolic rates
            a) Fever
            b) Respiratory distress syndrome
            c) Seizures
          (ii) Ketoacidosis
          (iii) Interference with normal metabolism
          (iv) Loss of bicarbonate
          (v) Acute and chronic renal failure
      (b) Signs and symptoms
          (i)   Increased heart rate
          (ii) Dysrhythmias
          (iii) Cold, clammy skin (mild to moderate acidosis)
          (iv) Warm, dry skin (severe acidosis)
          (v) Changes in level of consciousness (from confusion to stupor to coma)
      (c) Treatment
          (i)   Treat underlying cause
          (ii) Sodium bicarbonate replacement
          (iii) Potassium replacement
          (iv) Mechanical ventilation
   iv.   Metabolic alkalosis
      (a) Causes
          (i)   Volume depletion
      (b) Signs and symptoms
          (i)   Dysrhythmias
          (ii) Increased heart rate
          (iii) Changes in level of consciousness (confusion to stupor)
          (iv) Muscular weakness
      (c) Treatment
          (i)   Treat underlying cause
          (ii) Administer fluids with sodium chloride and potassium
          (iii) Isotonic saline
          (iv) Histamine H_2 receptor antagonist (cimetidine)
E. Body temperature
  1. Infants and children
    a. Heat loss occurs by:
      i.   Evaporation—skin becomes wet; evaporative heat loss can occur
      ii.   Radiation—heat transfers from body surface to surfaces in room not in direct contact with body

   iii. Conduction—air currents pass over skin
    (a) Can be caused by cold diapers and blankets
  2. Assessment of infants
   a. May exhibit mottling
    i. Due to immature temperature-regulating mechanism
  3. Measurement of temperature
   a. Methods
    i. Axillary
     (a) For infants and children <4 to 6 years of age
     (b) For uncooperative, immunosuppressed, neurologically impaired
     (c) For patient who has undergone oral surgery
     (d) Reading is approximately 1 degree lower than the body's core temperature
    ii. Oral
     (a) For children >6 years of age
     (b) Avoid liquids 30 minutes prior to oral temperature assessment
     (c) Inaccurate readings may be caused by oral intake, oxygen administration, nebulizer treatments, and crying
    iii. Rectal
     (a) Taken only when no other route is feasible
    iv. Digital
     (a) May be used for oral, axillary, or rectal readings
     (b) Disposable covers over probe prevent cross-contamination
    v. Tympanic
     (a) Frequently used for pediatric patients
     (b) Provides quick measurement
     (c) Temperature correlates with oral and rectal readings
     (d) Placing traction on pinna to expose tympanic membrane increases accuracy of reading
   b. Documentation
    i. Important to document method used to obtain reading
    ii. Provides health-care professional with consistent measurement when evaluating fluctuations in temperature
  4. Hypothermia
   a. Child has difficulty maintaining temperature
    i. Due to body being stressed from illness or injury
   b. Occurs rapidly in child due to:
    i. Increased body surface area
    ii. Decreased mass
    iii. Lack of insulating subcutaneous fat
    iv. Infants less than 6 months lack involuntary shivering mechanism
   c. Potential causes of hypothermia
    i. Vasodilating anesthetic agents (halothane, isoflurane, enflurane)
    ii. Muscle relaxants
    iii. Environmental causes (cool environment of operating room)
    iv. Administration of cool intravenous fluids
   d. Danger to small child
    i. Increased oxygen consumption
    ii. Increased vasoconstriction
     (a) Results in hypoxemia, hypoglycemia and metabolic acidosis
     (b) Depletes metabolic energy stores
     (c) Causes fluid and electrolyte imbalance

e. Must be kept warm to minimize heat loss and prevent hypothermia
  i.   Body temperature decreases in operating room due to cooler temps
  ii. Room temperature should be maintained as warm as 85°F (29°C)
  iii. Continuous monitoring during anesthesia period
  iv. Other precautionary measures
     (a) Warm blankets
     (b) Warm air devices
     (c) Radiant heat lamps
     (d) Wrapping head
     (e) Heated humidification of inspired gases
     (f) Drapes must permit some evaporative heat loss to maintain equalization of body temperature
     (g) Solutions should be warmed
        (i) Skin preps
        (ii) Irrigation solutions

5. Hyperthermia
  a. Core temperature greater than 104°F (40°C)
  b. Causes
     i.   Fever
     ii. Dehydration
     iii. Infection
     iv. Decrease in sweating from atropine administration
     v.   Environmental causes (warm operating room)
     vi. Excessive drapes
     vii. Medications that disturb temperature regulation such as general anesthetics (malignant hyperthermia [MH])
        (a) Refer to Chapter 23 for complete information on MH

F. Respiratory assessment
  1. High priority due to impact of ineffective ventilation on cardiac function
  2. Majority of cardiac arrhythmias and arrests related to respiratory failure
  3. Airway problems most common on emergence and immediate postoperative period
  4. Anatomic differences
     a. Large tongue in proportion to mouth size; potential for airway obstruction
     b. Shorter neck; potential for compromised airway and difficult intubation
     c. Normal narrowing of trachea at cricoid cartilage ring
        i.   Provides an anatomic cuff when tracheal intubation is used
        ii. Cuffed endotracheal tubes not used for children under 9 years of age due to anatomic cuff
        iii. Smaller endotracheal tube used to eliminate risk of stenosis
     d. Smaller airway opening
        i.   Reduction in airway radius causes potential increase in airflow resistance
        ii. Small amount of mucous, edema or foreign body may cause airway obstruction significant to compromise gas exchange
     e. Infant is obligatory nose breather; difficult breathing through mouth
     f. Infants and young children use abdominal muscles to inhale
     g. Cartilage of larynx easily compressed
        i.   Can cause narrowing of airway
        ii. Occurs when neck is flexed or extended
        iii. More susceptible to spasm
     h. Epiglottis is short, stiff, U-shaped
        i.   Difficult intubation
        ii. Swelling narrows opening; potential for airway obstruction

    i. Tonsillar tissue normally enlarged until early school age

    j. Rib cage

      i.   Intercostal musculature poorly developed

      ii. Accessory muscles do not contribute to inspiration

      iii. Child more dependent on effective movement of diaphragm for ventilation

5. Assessment

    a. Evaluation of skin color

    b. Respiratory rate (normally higher than adult)

    c. Pattern of breathing

    d. Depth of respirations

    e. Quality of breath sounds

6. Measurement—Respirations

    a. Inform child of procedure; avoid excitement

    b. Observe respiratory rate and effort for one full minute

    c. Evaluate quality and symmetry of chest movement

    d. Allow infant or toddler to cry prior to performing comfort measures

      i.   Ensures deep breathing in child who cannot follow commands

      ii. May initiate coughing if secretions are present

    e. Observe for signs of respiratory distress

      i.   Increased heart rate one of first signs

      ii. Grunting

      iii. Stridor

      iv. Wheezing

          (a) Inspiratory

          (b) Expiratory

      v.   Croupy cough

      vi. Flared nostrils

      vii. Sternal retractions

      viii. Increased work of breathing

      ix. Cyanosis

      x.   Apneic periods

    f. Increased respiratory rate

      i.   Response to respiratory distress is an increase in respiratory rate

      ii. Potential causes include:

          (a) Respiratory distress

          (b) Excess fluid volume

          (c) Pain

          (d) Hypothermia

          (e) Elevated temperature

    g. Decreased respiratory rate

      i.   Potential causes include:

          (a) Administration of anesthetic agents

          (b) Administration of opioids; decreased respiratory rate may be compensated by increased depth of respirations

          (c) Pain

7. Abnormal Respiratory Findings

    a. Depressed respiratory rate

      i.   Causes

          (a) Anesthesia

          (b) Narcotic/barbiturate/sedative administration

          (c) Hypothermia

    ii.   Signs and symptoms
        (a) Shallow, slow, or absent respirations
    iii. Nursing interventions
        (a) Stimulate patient
        (b) Oxygen administration
        (c) Chin lift
        (d) Insertion of oral airway
        (e) Suction
        (f) Notify anesthesiologist/surgeon

b. Stridor
    i.   Definition
        (a) Shrill, harsh sound
        (b) Heard during inspiration, expiration, or both
        (c) Produced by air flowing through a narrowed segment of the respiratory tract
    ii.   Causes
        (a) Tracheal irritation
        (b) Edema
    iii. Signs and symptoms
        (a) Crowing respirations
    iv. Nursing interventions
        (a) Administer humidified oxygen
        (b) Elevate head of bed
        (c) Notify anesthesiologist/surgeon
        (d) Physician may order racemic epinephrine

c. Croup
    i.   Definition
        (a) Term used to describe a group of conditions
        (b) Characterized by inspiratory stridor, croupy cough, hoarseness, and varying degrees of respiratory distress
    ii.   Causes
        (a) Irritation caused by intubation
        (b) Endotracheal tube too large
        (c) Traumatic or repeated intubations
        (d) Coughing with endotracheal tube in place
        (e) Change of patient position while intubated
        (f) Surgical procedure greater than one hour in duration
        (g) Surgical trauma
    iii. Signs and symptoms
        (a) Usually occur soon after extubation—usually within 1 hour
        (b) May intensify within 4 hours
        (c) Completely resolved in 24 hours
        (d) Signs
            (i)   Stridor
            (ii) Thoracic retractions
            (iii) Hoarseness
            (iv) Croup-like cough
            (v) Varying degrees of obstruction cause varying degrees of distress
    iv. Nursing interventions
        (a) Humidified oxygen
        (b) Elevate head of bed

        (c) Notify anesthesiologist/surgeon

        (d) Physician may order racemic epinephrine; dexamethasone; reintubation if airway severely compromised; hydration

        (e) Calm child

           (i) Judicious use of narcotics

           (ii) Parental presence

        (f) Consider overnight admission; edema may rebound after administration of racemic epinephrine

  d. Laryngospasm

    i. Definition

        (a) Approximation of true vocal cords or both true vocal cords and false cords

    ii. Cause

        (a) Inadequate depth of anesthesia with sensory stimulation

           (i) Secretions

           (ii) Manipulation of airway

           (iii) Surgical stimulation

        (b) Irritant trigger

    iii. Signs and symptoms

        (a) Use of accessory muscles

           (i) Always auscultate lungs since "rocking motion of chest" may be misinterpreted

        (b) Partial to complete obstruction

    iv. Nursing interventions

        (a) Administer 100% oxygen

        (b) Continuous positive pressure by mask

        (c) Notify anesthesiologist/surgeon; may administer muscle relaxants

        (d) Remove stimulus

        (e) Jaw thrust

  e. Bronchospasm

    i. Causes

        (a) Pre-existing airway disease (asthma)

        (b) Allergy/anaphylaxis

        (c) Histamine release

        (d) Aspiration

        (e) Mucous plug

        (f) Foreign body

        (g) Pulmonary edema

    ii. Signs and symptoms

        (a) Increased respiratory rate

        (b) May have mild, moderate, or severe dyspnea

        (c) Intercostal retractions

        (d) Inspiratory and expiratory wheezing

    iii. Nursing interventions

        (a) Administer oxygen

        (b) Suction secretions; remove foreign body

        (c) Notify anesthesiologist/surgeon

        (d) Physician may order:

           (i) Inhaled bronchodilators (nebulized albuterol or metaproterenol)

           (ii) Terbutaline

           (iii) Epinephrine

           (iv) Antihistamine

Table 15–11 • NORMAL VITAL SIGNS BY AGE

AGE	TEMPERATURE* FAHRENHEIT	TEMPERATURE* CELSIUS	PULSE RATE (BPM)	RESPIRATORY RATE (BREATHS/MIN)	BLOOD PRESSURE (MMHG)
Newborn	98.6–99 (axillary)	36–37.2 (axillary)	120–160	30–60	Systolic: 46–92 Diastolic: 38–71
3 years	97.5–98.6 (axillary)	36.4–37	80–125	20–30	Systolic: 72–110 Diastolic: 40–73
10 years	97.5–98.6 (oral)	36.4–37 (oral)	70–110**	16–22	Systolic: 83–121 Diastolic: 45–79
16 years	97.5–98.6 (oral)	36.4–37 (oral)	55–90	15–20	Systolic: 93–131*** Diastolic: 49–85

*The normal range of the child's temperature will depend on the method used. Temperatures are subject to circadian rhythms in all ages.
**After age 12 years, a boy's pulse is 5 bpm slower than a girl's.
***After age 14 years, blood pressure in boys is higher than in girls.
From Ashwill, J.W., Droske, S.C. (1997). *Nursing Care of Children*. Philadelphia: Saunders, p. 212.

          (v) Dexamethasone
          (vi) Support ventilation; reintubation
      (e) Consider overnight admission
   f. Airway obstruction
      i.   Causes
         (a) Tongue
         (b) Soft tissue edema
         (c) Retained packs/sponges
      ii. Signs and symptoms
         (a) Use of accessory muscles
         (b) Nasal flaring
         (c) Abdominal/diaphragmatic contractions
         (d) Decrease in inhaled air
     iii. Nursing interventions
         (a) Administer oxygen
         (b) Chin lift
         (c) Suction
         (d) Notify anesthesiologist/surgeon
G. Cardiovascular assessment
  1. Vital signs
    a. Measure vital body functions
    b. Provide basis for decisions concerning overall health of child
    c. Vary depending on state of the child (see Table 15–11)
      i.   Resting vital signs (sleeping)
      ii. Awake vital signs (crying)
  2. Anatomy
    a. Chest wall thin in infants and young children
      i.   Less subcutaneous fat and muscle tissue than older child
      ii. Potential to auscultate innocent murmurs
  3. Heart rate
    a. Regulated by autonomic nervous system
    b. Increased heart rate results in increase in cardiac output
    c. Decreased heart rate results in decreased cardiac output

4. ECG monitoring
   a. T waves in infants much larger because electrodes are situated much closer to the heart
   b. May be same size as QRS complex
   c. Accurate assessment necessary to avoid erroneous or double counting
   d. Monitor in lead II for best P wave configuration
   e. Lead placement
      i. Place on extremities to decrease artifact from breathing
      ii. Do not place leads on bony prominence
      iii. To decrease potential of trauma on fragile ribs, snap leads to electrodes before placing on child
5. Measurement—Pulse
   a. Apical pulse rate recommended for infants and children <2 years of age
   b. Assess prior to administering medications
   c. Inform child of procedure
   d. Allow child to play with stethoscope
   e. Radial pulse may be used for children >2 years of age
6. Measurement—Blood pressure
   a. Choose appropriate cuff size
      i. Based on midpoint limb circumference
      ii. Inappropriate size will cause blood pressure to be artificially elevated or decreased
   b. Measure in same extremity with patient in same position for increased consistency
   c. Inform child of procedure
7. Assessment findings
   a. Cyanosis, tachypnea
      i. Sign of impending respiratory failure
      ii. Indication of cardiovascular compromise and possible hemodynamic instability
   b. Tachycardia
      i. Normal method of increasing cardiac output
      ii. Possible causes include:
         (a) Decreased perfusion due to impending shock
         (b) Elevated temperature
         (c) Pain
         (d) Early respiratory distress
         (e) Administration of medications (atropine, morphine, epinephrine)
   c. Bradycardia
      i. Of great concern in pediatric patient
      ii. Possible causes include:
         (a) Respiratory distress (late sign)
         (b) Hypoxia
         (c) Vagal response
         (d) Increased intracranial pressure
         (e) Administration of Prostigmin
   d. Hypertension
      i. Possible causes include:
         (a) Excess intravascular fluid
         (b) Carbon dioxide retention
         (c) Pain
         (d) Increased intracranial pressure
         (e) Administration of medications such as ketamine, epinephrine

e. Hypotension
  i.   Possible causes include:
      (a) Anesthetic agents such as halothane, isoflurane, enflurane
      (b) Administration of opioids
      (c) Late sign of shock
H. Postoperative assessment
  1. Airway (refer to respiratory assessment section on pages 277–281 for in-depth discussion)
    a. Respiratory rate
      i.   Pattern, depth, and quality of breath sounds
    b. Assess breath sounds
    c. Assess respiratory effort
      i.   Observe for dyspnea, tachypnea, wheezing, use of accessory muscles of ventilation, persistent coughing accompanied with frothy secretions
      ii. Tachypnea is often the first sign of respiratory distress in infant
      iii. Support airway
      iv. Increase oxygen delivery (humidified)
      v.   Bag-valve mask
      vi. Prepare for possible endotracheal intubation
  2. Breathing
    a. Monitor oxygen saturation level
    b. Listen
      i.   Snoring indicates possible obstruction from the tongue
      (a) Chin-lift/jaw-thrust maneuver
      (b) Place on side
      (c) Position sitting up with tongue falling forward
      ii. Gurgling indicates possible secretions
      (a) Suction
  3. Circulation/perfusion
    a. Evaluate heart rate
      i.   Assess ECG rate and rhythm
    b. Assess distal perfusion (palpation of peripheral pulses)
    c. Evaluate blood pressure
    d. Assess skin color
  4. Check dressing if present
    a. Note and record amount of drainage if present
    b. Reinforce if necessary
    c. Inspect areas underneath bed linens to identify potential bleeding sites
  5. Assess for bleeding in areas without dressing
    a. Throat following tonsillectomy, oral/dental procedures
    b. Genitourinary area
  6. Inspect intravenous site
    a. Secure intravenous by wrapping area with gauze to prevent removal by infant, toddler, or small child
    b. Assess and regulate infusion rate
  7. Assess skin color and integrity
    a. Observe for any abnormalities that may not have been present preoperatively; e.g., scratches, bruises
    b. Wash antiseptic from skin (e.g., Betadine)
  8. Assess level of consciousness
    a. Reactive, unreactive, restless, responsive, combative, cooperative, etc.
    b. Restrain if necessary
    c. Pad side rails to prevent injury

9. Pain
    a. Myths
        i.   Children do not feel pain
        ii. Children will not remember having pain
        iii. A child is not in pain if he/she can be distracted or is sleeping
        iv. A child can tolerate pain better than an adult can
        v.   Medication should not be given to a child unless he/she exhibits obvious signs of pain
        vi. A child cannot tell you where it hurts
        vii. It is best to medicate children using the intramuscular route
        viii. Addiction is a dangerous side effect of pain management in the pediatric patient
    b. Physiologic changes
        i.   Observe for:
            (a) Increased heart rate
            (b) Increased blood pressure
            (c) Increased respiratory rate
            (d) Decreased oxygen saturation
            (e) Flushed skin
            (f) Restlessness
            (g) Sweating
            (h) Dilated pupils
        ii. Above physiologic changes are mimicked when child exhibits fear and anxiety
        iii. Assess further to determine cause of physiologic changes
    c. Assessment
        i.   Assess according to developmental level (see Table 15–12)
        ii. Consider child's previous pain experiences
            (a) Obtain history from parent/child
            (b) Identify child's normal response to pain
            (c) Identify child's normal words to communicate pain
        iii. Assessment tools
            (a) Used to obtain more objective data related to pain assessment
            (b) Types
                (i) Self-report
                (ii) Behavioral instruments
            (c) Benefits
                (i) Gives child an effective means to communicate the pain he/she is feeling
                (ii) Allows consistent means for child to express pain level
            (d) Examples
                (i) Oucher or Faces pain-rating scale
                    a) Consists of drawings or pictures of faces ranging from smiling to crying
                (ii) Numeric scale
                    a) Usually a line with numbers (0 to 10) with 0 meaning no pain and 10 meaning the worst possible pain
                (iii) Poker chip tool
                    a) Uses four poker chips, with each chip representing a little bit of pain; child is asked to take as many chips as he/she has pain

Table 15–12 • ASSESSMENT OF PAIN ACCORDING TO DEVELOPMENTAL LEVELS

Neonate and Infant
- Changes in facial expression, including frowns, grimaces, expressions of surprise, and facial flinching
- Increases in blood pressure and heart rate and decrease in arterial saturation
- High-pitched, tense, harsh, crying
- General or total body response in neonate and young infant that becomes more purposeful as infant matures
- Extremities may thrash about; some infants exhibit tremors
- Older infants rub painful area, pull away, or guard the involved part

Toddler
- Loud crying
- Verbalizes words that indicate discomfort ("ouch," "hurt," "boo-boo")
- Attempts to delay procedures perceived as painful
- Generalized restlessness
- Guards the site
- Touches painful area
- May run from nurse

Preschooler
- May think he/she is being punished for some deed or thought
- Cry, kick
- Describe location and intensity of pain ("ear hurts bad")
- Regression to earlier behaviors (loss of bladder and bowel control)
- Withdrawal
- Deny pain to avoid possible injection
- May have been told to be "brave" and deny pain even though it is present

School-Age
- Able to describe pain
- Fears bodily harm
- Has an awareness of death
- Stiff body posture
- Withdrawal
- Procrastinates or bargains in order to delay procedure

From Ashwill, J.W., Droske, S.C. (1997). *Nursing Care of Children*. Philadelphia: Saunders, p. 517.

        (iv) Word Graphic Rating Scale
            a) Uses descriptive words on a scale; child is asked to identify the degree of pain
    d. Postoperative pain
      i.   Treatment plans begin preoperatively
        (a) Age-appropriate education prior to procedure
        (b) Discussion of proposed plan
        (c) Hands-on play with medical equipment
      ii. Intraoperative treatment
        (a) Regional blocks
        (b) Analgesics administered intraoperatively
      iii. PACU
        (a) Analgesics, opioid administration
          (i) Orally
          (ii) Intravenously, through existing line—intermittent or continuous infusion

(iii) Combination therapy
  a) Opioids, with acetaminophen or nonsteroidal antiinflammatory drugs
(iv) PRN dosing not recommended—results in inadequate pain relief
(v) Patient-controlled analgesia (PCA)
  a) Allows for timely administration of medication improving analgesic efficacy
  b) Allows for the patient to participate in self care
  c) Patients individually selected for PCA based on manual dexterity and conceptual understanding
(b) Assess at regular intervals
(c) Assess during vital sign checks
(d) Whenever possible administer medications through a noninvasive route, orally, or an existing intravenous line
iv. Nursing considerations
  (a) Administer analgesics as prescribed
  (b) Avoid waiting until child experiences severe pain before medicating
  (c) Avoid palpating surgical site unless necessary
  (d) Medicate prior to performing nursing activities that could be painful (dressing change, deep breathing, ambulation)
  (e) Involve parents in process
v. Nonpharmacologic interventions for pain management
  (a) Provide distraction (playing, singing, taking a deep breath, blowing bubbles, watching TV, reading)
  (b) Provide relaxation opportunities (hold baby in comfortable position, rock, assist child to get into a comfortable position, ask child to take a deep breath and hold it—then to go "limp as a rag doll" while exhaling slowly)
  (c) Behavioral contracting
    (i) Set up a reward system using stars or tokens (for younger children)
    (ii) Use a written contract (for older children) that includes measurable goals and identified rewards
  (d) Guided imagery (child describes the details of a pleasurable experience; concentrates on pleasurable experience during painful procedure)
e. Medications (see Chapter 24)
10. Thermoregulation
  a. Assess temperature on admission, every hour, and at discharge (may vary according to facility policy)
    i. Hypothermia
      (a) Implement warming measures
    ii. Hyperthermia
      (a) Potential for malignant hyperthermia
I. Discharge
  1. Process
    a. Planning usually begins before admission
    b. Encourage parental participation in child's care
    c. Encourage child to participate in own care based on physical and developmental abilities
      i. Involvement helps maintain and improve coordination, muscle tone, and circulation

  ii. Fosters positive self-esteem and self control

  iii. Assists child to view hospitalization in a more positive manner

 d. Seek child's input when developing plan of care

2. Criteria

 a. Facility-specific criteria

3. Instructions

 a. Procedure-specific

 b. Anesthesia

  i. Written instruction on how to contact anesthesia department should questions arise regarding anesthesia-related concerns or complications

  ii. Two adults to accompany child on discharge; one to drive and one to attend to needs of the child

  iii. Child safely secured in restraint device appropriate for age

4. Nurse's role

 a. Clarify misconceptions for both parent and child

 b. Encourage child to talk about experience

 c. Review necessary information, including, but not limited to:

  i. Necessary physical care

   (a) Encourage child and/or parent participation

   (b) Return demonstration assists in verifying child and/or parental understanding

  ii. Necessary equipment and/or supplies needed to care for child (crutches, dressings, etc.)

  iii. Instructions on activities of daily living (play activities, sports, return to school)

  iv. Diet

  v. Medication administration

  vi. Potential complications

   (a) Expected

   (b) Unexpected

  vii. Emergency contact information

  viii. Follow-up appointment with physician

  ix. Necessary home health agency referrals

  x. Assessment of parental capability to meet child's needs

 d. Reinforce physician's instructions

 e. Allow time for questions and answers

 f. Provide written instructions

5. Postoperative telephone evaluation

 a. Usually performed the day after surgery

 b. Assess patient's progress

 c. Identify postoperative complications

 d. Evaluate need for referral to physician

 e. Answer questions or concerns

 f. Reinforce discharge instructions

Bibliography

1. Ashwill, J.W., Droske, S.C. (1997). *Nursing Care of Children Principles and Practice.* Philadelphia: Saunders.

2. Asprey, J.R. (1994). Postoperative analgesic prescription and administration in a pediatric population. *J Pediatric Nursing*, 9(3):150–157.

3. Band, E.B., Weisz, J.R. (1988). How to feel better when it feels bad: Children's perspectives on coping with everyday stress. *Dev Psychol*, 24:247–253.

4. Behrman, R.E., Kliegman, R.M., Arvin, A.M. (1996). *Nelson Textbook of Pediatrics*, 15th ed. Philadelphia: Saunders.

5. Behrman, R.E., Kliegman, R.M. (1994). *Nelson Essentials of Pediatrics,* 2nd ed. Philadelphia: Saunders.

6. Bell, C., Kain, Z.N. (1997). *The Pediatric Anesthesia Handbook,* 2nd ed. St. Louis, MO: Mosby.

7. Betz, C.L., Hunsberger, M., Wright, S. (1994). *Family-Centered Nursing Care of Children,* 2nd ed. Philadelphia: Saunders.

8. Broyles, B.E. (1997). *Clinical Companion for Ashwill and Droske Nursing Care of Children Principles and Practice.* Philadelphia: Saunders.

9. Burden, N. (1993). *Ambulatory Surgical Nursing.* Philadelphia: Saunders.

10. Dox, I.G., Melloni, B.J., Eisner, G.M. (1994). *Melloni's Illustrated Medical Dictionary,* 3rd ed. Pearl River, NY: Parthenon.

11. Fiorentini, S.E. (1993). Evaluation of a new program: Pediatric parental visitation in the PACU. *J Post Anesth Nurs,* 8(4):249–256.

12. Fossum, S.R., Knowles, R. (1995). Perioperative oxygen saturation levels of pediatric patients. *J Post Anesth Nurs,* 10(6):313–319.

13. Frederick, C., Reining, K. (1995). Essential components of growth and development. *J Post Anesth Nurs,* 10(1):12–17.

14. Hanna, D. (1995). Guidelines for pulse oximetry use in pediatrics. *J Pediatric Nurs,* 10(2):124–126.

15. Keller, V.E. (1995). Management of nausea and vomiting in children. *J Pediatric Nursing,* 10(5):280–286.

16. Maligalig, R.M.L. (1994). Parents' perceptions of the stressors of pediatric ambulatory surgery. *J Post Anesth Nurs,* 9(5):278–282.

17. Sieving, R., Zirbel-Donisch, S. (1990). Development and enhancement of self-esteem in children. *J Pediatric Health Care,* 4(6):290–296.

18. Wong, D. (1995). *Nursing Care of Infants and Children,* 5th ed. St. Louis, MO: Mosby.

REVIEW QUESTIONS

1. The following description identifies the developmental approach of the hospital child in what age group?
   Description of approach:
   Involve parents in care
   Anticipate temper tantrums when frustration level is high
   Encourage independence (e.g., undressing self)
   Approach with positive attitude ("I am going to give you your medicine")
   Expect regression
   Follow home routines

   A. Preschooler
   B. School-age
   C. Toddler
   D. Infant

2. The following suggested approach to communication describes which age group?
   Suggested approach:
   Seek opportunities to offer choices
   Use play to explain procedures and activities
   Speak in simple sentences
   Use pictures, storybooks, puppets
   Describe activities and procedures as they are about to be performed
   Be concise; limit explanations to less than 5 minutes
   Begin preparation 1 to 3 hours prior to procedure

   A. Preschooler
   B. School-age
   C. Toddler
   D. Infant
   E. Adolescent

3. When approaching a child to administer medication intramuscularly, it is best to say

   A. "I'm going to give you a little shot"
   B. "This is going to hurt a little—just like a bee sting"
   C. "I'm going to give you an injection in your bottom"
   D. "I'm going to give you a little medicine under your skin"
   E. "This is just going to be a little stick"

4. Which of the following are true regarding fluid and electrolyte balance in infants?
   (1) Infants have a decreased ability to concentrate urine
   (2) Infants have a high peristalsis
   (3) Infants have an immature lower esophageal sphincter making them prone to gastroesophageal reflux
   (4) Infants have a harder time compensating for acidosis due to decreased ability to acidify urine

   A. 1, 4
   B. 1, 3, 4
   C. 1, 2, 4
   D. None of the above
   E. All of the above

5. When assessing the infant for pain, the nurse will note which of the following?
   (1) Changes in facial expressions, including frowns, grimaces, expressions of surprise, and facial flinching
   (2) Thrashing of extremities
   (3) High-pitched, tense, harsh crying
   (4) Increase in blood pressure and heart rate
   (5) Increase in oxygen saturation

   A. 1, 3, 4
   B. 1, 2, 4
   C. 2, 3, 4, 5
   D. 1, 2, 3, 4
   E. All of the above

6. Response to hospitalization varies according to
   (1) Developmental age
   (2) Presence of support system
   (3) Consistency of care providers
   (4) Past exposure to hospital

   A. 1, 4
   B. 1, 2,
   C. 1, 2, 3
   D. 1, 2, 4
   E. All of the above

7. The nursing goals of the preoperative assessment include all of the following except
   A. To decrease the child's anxiety level
   B. To review preoperative lab results
   C. To assist the family in developing a plan of care
   D. To review time frames (preoperatively, intraoperatively, and postoperatively)
   E. To establish a trusting relationship with the child

8. Periorbital edema
   (1) Is a sign of dehydration
   (2) Is a sign of hypervolemia
   (3) May be more prominent on dependent side (side child is lying on)
   (4) May present before alteration in vital signs are noted
   (5) Is a late sign of hypovolemia

   A. 1, 4
   B. 2, 4
   C. 2, 3, 4
   D. 1, 3, 5
   E. 2, 4, 5

9. Causes of croup in the pediatric patient include
   (1) Irritation caused by intubation
   (2) Inserting an endotracheal tube that is too large
   (3) Coughing with an endotracheal tube in place
   (4) Change of patient position while intubated
   (5) Undergoing a surgical procedure that is greater than one hour in duration
   (6) Surgical trauma

   A. 1, 2
   B. 1, 3
   C. 1, 3, 5
   D. 2, 3, 4
   E. All of the above

10. All of the following are myths associated with pediatrics and pain except

    A. Children do not feel pain
    B. The physiologic changes associated with pain are mimicked when a child exhibits fear and anxiety
    C. A child is not in pain if he/she can be distracted or is sleeping
    D. A child cannot tell you where it hurts
    E. It is best to medicate children using the intramuscular route

ANSWERS TO QUESTIONS

1. C
2. A
3. D
4. E
5. D

6. E
7. B
8. C
9. E
10. B

16

The Adolescent Patient

Donna M. DeFazio Quinn
Elliot 1-Day Surgery Center
Manchester, New Hampshire

I. Growth and Development
  A. Definition
    1. Eleven to 21 years of age
    2. Transition from childhood to adulthood
      a. Biological changes
      b. Psychosocial changes
    3. Three stages
      a. Early adolescence
      b. Middle adolescence
      c. Late adolescence
  B. Early adolescence
    1. Ten to 13 years of age
    2. Period of growth acceleration
      a. Increase in appetite in response to rapid growth
    3. Biological development
      a. Girls
        i. Development of breast tissue
        ii. Begin to put on fat
        iii. Slightly taller and heavier than boys
        iv. Beginning of hair growth
          (a) Pubic
          (b) Axillary
        v. Menarche
      b. Boys
        i. Enlargement of testes
        ii. Gynecomastia
        iii. Spermatogenesis
    4. Motor development
      a. Increase in gross muscle mass
      b. Increase in fine motor coordination
      c. Prone to ligament tears
      d. Awkward, gangly period

Objectives

1. Discuss biological and psychosocial development of early, middle, and late adolescence.
2. Identify three stressors associated with hospitalization.
3. List five nursing interventions used to approach the hospitalized adolescent.
4. Discuss five nursing interventions to communicate effectively with an adolescent.
5. Identify five educational strategies used to educate the adolescent.
6. Describe four signs that the nurse might observe that may indicate the adolescent is in pain.

5. Psychosocial development
    a. Erikson
        i. Stage of identity versus role confusion (12 to 18 years of age)
            (a) Corresponds to Freud's genital stage
            (b) Characterized by rapid physical changes
            (c) Become preoccupied with appearance (how they look to others)
    b. Freud
        i. Genital stage (age 12 and older)
            (a) Begins with puberty
            (b) Reproductive system and sex hormones mature
            (c) Genital organs become major source of sexual tensions and pleasures
            (d) Also period of forming relationships and preparing for marriage
    c. Other characteristics
        i. Shy, awkward
        ii. Adjusting to middle school
        iii. Move from operational thinking to formal, logical operations
            (a) Ability to manipulate abstractions
            (b) Able to reason from principles
            (c) Able to weigh multiple points of view according to varying criteria
            (d) Able to think about the process of thinking
        iv. More at ease with same sex
            (a) Tend to move away from family
            (b) Increased activity with peers
            (c) Conformity
            (d) Cliques
        v. Increase in self consciousness
            (a) Meticulous about their appearance
            (b) Feel everyone is looking at them
        vi. Low self esteem
        vii. Increase in rebellious behavior
        viii. Increase in independence
        ix. Increase in sexual interest
            (a) Interest is greater than sexual activity
            (b) Often have questions about sexual changes they are experiencing
C. Middle adolescence
    1. Fourteen to 16 years of age
    2. Biological development
        a. Girls
        b. Increase in height
            i. Increase in breast size
            ii. Increase in growth of pubic hair
            iii. Sexual maturation occurs
            iv. Develop hips
            v. Growth acceleration declines
            vi. Appetite decreases
        c. Boys
            i. Change in voice
                (a) Larynx enlarges
            ii. Muscle mass enlarges followed by increase in strength
            iii. Widening of shoulders
            iv. Growth of facial hair
            v. Rapid increase in height

      vi. Increase in appetite
      vii. Increase in size of genitalia
      viii. Gynecomastia decreases
   d. Both sexes
      i.   Increase in acne
      ii. Development of sweat glands (increase in body odor)
      iii. Completion of dentition
      iv. Sensory and language development complete
      v.   Capacity of cardiovascular pump increases
         (a) Heart size doubles
         (b) Blood pressure, blood volume, and hematocrit increase
      vi. Lung capacity doubles
      vii. Physiological increase in sleepiness
3. Motor development
   a. Increase in physical endurance
   b. Increased skill in sports
   c. Increase in fine and gross muscle coordination
   d. Increase in fine motor skill activities
4. Psychosocial development
   a. Increased conflicts with parents
   b. Mood swings
      i.   Impulsive
      ii. Impatient
      iii. Narcissistic
      iv. Moody
   c. Tests established limits
   d. Privacy very important
   e. Peer group very important
   f. Abstract thoughts increase
      i.   Tend to question and analyze everything
      ii. Become more self-centered
5. Sexual development
   a. Sexual experimentation begins
   b. Degree of sexual activity varies
   c. Begin to sort out sexual identity
      i.   Beliefs regarding love, honesty, and propriety
   d. Choose either celibacy, monogamy or polygamous experimentation
   e. Knowledgeable regarding risk of pregnancy, AIDS, and other sexually transmitted diseases
      i.   Knowledge does not necessarily control behavior
6. Development of self concept
   a. Period of experimentation
      i.   Peers less important
      ii. Change style of dress
      iii. May change group of friends
   b. Deal with inner turmoil
7. Development of relationships
   a. Parental relationship strained
      i.   May become distant
      ii. Dating may become source of conflicts
   b. Physical attractiveness still important
   c. Popularity is critical for peer relationships and self-esteem

        d. Begin to identify career path
           i.   Life skills
           ii.   Opportunities
        e. Positive role models crucial at this stage of development
    D. Late adolescence
      1. Seventeen to 20 years of age or beyond
      2. Biological development
        a. Growth slows
        b. Physically mature
        c. Structure and reproductive growth almost complete
        d. No neurodevelopmental changes apparent
        e. Cardiopulmonary capacity relatively mature
      3. Psychosocial development
        a. Aware of own strength and limitations
        b. Establishes own value system
        c. Cognition tends to be less self-centered
        d. Ability to think abstractly
        e. Able to express thoughts and feelings about various aspects of life
           i.   Justice, patriotism, history
        f. Idealistic about love, social issues, ethics, and lifestyles
        g. Conformity less important
        h. More consistency of emotions
        i. Able to control anger
        j. Turbulence with parents decreases
        k. Prepares to leave home
        l. Social relationships more mature
      4. Sexual development
        a. More commitment to intimate relationships
        b. Form stable relationships and attachments
        c. More realistic concept of partner's role
      5. Self concept
        a. More secure body image and gender-role definition
        b. Sexual identity secured
        c. Self esteem increases
           i.   More stable body image
           ii.   Comfortable with physical growth
        d. Social roles defined and articulated
           i.   Career decisions become pressing
           ii.   Self-concept increasingly tied to role in society (students, workers, parents)
      6. Relationships
        a. Separation from parents complete (emotional and physical)
        b. Gained independence from family
        c. Peer group not so important as individual friendships
        d. Relationships are characterized by giving and sharing
        e. Testing possibility of permanent male–female relationship
II. Stressors Associated with Hospitalization
    A. Separation anxiety
      1. May or may not want parents involved
      2. May become more dependent on parents
      3. Separation from friends increases anxiety

B. Fear of injury or pain
  1. Fear how illness is viewed by peers
     a. Activity limitations
     b. Appearance
  2. May refuse to cooperate if treatment does not fit into lifestyle
  3. May project image of "calm and cool" even though they are terrified
  4. May question everything or appear confident in that they know it all
  5. Able to describe degree of pain
C. Loss of control
  1. May resist dependence
  2. Wants to be in control
  3. May react to loss of control with anger, withdrawal, uncooperativeness, and refusal to follow rules
  4. A planned procedure (scheduled surgery) allows a greater sense of control than an unplanned (emergency) procedure
  5. Often feel isolated and unable to obtain adequate support

III. **Interventions to Minimize Stress**
A. Preparation
  1. Give information about proposed procedure
     a. Adolescent very anxious regarding self image and identity
     b. Information will help to reduce psychological stress and elicit more cooperation
        i.   Explain tests/procedures
        ii. Provide information on how the adolescent will feel during certain tests/procedures
        iii. Provide information regarding when results of tests will be known
        iv. Discuss approximate length of time in each phase of hospitalization (preadmission, operating room, PACU, etc.)
        v.   Discuss impact of procedure on daily living (expected return to school, driving, etc.)
        vi. Adolescent more accepting of information provided by health-care professional rather than parent
     c. May be concerned regarding cause of illness (need for surgery); provide necessary information
  2. Allow choices when possible
     a. Induction of anesthesia
     b. Parental presence
  3. Intraoperative
     a. Monitoring devices that will be applied (ECG, pulse oximeter, B/P)
     b. Sensations from anesthetics administered
     c. Endotracheal intubation after "asleep" or loss of consciousness obtained
     d. Only surgical area exposed; respect adolescent's privacy
        i. Sterile drapes applied
        ii. Only area exposed to staff view is operative area
     e. Will remain unconscious throughout procedure; will not talk or do anything to cause them embarrassment

IV. **Developmental Approach to the Hospitalized Adolescent**
A. Nursing interventions
  1. Provide privacy
  2. Avoid stereotyping adolescent as difficult and unmanageable
  3. Adolescent reacts to not only information given, but also manner in which it is delivered

  4. Encourage wear of normal street clothes when possible
  5. Encourage questions regarding appearance and the effects of the current illness/surgery on the adolescent's future
  6. Incorporate scientific and medical terminology into explanations and preparations for procedures
  7. Provide adolescent with body outlines, diagrams, etc., when explaining procedures; include rationale
  8. If possible, utilize special area on unit reserved for adolescents
  9. Introduce adolescent to other adolescents on unit
  10. Encourage peer communication if length of stay is prolonged
      a. Telephone
      b. Visitation by peers
  11. Assist parents with communicating to adolescent
      a. Offer support
      b. Provide with growth and development information
  12. Approach adolescent with caring, understanding, and acceptance
B. Cause and effect
  1. Puts into perspective why adolescents think and act the way they do
  2. Adolescent uses formal rules of logic and evidence to assess cause and effect
  3. Understands why something happens the way it does
C. Handling emotion
  1. Uses a range of modalities from sophisticated verbal or written expression to motoric activity
  2. May regress in behavior
  3. Thoughts, feelings, fears may be shared with friends, especially peers
D. Major fears and worries
  1. Uncertainty about self as a person
  2. Concerned about whether or not body, thought, and feelings are normal
  3. Nursing interventions
      a. Involve in decision making
      b. Give information sensitively
      c. Explore tactfully what is known or unknown
          i. Fearful that nurse may think they are "dumb"

V. Legal Issues
A. Consent of minors
  1. Governed by state laws
  2. Exemptions to parental consent for medical treatment
      a. Emancipated minors
          i. Live away from home
          ii. No longer subject to parental control
          iii. Economically self-supporting
          iv. Married
          v. Member of military service
      b. Emergencies
          i. May be treated without parental consent during medical emergency
              (a) Physician judgment
              (b) Delay would jeopardize health or life of minor
      c. Mature minor rule
          i. Emerging trend in law
          ii. Recognizes minor is mature to understand nature of illness and risks and benefits of therapy
          iii. Should receive treatment at their own request

VI. Guidelines for Communicating with the Adolescent

See Table 16–1.

- A. Build a foundation
  1. Spend time together
  2. Encourage expression of ideas and feelings
     - a. May talk quite freely when given opportunity
     - b. Have language and culture all their own
     - c. More willing to discuss concerns with an outsider
     - d. Occasionally will answer in monosyllables
       - i.   Opposed to contact with nurse
       - ii. May not feel safe enough to reveal themselves
       - iii. May not want to communicate in front of parents
  3. Respect adolescent's views
  4. Tolerate differences
  5. Praise good points
  6. Respect adolescent's privacy
     - a. Maintain confidentiality of information provided
     - b. Issues regarding pregnancy, sexual activity, substance abuse
  7. Set a good example
- B. Communicate effectively
  1. Give undivided attention
  2. Be alert for signals indicating readiness to talk
  3. Listen, listen, listen
  4. Be courteous, calm, and open-minded
  5. Try not to over react to anything the adolescent says or does
  6. Avoid passing judgment or criticizing

VII. Physical Assessment of the Adolescent

- A. Approach
  1. Best to use straightforward approach
  2. Avoid being condescending
  3. Involve in decision of who should be present for exam
- B. Technique
  1. Move from head to toe
  2. Perform genital exam in the middle of exam
     - a. Allow ample time for questions and answers
  3. Assure adolescent regarding normal growth and development
  4. Answer questions or concerns regarding what is happening to their body
  5. Drape appropriately to preserve dignity
- C. Nursing considerations
  1. Admission to hospital or ASC may be viewed as a threat to adolescent's independence; results in loss of control
  2. May react by not cooperating or withdrawing
  3. May resent dependency on others and have difficulty accepting restrictions
     - a. Identify NPO status
     - b. Explain consequences of not telling the truth regarding NPO status
  4. Involve in decision making and planning
  5. Accept childish methods of coping
  6. Provide support
  7. Give explanations and consequences

Table 16–1 • DEVELOPMENTAL MILESTONES AND THEIR RELATIONSHIP TO COMMUNICATION APPROACHES

DEVELOPMENT	LANGUAGE DEVELOPMENT	EMOTIONAL DEVELOPMENT	COGNITIVE DEVELOPMENT	SUGGESTED COMMUNICATION APPROACH
Adolescent (12 years and older) The adolescent is able to create theories and generate many explanations to situations; beginning of communicating like an adult.	Able to verbalize and comprehend most adult concepts.	Beginning to accept responsibility for own actions. Perceptions of "imaginary audiences." Needs independence. Competitive drive. Strong need for group identification. Frequently has small group of very close friends. Questions authority. Strong need for privacy.	Able to think logically and abstractly. Attention span extends up to 60 minutes.	Engage in conversations about adolescent's interests. Use photographs, books, diagrams, charts, videos to explain. Use collaborative approach and foster/support independence. Introduce preparatory materials up to 1 week in advance of event. Be respectful of privacy needs.

From Ashwill, J.W., Droske, S.C. (1997). *Nursing Care of Children*. Philadelphia: Saunders, pp. 193-194.

VIII. Preoperative, Intraoperative, and Postoperative Considerations

Refer to Chapter 7 and Chapter 8 for complete information.

   A. Preoperative interview
      1. Role of family
         a. Identify importance of family to adolescent
         b. Ascertain if adolescent wants parent(s) present
         c. Questions might not be answered in presence of parents
         d. Allow parents to accompany adolescent to holding area if requested
         e. Inform parents of necessity to remain at facility
      2. Employ communication techniques to ensure a full understanding of procedure by adolescent
      3. Answer all questions truthfully and honestly
      4. Provide for privacy
         a. Conduct procedures that violate privacy only after induction of anesthesia (hair removal, skin prep, insertion of urinary catheters, etc.)
      5. Allow choices when possible
         a. Type of anesthesia induction
         b. Site of intravenous
   B. Guidelines for preoperative preparation
      1. Adolescent capable of abstract thought and reasoning
         a. Supplement explanations with reasons
         b. Explain long-term consequences of procedure
         c. May fear death and disability
         d. Encourage questions regarding fears, options, and alternatives
      2. Conscious of appearance
         a. Provide privacy
         b. Discuss how procedure may affect appearance (visible scar, correction of deformity)
         c. Emphasize physical benefits of procedure
      3. Adolescent very concerned with present
         a. Immediate effects of procedure more important than future benefits
      4. Adolescent striving for independence
         a. Involve in decision making
         b. Impose few restrictions
         c. Suggest methods for maintaining control
         d. Accept regression to more childish ways of coping
         e. May have trouble accepting new authority figures and may resist complying with procedures (NPO guidelines)
      5. Need for support
         a. May show false bravery to nurse
         b. Very anxious but may not be able to verbalize concerns
   C. Admission assessment
      1. Necessary to anticipate postoperative complications
         a. Assess cardiac, respiratory, and neurologic functions
         b. Recent or current cold, chest sounds
      2. Observe verbal and nonverbal behavior prior to surgery
      3. Vital signs, including temperature
      4. Allergies and sensitivities, including latex
      5. Use of alcohol, tobacco, recreational drugs

6. Sexual assessment
   a. Use of birth control
   b. Possible pregnancy
7. Educate (refer to Chapter 9 for complete information; see Table 16–2)
   a. What is going to happen
   b. Time frames
   c. Postoperative routine in PACU
      i.   Oxygen
      ii. Position
      iii. Dressing checks
      iv. Intravenous
      v.   Pain assessment and treatment

Table 16–2 • EDUCATIONAL STRATEGIES ACCORDING TO AGE OF CHILD

DEVELOPMENTAL CHARACTERISTICS OF CHILD	EDUCATIONAL STRATEGIES
Adolescent	
Struggling with identity versus role confusion; trying to answer the question "Who am I?"	Include a clear explanation about how the body is affected by an illness or treatment
Concerned about body image	Anticipate feelings of anger and grief in response to change in body image
	Assist patient to identify ways to adapt to experienced changes
Peers extremely important	Invite peers with similar experiences to teach an adolescent
	Education sessions with a group of peers
Independence versus dependence	Give adolescent some control over when teaching sessions will be held, methods of learning that are preferred; encourage collaborative decision making
Is struggling with autonomy	
Wants to be autonomous but still needs some dependence	
Able to think abstractly and understand complex language; can verbalize fears	Scientific names (with explanations) can be used to describe illnesses, procedures, and techniques; use diagrams, literature, and pamphlets; encourage verbal expression of fears; explain what symptoms are expected in an illness and when it will be necessary to seek further advice
Need for privacy	Explore with adolescent whether he or she wants parents involved in educational sessions; teach parents separately if adolescent prefers
Coping behaviors now well-established	Involving the adolescent in planning can facilitate coping; assess adolescent's coping resources and provide opportunity for expression of anxieties; provide information honestly; recognize that regression is common during stress and therefore adapt teaching accordingly; increase amount of teaching according to adolescent's readiness

Adapted from Betz, C.L., Hunsberger, M., Wright, S. (1994). *Family-Centered Nursing Care of Children.* Philadelphia: Saunders, pp. 810–811.

D. Intraoperative
  1. Provide reassurance prior to induction
    a. Hold hand
    b. Offer support
    c. Assure preservation of privacy and dignity
    d. Provide for patient safety
E. Postoperative
  1. Respiratory assessment
    a. Monitor rate and depth of ventilation
    b. Monitor oxygen saturation
    c. Observe for tongue obstruction
    d. Observe for respiratory depression due to narcotics and muscle relaxants
  2. Cardiovascular assessment
    a. Assess vital signs/perfusion
    b. Heart rate: 60–90 BPM (awake); 50–90 BPM (sleeping)
    c. Blood pressure: 112–128 mm Hg systolic; 66–80 mm Hg diastolic
  3. Thermoregulation
    a. Respond to cold environment by increasing metabolism
      i.   Leads to increase in oxygen consumption
    b. Hypothermia
      i.   Monitor vital signs including core temperature, pulse, respiratory rate, degree of emergence from anesthesia, continuous ECG (dysrhythmias and cardiovascular depression associated with hypothermia)
    c. Hyperthermia
      i.   Malignant hyperthermia
  4. Emergence delirium
    a. Description
      i.   Dissociative state
      ii.   No response to verbal commands
      iii. Appears confused and disoriented
      iv.   Generalized purposeless movements
      v.   Lasts 30 seconds to 5 minutes
    b. Nursing interventions
      i.   Protect from injury
      ii.   Generally will fall back to sleep and reawaken without recollection
      iii. Avoid stimulation—provide quiet environment
    c. Causative factors
      i.   Preoperative anxiety
      ii.   Postoperative pain
      iii. Hypoxia
      iv.   Hypotension
      v.   Urinary distention
  5. Assessment of pain
    a. Perceive pain on three levels
      i.   Physical
      ii.   Emotional
      iii. Mental
    b. Able to understand cause and effect of pain
      i.   Can describe pain
      ii.   Can describe their feeling regarding pain
      iii. Can describe strategies that have helped with past experiences of pain

   c. Not unusual for adolescent to deal with pain through regressive behavior

     i. Increased dependence on parent

     ii. Expects the nurse to know they are in pain—should not have to ask for pain medication

   d. Observed signs include:

     i. Increased muscle tension

       (a) Facial grimacing

       (b) Muscle rigidity

     ii. Withdrawal

       (a) Decreased interest in environment and usual activities

     iii. Decreased motor activity

       (a) Reluctant to move

     iv. Verbalizes with words such as "ache," "sore," "pounding," etc., to describe pain

       (a) May grunt, groan, or sigh

       (b) Rarely cries or screams

         (i) Physical resistance and aggression are unusual unless the adolescent is totally unprepared for the procedure

         (ii) Very concerned with maintaining composure and are embarrassed and ashamed if they lose control

       (c) Describes pain intensity and quality

       (d) May hesitate to disclose pain unless they are sure nurse is willing to listen

   e. Assessment tools

     i. Self report

       (a) Visual analog scale (VAS)

         (i) Mark on a line (no pain to worst pain) a point that corresponds to their pain level

       (b) Verbal numerical score

         (i) Choose a number from 0 to 10 (0 = no pain, 10 = worst pain imaginable) that corresponds to their pain level

     ii. Adolescent Pediatric Pain Tool (APPT)

       (a) Patient draws on front and back of body outlines to locate pain

       (b) Indicates pain intensity on a Word Graphic Rating Scale

       (c) Circles words that describe the quality of pain

   f. Pharmacologic interventions

     i. Nonsteroidal antiinflammatory drugs (NSAIDs)

       (a) Oral

         (i) For mild to moderate pain

         (ii) Can be administered preoperatively

         (iii) Contraindicated in patients with renal disease and those at risk of or with actual coagulopathy

         (iv) May mask fever

         (v) Can be given in conjunction with opioid

       (b) Parenteral

         (i) Ketorolac

           a) For moderate to severe pain

           b) May be useful when opioids contraindicated

     ii. Opioids—for moderate to severe pain

       (a) Oral

         (i) May be as effective as parenteral in appropriate doses

         (ii) Administer as soon as oral intake tolerated

         (iii) Route of choice

    (b) Intramuscular
       (i)   Painful
      (ii) Absorption unreliable
     (iii) Avoid IM route if possible
    (c) Subcutaneous
       (i)   Preferred route to IM
      (ii) Painful
     (iii) Absorption unreliable
     (iv) Avoid SC route if possible
    (d) Intravenous
       (i)   Preferred route after major surgery
      (ii) Can be administered continuous or intermittently
     (iii) Used for patient-controlled analgesia (PCA)
     (iv) Increased risk for respiratory depression
    (e) PCA
       (i)   Provides steady level of analgesia
      (ii) Not routinely used in outpatient setting
    (f) Epidural/intrathecal
       (i)   Provides good analgesia
      (ii) Increased risk of respiratory depression
     (iii) May have delayed onset
     (iv) Requires careful monitoring
      (v) Not routinely used in outpatient setting

   iii. Local anesthetics
    (a) Limited indications
    (b) Provides effective regional analgesia
    (c) Limited duration of action
    (d) May be used for orthopedic procedures
       (i)   Arthroscopy
      (ii) Anterior cruciate ligament repairs
     (iii) Other joint procedures
          a) Shoulder
          b) Elbow
          c) Wrist
          d) Foot
          e) Ankle
     (iv) General surgery
          a) Injected into incisional area

g. Dosage
    i.   Acetaminophen (Tylenol)
    (a) Dose
    (b) 10–15 mg/kg orally, q 4 hours
    (c) Comments
       (i)   Can be given rectally
      (ii) Lacks peripheral antiinflammatory activity of NSAIDs
     (iii) Does not inhibit platelet function
     (iv) Maximum of 60 mg/kg per day
   ii.   Aspirin
    (a) Dose
       (i)   10–15 mg/kg orally, q 4 hours

   (b) Comments

    (i) Contraindicated in presence of fever or other viral diseases

    (ii) Inhibits platelet aggregation

    (iii) May cause postoperative bleeding

    (iv) Associated with Reye syndrome

  iii. NSAIDs

   (a) Ketorolac

    (i) Dose

     a) 0.75–1.0 mg/kg intravenous route—administer slowly, q 6 hours prn

     b) 1.0 mg/kg intramuscularly, q 6 hours prn

    (ii) Comments

     a) Only NSAID approved for parenteral analgesia

     b) Limit use to 48–72 hours

   (b) Ibuprofen

    (i) Dose

     a) 10 mg/kg orally, q 6–8 hours

    (ii) Comments

     a) Available as oral suspension

     b) Available as several brand names and generic

   (c) Naprosyn

    (i) Dose

     a) 5 mg/kg orally, q 12 hours

    (ii) Comments

     a) Longer half life than other NSAIDs

  iv. Opioids

   (a) Fentanyl

    (i) Dose

     a) 1.0 µg/kg, intravenous bolus q ½ hour

     b) 1–2 µg/hour, intravenous infusion

    (ii) Comments

     a) Rapid onset

     b) Short duration

     c) Useful for painful procedures

     d) Potential for respiratory depression; monitor closely

   (b) Morphine

    (i) Dose

     a) 0.2–0.4 mg/kg orally, q 4–6 hours

     b) 0.1 mg/kg intravenously, q 2 hours

    (ii) Comments

     a) Observe for respiratory depression

     b) Common side effects include nausea and vomiting and histamine release

   (c) Meperidine

    (i) Dose

     a) 1–5 mg/kg intramuscularly, q 3–5 hours

     b) 1.0 mg/kg intravenous bolus, q 2 hours

    (ii) Comments

     a) Observe for respiratory depression

     b) Dizziness, nausea, and vomiting common in ambulatory patient

(d) Codeine
  (i) Dose
      a) 1.0 mg/kg orally, q 3 hours
  (ii) Comments
      a) Monitor for respiratory depression
      b) Dizziness, nausea, vomiting, and hypotension more frequent in ambulatory patient
      c) Dose may be limited due to nausea and vomiting
(e) Oxycodone (Percocet, Percodan, Tylox)
  (i) Dose
      a) 0.2 mg/kg orally, q 3–4 hours
  (ii) Comments
      a) Suppresses respirations
      b) Dizziness, nausea, vomiting, and hypotension more common in ambulatory patient
(f) Hydrocodone (Lortab, Larcet, Vicodin)
  (i) Dose
      a) 0.2 mg/kg orally, q 3–4 hours
  (ii) Comments
      a) Suppresses respirations
      b) Dizziness, nausea, vomiting, and hypotension more common in ambulatory patient

6. PACU Phase I considerations
  a. Safety
    i.   Side rails up
    ii. When adolescent wakes up out of control
      (a) Speak in strong voice
      (b) Orient to place
      (c) Explain foul language is unacceptable in PACU environment
  b. Prevent complications
  c. Transport from OR to PACU
    i.   Safely
    ii. Position on side
    iii. Safety strap in place
    iv. Oxygen administered
  d. Length of stay
    i.   No general rule
    ii. Institutional policy
    iii. Utilize discharge criteria rather than time
  e. Replacing fluid deficits
    i.   Properly hydrated
  f. Equipment
    i.   Generally same as adult
7. PACU Phase II Considerations
  a. Pain management
  b. Patient and family anxiety
    i.   Maintain calm, reassuring manner
    ii. Provide privacy
    iii. Encourage expression of feelings
    iv. Give encouragement and positive feedback
    v.   Encourage parental presence if approved by patient

    c. Discharge criteria
       i.   Individual criteria established by facility
       ii.   Comply with standards (ASPAN, state, and regulatory agencies)
    d. Discharge instructions
       i.   Follow-up visit with surgeon
       ii.   Provide information regarding procedure findings
       iii. Provide instructions regarding home care
           (a) Activity
           (b) Diet
           (c) Procedure-specific instructions
           (d) Drug and food interaction sheet
       iv. Enforce importance of compliance with postoperative instructions
       v.   Parental involvement as requested by adolescent
           (a) If not involved, be sure to review information with parents separately to insure their understanding of postoperative instructions
       vi. Instructions on how to contact anesthesia department or surgeon in case of emergency

Bibliography

1. Ashwill, J.W., Droske, S.C. (1997). *Nursing Care of Children Principles and Practice.* Philadelphia: Saunders.
2. Asprey, J.R. (1994). Postoperative analgesic prescription and administration in a pediatric population. *J Pediatric Nursing,* 9(3):150–157.
3. Band, E.B., Weisz, J.R. (1988). How to feel better when it feels bad: Children's perspectives on coping with everyday stress. *Dev Psychol,* 24:247–253.
4. Behrman, R.E., Kliegman, R.M., Arvin, A.M. (1996). *Nelson Textbook of Pediatrics,* 15th ed. Philadelphia: Saunders.
5. Behrman, R.E., Kliegman, R.M. (1994). *Nelson Essentials of Pediatrics,* 2nd ed. Philadelphia: Saunders.
6. Bell, C., Kain, Z.N. (1997). *The Pediatric Anesthesia Handbook,* 2nd ed. St. Louis: Mosby.
7. Betz, C.L., Hunsberger, M., Wright, S. (1994). *Family-Centered Nursing Care of Children,* 2nd ed. Philadelphia: Saunders.
8. Broyles, B.E. (1997). *Clinical Companion for Ashwill and Droske Nursing Care of Children Principles and Practice.* Philadelphia: Saunders.
9. Burden, N. (1993). *Ambulatory Surgical Nursing.* Philadelphia: Saunders.
10. Dox, I.G., Melloni, B.J., Eisner, G.M. (1994). *Melloni's Illustrated Medical Dictionary,* 3rd ed. Pearl River, NY: Parthenon.
11. Fiorentini, S.E. (1993). Evaluation of a new program: Pediatric parental visitation in the PACU. *J Post Anesth Nurs,* 8(4):249–256.
12. Frederick, C., Reining, K. (1995). Essential components of growth and development. *J Post Anesth Nurs,* 10(1):12–17.
13. Maligalig, R.M.L. (1994). Parents' perceptions of the stressors of pediatric ambulatory surgery. *J Post Anesth Nurs,* 9(5):278–282.
14. Savedra, M.C., Tesler, M.D., Holzemer, W.L., Ward, J.A. (1989). *Adolescent Pediatric Pain Tool (APPT): Preliminary User's Manual.* San Francisco: University of California.
15. Sieving, R., Zirbel-Donisch, S. (1990). Development and enhancement of self-esteem in children. *J Pediatric Health Care,* 4(6):290–296.
16. Wong, D. (1995). *Nursing Care of Infants and Children,* 5th ed. St. Louis: Mosby.

REVIEW QUESTIONS

1. In which stage of adolescence do the following occur
   —Period of growth acceleration
   —Period of biologic development
   —Period of motor development in which there is an increase in muscle mass and fine motor coordination
   —Increase in self consciousness
   —Low self-esteem
   —Increase in sexual interest
   —Stage where the adolescent moves from operational thinking to formal, logical operations

   A. Early adolescence
   B. Middle adolescence
   C. Late adolescence
   D. Normal adolescence

2. Stressors associated with hospitalization for the adolescent include
   (1) Separation anxiety
   (2) Fear of injury
   (3) Fear of pain
   (4) Loss of control

   A. 2, 4
   B. 2, 3
   C. 1, 3, 4
   D. All of the above

3. With regard to consent from minors, all of the following are true except

   A. Emancipated minors are exempt from parental consent
   B. Treatment may be given without parental consent during an emergency
   C. Federal laws govern a minor's ability to consent for own treatment
   D. The mature minor rule recognizes that the minor is mature to understand the nature of the illness and risks and benefits associated with treatment

4. The emotional development of the adolescent includes all of the following except

   A. Demonstrates purposeful attention-seeking behaviors
   B. Needs independence
   C. Questions authority
   D. Begins to accept responsibility for own actions

5. Cognitive development of the adolescent includes

   A. Able to think logically and abstractly
   B. Begins to identify cause-and-effect relationships
   C. Magical thinking becomes prominent
   D. Becomes very oriented to "rules"

6. Suggested communication approaches for dealing with the adolescent include all of the following except

   A. Engage in conversations about adolescent interests
   B. Use collaborative approach
   C. Use medical play techniques
   D. Use photographs, books, diagrams, charts, and videos to explain

7. To assist the adolescent with coping behaviors
   (1) Involve the adolescent in planning care
   (2) Provide opportunities for expression of anxieties
   (3) Devise games that contain content to be learned
   (4) Provide information honestly
   (5) Increase amount of teaching according to adolescent's readiness

   A. 1, 2, 4
   B. 1, 2, 4, 5
   C. 2, 3, 4, 5
   D. 1, 2, 3, 5

8. Nursing interventions during emergence delirium include

   A. Stimulating the patient to breathe
   B. Protecting the patient from injury
   C. Orienting the patient
   D. Taking the patient's vital signs

9. The adolescent responds to pain by
   (1) Exhibiting regressive behavior
   (2) Increasing dependence on parents
   (3) Exhibiting decreased interest in environment and usual activities
   (4) Expecting the nurse to know he/she is in pain

   A. 1, 4
   B. 2, 3
   C. 1, 2, 3
   D. All of the above

10. The preferred route of administration of opioids to the adolescent who has undergone an outpatient procedure is

    A. Intravenous
    B. Intramuscular
    C. Oral
    D. Subcutaneous

ANSWERS TO QUESTIONS

1. A	6. C
2. D	7. B
3. C	8. B
4. A	9. D
5. A	10. C

The Adult Patient

Vallire D. Hooper
Medical College of Georgia
Augusta, Georgia

I. **Definitions**
  A. Growth
    1. Increase in body size
    2. Change in structure, function, or complexity of body cell content and metabolic and biochemical processes
    3. Occurs up to some point of optimum maturity
  B. Development
    1. Growth responsibility arising at a certain time in the course of development
      a. Successful achievement
        i.   Satisfaction
        ii.   Continued success in future tasks
      b. Failure
        i.   Unhappiness
        ii.   Disapproval by society
        iii. Difficulty with later developmental tasks and functions
  C. Maturation and learning
    1. Maturation: emergence of genetic potential for changes in form, structure, complexity, integration, organization, and function
    2. Learning
      a. The process of gaining specific knowledge or skill
      b. Acquiring habits and attitude
      c. Results from experience, training, and behavioral changes
    3. Adequate maturation must be present for learning to occur
II. **Stages of Adulthood**
  A. Young adulthood

Objectives

1. Identify developmental issues associated with each stage of adulthood.
2. Define health, wellness, and illness.
3. List three types of health/illness behaviors.
4. Identify the effects of the stress response on the body's adaptation to surgery.
5. List three characteristics unique to the adult learner.

1. Definitions
   a. Young-young adult: 25–30 years of age
   b. Old-young adult: 30–45 years of age
2. Developmental issues
   a. Settling down
   b. Developing a more conservative, traditional viewpoint
   c. Must enter and successfully manage multiple new roles simultaneously
      i. Work
      ii. School
      iii. Marriage
      iv. Home
      v. Child-rearing
   d. Primary tasks
      i. Finding an occupation
      ii. Staying in one place
      iii. Establishing a new family
3. Socio-cultural issues
   a. Born in the 1950s, 1960s, and 1970s
   b. Consistent positive influences
      i. Continuous economic growth
      ii. Abundance of material goods and technology
      iii. Rapid social changes
      iv. Sophisticated medical care
   c. Constant threats
      i. Nuclear war
      ii. Pollution
      iii. Overpopulation
      iv. Loss of natural resources
   d. Instant media coverage makes the world small and outer space a not-so-distant place
   e. Other influences
      i. Changes in women's roles
      ii. Decreasing birth rates
      iii. Increasing longevity
4. Issues affecting response to ambulatory surgery (see Table 17–1)

Table 17–1 • DEVELOPMENTAL ISSUES AS RELATED TO AMBULATORY SURGERY

ISSUES AFFECTING AMBULATORY SURGICAL EXPERIENCE	
YOUNG ADULTHOOD	**MIDDLE AGE**
Little or no insurance coverage	Physical condition often better indicator of surgical/anesthesia response than chronological age
Needs to return to work or school as soon as possible	More financially stable
May need help with care of home, children, or parents	Better insurance coverage
May expect sophisticated medical technology to be able to fix anything with very little "down" time	May be balancing many professional, civic, and family responsibilities

B. Middle age
  1. Definition
    a. Covers ages 45 to 65
      i.   Consider the physiologic age/condition of the body
      ii. Also consider psychological age: how old the person acts and feels
    b. Age divisions
      i.   Early middle age: 40–55
      ii. Late middle age: 56–64
    c. Social class will affect age assignment
      i.   Poorer person will perceive prime or midpoint as occurring at an
           earlier age
  2. Developmental/socio-cultural issues
    a. Becoming one of the largest segments of the population
      i.   Earn the most money
      ii. Pay a major portion of the bills and taxes
    b. Yield much power in:
      i.   Government
      ii.   Politics
      iii. Education
      iv.   Religion
      v.   Science
      vi.   Business
      vii. Communication
    c. Common experiences
      i.   Good physical and mental health
      ii.   Personal freedom
      iii. Good command of self and the environment
  3. Issues affecting response to ambulatory surgery (see Table 17–1)
III. **Health, Wellness, and Illness**
  A. Definitions
    1. Health
      a. Defined by the World Health Organization (WHO), 1947, as a state of
         complete physical, social, and mental well-being; not merely the absence of
         disease
      b. Is often described on a continuum of wellness and illness
    2. Wellness
      a. The ability to adapt, relate effectively, and to function at near maximum
         capacity
      b. Need to examine functioning in four areas
        i.   Physiologic factors: structures and functions of the body
        ii. Psychologic factors: self-concept as affected by various demographic
             variables
             (a) Age
             (b) Sex
             (c) Race
             (d) Education
             (e) Economic status
             (f) Other
        iii. Sociocultural factors
             (a) Interrelationships with others
             (b) Environmental factors
             (c) Lifestyle
        iv. Developmental factors: related to completion of developmental tasks

3. Disease and illness
   a. Disease
      i.   A state of nonhealth
      ii. Biological dysfunction is present
      iii. Major focus of the medical model
      iv. Can be legitimized by the health-care provider
   b. Illness
      i.   The patient's personal perspective of the disease state
      ii. Related to the psychosocial impact of the disease on the individual
      iii. Individual influences on perception of illness severity
           (a) Personality
           (b) Demographic characteristics
           (c) Presence of support systems
B. Health care and prevention
   1. Levels of health care
      a. Health promotion: activities to improve or maintain optimum health
      b. Disease prevention: actions to prevent disease or disability
      c. Diagnosis and treatment: emphasizes early recognition and treatment of health problems
      d. Rehabilitation: designed to limit incapacities due to health problems as well as to prevent recurrences
   2. Levels of prevention
      a. Primary prevention: ways to prevent illness
      b. Secondary prevention: early identification and treatment of health problems
      c. Tertiary prevention: activities designed to return the physically or emotionally compromised person to the highest possible level of health
   3. The ambulatory arena is now involved in all levels of health care and prevention

IV. **Health/Illness Behavior**
A. Health behavior
   1. Activities undertaken by those believing themselves to be healthy
   2. Purpose is to prevent disease or detect it in an asymptomatic stage
   3. Examples
      a. Breast self exam (BSE)
      b. Regular exercise
      c. Prudent heart living
      d. Routine check-ups
      e. Ambulatory procedures
         i.   Routine screening colonoscopy
         ii. Follow-up cardiac catheterization in nonsymptomatic patient
B. Illness behavior
   1. Activities carried out in response to a set of symptoms by those who feel ill
   2. Allows the individual to determine his/her state of health and need for treatment
   3. Limited to health-seeking behavior to identify and/or assess the changes occurring or to search for a solution
   4. Influences affecting illness behavior
      a. Recurrence of symptoms
         i.   The more frequent or severe the symptoms, the more likely that outside help will be sought
      b. Visibility and consequences
         i.   The more apparent the symptoms, the more illness behavior exhibited

      ii.   If the disorder is attached to stigma, the individual will be less likely to seek help

      iii. Help will usually be sought for life-threatening symptoms

    c. Perceived seriousness or severity

      i.   Disorders perceived as serious lead to earlier illness behavior

      ii.   Influences on perception of symptom severity

         (a) Social class

         (b) Health belief system

         (c) Hierarchy of other needs and desires

    d. Availability of treatment and the medical care system

      i.   Distance, costs, convenience, time, effort, and fear of outcome affect willingness to seek help

      ii.   Individual subordination by the health-care system also affects willingness to seek treatment

    e. Knowledge and significance of symptoms

      i.   Lack of knowledge of symptom significance often influences the individual to seek help

    f. Cultural and social expectations

      i.   Cultural and ethnic backgrounds affect symptom interpretation and notion of when it is acceptable to seek health care

      ii.   Lower classes are more influenced by symptoms interfering with important roles

      iii. The elderly use more health-care services

      iv. Women seek medical attention more frequently than men

C. Sick role behavior

  1. Activities undertaken by individuals who consider themselves ill for the purpose of getting well

  2. Is learned and influenced by evaluation and legitimization from others

  3. Is assumed when one accepts being ill, initiates some form of action, and demonstrates a desire to be well again

  4. Four major role components, divided into rights and obligations

    a. Rights

      i.   Exemption from normal responsibilities

         (a) Dependent on the nature and severity of the illness

         (b) Requires validation or legitimization by others and the physician

         (c) Once legitimized, person is obligated to avoid responsibilities

      ii.   Right to be cared for

         (a) Person is not expected to recover by an act of will or decision

         (b) Is not responsible for becoming sick and therefore has a right to be cared for

         (c) Physical dependency and the need for emotional support are acceptable

    b. Obligations

      i.   Obligation to want to become well

         (a) Being ill is seen as undesirable

         (b) The sick role can result in secondary gains

         (c) Motivation to recover is of primary importance

      ii.   Obligation to seek and cooperate with technically competent help

         (a) The individual needs the technical expertise that health-care professionals can provide

         (b) Cooperation with these professionals for the goal of getting well is mandatory

    5. Ambulatory implications
      a. Patient may need to be educated that sick role behavior is acceptable and often expected following ambulatory procedures
      b. Ambulatory procedures often reduce the amount of time spent in the sick role

V. Stress Response Syndrome

  A. Definitions
    1. Stress
      a. A socio-psychophysiological phenomenon
      b. A composite of intellectual, behavioral, metabolic, and other physiological responses to a stressor or stressors of internal or external origin
      c. Influenced by environmental, psychologic, and social factors
      d. Uniquely perceived by the individual
    2. Stressors (stress agents)
      a. May be internal or external
      b. Examples
        i.   Cold
        ii.   Heat
        iii. Infectious organisms
        iv. Disease processes
        v.   Fever
        vi. Pain
        vii. Imagined events
        viii. Intense emotional involvement
    3. Stress response
      a. Initiated in response to a stressor
      b. Is protective and adaptive by nature
      c. Regulated by the nervous and endocrine systems
        i.   Sympathetic nervous system (SNS)
        ii.   Pituitary gland
        iii. Adrenal gland
      d. The magnitude of the response depends on the perceived severity of the threat
    4. Survival depends on one's ability to balance between stressors and adaptive capacities

  B. General adaptation syndrome (GAS)
    1. Developed by Hans Selye
    2. Most widely accepted and frequently used physiologic theory of stress and adaptation
    3. Three stages
      a. Alarm stage
        i.   Begins with the first exposure to the stressor
        ii.   Fight or flight mechanism (SNS) is activated
          (a) Heart rate increases
          (b) Cardiac output (CO) increases
          (c) Stroke volume increases
          (d) Peripheral vasoconstriction
          (e) Increased perspiration
          (f) Gastrointestinal upset
        iii. In most situations, the body's defensive forces are mobilized to deal with the stressor
        iv. Death can occur in this stage if the stressor is strong enough to result in exhaustion of the body's adaptive mechanisms and energy supply

    b. Stage of resistance or adaptation
       i.   Reflects "adaptation" as the body fights back
       ii.   Psychologic mobilization occurs
       iii. Influences on ability to adapt
          (a) Physical functioning
          (b) Coping skills
          (c) Total number of stressors experienced
    c. Stage of exhaustion
       i.   A progressive breakdown of compensatory mechanisms and homeostasis
       ii.   Occurs only if the stress becomes overwhelming, is not removed, or if the individual is ineffective in coping with it
       iii. All energy for adaptation is exhausted
       iv. Physiologic and psychologic collapse will ensue

C. Physiologic responses to stress
  1. The initial response is stimulated by the central nervous system (CNS)
  2. Information is then forwarded to the hypothalamus which integrates and coordinates the homeostatic adjustments
  3. Hypothalamus stimulates the autonomic nervous system (ANS) and the anterior and posterior pituitary
  4. The physiologic responses to hypothalamic stimulation and their affects on the surgical patient are listed in Table 17–2

D. Psychosocial responses to stress
  1. Primary theory is the stress-appraised event theory by Lazarus
    a. Looks at stress and adaptation from the viewpoint of cognition, perception, and transaction
       i.   The way the individual interprets the situation will determine if he/she perceives it as stressful
    b. Positive and negative events can result in stress
    c. Emphasis is on the process or dynamics of what is happening
  2. Cognitive appraisal
    a. The mental process used by the person to assess an event in relation to his/her well-being and available coping resources and options
    b. Evaluative forms
       i.   Irrelevant appraisal
          (a) Occurs if the event is considered to be of no concern or impact on the current level of well-being
       ii.   Benign–positive appraisal
          (a) Occurs if the event is considered as indicative of a positive state of affairs
          (b) The event shows that all is well
       iii. Stressful appraisal
          (a) Occurs with a negative evaluation of the present or future state of well-being
          (b) Occurs in three forms
             (i)   Harm–loss: damage or injury has already taken place
             (ii) Threat: harm or loss has not yet occurred but is expected
             (iii) Challenge
                a) The possibility for growth or mastery is perceived
                b) The opportunity for gain outweighs the possible risk of harm
  3. Coping modes
    a. Defined as those efforts used to manage the environmental and internal demands exceeding personal resources. Mobilized in response to an event perceived as stressful

Table 17–2 • PHYSIOLOGICAL RESPONSES TO HYPOTHALAMIC STIMULATION

RESPONDING ORGAN/SYSTEM	ORGAN/SYSTEM ACTION	PHYSIOLOGICAL RESPONSE	SURGICAL ADAPTATION	SURGICAL MALADAPTATION
Autonomic Nervous System (ANS)	Simulates the SNS to stimulate: Exocrine glands	Sweating	No impact	No impact
	Epinephrine and Norepinephrine release	Decreases insulin and increases glucagon releases: See net increase in blood glucose and protein and fat catabolism	Increased amino acids for wound healing Increased wound healing Increased energy available Increased blood sugar Increased energy available for adaptation	Negative nitrogen balance that may negatively impact tissue repair unless reversed Development of excessive scar tissue and adhesions Increased blood sugar is detrimental to diabetics Increased heat loss may result in hypothermia, shivering, and increased oxygen demand
		Constriction of vascular smooth muscle: Increase in BP	Shifts blood away from periphery to the vital organs Decreases blood loss by increasing clotting	May decrease renal perfusion Increased thrombus formation
		Cardiopulmonary responses: Increased heart rate and contractility Bronchodilatation	Increased myocardial perfusion Increased oxygen and perfusion to vital organs Increased oxygen exchange Improved ventilation	Increased work load for heart: May lead to heart failure Hypertension No maladaptation as a result of bronchodilatation

	Kidneys are stimulated to release renin: Converted to aldosterone by angiotensin II Aldosterone results in sodium and water retention at the renal tubules See increased blood volume	Increased blood volume helps to reduce hypovolemia: Maintenance of blood pressure and cardiac output	Hypervolemia Hypertension Circulatory overload Heart failure
Anterior Pituitary	Releases adrenocorticotropin hormone (ACTH): Stimulates the adrenal cortex to release aldosterone and cortisol Aldosterone results in increased blood volume Cortisol results in an increase in blood glucose and protein and fat catabolism	Increased blood sugar Increased wound healing Increased energy Increased antiinflammatory response	Prolonged antiinflammatory response may lead to infection See above for other maladaptive responses
Posterior Pituitary	Stimulates the release of vasopressin/antidiuretic hormone (ADH) Causes sodium and water retention at the renal tubules: Results in increased blood volume	See above	See above

    b. Accomplished by eight coping modes
      i. Escape–avoidance
        (a) Wishful thinking and other behavioral efforts to escape or avoid the problem
      ii. Confrontive
        (a) Aggressive efforts to alter the situation
        (b) Involves some degree of hostility and risk taking
      iii. Distancing
        (a) Attempt to detach from the situation and thus minimize the significance
      iv. Self-control
        (a) Strive to regulate one's feelings and actions
      v. Seeking social support
        (a) Seek information, tangible and emotional support
      vi. Accepting responsibility
        (a) Acknowledge one's own role in the problem
        (b) Attempt to rectify the situation
      vii. Planful problem solving
        (a) Deliberate and analytical approach to altering the situation
      viii. Positive reappraisal
        (a) An effort to focus on the positive side or opportunity for personal growth

E. Behavioral responses to stress
  1. Anger, hostility, antagonism, noncompliance
  2. Depression, apathy, crying, inability to concentrate, depression
  3. Grief, shock, denial, withdrawal
  4. Acceptance, information seeking, planning, decision making

F. Factors affecting response to stressors
  1. Nature of specific stressors encountered
  2. What the stressors mean to the patient
    a. May differ based on past experience and development
    b. Ill patients may become less mature, less discriminating, and less reality oriented
  3. Patient's characteristic mode of coping with stress
    a. Depends on personality
    b. Threat of hospitalization/surgery may be responded to by:
      i. An aggressive manner
      ii. Resignation
      iii. Seeking constant information
  4. Patient's current psychologic resources
    a. Determines the person's resiliency and ability to endure the stress without decompensation
    b. Affected by:
      i. Level of self-esteem and social support
      ii. Presence or absence of any underlying depression or chronic anxiety
  5. Hardiness factor
    a. A personality characteristic
      i. A sense of control over one's life
      ii. Involvement and commitment to productive activities
      iii. Anticipation of change as an exciting positive challenge
    b. Acts as a buffer between stress and illness

VI. Stress Management
  A. Assessment of current level of stress
  B. Intervention
    1. Physical relaxation/stress management
      a. Progressive relaxation
      b. Acupuncture/acupressure
      c. Biofeedback
      d. Massage
      e. Therapeutic touch
    2. Cognitive methods of relaxation/stress management
      a. Thought stopping
      b. Positive self-talk
      c. Assertive communication training
      d. Laughter, humor, play, tears
      e. Guided imagery
    3. Time and resource management
    4. Other nursing interventions
      a. Acknowledge individual feelings and behaviors
      b. Develop trusting relationship
      c. Involve family/significant others
VII. Health Promotion and Prevention
  A. Activities designed to improve or maintain optimum health
  B. Likelihood to participate in such behaviors is influenced by internal and external cues
    1. Internal cues include bodily states such as feeling good or energetic
    2. External cues
      a. Interactions with significant others
      b. Impact of media communication
      c. Visual stimuli from the environment
  C. Strategies include:
    1. Physical/physiologic
      a. Proper nutrition
      b. Balance of exercise/rest
      c. Cessation of destructive health habits (smoking, alcohol, or drug abuse)
      d. Health screening
    2. Emotional
      a. Effective communication
      b. Promotion of self-esteem, self-confidence, security
      c. Anxiety reduction measures
      d. Crisis resolution
    3. Cognitive
      a. Coping methods
      b. Visualization/imagery
      c. Health education
    4. Social
      a. Family, friend, peer relations
      b. Group associations and processes
      c. Maintenance of cultural ties
    5. Spiritual/moral
      a. Values clarification
      b. Acknowledgment of meaning and purpose of life
      c. Establishment of belief system
      d. Establishment of moral and ethical behaviors

VIII. Preoperative Health History Interview
   A. Should focus on age-specific issues in addition to general preoperative assessment and preparation
   B. Young adulthood
      1. Generally a healthy population
      2. Pertinent health problems include:
         a. Upper respiratory infection
         b. Influenza
         c. Essential hypertension
         d. Mitral valve prolapse
         e. Iron deficiency anemia
         f. Simple diarrhea
         g. Cystitis
         h. Acute pyelonephritis
         i. Chronic fatigue syndrome
         j. Acquired immunodeficiency syndrome (AIDS)
         k. Hepatitis B
         l. Cervical, breast, and testicular cancer
   C. Middle age
      1. Variety of health problems may begin to develop
      2. Pertinent health problems include:
         a. Sinusitis
         b. Hiatal hernia
         c. Duodenal peptic ulcer disease
         d. Angina pectoris
         e. Secondary hypertension
         f. Hyperthyroidism
         g. Hyperuricemia or gout
         h. Diabetes type II
         i. Acute and chronic prostatitis
         j. Lumbosacral strain
 IX. Health Teaching–Learning
   A. Teaching is a critical nursing intervention that is crucial to successful outcomes in the ambulatory setting
      1. Teaching and learning processes are related
      2. Teaching–learning process is easily integrated into the nursing process
   B. Definitions
      1. Learning
         a. Process of acquiring wisdom, knowledge, or skill
         b. Overt changes in behavior may be observed
      2. Teaching
         a. Process of sharing knowledge and insight
         b. Facilitating another to learn knowledge, insight, and skills
      3. Health education
         a. Transmits information, motivates, and helps people adopt and maintain healthful practices and lifestyles
         b. Is concerned with the environment, professional training, and research to maintain and evaluate the process
         c. Traditionally focuses on what the professional thinks is good or needed by the patient
         d. Positive approaches are generally more effective than fear

C. Phases of the teaching–learning process
  1. Assessment
      a. Begins with an assessment of the nurse's teaching abilities
      b. Gather information about the patient, his/her learning needs, and his/her readiness to learn
          i.   Patient's level of understanding, ability to comprehend, and any obstacles to learning (sensory losses, language barriers) should be identified during the general psychosocial assessment
          ii. Assessment should also include patient's interest level, attentiveness, and current understanding about upcoming procedure
      c. A realistic teaching plan should be established based on:
          i.   Patient's current level of knowledge
          ii. Nurse's ability to provide the new information needed by the patient
          iii. A plan to identify and dispel patient misconceptions should also be included
  2. Diagnosis
      a. Diagnose the patient's learning needs
      b. Set teaching priorities
  3. Planning
      a. Set goals with the patient
      b. Determine behavioral objectives
      c. Select teaching and evaluation methods
          i.   Content and type of information
          ii. Type of media used
          iii. Who will be involved
          iv. The environment and time frame in which it will be provided
  4. Intervention
      a. Use appropriate strategies for instruction
  5. Evaluation
      a. Evaluate patient outcomes
      b. Revise and reevaluate as needed
D. Characteristics of the adult learner
  1. Readiness to learn is determined by life tasks, roles, and immediate problems
  2. Application of learning is related to the relevancy of the problems
  3. Orientation to learning is independent and self-directed
  4. Value of experiences
      a. Experiences are internalized
      b. Experiences provide a foundation for further learning
      c. May contribute to resistance to change
  5. Rate of learning
      a. Resistant to learning nonrelevant material
      b. Aging process increases time needed to complete some learning tasks
  6. Barriers to learning
      a. Family, work, or community responsibilities may compete with learning time and energy
      b. Anxieties about self-image may also threaten ability to learn
  7. Cultural differences
      a. Unique beliefs should be respected
      b. Use interpreters and/or audiovisual aids for persons who do not speak English
      c. Be knowledgeable of cultures, ethnic groups, and religions commonly encountered in your environment

    8. Educational background
      a. Identify level of formal education attained by the patient
      b. Remember that level of formal education does not equate with one's ability to learn
      c. Determine patient's reading level
      d. Determine patient's health knowledge
      e. Determine patient's feelings about education and learning
      f. Use pictures for patients with low literacy skills

E. Domains of learning
    1. Cognitive: concerns the learner's knowledge and understanding
    2. Affective: concerned with the learner's attitudes, emotions, and ways of adjusting to an illness
    3. Psychomotor: concerned with motor skills

F. Goals of teaching
    1. To forewarn or provide information
    2. To teach skills (Foley care, dressing changes, etc.)
    3. Assist in decision making and planning
    4. Family involvement in patient care
    5. Reinforcement of existing knowledge
    6. Explain procedures, follow-up, and medications
    7. Discuss future events, expectations
    8. Advice about home health follow-up, home management
    9. Encourage change, provide alternative behaviors or thoughts

G. Maximizing teaching–learning effectiveness
    1. Allow sufficient time
    2. Choose appropriate time and environment
    3. Confirm patient readiness
      a. Preoperative: admission details are taken care of
      b. Postoperative: pain controlled, stable, awake, family present
    4. Actively involve the learner
    5. Use creativity in approaches
    6. Encourage learner to contribute to ideas
    7. Use humor or novelty to help learner relax and retain the content
    8. Organize material logically and present it in manageable amounts
    9. Highlight or point out important information
    10. Differentiate between similar concepts and contrasting information
    11. Allow practice as much as possible, giving constructive feedback

H. Common barriers to effective teaching–learning
    1. Providing false reassurance
    2. Invading privacy
    3. Minimizing or ignoring feelings
    4. Not listening
    5. Giving wrong information
    6. Violating trust relationship
    7. Noisy environment
    8. Lack of privacy
    9. Physiologic distraction (pain, nausea, vomiting, etc.)

Bibliography

1. Black, J.M., Matassarin-Jacobs, E. (1997). *Medical-Surgical Nursing*, 5th ed., p. 451. Philadelphia: Saunders.
2. Burden, N. (1993). Preparing the patient. In Burden, N., ed. *Ambulatory Surgical Nursing*, p. 152. Philadelphia: Saunders.
3. Burrell, L.O. (1997). Contemporary nursing practice. In Burrell, L.O., Gerlach, M.J.M., Pless, B.S., eds., *Adult Nursing: Acute and Community Care*, 2nd ed., p. 3. Stamford, CT: Appleton & Lange.
4. Lambert, V.A., Lambert, C.E., Gugino, H.S. (1997). Crisis & stress. In Burrell, L.O., Gerlach, M.J.M., Pless, B.S., eds., *Adult Nursing: Acute and Community Care*, 2nd ed., p. 74. Stamford, CT: Appleton & Lange.
5. Lewis, P., Lubkin, I. (1995). Illness roles. In Lubkin, I.M., ed., *Chronic Illness: Impact and Interventions*, 3rd ed., p. 74. Boston: Jones and Bartlett.
6. Lindsey, A.M., Carrieri, V.K. (1986). Stress response. In Carrieri, V.K., Lindsey, A.M., West, C.M., eds., *Pathophysiological Phenomena in Nursing: Human Responses to Illness*, p. 301. Philadelphia: Saunders.
7. Litwack, K. (1995). The adult patient. In Litwack, K., ed. *Core Curriculum for Post Anesthesia Nursing Practice*, 3rd ed., p. 47. Philadelphia: Saunders.
8. McCance, K.L., (1990). Stress and disease. In McCance, K.L., Huether, S.E., eds., *Pathophysiology: The Biologic Basis for Disease in Adults and Children*, p. 279. St. Louis: Mosby.
9. Murray, R., Pinnell, N., McDowell, P. (1993). Health promotion strategies. In Murray, R.B., Zentner, J.P., eds., *Nursing Assessment and Health Promotion: Strategies Through the Life Span*, 5th ed., p. 656. Norwalk, CT: Appleton & Lange.
10. Murray, R., Pinnell, N., Zentner, J. (1993). Basic considerations in health and illness. In Murray, R.B., Zentner, J.P., eds., *Nursing Assessment and Health Promotion: Strategies Through the Life Span*, 5th ed., p. 634. Norwalk, CT: Appleton & Lange.
11. Murray, R., Pinnell, N., Zentner, J., et al. (1993). Assessment and health promotion for the young adult. In Murray, R.B., Zentner, J.P., eds., *Nursing Assessment and Health Promotion: Strategies Through the Life Span*, 5th ed., p. 426. Norwalk, CT: Appleton & Lange.
12. Murray, R., Zentner, J. (1993). Assessment and health promotion for the middle-aged person. In Murray, R.B., Zentner, J.P., eds., *Nursing Assessment and Health Promotion: Strategies Through the Life Span*, 5th ed., p. 500. Norwalk, CT: Appleton & Lange.
13. White, N., Lubkin, I. (1995). Illness trajectory. In Lubkin, I.M., ed., *Chronic Illness: Impact and Interventions*, 3rd ed., p. 51. Boston: Jones and Bartlett.

REVIEW QUESTIONS

1. Your diagnostic laparoscopic patient is concerned about returning to work, and finding care for her two children, ages 4 and 2, while she is recovering. Her husband is currently in graduate school and is not of much help at home. Your patient is most likely in what age group?

   A. Late adolescence
   B. Young adulthood
   C. Middle age
   D. Young old

2. The ability to adapt, relate effectively, and to function at near maximum capacity is defined as

   A. Health
   B. Illness
   C. Wellness
   D. Disease

3. Your 45-year-old patient states that he quit smoking 10 years ago, exercises at least five times a week, and eats a low-fat diet. These activities are examples of what type of behavior?

   A. Health
   B. Preventive
   C. Illness
   D. Rehabilitative

4. The major role components of the sick role include all of the following except

   A. Exemption from all responsibilities
   B. Right to be cared for
   C. Obligation to want to become well
   D. Obligation to seek and cooperate with technically competent help

5. Activation of the sympathetic nervous system results in all of the following except

   A. Increased heart rate
   B. Increased cardiac output
   C. Increased stroke volume
   D. Increased vasodilatation

6. A patient scheduled to undergo a needle breast biopsy comes for her preoperative visit with a current article on breast cancer and a list of questions to ask. This is an example of what type of coping mode?

   A. Escape–avoidance
   B. Self-control
   C. Seeking social support
   D. Accepting responsibility

7. Cognitive methods of stress management include all of the following except

   A. Thought stopping
   B. Biofeedback
   C. Laughter
   D. Guided imagery

8. Your 55-year-old male outpatient is 40 pounds overweight and leads a sedentary lifestyle. A common health problem for this age group would be

   A. Mitral valve prolapse
   B. Iron deficiency anemia
   C. Chronic fatigue syndrome
   D. Diabetes type II

9. Setting goals with the patient to determine his/her preoperative learning needs is an example of what phase of the teaching–learning process?

   A. Assessment
   B. Diagnosis
   C. Planning
   D. Intervention

10. A patient is able to demonstrate how to discontinue his/her Foley catheter using a model. This is an example of what learning domain?

   A. Behavioral
   B. Cognitive
   C. Affective
   D. Psychomotor

ANSWERS TO QUESTIONS

1. B
2. C
3. A
4. A
5. D

6. C
7. B
8. D
9. C
10. D

18

The Elderly Patient

Joyce C. Hadley
Inova Health Systems
Falls Church, Virginia

I. **General Considerations (Nursing Impact)**
  A. Demographics
    1. Life expectancy
      a. Female 78 years
      b. Male 74 years
    2. Population
      a. Currently about 12.5% of the population
      b. Expect 35 million to be over 65 by year 2000
      c. Projected: over 66 million elders by year 2030
      d. Reasons for increased longevity of humans include:
        i. General health improvement
        ii. More and better health care
        iii. Improved sanitation efforts worldwide
  B. Define elderly
    1. Young-old: 65–75 years
    2. Old: 75–85 years
    3. Old-old: over 85 years
  C. Physiologic age versus chronological age
    1. Functional age is impacted by:
      a. Chronic disease processes
      b. Personal attitudes/outlook
      c. Family and friends network
    2. Persons over 70 years may have productive, vigorous lives, while significantly younger persons may lead more restricted lives due to depression, chronic illness, or lack of support systems
II. **Physiologic Changes of Aging**
  A. Central nervous system

Objectives

1. Discuss the demographics of the elderly patient.
2. Identify the physiologic changes characteristic of elderly patients.
3. Explain the impact of surgical intervention upon the elderly patient.
4. Weigh the advantages/ disadvantages of ambulatory surgery for the elderly.
5. Discuss appropriate interventions by the ambulatory surgery nurse.
6. Identify elder abuse issues.

1. Neurogenic atrophy and reduction of peripheral nerve fibers
   a. Decreased blood flow and CNS activity
      i.   Causing slower reaction times
      ii. Reduced ability to cope with body stressors
      iii. Diminished ability to respond to demands on cardiovascular systems
      iv. Prolonged emergence from pharmacologic interventions (e.g., benzodiazepines) and decreased pain perception
   b. Decreased cognitive function
      i.   Loss of memory and decreased understanding
      ii. Lengthening of learning speed
      iii. Higher risk of confusion
      iv. Short attention span
      v.   Decreased sensory abilities
           (a) Impaired hearing acuity
               (i) Men especially lose high-frequency sounds
               (ii) Vestibular changes may also alter balance and/or cause vertigo
           (b) Visual precision is reduced
               (i) Lenses fail (as in cataracts)
               (ii) Glaucoma
           (c) Impaired temperature regulation
           (d) Decreased tactile perception
           (e) Acuity of smell diminished
               (i) May impair hygiene
   c. Nursing implications
      i.   Allow additional time to assimilate information and give responses
      ii. Encourage use of sensory aids
           (a) Hearing aids
           (b) Visual aids
               (i) Glasses
               (ii) Magnifying glass
      iii. Include family member/responsible adult in instructions
      iv. Verbal communication
           (a) Face patient when speaking
           (b) Raise speaking volume, not pitch
           (c) Speak slowly and clearly
      v.   Observe for prolonged or toxic effects of drugs
      vi. Encourage lower doses
      vii. Safety measures
           (a) Hand rails
           (b) Other assistive devices
               (i)   Canes, walkers, nonslip shower chairs
               (ii) Nonskid footware
               (iii) Physical support by caretaker
           (c) Observation
B. Cardiovascular system
   1. Most changes are due to arteriosclerotic changes
   2. Loss of tissue elasticity
      a. Organ perfusion decreases
         i.   Myocardium
         ii. Decreases optimal regulation of all body systems
      b. Peripheral circulation impaired
         i.   Lowers tolerances to stress responses (heart workload increases)

      ii. Along with decreased collagen, increases difficulty of venipuncture
        (a) Aging collagen makes tough "rolling" veins
        (b) Loss of elasticity likely to cause bleeding around site during and after venipuncture
      iii. Higher risk for bruising
      iv. Increases peripheral vascular resistance
        (a) Which restricts left ventricular ejection
        (b) Therefore promotes cardiac hypertrophy
      v. Potential for orthostatic hypotension
    c. Increased susceptibility to clotting disorders
      i. Stroke
      ii. Thrombosis
      iii. Embolism
  3. Cardiac conduction system
    a. Conduction deficits
      i. Heart rate slows
      ii. Dysrhythmias and blocks occur more frequently
  4. Pump effectiveness diminishes
    a. Due to atrophy of myocardial fibers
    b. Decrease in cardiac output
    c. Slower circulation time
    d. Prolonged onset of action and clearing times for drugs
  5. Nursing considerations
    a. Observe responses to medications
      i. Allow adequate time for response before repeating
      ii. Use lower range of medication dosage and encourage team to utilize lower dosages
    b. Monitor for cardiac inadequacy
      i. Lungs
        (a) Provide adequate oxygenation
          (i) Encourage deep breathing
        (b) Watch for fluid overload while ensuring adequate hydration
      ii. Heart
        (a) Assess heart sounds
        (b) Cardiac monitoring for arrhythmias
        (c) Assess lung sounds
        (d) Avoid extremes of blood pressure
          (i) Watch for orthostatic changes
          (ii) Encourage slow position changes
        (e) Vascular considerations
          (i) Gentle venipunctures
          (ii) Avoid tourniquets where possible
            a) Minimize use of automatic blood pressure devices
          (iii) Adequate pressure on sites post venipuncture or catheter removal
          (iv) Encourage early ambulation
C. Respiratory system
  1. Airway
    a. Edentia
      i. Impacts patency of airway
      ii. Creates difficulty in intubation
  2. Decreased elasticity of tissues
    a. Alveolar level

        i. Alteration in structure (loss of alveolar surface)

        ii. Leads to diminished lung function

           (a) Reduces recoil of lungs

           (b) Reduces functional vital capacity

           (c) Increases vital capacity

           (d) Increases residual volume

        iii. Alterations in carbon dioxide and oxygen levels caused by diminished lung functions, ultimately leads to "senile emphysema"

    b. Chest wall

        i. Stiffness due to arthritic or calcification of cartilage

           (a) Inhibits chest expansion, therefore decreases functional residual capacity

        ii. Decreased muscle strength restricts

           (a) Adequacy of respiratory effort (harder to deep breathe!)

           (b) Cough

           (c) Action of diaphragm

    c. Decreased effectiveness of cough mechanisms

        i. Reduced elasticity of lungs

        ii. Anesthesia, analgesia blunt normal responses

        iii. Operative pain may decrease effectiveness of cough even more as the patient "splints" to avoid pain

    d. Secretions

        i. Increase

        ii. Potential for aspiration

  3. Nursing considerations

    a. Airway

        i. Assess airway constantly

        ii. Protect unconscious airway

           (a) Suction oropharynx prn

           (b) Support/position

        iii. Provide appropriate airways and oxygen delivery supplies

        iv. Returning dentures can help support the airway

    b. Secretions/effective cough

        i. Position:

           (a) With head elevated when possible

           (b) To maximize chest expansion

        ii. Encourage coughing and deep breathing

        iii. Assure reflexes have returned prior to administering oral fluids

    c. Oygenation

        i. Monitor oxygen saturation (e.g., pulse oximeter)

        ii. Support with oxygen as necessary

    d. Pain

        i. Alleviate pain

        ii. Employ anxiety and stress-reduction tactics

D. Musculoskeletal system

  1. Musculoskeletal tissues are able to change in response to altered functional demands; changes in the elderly are related to (Bejelle, 1996):

    a. Decline of function

    b. Reduced physical demands

  2. Atrophy and denervation of muscle mass

    a. Loss of strength

    b. Reduced requirement for regional anesthesia dosage

3. Osteoporosis
   a. Definition: inappropriately low bone mass for age, gender, and race
   b. Peak bone mass around 30–40 years of age
   c. Mineral content of bone (bone density) decreases
      i.   After 40 years of age
      ii. 0.5% per year for men
      iii. About 1.0% per year for women
   d. Risk factors
      i.   Age
      ii. Female
      iii. Low body weight
      iv. Caucasian race
      v.   Cigarette smoking
   e. Degeneration of bone causes:
      i.   Pathologic changes
         (a) Vertebral degeneration
            (i) Kyphoscoliosis
               a) Limits chest expansion/capacity
               b) Limits success in establishing spinal or epidural injection
         (b) Compression fractures
         (c) Increased potential for pathologic fracture
         (d) Higher incidence of traumatic fractures (falls especially)
4. Osteoarthritis
   a. Specific cause unknown, but there is demonstrated relationship with:
      i. Advancing age
      ii. Wear and tear of joints throughout lifespan
   b. Structural changes in the joint
      i. Probably starts in cartilage
      ii. Leads to:
         (a) Reduced mobility of joint
            (i) Difficult ambulation
            (ii) Potential for falls
         (b) Pain
         (c) Less flexibility
5. Nursing considerations
   a. Careful positioning throughout perioperative experience
      i.   Support for back
      ii. Alignment
      iii. Protection of bony processes
   b. Observe for prolonged or toxic effects of regional agents
   c. Provide for pain relief
   d. Assist patient with physical tasks related to strength
      i.   Moving
      ii. Ambulation
      iii. Exercise
         (a) Gentle movement
         (b) Encourage frequent activity
   e. Safety concerns
      i.   Concerted fall-prevention program
         (a) Support when walking: cane, walker, rails
         (b) Treaded (skid-resistant) footware
         (c) Education for patient and caretakers

E. Renal/genitourinary systems
  1. Age-related renal physiological changes include reduced glomerular mass, impaired perfusion, and diminished function
     a. Impaired salt-conservation system
        i.   Diminished thirst perception
        ii. Potential for dehydration
        iii. Hypokalemia and hyponatremia
     b. Reduced glomerular filtration rate
        i.   Slowed clearance of renally excreted drugs (e.g., long-acting barbiturates, digoxin, atropine)
        ii. Decreased metabolism of drugs excreted by the kidneys
     c. Renal concentrating and diluting capability is impaired
        i.   Altered responses to ADH regulation and utilization
  2. Lower urinary tract dysfunction
     a. Reduced muscle tone
     b. Impaired sphincter activity
     c. Reduced bladder capacity
     d. Heightened incidence of incontinence
  3. Females
     a. Relaxation of pelvic musculature
        i.   Bladder and vaginal prolapse
        ii. Impinges on urethra
             (a) Obstructs emptying bladder
             (b) Increases "dribbling" incontinence
     b. Hormonal changes
        i.   Raises potential for urinary tract infection
  4. Males
     a. Prostatic enlargement
        i.   Inhibits free-flow of urine
        ii. Starting urine stream often difficult
  5. Nursing implications
     a. Observe for fluid imbalance
        i.   Monitor intake and output
        ii. Encourage oral fluids postoperatively
     b. Observe for effects of electrolyte imbalance
        i.   Monitor and/or observe for cardiac dysrhythmias, ECG changes
        ii. Consider that hyponatremia may be a cause of confusion
     c. Observe for prolonged medication effect
        i.   Use lower dosage range of medications and encourage smaller medication dosage by team
        ii. Provide support for toileting needs
             (a) Toilet frequently
                 (i)   Offer urinal/bedpan
                 (ii) Assist to bathroom
                 (iii) Facilitate genitourinary hygiene
             (b) Provide protection for bedding and clothing
             (c) Reassure/support emotionally
             (d) Regard privacy to diminish embarassment
  6. Gastrointestinal system concerns around the surgical event
     a. Gastrointestinal dysfunction due to impaired muscle function
        i.   Esophageal and/or gastric reflux
             (a) Poor or absent closure of sphincters

(b) Hiatal hernia

(c) Effects

    (i)   Esophagitis

    (ii) Swallowing difficulty

    (iii) Increased potential for aspiration

ii.   Stomach

    (a) Ulcers may cause chest pain

iii. Motility disorders (reduced peristaltic action)

    (a) Gastric emptying

        (i)   Gastric distention

        (ii) Vomiting

    (b) Intestinal emptying

        (i)   Constipation

        (ii) Intestinal distention

iv. Hepatic changes

    (a) Liver becomes more fatty (especially with increased alcohol consumption)

    (b) Blood flow is reduced

    (c) Effects:

        (i)   Reduced ability to metabolize drugs

        (ii) Agents cleared by liver remain longer in bloodstream

b. Nursing considerations

    i.   Careful administration of oral fluids/food

        (a) Start with small amounts

        (b) Begin when sitting up if possible

    ii. Elevate head of bed for most effective gastric emptying

    iii. Consider ulcers with complaint of chest pain

    iv. Observe for prolonged or toxic drug effects

7. Integumentary system

    a. Decrease in fat layers of skin

        i.   Inhibits thermoregulation

        ii. Decreased protection from trauma

    b. Loss of elasticity causes wrinkled, loose, more easily torn skin

    c. Reduced blood supply

        i.   Adds to atrophy of tissue

    d. Sebaceous gland function diminishes, causing dry skin

    e. Diminished skin pigmentation

8. Nursing considerations

    a. Provide warmed blankets and warm environment during and after operative event

    b. Protect skin with:

        i.   Proper positioning

        ii. Padding on bony prominences

        iii. Use paper or other nontearing skin tape

    c. Remember, loss of pigmentation mimics pallor

        i.   Don't rely on skin color to assess for anemia or cardiac distress

III. Psychosocial Considerations for the Elderly

A. Maintain/promote autonomy

    1. Independence

        a. Encourage performance of self-care

  b. Address issues of concern
   i. Advance directives
   ii. Quality-of-life issues
  c. Talk with, not "around," the patient
  d. Inquire about preferences
   i. Name use (e.g., "What do you prefer that I call you?")
   ii. Time schedules (eating, sleeping, etc.)
 2. Competence
  a. Reduced ability to provide self-care leads to depression/reduced self-worth
  b. Abilities to perform may alter with time of day, health status, and life events
  c. Elders require more practice with new skills
  d. Repetition and clarification enhance learning
B. Encourage self-acceptance
 1. **Maintain patient dignity**
 2. Invite expression of fears
  a. Death/dying
  b. Change in body image/function
 3. Review coping mechanisms
 4. Present patient with decision alternatives when possible
C. Time concept is altered
 1. Employ tactics for time orientation
  a. Time perception/elapsed time
  b. Past, present, and future
D. Social awareness
 1. Elders are experiencing life role changes
  a. May outlive friends/family (especially old-old)
  b. Caregivers become the patient (drastic role change when other party is already ill/debilitated)
 2. Encourage participation of significant others
IV. **Elder abuse (usually related to family or other caregiver)**
 A. Types
  1. Material/financial
  2. Physical
   a. Sexual
   b. Beating/slapping/kicking
   c. Neglect
    i. Passive
    ii. Active (especially old-old)
    iii. Self
   d. Emotional
   e. Verbal
    i. Threatening physical abuse or isolation
    ii. Humiliation/intimidation
   f. Withholding (e.g., care, food, company)
 B. Detection
  1. Physical assessment/evidence of bodily harm
   a. Bruises
   b. Skin tears
   c. Burns
   d. Evidence of restraint
  2. Emotional abuse (difficult to assess)
   a. Fear of violence
   b. Social isolation

C. Mandatory reporting
   1. Different laws in each state
D. Resources
   1. Adult protection programs
   2. Domestic violence programs
   3. Services
      a. Financial advocacy
      b. Social advocacy
      c. Religious groups
V. **Special Concerns for the Elderly Around the Ambulatory Surgical Event**

| **NOTE:** These considerations are *adjunct* to the usual adult concerns. |

A. Advantages of ambulatory surgery for the elderly
   1. Decrease risk of nosocomial infections
      a. Wound infections
      b. Respiratory infections
   2. Decreased incidence of mental confusion
      a. Environment less disruptive
      b. Decreased disruption in personal routine
   3. Minimized length of stay away from home environment
   4. Cost effectiveness
B. Disadvantages of ambulatory surgery for the elderly
   1. Compliance to the plan of care
      a. Diminishing abilities
         i. Cognitive (e.g., forgetfulness)
            (a) Unable to complete care regime
            (b) Unable to cope with changes in routine
               (i) New medication protocols
               (ii) Care related to procedure
         ii. Physical
            (a) Diminished stamina/strength for self-care
            (b) Increased potential for falls
            (c) Unaware of wound contamination
      b. Lack of support system at home
         i. Transportation issues and other logistical issues
         ii. Financial concerns (unable to obtain medications, supplies)
         iii. Lack of caregiver/significant other
         iv. Reduced or nonexistent circle of friends (especially in the old-old)
C. In physician's office
   1. Insure involvement of significant other in information/instructions
   2. Provide directions to facility
      a. Written/verbal
      b. Include maps
   3. Give clear parking directions
   4. Remind patient and significant other to keep list of current medications and take it to interview
   5. Explain processes of:
      a. Preadmission interview (as required)
      b. Laboratory and diagnostic testing

        c. Importance of adherence to instructions

           i.   NPO and other preop intake information

           ii. Transportation arrangements

    D. Preadmission interview special considerations for the elderly

---

NOTE: If preadmission interview is not possible, initiate telephone contact and (a.) review preoperative instructions and (b.) investigate potential health history concerns.

---

    1. Provide adequate time for interview and assessment

    2. Physical status assessment, especially note:

       a. Sensory limitations

       b. Restriction of mobility

       c. Use of any prosthetic devices

    3. Assess mental status

       a. Include significant other

       b. Seek cues about changes during stressful events

    4. Provide verbal and written preoperative instructions in large print

       a. Arrival time

       b. Appropriate clothing

       c. How to handle routine medications (take/omit)

    5. Assure transportation and home-support concerns are addressed prior to the surgical event

    6. Review patient expectations of postoperative period

       a. Pain

       b. Physical limitations

  E. Preoperative admission

    1. Verify transportation and home-support arrangements

    2. Review instructions clearly and slowly

    3. Verify NPO status, including medications taken or omitted

    4. Secure belongings (and reassure of postoperative return)

    5. Provide for elder adaptations

       a. Special positioning (e.g., extra pillows for "stiff neck")

       b. Protect fragile skin and tissues

       c. Keep sensory aids and dental prostheses with patient as long as possible

    6. Be gentle!

    7. Facilitate alternatives to decrease medication needs

       a. Family presence

       b. Comfort measures

       c. Touch

       d. Relaxation

    8. Observe closely for medication effects

       a. Prolonged

       b. Untoward

    9. Communicate special needs to OR team and anesthesia personnel

  F. Intraoperative considerations for the elderly

    1. Sensory

       a. Avoid loud noises

          i.   Music

          ii. Conversation not including the patient

       b. Allow patient to keep sensory aids if possible

       c. Maintain voice, tactile, or visual contact with awake patient

2. Environment
   a. Remember thermostatic needs
      i.   Increased risk when core body temperature falls below 96.8°F (36°C)
   b. Protective measures
      i.   Raise room temperature
      ii. Use warming blankets/devices
      iii. Warm anesthetic gases/solutions/IV fluids
      iv. Cover patient's head
3. Positioning
   a. Change slowly and gently; avoid extremes
   b. Lift patient! Do not pull!
   c. Support back of neck (prevent discomfort from kyphosis/arthritis, for example)
   d. Pad and support to protect pressure points
4. Circulation: remember that hypotension and slowed circulation predispose patient to thrombus formation and emboli
   a. Use antiembolitic stockings or sequential compression devices
      i.   Especially high-risk patient
      ii. Prolonged (>2 hours) procedures
   b. Observe for points of pressure that might inhibit blood flow to extremities
5. Nurse-monitored local anesthesia; monitoring notes
   a. Elders do not tolerate fluid/blood loss well
      i.   When patient approaches hypovolemia, small changes can have large impact
      ii. Monitor fluid loss and output carefully
   b. Impending crisis may be indicated by fluctuations in cardiac rate and rhythm
G. PACU Phase I
   1. Prevention/reduction of morbidity and mortality
   2. Airway/ventilation
      a. Promote optimal gas exchange
         i.   Encourage deep breathing/coughing
         ii. Facilitate optimal chest expansion; elevate head of bed
         iii. Provide oxygen support
      b. Observe for compromised function
         i.   Monitor cardiovascular and respiratory status
         ii. Increased potential for aspiration due to swallowing dysfunction
         iii. Potential for untoward or extended drug effects
            (a) Increase in fat deposits increases potential for harboring fat-soluble drugs
            (b) Decreased kidney and liver functions
   3. Fluid status
      a. Maintain or establish fluid *balance*
         i.   Regard pre- and intraoperative deficits
         ii. Monitor/treat nausea and/or vomiting
         iii. Observe intake and output fluids
            (a) Avoid overload, especially by intravenous route
            (b) Note diminished output
   4. Physical activity ("stir-up regime") and appraisal
      a. Encourages adequate circulation and ventilation
      b. Promotes mobilization
         i.   Assess for orthostatic hypotension

        ii. Beware of fast movement
           (a) Balance attained more slowly
           (b) Joints/muscles often altered in aging process
     c. Allows for observation of neuromuscular status
  5. Psychological and sensory status
     a. Reorientation
        i. Reinforce verbal and tactile contact
        ii. Avoid sensory overload
           (a) Care unit noises can be loud, constant, and frightening
           (b) Return assistive/prosthetic devices as soon as possible
           (c) Avoid restraint use
       iii. Facilitate presence of significant others as appropriate to encourage reorientation
       iv. In event of mental dysfunction:
           (a) Consider action of anesthesia agents and other medications as cause
           (b) Rule out hypoxemia as cause of agitation/confusion
           (c) Remember, if confusion/dysfunction was present before surgery, it will probably be present after surgery
  6. Skin
     a. Thermoregulation
        i. Keep warm or rewarm
        ii. Normothermia promotes cardiovascular stability
     b. Prevent damage
        i. Avoid excess tape application
           (a) Remove excess tape/ECG lead pads and skin prep solutions to minimize irritation
        ii. Avoid automatic (noninvasive) blood pressure devices when possible
           (a) If necessary to use, protect with soft wrapping
       iii. Keep skin dry
           (a) Observe for dribbling or other incontinence
           (b) Toilet early, remembering bladder shrinkage, decreased sphincter tone
     c. Potential for infection
        i. Dress wound appropriately
        ii. Aged body may have decreased healing capability
     d. Pain management
        i. Be aware of:
           (a) Drug interactions
           (b) Titrate narcotics ("Begin low, go slow")
              (i) Pain increases myocardial oxygen demand
              (ii) Consider decreased sensory response to pain
              (iii) Consider patient may be stoic/not inclined to admit to pain
           (c) Residuals of preoperative and anesthetic agents may be present

VI. PACU Phase II
  A. Physical status
    1. Assure safety
      a. Ambulate carefully
        i. Sit on edge of stretcher to gain balance
        ii. Provide physical support for walking
           (a) Use orthopedic/prosthetic devices as necessary
           (b) Lower stretcher
           (c) Step-stool with caution (they tip!)
        iii. Encourage, while allowing patient to find own pace of movement

b. Return all sensory aids prior to ambulation

c. Monitor neuromuscular status

2. Psychological interventions

    a. Promote wellness concept

        i.   Return clothes and belongings promptly

        ii. Reunite with family members/responsible adult/significant others

    b. Communicate with patient expecting:

        i.   Slower thought processes, movements, and responses

        ii. **Old** does not mean stupid!

3. Home preparation

    a. Include support persons when reviewing home instructions

    b. Verify plans for home support

        i.   Ascertain patient/family/responsible adult's understanding of and ability to comply with discharge instructions

        ii. Elderly caring for elderly may not be adequate or responsible

        iii. Arrange time and place for postoperative contact

            (a) Recovery issues evaluation

                (i)   Consider tool easily understood by patient

                (ii) Introducing a likert-type scale to patient prior to surgery would be beneficial

                (iii) Discuss possible topics of postoperative telephone contact

    c. Instruct on return to normal preoperative medication regime

    d. Instructions

        i.   Avoid sedating medications

        ii. Provide clear verbal instructions

        iii. Provide large print written instructions

            (a) Large *simple* diagrams or pictures

        iv. Ascertain understanding (patient and other care providers as necessary)

            (a) By demonstration

            (b) Return demonstration

        v.   Repeat instructions

VII. After Discharge: Phase III, Extension of Care

A. Nursing interventions

1. Postoperative patient contact by *telephone*

    a. Prior to contact

        i.   Review patient data

        ii. Have scale available to assist patient in symptom evaluation; examples:

            (a) Visual analog scale

            (b) Numerical scale

                (i)   Horizontal or vertical

                (ii) Usually 1–10 or 1–5

            (c) Faces scale

                (i)   Pediatric (happy to sad faces)

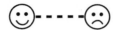

                (ii) Other depictions of faces

    b. Telephone contact

        i.   Have prepared questionnaire available

            (a) Amend questions as issues arise

  ii. Interpersonal concerns
   (a) Identify self: speak slowly and clearly
   (b) Express concern and interest
  iii. Obtain data on physical condition
  iv. Inquire about expected/unexpected symptoms, which might include:
   (a) Nausea/vomiting
   (b) Pain
   (c) Fatigue
   (d) Fever
   (e) Impaired movement
   (f) Bleeding
   (g) Dizziness

> **NOTE:** Oberly, Allen, and Lynkowski (1994) concluded " . . . the most important information to teach patients is how to cope with pain and fatigue and what to expect during the postoperative course. Patients require guidelines against which they can gauge their progress."

  v. Identify actual/potential complications
  vi. Verify patient's compliance with instructions
   (a) Validate with significant other/adult care provider if necessary
 c. Initiate follow-up as required
  i. Quality improvement monitors
  ii. Second follow-up call if necessary
  iii. Physician referral if necessary
  iv. Make other service referrals as indicated
   (a) Support groups related to particular condition (diabetes/cancer/ smoking cessation)
   (b) Community resources
    (i) Meals on Wheels
    (ii) Visiting nurses/social workers
    (iii) Other senior citizens groups
    (iv) Religious groups/visitation, etc.
2. Other settings for Phase III care (see Chapter 20)
 a. Hospital-based 23-hour care units
 b. Ambulatory center non-hospital 23-hour units
 c. Recovery care centers
 d. Home care with home care nursing personnel

Bibliography

1. Allen, A. (1993). Caring about the elderly: Opportunities and obligations. *J Post Anesth Nurs.* 8(2): 131–133.
2. Bejelle, A. (1996). Rheumatic diseases. In Birren, J.E., ed., *Encyclopedia of Gerontology*, p. 451. Los Angeles: Academic Press.
3. Burden, N. (1993). *Ambulatory Surgical Nursing.* Philadelphia: Saunders.
4. Birren, J. (ed.). (1996). *Encyclopedia of Gerontology.* San Diego: Academic Press.
5. Cassel, C.K. et al. (eds). (1997). *Geriatric Medicine,* 3rd ed. New York, Springer.
6. Clyne, M., Forlenza, M. (1997). Consumer-focused preadmission testing: A paradigm shift. *J Nurs Care Qual*, 11(3):9–15.
7. Drain, C. (1994). *The Post Anesthesia Care Unit.* Philadelphia: Saunders.
8. Ferrara-Love, R. (1997). *Geriatric Considerations for the Ambulatory Surgery Patient.* Presentation: "Issues for a New Millennium." Conference co-sponsored by Chesapeake Bay Society of PeriAnesthesia Nurses and ASPAN. Stevensville, MD.
9. Gibson, J.R., Jr., Mendenhall, M.K., Axel, N.J. (1985). Geriatric anesthesia: Minimizing the risk. *Geriatr Clin North Am*, 1:313–321.
10. Hazen, S.E., Larsen, P.D., Martin, J.L.H. (1997). General anesthesia and elderly surgical patients. *AORN J*, 65(4):815–822.

11. Lancaster, K.A. (1997). Patient teaching in ambulatory surgery. In Greenfield, E., DeFazio Quinn, D. eds., *Nursing Clinics of North America*, 32(2).

12. Linden, I., Engberg, I.B. (1994). Nursing discharge assessment of the patient post-inguinal herniorrhaphy in the ambulatory surgery setting. *J Post Anesth Nurs*, 9(1):14–18.

13. Litwack, K. (1995). *Post Anesthesia Care Nursing*, 2nd ed. St. Louis: Mosby.

14. Lynch, S.H. (1997). Elder abuse: What to look for, how to intervene. *AJN*, 97(1):27–33.

15. Oberle, K., Allen, M., Lynkowski, P. (1994). Follow-up of same day surgery patients. *AORN*, 59(5):1016–1025.

16. Worfolk, J.B. (1997). Keep frail elders warm! *Geriatric Nursing*, (J) 18(1).

REVIEW QUESTIONS

1. Preadmission preparation of the geriatric patient should include

   A. Minimum of two preadmission assessment visits
   B. Explicit directions to preadmission assessment site and hospital
   C. Action of drugs to be administered during surgery
   D. Awareness of policies on visiting

2. Which of the following makes awareness of geriatric concerns most important to the ambulatory surgery nurse?

   A. Diminishing need for special care for the elderly
   B. Projection of increased longevity of world population
   C. Changing attitudes toward aging
   D. Improved public support of health systems for the elderly

3. A person of 77 years is considered

   A. Young-old
   B. Average-old
   C. Old
   D. Old-old

4. Decreased cognitive function in elders is caused by

   A. Diminished reading and mental activity capabilities
   B. Decreased blood flow and atrophy of CNS tissues
   C. Reduction in visual precision
   D. Changing response to pharmacologic effects of testosterone/estrogen

5. Due to generalized changes, such as loss of tissue elasticity and decreased collagen, the nurse may expect which of the following?

   A. Impaired peripheral circulation
   B. Difficulty starting IVs due to "rubbery" veins
   C. More bleeding at venipuncture sites
   D. All of the above

6. Cardiac pump effectiveness in elders is diminished by

   A. Atrophy of myocardial fibers
   B. Faster circulation time
   C. Lowered peripheral resistance
   D. Increased cardiac output

7. Special concerns of the elderly patient during the preadmission interview may include

   A. Scheduling/timing
   B. Logistical information
   C. Outcomes
   D. All of the above

8. A very important reason to return dental prostheses to a patient as soon as possible is

   A. To support conversation/communication
   B. To support/maintain the patient's airway
   C. To enhance self-image and return to normalcy
   D. All of the above

9. To encourage adequate circulation and ventilation

   A. Encourage visitation in Phase II
   B. Return clothing as soon as possible
   C. Utilize stir-up regime
   D. Offer oxygen supplement

10. Which of the following act **most** to prolong effect of drugs in elderly patients?

   A. Decreased renal, cardiac, and hepatic blood flow
   B. Increased cardiac output and hepatic blood flow
   C. Increased renal, cardiac, and hepatic blood flow
   D. Decreased cardio-hepatic compliance

11. Verification of home-support plans should be included in which phase of the perianesthesia scenario?

   A. During preoperative assessment appointment
   B. Before procedure
   C. After procedure
   D. All of the above

12. Which speaking technique is least helpful when dealing with hearing-impaired patients?

   A. Speaking louder
   B. Speaking clearly
   C. Raising pitch of voice
   D. Keeping your face in patient's view

13. Elder abuse

   A. Is uncommon in our society
   B. Always requires reporting to state authorities upon discovery
   C. Usually has extreme physical symptoms
   D. Is often committed by family caregivers

14. Osteoporosis does not increase potential for

   A. Falls/fractures
   B. Kyposis
   C. Reduced lung expansion
   D. Rheumatoid arthritis

15. Elders are at increased risk to develop aspiration pneumonia related to

   A. Poor ejection fractions
   B. Poor or absent closure of sphincters
   C. Kyphoscoliosis
   D. None of the above

ANSWERS TO QUESTIONS

1. B	9. C
2. B	10. A
3. C	11. D
4. B	12. C
5. D	13. D
6. A	14. D
7. D	15. B
8. D	

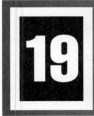

The Mentally and Physically Challenged Patient

Gwen D. Williams
Our Lady of Lourdes Regional Medical Center
Lafayette, Louisiana

NOTE: The intent of this chapter is to cover only those nursing interventions specific to the stated disease or illness. Refer to Chapter 7 and Chapter 8 for complete information.

I. The Mentally Challenged Patient
  A. Communication
    1. An act by means of which one person conveys to another his/her ideas, thoughts, needs, or feelings
    2. To communicate, a person must have some communication channel open to him/her to convey information to those around him/her
    3. Communication involves:
      a. Getting information to the brain
      b. Processing the information, **and then**
      c. Transmitting the brain's response
    4. For the mentally or physically challenged patient, normal channels of communication may not be available
  B. General information
    1. Mental ability may be impaired from birth or acquired as a result of disease or injury
    2. Level of impairment
      a. Mild
        i. Slow learner
        ii. Rarely asks questions
        iii. Answers questions with a minimum of words
        iv. Can usually function at a 10-year-old level

Objectives

1. Identify three degrees of mental retardation and the level of function associated with each.
2. Identify techniques to reduce apprehension and facilitate learning for the visually impaired patient.
3. Identify techniques to reduce apprehension and facilitate learning for the hearing impaired patient.
4. Identify techniques to facilitate learning for the patient with aphasia.
5. Identify characteristics associated with certain physical disabilities and incorporate these differences in developing a plan of care.

  b. Moderate
    i.   Has little or no speech
    ii. Understands and can follow simple commands
    iii. Can learn simple tasks; may need supervision to perform
    iv. May be able to function at 2- to 6-year-old level
  c. Severe/profound
    i.   May learn to perform simple self-care tasks with supervision
    ii. Shows basic emotional response
    iii. May function at 0- to 2-year-old level
3. Special considerations
  a. Cognitive functions
    i.   Degree of impairment will determine method of instruction
    ii. Understands simple words and phrases
    iii. Tends to have:
       (a) Short attention span
       (b) Decreased retention capability
       (c) Decreased sensory capability
    iv. Becomes confused and distracted easily
    v. Fearful of changes in environment, loss of familiar routine
    vi. Unable to understand complex words
  b. Mental status
    i.   May be agitated
    ii. May show aggression
    iii. May not exhibit any response
  c. Sensory function
    i.   May have visual or auditory deficits
    ii. Understands simple words and phrases
    iii. May need information repeated
    iv. Benefits from demonstration
    v. May need extra time to answer question
  d. Communication problems
    i.   Poor articulation, especially consonants
    ii. More inarticulate when upset, frustrated, or discussing emotionally charged area
    iii. May use words that he/she does not really understand
    iv. May need extra time to formulate answers
    v. May use sign language, read lips
    vi. May use nonverbal forms of communication
4. When providing information:
  a. Determine the patient's strengths and weaknesses
  b. Communicate slowly and clearly
  c. Be sensitive to nonverbal communication
  d. Show respect to the patient
  e. Don't talk down to the patient
  f. Remain calm, relaxed, and unhurried
  g. Use the name to which the patient is accustomed
  h. Encourage and allow patient independence
  i. Include family/caregiver in planning care and instructions as appropriate
  j. Demonstration may be more effective than verbal explanations
  k. Provide frequent reinforcement
C. Preoperative preadmission interview
  1. General overview

    a. An in-person interview is preferable to a telephone interview
       i. Nonverbal communication may be as important as verbal communication
      ii. May be the only way to communicate with the person
    b. Allow adequate time for the interview and assessment
    c. Determine the patient's functional ability
       i. Developmental assessment if appropriate
      ii. Question the family/caregiver about the patient's abilities
    d. Determine the patient's and the family's/caregiver's knowledge of the proposed procedure
2. Develop a plan of care based on the patient's/caregiver's knowledge and needs
3. Assess:
    a. Abilities, special needs
    b. Family's/caregiver's successful management techniques
    c. Use of assistive devices, i.e., glasses, braces, hearing aid
    d. Willingness of family/caregiver to participate in preoperative preparation and postoperative care
    e. Effective means of communication
4. Complete health history
    a. Etiology of disability
    b. Past surgical history
    c. Anesthetic complications for patient or family
    d. Past illnesses
       i. Frequent respiratory infections
      ii. Ability to handle illness-related stress
     iii. Length of recuperative period
     iv. History of renal problems
      v. Normal bowel function
     vi. Other health problems
    e. Current illnesses
       i. Congenital heart defect
      ii. Diabetes insipidus
     iii. Seizures
     iv. Other
    f. Medications
       i. Behavior changes caused by medications
      ii. Previous response to medications
     iii. Current medication use
         (a) Prescription
         (b) Over the counter
         (c) Herbal preparations
    g. Allergies, including latex
    h. Nutritional requirements/modifications
       i. Preferences
      ii. Food consistency
     iii. Special dietary restrictions
     iv. Ability to swallow
      v. Ability to eat independently
     vi. Obesity
    i. Usual behavior
       i. Patient's interaction with people and environment
      ii. Orientation to time and place

      iii. Emotional stability

      iv. State of consciousness

      v. Language ability

5. Physical assessment

  a. Vital signs and oxygen saturation (vital signs usually within expected range for size and age)

    i. Past history of vital sign instability

    ii. Past tendency for pronounced temperature deviations

  b. Heart and lung assessment

  c. Peripheral pulse assessment if indicated

  d. Other assessment based on history and proposed procedure

  e. Variations in general appearance

    i. Color may provide clues to other illnesses

      (a) Pallor may indicate anemia

      (b) Uneven coloring and/or mottling may indicate poor neural functioning of the autonomic system

      (c) Excessive pigmentation (freckles) could indicate pathology

      (d) Multiple café au lait spots indicate neurofibromatosis (von Reckinghausen's disease)

      (e) Port-wine stain on the face along the trigeminal nerve may indicate Sturge-Weber syndrome

  f. Differences in skin temperature

  g. Skin turgor

  h. Defects of the craniofacial area

  i. Joint deformities

    i. Pain on movement

    ii. Muscle strength

    iii. Involuntary movements

    iv. Altered stance, gait, or posture

  j. Deficits in hearing or vision

6. Psychosocial assessment

  a. Anxiety

    i. Explain what will happen in simple terms, what to expect preoperative and immediate postoperative, preoperative medications to decrease anxiety, intravenous (may benefit from the use of EMLA cream applied at least one hour prior to intravenous insertion), family waiting area, discharge criteria, postoperative pain control

    ii. Determine the patient's regular schedule and incorporate that schedule into the hospital routine whenever possible

    iii. Encourage the patient to bring some familiar comfort item(s) from home

    iv. Demonstrate preoperative preparation or postoperative exercises and/or treatments; have the patient/caregiver do a return demonstration

    v. Determine the patient's/caregiver's expectations resulting from the procedure

    vi. Be alert to nonverbal communication

  b. Support system

    i. Arrangements made for safe transportation to and from the hospital

    ii. Ensure competent adult to assist with care after discharge

    iii. Include family/caregiver in the pre- and postoperative preparations

7. Preoperative instructions

  a. NPO requirements

  b. Medications to take or hold

  c. What to bring to the hospital

      d. Where to report the day of surgery

      e. Time of arrival

      f. Preoperative preparations or procedures

      g. Pain scale (modify to suit patient's learning ability)

      h. Responsible adult to assist with care after discharge

      i. Safe transportation home

      j. Other instructions as determined by individual facility

   8. Make referrals as necessary

   9. Document and communicate special needs to the perianesthesia staff

 10. Preoperative testing as ordered

D. Admission

   1. Review data collected during preadmission interview

   2. Verify compliance with preoperative instructions

      a. NPO status

      b. Medications taken/held

      c. Preoperative preps or procedures done

   3. Verify safe transportation home and competent adult help at home

   4. Physical assessment

      a. Vital signs, oxygen saturation, temperature

      b. Lab values within acceptable range

      c. Lung and heart assessments

      d. Peripheral pulse assessment if indicated

      e. Additional assessments as indicated by history and proposed procedure

   5. Provide emotional support to patient and/or caregiver

   6. Allow patient to use assistive devices as long as possible

   7. Use measures to decrease anxiety

      a. Maintain a calm, unhurried, and accepting attitude

      b. Provide comfort measures

      c. Allow family/caregiver to remain with the patient as long as possible

      d. Use the name with which the patient is familiar

      e. Administer medication for anxiety if necessary

   8. Administer preoperative medications as ordered

   9. Observe for desired and adverse reactions to medication

 10. Allow patient to bring comfort item to surgery if desired, and permitted

 11. Communicate the patient's special needs to the surgical and anesthesia team members

E. Intraoperative

   1. Whenever possible, meet the patient beforehand

      a. Patient will recognize and be comforted by a familiar face in an unfamiliar and frightening environment

   2. Review collected data

   3. Provide emotional support

   4. Use the name with which the patient is familiar

   5. Reassure the patient you are with him/her; touch patient if it will provide comfort

   6. Maintain normothermia

      a. Keep the room at a comfortable temperature

      b. Keep the patient covered as much as possible

      c. Provide warmed blankets or heating devices

      d. May need warmed gases and/or intravenous fluids

   7. Whenever possible, allow patient to keep his/her hearing aid, glasses, contact lenses, etc.

8. If a comfort item was brought, allow the patient to keep it
9. Protect bony prominences by positioning and use of padding
10. When moving the patient, lift rather than pull, if joint deformities are present
11. Communicate the patient's special needs to the PACU staff

F. Postoperative PACU Phase I
1. On arrival, the patient may be agitated, disoriented, or combative
2. Review collected data
3. Routine care per PACU protocol
4. Use the name with which the patient is familiar
5. Provide reassurance
6. Allow him/her to use assistive devices as soon as possible
7. If allowed, have a family member/caregiver with the patient
8. Allow use of comfort item if sent with patient
9. Monitor vital signs, oxygen saturation, temperature per protocols
10. Administer medication for pain or nausea if necessary
11. Observe for desired and adverse reactions to medications
12. Provide care based on pre-existing medical condition and procedure
13. Observe for reversal of, or adverse reaction to, anesthetic agents
14. Use restraints for safety and protection only as a last resort to prevent injury
15. Minimize risk of aspiration
    a. Observe for return of gag and swallowing reflexes
    b. Elevate the head of the bed if allowed
    c. Suction as necessary
    d. Position on side if not contraindicated
16. Maintain normothermia
    a. Keep room at comfortable temperature
    b. Keep the patient covered as much as possible
    c. Provide warmed blankets or heating devices
    d. May need warmed gases and/or intravenous fluids
17. Reorient patient to surroundings
18. Communicate patient's special needs to Phase II team

G. PACU Phase II
1. The patient may return to Phase II directly from the operating room and may be disoriented, combative, or agitated
2. Review collected data
3. Routine care per protocol
4. Allow family/caregiver to be with patient as soon as possible
5. Allow use of assistive devices as soon as possible
6. Reorient to surroundings
7. Monitor vital signs, oxygen saturation, temperature
8. Provide care based on pre-existing medical condition and procedure
9. Minimize risk of aspiration; nursing interventions as above
    a. Use caution when giving liquids or solids
10. Administer medications as ordered
11. Observe for desired or adverse reactions to medications
12. Maintain normothermia
13. Provide reassurance to patient as well as family/caregiver
14. Verify competent adult to care for patient at home
15. Verify safe transportation home
16. Include family/caregiver when reviewing instructions; if a procedure is to be done at home, have the patient/caregiver do a return demonstration
17. Provide written instructions, using large type if necessary; may be necessary to use a tape recorder if reading skills are inadequate

18. Obtain a phone number to reach the patient/caregiver for postoperative follow-up phone call

H. Post discharge
1. Contact patient/caregiver within 24 hours of discharge
2. Identify yourself and state purpose of the call
3. Obtain information (to include, but not limited to):
    a. Compliance with postoperative instructions
    b. Unrelieved pain/nausea
    c. Unexpected or excessive bleeding or swelling
    d. Elevated temperature
    e. Redness or drainage from the operative site
    f. Other adverse occurrences

PHYSICAL DISABILITIES

Physical disabilities may be manifest in many different ways. Persons with similar deficits will cope in different ways. It is important to treat each person as an individual, determining his/her method of coping and functional ability, and develop the plan of care based on the patient's needs.

The information presented will assist the nurse in caring for the patient with a specific disability. The reader is referred to Chapters 8 and 9 for complete assessment information.

II. **Visual Impairment**
    A. General information
        1. May have limited vision, light perception, or total blindness
        2. If hemiplegic, may have loss of half of visual field in each eye
        3. May have other disabilities
        4. Unless hard of hearing, do not raise voice
    B. Preoperative preadmission interview
        1. Identify yourself and state purpose of visit
        2. Provide a safe environment
            a. If moving to another area, offer arm to patient
            b. Identify barriers
            c. Inform patient of what will happen
            d. Assure patient his/her needs will be communicated to perianesthesia team members
        3. Identify level and duration of disability
            a. Totally blind
            b. Partial vision
            c. Light perceptive
        4. Determine patient's and family's knowledge of proposed procedure
        5. Develop plan of care based on patient's needs and knowledge
        6. Assess:
            a. Abilities, special needs, method of communication
            b. Use of glasses, contacts, Braille, other assistive devices
            c. Other disabilities
        7. Complete health history
            a. Per protocols
        8. Physical assessment
            a. Based on patient's history and proposed procedure
            b. Additional assessment per protocol

9. Psychosocial assessment
   a. Family status
      i. Has competent adult who can assist after discharge
      ii. If primary caregiver for another person, have arrangements been made for someone to provide care for that person?
      iii. Safe transportation to and from the hospital
   b. Anxiety
      i. Explain what will happen preoperative and immediately postoperative, administration of preoperative medications, intravenous, family waiting area, discharge criteria, postoperative pain control
10. Preoperative teaching
    a. Per protocols
11. Special diet
12. Preoperative tests as ordered
13. Referrals as necessary
14. Document and communicate patient's special needs to perioperative team members
15. May be necessary to provide tape recording of preoperative instructions

C. Admission
1. Review data collected during preadmission interview
2. Utilize communication technique patient is comfortable with; provide interpreter if necessary
   a. Verbal only
   b. Braille
   c. Gestures
   d. Combination of methods
3. Lab values within accepted range
4. Get patient's attention before speaking
5. Promote sense of independence
6. Provide description of new surroundings
7. Allow time and opportunity for patient to explore new environment
8. Include patient in discussions about his/her procedure
9. Maintain normal voice volume
10. Verify compliance with preoperative instructions
11. Verify safe transportation home and competent adult caregiver available
12. Physical assessment
    a. Per protocol
    b. Additional assessment as indicated based on procedure and patient's health status
13. Provide emotional support to patient and family
    a. Maintain calm and unhurried attitude
    b. Allow family to remain with patient as long as possible
    c. Allow use of assistive devices as long as possible
    d. Inform patient that communication device will be returned as soon as possible
    e. Administer medication for anxiety if necessary
14. Administer other preoperative medications as ordered
15. Observe for desired and adverse medication reactions
16. Communicate patient's special needs to surgery and anesthesia team members

D. Intraoperative
1. Whenever possible, meet patient before taking him/her to the OR
   a. Patient will recognize and be comforted by a familiar voice in an unfamiliar and frightening environment

2. Review collected data
3. Let the patient know what will be done before touching him/her
4. Avoid confusion and too many people speaking at once
5. If patient is elderly, lift rather than pull, to move patient to decrease chance of injury
6. Communicate patient's special needs to PACU team members

E. Postoperative PACU Phase I
1. Review collected data
2. Speak softly to patient
3. Touch patient gently to get his/her attention
4. Provide interpreter if necessary
5. Resume use of assistive devices if possible
6. Reorient patient to surroundings
7. Maintain calm, quiet environment to decrease confusion
8. Routine PACU care per protocols
9. Reunite patient and family as soon as possible
10. Communicate patient's special needs to Phase II team

F. PACU Phase II
1. The patient may return to Phase II directly from the OR
2. Review collected data
3. Speak softly and gently touch patient to get his/her attention
4. Resume use of assistive devices as soon as possible
5. Maintain safe environment
6. Reorient patient to surroundings
7. Routine PACU care per protocol
8. Verify safe transportation home
9. Verify competent adult help at home
10. Provide clear discharge instructions; provide written copy of instructions for caregiver; may need to provide tape recording of instructions
11. Obtain phone number to reach patient for postoperative follow-up phone call
12. Instruct caregiver on assessment necessary of the operative site

G. Post discharge
1. Make follow-up call within 24 hours of discharge
2. Identify yourself and state purpose of call
3. Obtain information (to include, but not limited to):
   a. Compliance with postoperative instructions
   b. Unrelieved pain or nausea
   c. Unexpected or excessive bleeding or swelling
   d. Temperature elevation
   e. Redness or purulent drainage from operative site
   f. Other adverse occurrences

III. Hearing Loss

A. Hearing loss may range from slight to complete
B. Preoperative
1. Determine degree and duration of disability
2. Determine the patient's method of communication
   a. Hearing aid
   b. Lip reading
   c. Sign language
   d. Written messages
   e. Alphabet, picture, word or phrase board
   f. Combination of methods

     3. Provide interpreter if necessary

     4. Provide a quiet, distraction-free environment

     5. Get patient's attention before speaking

     6. Speak slowly and distinctly

     7. Sit or stand directly in front of the patient

     8. Keep mouth visible when speaking

     9. Provide adequate lighting

    10. Maintain comfortable voice volume

    11. Include family member in preoperative visit if possible; include patient when discussing his/her procedure

    12. Repeat or reinforce information if necessary

  C. Preadmission interview

     1. An in-person interview facilitates the patient's participation, especially if he/she relies on lip reading or gestures

     2. Provide adequate time for interview and assessment

     3. Utilize patient's method of communication or provide an interpreter if necessary

     4. Determine the patient's and family's knowledge of the proposed procedure

     5. Develop a teaching plan based on patient's and family's knowledge and needs

     6. Assess

       a. Abilities and special needs

       b. Willingness of family to participate in preparation and postoperative care

       c. Use of hearing aid or other assistive devices

     7. Complete health history

       a. Per protocol

     8. Physical assessment

       a. Per protocol

       b. Additional assessment based on history and proposed procedure

     9. Psychosocial assessment

       a. Anxiety

         i. Provide explanation of what will happen prior to surgery and immediately postoperative, administration of preoperative medications, intravenous, family waiting, discharge criteria, postoperative pain management

         ii. Explain that family can be with patient as long as possible before surgery and as soon as possible after surgery

        iii. Hearing aid and/or assistive devices will be used as long as safely possible before surgery, and returned as soon as possible after surgery

        iv. Determine patient's and family's expectations resulting from surgery

         v. Be alert to nonverbal communication

        vi. If patient is primary caregiver of another person, have arrangements for help been made while patient recovers?

       b. Support system

         i. Arrangements made for safe transportation to and from hospital

         ii. Arrangements made for competent adult help after discharge

    10. Preoperative teaching

       a. Per protocol

    11. Referrals made as necessary

    12. Preoperative tests as ordered

    13. Document and communicate special needs to other members of perioperative team

  D. Admission

     1. Review data collected in preadmission

2. Lab values within accepted range
3. Utilize communication technique for hearing impairment
   a. Know patient's method of communication
      i. Hearing aid
      ii. Lip reading
      iii. Sign language
      iv. Written messages
      v. Alphabet, picture, word or phrase board
      vi. Other method
   b. Provide interpreter if necessary
   c. Get patient's attention before speaking
   d. Speak slowly and distinctly
   e. Remain in patient's line of sight
   f. Have your mouth visible when speaking to patient
   g. Direct conversation to patient, even if interpreter present
   h. Speak in comfortable voice volume
   i. Repeat or rephrase information if necessary
   j. Include family whenever possible
4. Verify compliance with preoperative instructions
5. Verify safe transportation home and competent adult help at home
6. Physical assessment
   a. Per protocol
7. Provide emotional support for patient and family
   a. Maintain calm and unhurried attitude
   b. Allow family to remain with patient as long as possible
   c. Inform patient that hearing aid or communication device will be returned as soon as possible after surgery
8. Administer preoperative medication as ordered
9. Observe for desired and adverse medication reactions
10. Communicate patient's special needs to surgical and anesthesia team members

E. Intraoperative
   1. Whenever possible, meet the patient before taking him/her to surgery
      a. Patient will recognize and be comforted by a familiar face in an unfamiliar and frightening environment
   2. Review collected data
   3. Get the patient's attention before speaking to him/her
   4. Look directly at patient
   5. If possible, avoid covering face with mask when speaking to patient
   6. Allow use of hearing aid, communication, or other assistive devices if possible; use gestures or written messages if necessary
   7. Speak slowly and distinctly
   8. Communicate patient's special needs to PACU team members

F. Postoperative PACU Phase I
   1. Review collected data
   2. Approach patient in his/her line of sight
   3. Gently touch patient to get his/her attention
   4. If protective lubricant used, clear from patient's eyes
   5. Return hearing aid or other assistive devices as soon as possible
   6. Speak slowly and distinctly
   7. Remain in patient's line of vision when speaking
   8. Keep your mouth visible when speaking
   9. Postoperative assessment per protocol

10. Reorient patient to surroundings
11. Reunite patient with family as soon as possible
12. Communicate patient's special needs to Phase II team

G. PACU Phase II
   1. The patient may return to Phase II directly from surgery
   2. Review collected data
   3. Return hearing aid and assistive devices as soon as possible
   4. Reunite patient with family as soon as possible
   5. Approach patient in his/her line of sight
   6. Gently touch patient to get his/her attention
   7. Remain in patient's line of sight when speaking to him/her
   8. Reorient patient to surroundings
   9. Routine PACU assessments per protocol
   10. Verify competent adult to care for patient at home
   11. Verify safe transportation home
   12. Include family when reviewing postoperative instructions; if a procedure is to be done at home, have patient or family do a return demonstration
   13. Provide clear written instructions
   14. Obtain phone number to reach patient for postoperative follow-up phone call

H. Post discharge
   1. Make follow-up phone call within 24 hours of discharge
   2. Identify yourself and state purpose of call
   3. Complete post-discharge assessment per protocol

IV. **Aphasia**
   A. General information
      1. Aphasia affects a person's ability to communicate in one or more different ways
      2. Speak to the patient naturally, using short and simple sentences
      3. Encourage, but do not pressure, the patient to respond in whatever way he/she can
      4. Allow for differences in accuracy and articulation when soliciting patient's response
      5. Maintain a normal voice volume
      6. The patient can probably understand all or part of what is said
      7. Include patient in discussions about procedure
      8. Present a relaxed attitude by mannerisms, patience, and acceptance
      9. One person speaking at a time helps to decrease confusion
      10. Ask direct questions requiring one-word answers
      11. Encourage patient to write responses, if he/she can write and spell
      12. Encourage the use of gestures if that is the patient's most effective means to communicate

   B. Preoperative preadmission interview
      1. An in-person interview will be more effective than a telephone interview and will allow the patient a greater opportunity to participate
      2. Allow adequate time for the interview and assessment
      3. Determine the patient's ability to communicate
      4. Determine the patient's/family's knowledge of the proposed procedure
      5. Develop a teaching plan based on the patient's/family's knowledge and needs
      6. Assess:
         a. Use of assistive devices, i.e., glasses, hearing aid, story board, writing tablet/slate
         b. Effective means of communication

  7. Complete health history
    a. Per protocol
    b. Etiology and duration of disability
  8. Physical assessment
    a. Per protocol
    b. Additional assessment based on health status and proposed procedure
  9. Psychosocial assessment
    a. Anxiety
    b. Support system
      i. Who will provide transportation to and from the hospital
      ii. Who will assist the patient after discharge; is this person competent to perform/assist with postoperative care
      iii. If the patient is the primary caregiver for another person, have arrangements for help been made while patient recovers?
  10. Preoperative teaching
    a. Per protocol
  11. Preoperative tests as ordered
  12. Referrals as necessary
  13. Document and communicate patient's special needs to perioperative team members
C. Admission
  1. Review data collected in preadmission
  2. Verify safe transportation to home and competent adult help at home
  3. Confirm that preoperative instructions/preparations were followed
  4. Physical assessment
    a. Per protocol
    b. Additional assessment based on patient's condition and proposed procedure
  5. Provide emotional support
  6. Allow use of assistive devices as long as possible
  7. Administer preoperative medications as ordered
  8. Follow up on referrals if any were needed
  9. Communicate special needs to the surgery and anesthesia team members
D. Intraoperative
  1. If possible, meet the patient beforehand
  2. Review collected data
  3. Provide emotional support
    a. Reassure the patient that you are with him/her
  4. Allow the patient to continue to use assistive devices as long as possible
  5. Communicate the patient's special needs to the PACU team
E. Postoperative PACU Phase I
  1. Review collected data
  2. Routine PACU care per protocol
  3. May be at higher risk for aspiration
    a. Observe for return of swallowing and gag reflexes
    b. Position on side, if allowed, until return of gag and swallowing reflexes
    c. Elevate head of bed after return of reflexes if not contraindicated
    d. Suction as needed
  4. Reduce apprehension
    a. Reorient to surroundings
    b. Provide means of communicating
    c. Return assistive devices as soon as possible
    d. Reunite patient and family as soon as possible

     5. Provide care related to procedure performed and based on pre-existing medical conditions

     6. Communicate patient's special needs to Phase II team

  F. PACU Phase II

     1. The patient may return to Phase II directly from the OR and may be disoriented

     2. Review collected data

     3. Allow family to be with patient as soon as possible

     4. Return assistive devices as soon as possible

     5. Reorient to surroundings

     6. Provide procedure-specific care and care related to pre-existing medical conditions

     7. Provide emotional support to patient and family

     8. Verify safe transportation and competent adult help at home

     9. Include family when reviewing postoperative discharge instructions; if a procedure is to be done at home, have the patient and/or family member do a return demonstration

    10. Provide written instructions, using large type printing if necessary; use of a tape recorder may help provide reinforcement of instructions

    11. Obtain a phone number to reach patient for postoperative follow-up phone call

  G. Post discharge

     1. Contact the patient/family member within 24 hours of discharge

     2. Identify yourself and state purpose of call

     3. Complete post-discharge assessment per protocol

V. Spinal Cord Injury

  A. General information

     1. Classification:

       a. Complete—Total paralysis and loss of sensation below the zone of injury, resulting in quadriplegia or paraplegia

       b. Incomplete—With partial preservation of function below the zone of injury

     2. Injury to:

       a. C1-C4—results in quadriplegia with complete loss of motor and sensory function from the neck down, and loss of respiratory function

       b. C5—results in quadriplegia and loss of all functions below the upper shoulder level; the phrenic nerve is intact but not the intercostal muscles

       c. C6—results in quadriplegia and loss of all functions below the shoulders and upper arms; will lack elbow, forearm, and hand control; phrenic nerve is intact but not the intercostal muscles

       d. C7—results in incomplete quadriplegia with loss of motor control to parts of the arm and hand, and loss of sensation below the clavicle and parts of the arms and hands; the phrenic nerve is intact but not the intercostal muscles

       e. C8—results in incomplete quadriplegia with loss of motor control to parts of the arms and hands, and loss of sensation below the chest and part of the hands; the phrenic nerve is intact but not the intercostal muscles

       f. T1 to T6—results in paraplegia with loss of motor function below the midchest, including the trunk muscles, and loss of sensation from the midchest downward, including the lower limbs; the phrenic nerve functions independently; there is some impairment of the intercostal muscles

       g. T6 to T12—results in paraplegia with loss of motor control and sensation below the waist; there is no interference with respiratory function

       h. L1 to L3—results in paraplegia with loss of most of the control of the legs and pelvic area, and loss of sensation to the lower abdomen and legs; there is no interference with respiratory function

      i. L3 to L4—results in incomplete paraplegia with loss of control and function of part of the lower legs, ankles, and feet; there is no interference with respiratory function

      j. L4 to S2—results in incomplete paraplegia with varying degrees of motor and sensory loss; can walk with braces or may use a wheelchair, and can be relatively independent

  3. May be at risk for:

    a. Cardiac arrhythmias and cardiac arrest

    b. Orthostatic hypotension (especially with an injury above level of T7)

    c. Autonomic hyperreflexia (possible only in an injury above the level of T6)

    d. Pain

    e. Skin breakdown

    f. Spasticity

B. Preoperative preadmission interview

  1. Identify the level and duration of the disability

  2. Determine patient's and family's coping strategies

  3. Develop a plan of care based on the knowledge and needs of the patient and family

  4. Assess:

    a. Abilities, special needs

    b. Use of assistive devices

    c. Willingness and ability of family to participate in preoperative preparation and postoperative care

  5. Medical history

    a. Previous history of:

      i. Cardiac arrhythmias and cardiac arrest

        (a) Electrolyte imbalance

        (b) Response to vagal stimulation

      ii. Orthostatic hypotension

        (a) History of hypotension when the head of the bed is raised or when the patient is gotten out of bed

      iii. Autonomic hyperreflexia

        (a) Previous response to noxious stimulation of the sensory receptors (examples of noxious stimuli may include: urinary calculi, severe bladder infections, acute abdomen, operative incisions)

      iv. Pain may be mild tingling to severe, intractable

      v. Spasticity

  6. Complete health history

    a. Etiology and duration of disability

    b. Previous surgical history

    c. Anesthetic complications for patient or family

    d. Past illnesses

    e. Pressure sores

    f. Current illnesses

    g. Bladder program

    h. Medications (prescription, over the counter, herbal preparations)

    i. Allergies

      i. Screen for latex sensitivity if on bladder program, or has indwelling catheter

  7. Physical assessment

    a. Per protocol

    b. Other assessment as indicated based on patient's medical history and proposed procedure

       8. Psychosocial assessment
         a. Support system
         b. Anxiety
           i. Be alert to nonverbal communication
       9. Special diet
     10. Preoperative instructions
         a. Per protocol
     11. Preoperative test as ordered
     12. Referrals as necessary
     13. Document and communicate the patient's special needs to the perioperative team members

C. Admission
   1. Review data collected in preadmission
   2. Use latex precautions if the patient is on a bladder program, or has indwelling catheter
   3. Verify compliance with preoperative instructions
   4. Safe transportation home and competent adult caregiver available after discharge
   5. Physical assessment
      a. Per protocol
      b. Lab values within acceptable range
        i. Electrolytes, especially potassium, and blood coagulation studies
      c. Other assessment as indicated by patient's health status and proposed procedure
   6. Provide emotional support to the patient and the family
      a. Allow family to remain with the patient as long as possible
      b. Allow use of assistive devices as long as possible
      c. Medicate for anxiety as ordered, if necessary
   7. Administer medications as ordered
   8. Observe for desired and adverse medication reactions
   9. Communicate patient's special needs to the OR and anesthesia care team members

D. Intraoperative
   1. Review data collected
   2. Use latex precautions if necessary
   3. Maintain normothermia
   4. Be aware of potential for:
      a. Cardiac arrhythmias
        i. Electrolytes, especially potassium, and blood coagulation studies, within acceptable range
        ii. Avoid excessive vagal stimulation
      b. Autonomic hyperreflexia (may be triggered by noxious stimuli such as a distended bladder or pain) characterized by:
        i. Hypertension
        ii. Superficial vasodilatation
        iii. Flushing
        iv. Profuse sweating
        v. Piloerection (gooseflesh) occurring above the level of injury; often seen in patients with upper thoracic and cervical injuries
      c. Pain, paresthesia, and hyperesthesia
      d. Spasticity (a state of increased tonus in a weak muscle) usually peaks 1½ to 2 years after the injury, with gradual regression

       i. May result from a slight touch on the skin

      ii. Aggravated by cold or staying in one position for a prolonged period of time

  5. Move patient with care, lifting rather than pulling

  6. Avoid pressure on bony prominences by positioning or use of padding

  7. Communicate patient's special needs to the PACU team

E. Postoperative PACU Phase I

  1. Review collected data

  2. Continue use of latex precautions if necessary

  3. Routine PACU care per protocol

  4. Keep patient warm

  5. Be aware that even slight touch could trigger spasticity

  6. Monitor for signs of autonomic hyperreflexia (may be triggered by noxious stimuli such as a distended bladder or pain)

    a. Paroxysmal hypertension

    b. Pounding headache

    c. Vasodilatation

    d. Flushing

    e. Profuse sweating

    f. Piloerection (gooseflesh)

  7. Potential for orthostatic hypotension exists if the patient has been bedridden

    a. Be cautious when elevating the head of the bed if the patient is a quadriplegic

    b. Most often seen with patients sustaining injury above the T7 level

  8. Monitor for reversal of, or adverse reaction to, the anesthetic agents

  9. Provide care based on the patient's medical condition and the procedure performed

  10. Administer medication for pain or nausea as ordered

  11. Observe for desired or adverse reactions to the medications

  12. Communicate the patient's special needs to the Phase II team members

F. PACU Phase II

  1. The patient may return to Phase II directly from the OR

  2. Review collected data

  3. Routine PACU Phase II protocol

  4. Keep patient warm without overheating

  5. Be aware that light touch on the skin may trigger spasticity

  6. Monitor for autonomic hyperreflexia

  7. Monitor for orthostatic hypotension if patient has been bedridden

    a. Be cautious when elevating the head of the bed of the patient who is a quadriplegic

    b. Most often seen with patients sustaining injury above the T7 level

  8. Provide care based on the patient's medical condition and the procedure performed

  9. Verify safe transportation home

  10. Verify competent adult caregiver at home

  11. Provide verbal and written discharge instructions

  12. Obtain a phone number to reach the patient for the follow-up phone call

G. Post discharge

  1. Contact the patient within 24 hours after discharge

  2. Identify yourself and state the nature of the call

  3. Complete post-discharge assessment per protocol

VI. Multiple Sclerosis (MS)

A. General information

1. Also known as disseminated sclerosis

2. Is a chronic, progressive, degenerative disease that affects the myelin sheath and conductive pathways of the central nervous system (CNS)

3. Predominately affects the central nervous system

4. Four categories

   a. Relapsing-remitting disease—attack comes on over a 1- to 2-week period and resolves over a 4- to 8-week period, after which the patient returns to a pre-attack baseline

   b. Relapsing-remitting progressive disease—does not return to baseline; accumulates stepwise in disability

   c. Chronic progressive disease—progressively worsening with no periods of stability; may also have superimposed acute attacks

   d. Stable MS—no clinical disease activity and no subjective worsening of condition over a previous 12-month period

5. Symptoms associated with MS

   a. Sensory—numbness, anesthesia, paresthesia, pain, decreased proprioception and sense of temperature, depth, and vibration

   b. Motor—paresis, paralysis, dragging of foot, spasticity, diplopia, bowel and bladder dysfunction (incontinence or retention)

   c. Cerebellar—ataxia, staggering, loss of balance and coordination, nystagmus, speech disturbances, tremors, vertigo

   d. Other symptoms—optic neuritis, impotence or decreased genital sensation, depression or euphoria, fatigue or decreased energy level

6. Symptoms of one episode may differ from other episodes

7. Factors that may trigger MS, or cause a relapse, include:

   a. Infections

   b. Trauma—accidental or planned (i.e., surgery)

   c. Pregnancy

8. Factors that may cause relapse in a previously diagnosed patient include:

   a. Undue fatigue or excessive exertion

   b. Overheating or excessive chilling or cold

   c. Emotional stress

   d. Fever

B. Preoperative preadmission assessment

1. An in-person interview may be more beneficial than a telephone interview

2. Patient may use some nonverbal forms of communication

3. Allow adequate time for interview and assessment

   a. Fatigue may be a factor

   b. Patient may need extra time to formulate questions and responses

4. Determine level and duration of disease

5. Provide comfortable environment

6. Determine patient's and family's understanding of disease process

7. Determine patient's response to physical and psychological stresses

8. Identify previous events triggering relapses

9. Determine patient's and family's knowledge of proposed procedure

10. Develop plan of care based on patient's and family's knowledge and needs

11. Assess

    a. Abilities, special needs

    b. Patient's successful management techniques

    c. Use of assistive devices

      d. Willingness and capability of family to participate in preoperative preparations and postoperative care
12. Complete health history
    a. Per routine protocol
    b. Include medications, previous response to medication, and current medication use (prescription, over the counter, herbal preparations)
    c. Allergies, including latex-sensitivity screening
    d. Special diet
13. Physical assessment
    a. Routine assessment per protocol
    b. Additional assessment based on patient's history and proposed procedure
14. Psychosocial assessment
    a. Anxiety
       i. Be alert to nonverbal communication
    b. Support system
15. Make referrals as necessary
16. Provide verbal and written instructions
17. Preoperative tests as ordered
18. Document and communicate special needs to the perianesthetic team
C. Admission
  1. Review information obtained in preadmission
  2. Provide comfortable physical environment
  3. Use measures to reduce stress
    a. Explain what will be happening
    b. Allow patient to verbalize concerns
    c. Allow family to be with patient as long as possible
    d. Allow use of assistive devices as long as possible
    e. Allow extra time for patient to answer, or formulate, questions
  4. Verify compliance with preoperative instructions
  5. Avoid undue fatigue; provide periods of rest
  6. Verify safe transportation home
  7. Verify competent adult help at home after discharge
  8. Physical assessment
    a. Per routine protocol
    b. Sensory deficit
    c. Motor deficit
    d. Cerebellar disturbances
    e. Peripheral pulse assessment if indicated
    f. Other assessment based on medical history and proposed procedure
  9. Provide emotional support for patient and family
10. Use measures to decrease anxiety
    a. Maintain a calm and accepting attitude
    b. Allow family to remain with patient as long as possible
    c. Allow use of assistive devices as long as possible
    d. Administer medication if necessary, as ordered
11. Administer preoperative medications as ordered
12. Observe for desired or adverse medication reactions
13. Provide safe environment
    a. Assist patient in getting out of bed
    b. Keep side rails up and bed in low position
14. Communicate patient's special needs to OR and anesthesia team

D. Intraoperative
1. When possible, meet patient before he/she is taken to the OR
2. Review collected data
3. Maintain latex precautions if necessary
4. Provide comfortable physical environment
   a. Protect patient from getting cold or overheated
5. Allow use of assistive devices as long as possible
6. Use measures to decrease anxiety
   a. Provide explanation of what will happen
   b. Allow patient to verbalize concerns; try to alleviate concerns
   c. Provide safe environment to reduce chance of injury
      i. Protect bony prominences with positioning or use padding
      ii. Use care when moving patient, lifting instead of pulling
7. Patient may be at increased risk for aspiration (if local anesthetic)
   a. Elevate head of bed if possible
   b. Suction as needed
   c. When possible, position on side
8. Communicate patient's special needs to PACU team
E. Postoperative PACU Phase I
1. Review collected data
2. Maintain latex precautions if needed
3. Routine PACU Phase I care
4. Provide care based on patient's medical history and procedure performed
5. May be at higher risk for aspiration
   a. Elevate head of bed if not contraindicated
   b. Suction as needed
   c. Observe for return of swallowing and gag reflexes
   d. Position on side if not contraindicated
6. Provide comfortable physical environment
   a. Do not allow patient to become chilled or overheated
7. Reduce stress
   a. Reorient patient to surroundings
   b. Medicate for pain or anxiety as necessary, as ordered
8. Prevent injury
   a. Reorient to surroundings
   b. Pad bed rails if necessary
   c. Use restraints for safety and protection, only as a last resort
   d. Medicate if necessary, as ordered
9. Observe for desired or adverse medication reactions
10. Communicate patient's special needs to Phase II team
F. PACU Phase II
1. Patient may return to Phase II directly from the OR
2. Review collected data
3. Maintain latex precautions if necessary
4. Patient may be at increased risk for aspiration
   a. Nursing interventions as above
5. Routine PACU Phase II care
6. Provide comfortable physical environment
7. Reduce stress
   a. Reorient patient to surroundings
   b. Reunite patient and family as soon as possible
   c. Allow use of assistive devices as soon as possible
   d. Medicate if necessary, as ordered

8. Prevent injury
   a. Nursing interventions as above
9. Avoid fatigue; provide periods of rest
10. Verify safe transportation home
11. Verify competent adult to help at home after discharge
12. Provide verbal and written discharge instructions; may need to provide an audio tape if patient has visual deficits
13. Demonstrate postoperative procedures to be done at home; have patient and/or family do return demonstration
14. Obtain phone number to contact patient for post-discharge follow-up call

G. Post discharge
1. Make follow-up phone call within 24 hours of discharge
2. Identify yourself and state purpose of call
3. Complete post-discharge assessment per protocol

VII. Traumatic Brain Injury
A. General information
1. May have:
   a. Motor impairment
      i. Spasticity
      ii. Weakness
      iii. Apraxia—the inability to perform a skilled motor act in the absence of paralysis
      iv. Paralysis
   b. Sensory impairment
      i. Impaired sense of position
      ii. Impaired spatial judgment
   c. Communication impairment
      i. Aphasia—inability to communicate
      ii. Dysarthia—defective articulation caused by motor deficits of the tongue or muscles used for speech
   d. Cognitive impairment
      i. Impaired abstract thinking
      ii. Impaired judgment
      iii. Impaired generalization and planning abilities
      iv. Impaired memory
      v. Decreased concentration ability

B. Preoperative preadmission assessment
1. An in-person interview may be more beneficial than a telephone interview; the patient may use some nonverbal forms of communication
2. Include family whenever possible
3. Allow adequate time for interview and assessment
4. Remember to include patient in the conversation when discussing procedure
5. Determine the level and duration of the disability
6. Determine the patient's and family's understanding of the proposed procedure
7. Develop a plan of care based on the knowledge and needs of the patient and family
8. Assess:
   a. Abilities, special needs
   b. Patient's and family's successful management techniques
   c. Use of assistive devices
   d. Willingness and ability of family to participate in preoperative preparation and postoperative care

9. Complete health history
   a. Etiology and duration of disability
   b. Past surgical history
   c. Anesthetic complications for patient or family
   d. Seizure activity
   e. Past illnesses
   f. Current illnesses
   g. Medications (prescription, over the counter, herbal preparations)
   h. Allergies, including latex
   i. Special diet
10. Physical assessment
    a. Per protocol
    b. Swallowing difficulty
    c. Other assessment as indicated by medical history and proposed procedure
11. Psychosocial assessment
    a. Anxiety
       i. Be alert to nonverbal communication
    b. Support system
    c. Make referrals as necessary
    d. Provide verbal and written preoperative instructions
12. Document and communicate special needs to the perioperative team members

C. Admission
1. Review data collected in preadmission
2. Verify compliance with preoperative instructions
3. Verify safe transportation home
4. Verify competent adult help at home after discharge
5. Physical assessment
   a. Per protocol
   b. Additional assessment as indicated by medical history and proposed procedure
6. Provide emotional support to patient and family
7. Allow use of assistive devices as long as possible
8. Use measures to decrease anxiety
9. Administer other medications as ordered
10. Observe for desired and adverse medication reactions
11. Communicate patient's special needs to the OR and anesthesia team members

D. Intraoperative
1. Review collected data
2. Whenever possible, meet the patient before transport to OR
3. Allow use of assistive devices as long as possible
4. Maintain normothermia
5. Protect bony prominences by positioning and use of padding
6. When moving patient, lift rather than pull
7. Communicate patient's special needs to PACU team members

E. Postoperative PACU Phase I
1. Review collected data
2. Routine PACU care per protocol
3. If swallowing difficulty exists, minimize risk for aspiration
   a. Observe for return of swallowing and gag reflexes
   b. Suction as needed
   c. Elevate the head of the bed if allowed
   d. Position on side if not contraindicated

4. Provide care based on medical history and procedure performed
5. Allow use of assistive devices as soon as possible
6. Reorient to surroundings
7. Communicate patient's special needs to Phase II team
F. PACU Phase II
   1. The patient may return to Phase II straight from the OR
   2. Review collected data
   3. Routine PACU care per protocol
   4. Verify safe transportation home
   5. Verify competent adult help at home after discharge
   6. Include family when reviewing discharge instructions; if a procedure will be done at home, have patient and/or family do a return demonstration
   7. Obtain a phone number to contact patient for postoperative follow-up
G. Post discharge
   1. Contact the patient within 24 hours after discharge
   2. Identify yourself and state the nature of the call
   3. Complete post-discharge assessment per protocol

VIII. Myasthenia Gravis
A. General information
   1. Myasthenia gravis is a chronic, progressive disease causing muscle weakness
   2. May have:
      a. Increased weakness of certain voluntary muscles
      b. Potential improvement of muscle strength with rest
      c. Dramatic improvement in muscle strength with use of anticholinesterase drugs
      d. Spasticity
      e. Difficulty swallowing
      f. Easily fatigued
      g. Difficulty with speech
      h. Respiratory insufficiency
      i. Bowel and bladder dysfunction
      j. Depression
      k. Eye muscle problems
      l. May develop myasthenia crisis, caused by under-medication or no cholinergic medications
         i. Acute respiratory difficulty
         ii. Acute motor weakness of voluntary muscles including those for swallowing, speaking, and moving parts of the body
      m. Exacerbation of symptoms can be caused by temperature extremes and emotional stress
B. Preoperative assessment interview
   1. Allow adequate time for interview and assessment
   2. Allow for periods of rest
   3. Include family in preoperative preparations whenever possible
   4. Determine patient's level of disability
   5. Determine patient's and family's understanding of myasthenia gravis
   6. Develop a plan of care based on patient's and family's knowledge and needs
   7. Assess:
      a. Patient's abilities and special needs
      b. Patient's successful management techniques
      c. Use of assistive devices
      d. Willingness and capability of family to participate in preoperative preparation and postoperative care

    8. Complete health history
      a. Length of time disease present
      b. Past surgical history
      c. Anesthetic complications for patient or family
      d. Past illnesses
      e. Current illnesses
      f. Medications (prescription, over the counter, herbal preparations)
      g. Allergies
      h. Special diet
    9. Physical assessment
      a. Per protocol
      b. Heart assessment
      c. Respiratory function assessment
      d. Muscle strength
      e. Peripheral pulse assessment if indicated
   10. Psychosocial assessment
      a. Anxiety
        i. Be alert to nonverbal communications
        ii. Determine patient's coping mechanisms
      b. Support system
   11. Referrals as necessary
   12. Provide verbal and written preoperative instructions
   13. Preoperative tests as ordered
   14. Document and communicate patient's special needs to the perianesthesia team
C. Admission
    1. Review data collected during preadmission interview
    2. Verify compliance with preoperative instructions
    3. Verify safe transportation home
    4. Verify competent adult help at home after discharge
    5. Physical assessment
      a. Per protocol
      b. Respiratory function assessment
        i. Auscultation
        ii. Observation
      c. Muscle strength
      d. Peripheral pulse assessment if indicated
      e. Additional assessment based on patient's history and proposed procedure
    6. Provide emotional support to patient and family
    7. Use measures to decrease anxiety
    8. Administer other medications as ordered
    9. Observe for unpredictable responses to any medications used
      a. Excessive sedation
      b. Decreased respirations
      c. Agitation
   10. Observe for desired medication reactions
   11. Communicate patient's needs to OR and anesthesia team members
D. Intraoperative
    1. If possible, meet patient before he/she goes to the OR
    2. Review collected data
    3. Potential for myasthenia crisis, manifested as
      a. Increased muscle weakness
      b. Respiratory distress
      c. Difficulty talking or swallowing

4. Potential for aspiration (if local anesthetic)
    a. Elevate head of bed if possible
    b. Suction as necessary
    c. Monitor for swallowing difficulty
5. At increased risk for infection
    a. Maintain aseptic technique
    b. Use care to avoid skin tears
        i. Protect bony prominences by positioning and padding
        ii. Use care when removing adhesive pads
        iii. Lift, rather than pull, when moving patient
6. Maintain normothermia
7. Use measures to reduce stress
    a. Explain what will happen
    b. Maintain calm attitude
    c. Allow patient to verbalize concerns and try to alleviate those concerns
    d. If patient is to have a local anesthetic, medication for anxiety may be necessary
        i. Observe for unpredictable responses to medications
            (a) Excessive sedation
            (b) Decreased respirations
            (c) Agitation
        ii. Allow use of assistive devices if possible
8. Protect eyes from injury
    a. Lubricant
    b. Tape eyelids closed
E. Postoperative PACU Phase I
    1. Review collected data
    2. Patient may be at risk for aspiration
        a. Observe for return of gag and swallowing reflexes
        b. Elevate head of bed if allowed
        c. Suction as necessary
        d. Watch for weakness in throat
            i. Difficulty speaking
            ii. Difficulty swallowing
        e. Position on side if not contraindicated
    3. Patient may be at risk for myasthenia crisis
        a. Maintain normothermia
        b. Medicate for pain and observe for:
            i. Excessive sedation
            ii. Decreased respirations
            iii. Agitation
        c. Observe for symptoms that may indicate crisis
            i. Acute respiratory distress
            ii. Acute motor weakness of voluntary muscles including those for swallowing, speaking, and moving parts of the body
        d. Assess muscle strength frequently
    4. Patient may be at greater risk for respiratory distress
        a. Auscultation of lungs
        b. Observe respiratory pattern and effort
        c. Monitor oxygen saturation
    5. Monitor vital signs and temperature
    6. Observe for reversal of, or adverse reaction to, anesthetic agents

   7. Use measures to decrease anxiety
   8. Administer other medications as ordered and monitor for desired or adverse effects
   9. Provide care based on medical history and procedure performed
   10. Allow use of assistive devices as soon as possible
   11. Reorient to surroundings
   12. Communicate patient's needs to PACU Phase II team
F. PACU Phase II
   1. The patient may return to Phase II directly from the OR
   2. Review collected data
   3. Patient may be at higher risk for aspiration
      a. Elevate head of bed
      b. Suction as necessary
      c. Assess for weakness of throat muscles
      d. Position on side if not contraindicated
      e. Exercise caution when giving fluids or solids
   4. Patient may be at risk for myasthenia crisis
      a. Maintain normothermia
      b. Medicate for pain and observe for:
         i. Excessive sedation
         ii. Decreased respirations
         iii. Agitation
      c. Observe for symptoms that may indicate an impending crisis
         i. Acute respiratory distress
         ii. Acute motor weakness of voluntary muscles including those used for swallowing, speaking, and moving part of the body
      d. Assess muscle strength frequently
      e. Reduce psychological stress
         i. Reorient patient to surroundings
         ii. Allow use of assistive devices as soon as possible
         iii. Allow family to be with patient as soon as possible
      f. Keep patient comfortable
         i. Have room at comfortable temperature
         ii. Medicate for pain or nausea and observe for desired or adverse medication reactions
         iii. Provide nourishment
         iv. Check for bladder distension
   5. May be at risk for respiratory distress
      a. Auscultate lungs
      b. Observe respiratory pattern and effort
      c. Monitor oxygen saturation
      d. Avoid fatigue
   6. Routine care per protocol
   7. Provide care based on patient's medical history and procedure performed
   8. Administer medications as ordered and observe for desired or adverse medication reactions
   9. Verify competent adult help at home after discharge
   10. Verify safe transportation home
   11. Include family when reviewing discharge instructions; if a procedure is to be done at home, have patient and/or family do return demonstration
   12. Provide verbal and written instructions
   13. Obtain phone number to reach patient for follow-up phone call

G. Post discharge
   1. Make follow-up phone call within 24 hours of discharge
   2. Identify yourself and state purpose of call
   3. Complete post-discharge assessment per protocol

IX. **Parkinson's Disease**
   A. General information
      1. Parkinson's disease is a chronic degenerative disease of insidious onset
      2. Characterized by:
         a. Motor impairment
            i. Tremors—improves at rest and is absent when asleep
            ii. Rigidity
            iii. Bradykinesia (slowness in starting and completing voluntary muscle activity)
            iv. Shuffling gait
            v. Tendency to accelerate walking and falling
         b. Postural and reflex changes
            i. Mask-like facial features
               (a) Appears to be expressionless
               (b) Stares straight ahead
               (c) Has decreased blinking of eyes
            ii. Imbalance
            iii. Stooped posture
         c. Speech changes
            i. Difficulty initiating speech
            ii. Difficulty coordinating expiration and articulation
         d. Autonomic symptoms
            i. Drooling
            ii. Excessive perspiration
            iii. Constipation
            iv. Orthostatic hypotension
            v. Dysphasia
         e. Changes in behavior and mental ability
            i. Dementia
            ii. Depression
            iii. Social withdrawal
            iv. Generalized apathy
         f. General weakness and muscle fatigue
         g. Hypersensitivity to heat
   B. Preoperative preadmission interview
      1. An in-person interview affords the opportunity to observe the patient's abilities and interaction with family members
      2. Allow adequate time for the interview and assessment
      3. Provide periods of rest
      4. Maintain a calm, accepting attitude
      5. Provide a comfortable environment
      6. Allow space for patient to move around if he/she has difficulty staying still
      7. Provide a safe environment
         a. Provide assistance with ambulation
         b. Do not leave patient unattended
      8. Speak to the patient and encourage him/her to respond in whatever manner he/she can
      9. Determine patient's functional ability

10. Include the family in preoperative preparation when possible
11. Determine the patient's and/or family's understanding of Parkinson's disease
12. Develop plan of care based on the patient's and family's knowledge and needs
13. Assess:
    a. Abilities and special needs of the patient
    b. Patient's and family's successful management techniques
    c. Use of assistive devices
    d. Willingness and ability of family to participate in preoperative preparation and postoperative care
14. Complete health history
    a. Length of time disease has been present
    b. Patient's abilities
    c. Past surgery
    d. Anesthetic complications for patient or family
    e. Past illnesses
    f. Current illnesses
    g. Medication use (prescription, over the counter, herbal preparations)
    h. Additional assessment per protocol
15. Allergies, including latex sensitivity
16. Physical assessment
    a. Vital signs and oxygen saturation
    b. Muscle strength
    c. History of dysphagia
    d. Heart and lung assessment
    e. Peripheral pulse assessment if indicated
    f. Additional assessment as indicated by medical history and proposed procedure
17. Cognitive assessment
    a. Memory loss
    b. Short attention span
18. Psychosocial assessment
    a. Anxiety
        i. Be alert to nonverbal communication
    b. Support system
        i. Arrangements made for safe transportation to and from the hospital
        ii. Competent adult help at home after discharge
        iii. Include family in preoperative preparation whenever possible
19. Make referrals as necessary
20. Provide verbal and written preoperative instructions
21. Document and communicate patient's special needs to the perianesthesia team members

C. Admission
   1. Verify information obtained in preadmission
   2. Verify compliance with preoperative instructions
   3. Verify safe transportation home
   4. Verify competent adult help at home after discharge
   5. Physical assessment
      a. Per protocol
      b. Muscle strength
      c. Swallowing problems
      d. Additional assessment as indicated by medical history and proposed procedure

6. Cognitive assessment
   a. Short-term memory loss
   b. Short attention span
7. Provide emotional support for family and patient
8. Use measures to decrease anxiety
9. Provide safe environment
   a. Assist patient in getting out of bed
   b. Keep side rails up and bed position low
   c. Do not leave patient unattended
10. Allow periods of rest
11. Maintain comfortable temperature
12. Communicate patient's special needs to surgery and anesthesia team members

D. Intraoperative
1. When possible meet patient before he/she goes to the OR
2. Review collected data
3. Potential for aspiration (if local anesthetic)
   a. Elevate head of bed if possible
   b. Suction as necessary
4. Avoid overheating
5. Allow use of assistive devices as long as possible
6. Protect bony prominences by positioning and padding
7. When moving patient, lift rather than pull
8. Communicate patient's needs to the PACU team members

E. Postoperative PACU Phase I
1. Review data collected
2. May be at increased risk for aspiration
   a. Elevate head of the bed if allowed
   b. Suction as necessary
   c. Observe for return of gag and swallowing reflexes
   d. Position on side if not contraindicated
3. Provide care based on medical history and procedure performed
4. Prevent overheating
5. Allow use of assistive devices as soon as possible
6. Reorient patient to surroundings
7. Communicate patient's special need to Phase II team members

F. PACU Phase II
1. Patient may return directly to Phase II from the OR
2. Review data collected
3. May be at increased risk for aspiration; nursing interventions as above
4. Reorient patient to surroundings
5. Allow use of assistive devices as soon as possible
6. Allow family to be with patient as soon as possible
7. Prevent overheating
8. Provide safe environment; nursing interventions as above
9. Include patient in conversations about his/her procedure
10. Encourage patient to take his/her time when asking or answering questions
11. Provide periods of rest
12. Provide care based on medical history and procedure performed
13. Verify safe transportation home
14. Verify competent adult help at home after discharge
15. Include family when reviewing discharge instructions; if a procedure is to be done at home, have patient and/or family do return demonstration

16. Provide verbal and written instructions
17. Obtain phone number to reach patient for postoperative follow-up phone call

G. Post discharge
   1. Contact the patient within 24 hours after discharge
   2. Identify yourself and state the nature of the call
   3. Complete post-discharge assessment per protocol

X. **Alzheimer's Disease**

A. General information
   1. Alzheimer's is a chronic neurological disorder
   2. Characterized by progressive and selective degeneration of neurons in the cerebral cortex and certain subcortical structures
   3. Sensory-perceptual alterations
      a. Loss of memory
      b. Lack of concentration
      c. Confusion
      d. Disorientation
      e. Lack of motivation
      f. Decreased problem-solving ability
      g. Depression
      h. Agnosia (inability to recognize common objects)
   4. Impaired motor function
      a. Difficulty with balance
      b. Problems with moving arms and legs
      c. Lack of coordination
      d. Spasticity
      e. Increased muscle tone
      f. Apraxia (inability to carry out a skilled act)
   5. Impaired communication
      a. Halting speech
      b. Inability to remember the necessary word
      c. Aphasia (unable to communicate)
   6. At risk for aspiration due to:
      a. Decreased level of consciousness
      b. Seizure activity
      c. Decreased cough and gag reflexes
      d. Impaired swallowing mechanism
   7. Lack of support system related to:
      a. Personality changes
      b. Altered behavior patterns
      c. Depression
      d. Inability to interact in an adult manner
      e. Delusions
      f. Socially unacceptable behavior

B. Preoperative preadmission interview
   1. The patient may not be able to provide information or participate in his/her own care
   2. Determine the patient's level of ability
   3. Determine the patient's and family's understanding of Alzheimer's
   4. Determine the family's willingness and ability to participate in preoperative preparation and postoperative care
   5. When possible, include the patient in discussions about his/her procedure

6. Determine the patient's and/or family's understanding of the proposed procedure
7. Develop a plan of care based on the patient's/family's knowledge and needs
8. Assess:
   a. Abilities and needs of the patient
   b. Patient's and family's successful management techniques
   c. Willingness and ability of the family to participate in preoperative preparation and postoperative care
   d. Use of assistive devices
   e. Effective method of communication
9. Complete medical history
   a. Level and duration of disability
   b. Swallowing problems
   c. History of aspiration
   d. Past surgical history
   e. Anesthetic complications of self or family
   f. Seizure activity
   g. Current medications (prescription, over the counter, herbal preparations)
   h. Present illnesses
   i. Past illnesses
   j. Allergies, including latex
   k. Special diet
10. Physical assessment
    a. Per protocol
    b. Additional assessment based on medical history and proposed procedure
11. Psychosocial assessment
    a. Support system
       i. Arrangements made for safe transportation to and from the hospital
       ii. Willingness and ability of an adult to assist with care after discharge
       iii. Include the family in pre- and postoperative preparation whenever possible
    b. Anxiety
       i. Be alert to nonverbal communication
12. Maintain a caring and accepting attitude
13. Keep instructions and information simple
14. Repeat information frequently and ask the patient to give information back
15. Provide a safe environment
    a. Provide assistance with ambulation
    b. Keep side rails up and bed in low position
    c. Do not leave the patient unattended
16. Provide verbal and written preoperative instructions
17. Preoperative testing as ordered
18. Document and communicate the special needs of the patient to the perianesthesia team
C. Admission
   1. Review data collected in preadmission
   2. Verify compliance with preoperative instructions
      a. May need to rely on family/caregivers for verification of compliance
   3. Verify safe transportation home
   4. Verify competent adult to care for patient at home

    5. Physical assessment
      a. Per protocol
      b. Additional assessment as indicated by the medical history and proposed procedure
    6. Provide emotional support for the patient and the family
    7. Allow the use of assistive devices as long as possible
    8. Use measures to decrease anxiety
      a. Maintain a calm, unhurried attitude
      b. Allow the family to remain with the patient as long as possible
      c. Administer medication for anxiety as ordered, if necessary and monitor for desired or adverse effects
    9. Provide a safe environment; nursing interventions as above
   10. Cognitive assessment
      a. Memory loss
      b. Confusion/disorientation
      c. Depression
   11. Keep explanations short, and repeat information frequently
   12. Communicate patient's special needs to the OR and anesthesia team members

D. Intraoperative
    1. Protect bony prominences by positioning or use of padding
    2. When moving patient, lift rather than pull
    3. Allow use of assistive devices as long as possible
    4. If local anesthetic, patient may be at risk for aspiration
      a. Elevate the head of the bed if possible
      b. Suction as needed
    5. Communicate the patient's special needs to the PACU team members

E. Postoperative PACU Phase I
    1. Review collected data
    2. May be at risk for aspiration
      a. Observe for return of swallowing and gag reflexes
      b. Elevate the head of the bed if possible
      c. Suction as needed
      d. Position on side if not contraindicated
    3. May be combative, confused
      a. Reorient patient to surroundings
      b. Use restraints for safety and protection only as a last resort
    4. Provide care based on medical history and procedure
    5. Administer medication as indicated for pain or nausea; monitor for desired or adverse effects
    6. Monitor for seizure activity
    7. Allow use of assistive devices as soon as possible
    8. Communicate patient's special needs to the Phase II team members

F. PACU Phase II
    1. Patient may return directly to Phase II from the OR
    2. Review data collected
    3. May be at risk for aspiration; nursing interventions as above
    4. Reorient patient to surroundings
    5. Administer medication as indicated for pain or nausea; monitor for desired or adverse effects
    6. Allow use of assistive devices as soon as possible
    7. Allow family to be with patient as soon as possible

8. Patient may be confused, combative
   a. Speak softly to patient, trying to reorient him/her
   b. Presence of family may help calm patient
   c. Medicate if necessary
   d. Use restraints for safety and protection only as last resort
9. Provide safe environment; nursing interventions as above
10. Include patient in discussions about his/her procedure
11. Encourage the patient to take his/her time asking or answering questions
12. Monitor for seizure activity
13. Provide care based on medical history and procedure
14. Verify safe transportation home
15. Verify competent adult help at home
16. Include the family when reviewing discharge instructions; if a procedure is to be done at home, have the patient and/or family do a return demonstration
17. Provide verbal and written discharge instructions
18. Obtain a phone number to contact the patient for a follow-up phone call
G. Post discharge
1. Contact the patient within 24 hours after discharge
2. Identify yourself and state the nature of the call
3. Complete post-discharge assessment per protocol

Bibliography

1. Antel, J.P. (1995). *Neurologic Clinics Multiple Sclerosis.* Philadelphia: Saunders, pp. 1–2, 174, 191, 197–207.
2. Benchol, R. (1986). Mentally retarded patients: Special needs before and after surgery. *AORN,* 44(5): 768–778.
3. Burden, N. (1993). *Ambulatory Surgery Nursing.* Philadelphia: Saunders, pp. 180, 210, 335, 353, 376, 384–387.
4. Cedarbaum, J.M., Gancher, S.T. (1992). *Neurologic Clinics Parkinson's Disease.* Philadelphia: Saunders, pp. 471–475.
5. Chipps, E., Clanin, N., Campbell, V. (1992). *Mosby's Clinical Nursing Series, Neurologic Disorders.* St. Louis: Mosby Year Book, pp. 211–213, 287.
6. Hickey, J.V. (1984). *Quick Reference to Neurological Nursing.* Philadelphia: Lippincott's Quick References, pp. 117–123, 341–342, 487–507.
7. Hirschberg, G.G., Lewis, L., Vaughn, P. (1976). *Rehabilitation: A Manual for the Care of the Disabled and Elderly.* New York: Lippincott.
8. Mansheim, P., Cohen, C.M. (1982). Communicating with developmentally disabled patients. *JPNMHS,* 20(6) 9–11.
9. Morrison, J. (1986). The special needs of the special patient. *RN,* (July) 49–54.
10. Mudge-Grout, C.L. (1992). *Mosby's Clinical Nursing Series, Immunologic Disorders.* St. Louis: Mosby Year Book, pp. 275–300.
11. Mumma, C.M. (1987). *Rehabilitation Nursing: Concepts and Practice, A Core Curriculum,* 2nd ed. Evanston, IL: Rehabilitation Nursing Foundation, pp. 125–130, 228–230, 237–239, 249–253, 258–265.
12. Sanders, D.B. (1994). *Neurologic Clinics Myasthenia Gravis and Myasthenic Syndromes.* Philadelphia: Saunders, pp. 244–253, 345–353, 361–382.
13. Snyder, M. (1983). *A Guide to Neurological and Neurosurgical Nursing.* New York: Wiley, pp. 379–383.
14. Whaley, L.F., Wong, D.L. (1991). *Nursing Care of Infants and Children,* 4th ed. St. Louis: Mosby Year Book.

REVIEW QUESTIONS

1. When providing information to a mentally retarded person

   A. Determine his/her strengths and weaknesses
   B. Address the family/caregiver, since he/she probably will not understand
   C. It is not necessary to do preoperative teaching
   D. Teaching should be done as far in advance as possible

2. When speaking to a mentally retarded person

    A. Provide detailed information
    B. Write everything down
    C. Don't talk down to the patient
    D. Speak in a loud voice; he/she is probably hard of hearing

3. When doing discharge planning for a person with a visual disability

    A. Assume he/she can do all self-care after discharge
    B. Assume that he/she can do no self-care after discharge
    C. Educate the adult caregiver to do wound assessment after discharge
    D. Provide written instructions

4. When caring for a hearing impaired patient in PACU

    A. Face the person when speaking
    B. Speak slowly and clearly
    C. Return hearing aid as soon as possible
    D. All of the above

5. When planning care for a person with aphasia, consider the following

    A. The patient cannot see
    B. The patient cannot hear
    C. The patient can probably understand all or part of what is said
    D. The patient will probably require around-the-clock care

6. When assessing the aphasic patient preoperatively

    A. Do not increase voice volume
    B. Present a relaxed attitude
    C. Use short, simple sentences
    D. All of the above

7. Spinal cord injury may result in

    A. Complete paralysis
    B. Incomplete paralysis
    C. Respiratory dysfunction
    D. All of the above

8. When preparing a patient with multiple sclerosis for surgery, the following must be considered

    A. The patient becomes fatigued easily
    B. The patient may have motor weakness
    C. Surgery could trigger a relapse
    D. All of the above

9. Myasthenia gravis may result in all of the following except

    A. Fatigue
    B. Respiratory difficulty
    C. Visual problems
    D. Paralysis

10. The patient with Parkinson's disease may have which of the following?

    A. Motor impairment
    B. Cognitive problems
    C. Speech changes
    D. All of the above

ANSWERS TO QUESTIONS

1. A
2. C
3. C
4. D
5. C

6. D
7. D
8. D
9. D
10. D

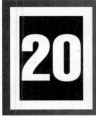

Home Support Network

Judy Ontiveros
St. Luke Medical Center
Pasadena, California

I. **Definition of Ambulatory Surgery Patient**
  A. "One who does not require hospital inpatient care" (Ferguson and Kaplan, 1966)
    1. Patient is able to walk and travel to his/her home after treatment
    2. Patient can safely care for him-/herself without aid from a professional care giver
    3. Patient is discharged with the intention of having his/her postoperative care provided by the patient and family/significant other
    4. Patient receives anesthesia that is tailored to a rapid discharge
      a. The use of premedication is often eliminated to prevent a prolonged stay
      b. Anesthesia techniques and medications provide for a quick induction, with a shorter duration of action and fewer side effects on the vital signs
  B. Ambulatory surgery is appealing to the patient
    1. There are fewer disruptions of normal daily activities
    2. There is less separation from family/significant others
    3. There is less time away from work
    4. There is less worry about financial outlay
  C. The patient and the family are active participants in the patient's plan of care
    1. The patient assumes responsibility for his/her own care
    2. Education is an integral part of the ambulatory surgery process

1. Define ambulatory surgery as it relates to discharge and follow up home care.
2. Describe alternative sources of care after discharge.
3. Know discharge criteria for the ambulatory surgery patient and the facets of continuing care post discharge.
4. Describe the unique aspects of home care and instructions for the pediatric patient.
5. Identify strategies to help the geriatric patient have a successful ambulatory surgery experience.
6. State the role of the home health nurse in ambulatory postoperative home care.

      a. Continuous process, beginning preoperatively until discharge and continuing with the follow-up phone contact

      b. Facilitates the preparation needed to meet the postoperative needs of the patient

      c. Teaches the patient and family when to seek additional advice if needed

      d. Discharge instructions contain information on how the patient and family monitor untoward symptoms

        i. Telephone numbers of the physician and hospital emergency are listed

      e. For the non-English–speaking patient, instruction must be given in the patient's native language to insure understanding

        i. If the center has a large number of non-English–speaking patients, the discharge instructions should be printed in patient's language

        ii. An interpreter in the facility is imperative if there is no family to interpret in the patient's language

        iii. Interpreter should be of the same sex as the patient if possible

        iv. Interpreter services may be obtained through ATT Language Line, 1-800-752-6096, if none else is available

D. Financial considerations

    1. Third-party payers may determine the types of surgical procedures that are done on an outpatient basis

      a. Patients may need additional care beyond the ambulatory care provision

      b. Referrals need to be made to home health agencies for follow-up care

      c. Specific guidelines need to be followed for funding from private insurance and government agencies

    2. Access to care for those without insurance

      a. Up-front cash payments may keep some from obtaining needed surgical intervention

      b. Alternative methods for health-care financing need to be explored

II. Discharge to Home Care

A. Patients may be discharged home under standardized discharge criteria

    1. Joint Commission for Accreditation of Healthcare Organizations (JCAHO) allows authorized personnel to discharge patients when discharge criteria has been established and is met by the patient

    2. Discharge instructions should include the following but are not limited to:

      a. Order from physician or anesthesiologist

      b. Stable vital signs

      c. No respiratory depression

      d. Oriented to time, person, place

      e. Minimal nausea and vomiting

      f. Minimal or controllable pain

      g. No bleeding or excessive drainage

      h. Able to void as related to procedure

      i. Able to ambulate commensurate with preoperative status

      j. Able to take fluids orally, as appropriate

      k. Responsible adult escort

      l. Written discharge instructions

B. Continuing care

    1. Patient is educated preoperatively and during course of care that he/she should not plan on resuming normal activities immediately after surgery

      a. Effects of medication impairs judgment; no important decisions for 24 hours following surgery

      b. No driving for 24 hours following surgery

      c. No alcohol for 24 hours following surgery

2. Discharge instructions should include the following, but are not limited to:
   a. Diet
   b. Activity restrictions
   c. Wound care
   d. Possible complications
   e. Prescriptions
   f. Follow-up care including doctor's visits, who to call in an emergency or if additional help is needed
3. Verbal instructions given to the patient and family with a written copy to be sent home
   a. Written copy is signed and kept as a part of the chart
   b. Medical record should contain documentation that instructions were given and understood
4. Return demonstration of care may be needed from patient or caregivers if care involves a physical activity associated with the procedure
5. Legal considerations—recurrent excuses for not seeking treatment postoperatively
   a. Patient did not know what to look for
   b. Patient did not know the significance of the symptoms experienced
   c. Patient did not know what to do or whom to contact
6. Medication instructions should be explicitly explained
   a. Reasons for noncompliance are:
      i.   Patient did not know when to take the medication
      ii. Patient did not know when *not* to take the medication
      iii. Patient did not know when to stop taking the medication
   b. Nurse should reinforce physician's teachings
   c. Instructions for taking medications should be written on discharge instruction sheet
C. Accessibility to emergency care
   1. Preadmission discharge planning
      a. Discharge-related procedure that needs to be planned for preoperatively
      b. Presence of a responsible adult to assist the patient home, receive patient's discharge instructions, and summon help if needed
      c. If there is a significant risk that the patient cannot reach the emergency facility, then discharge should be delayed
   2. Factors to be considered include:
      a. The operative procedure
      b. The patient's general health
      c. Risk factors that are determined preoperatively
      d. Patient's present status
      e. Accessibility of emergency facilities in the event of a complication
D. Patient satisfaction follow-up
   1. Feedback questionnaire may be given to the patient at discharge or mailed at a later date; feedback provided may include but are not limited to:
      a. Service received
      b. Postoperative complications
      c. Education—did they receive enough information regarding their surgical experience or procedure and how to care for themselves?
      d. Would they return to the facility?
      e. Provides an opportunity for additional comments or questions
   2. Follow-up phone call
      a. A call is placed to the patient 24–48 hours after discharge
         i.   Second call made next day if patient cannot be reached

        ii. Facility policy dictates how many noncontact calls are required—until patient reached or limit to two or three calls

    b. Assignment of calls

        i. Primary care approach—each nurse calls the patient he/she cared for

        ii. Shared duty—any nurse calls during the day during down time

        iii. Assigned duty—one nurse responsible to do the calls

    c. Primary focus is to evaluate the patient's general condition and how recovery is progressing

        i. Questions regarding care may be answered

        ii. The patient may be referred to the surgeon for concerns or the nurse may call the physician with care recommendations if appropriate

    d. The call should be documented on the chart

        i. Note patient's statement of progress

        ii. Note any problems that are occurring

           (a) Untoward signs or symptoms must be recorded accurately

           (b) If a problem is identified, the nurse has a duty to act on it in a timely manner

        iii. Note referrals given to physician or other source for follow-up care

    e. The questions in the above referenced survey may also be asked of the patient to determine patient satisfaction and the effectiveness of patient care at the facility

    f. Provide a positive marketing effect for the facility

    g. The ambulatory care experience is completed by the facility

        i. Nurse gains sense of satisfaction in job completed

        ii. Chart is completed with the follow-up documentation

        iii. Demonstrates compliance with accrediting bodies and community standards

        iv. Legal aspects

           (a) Potential liabilities addressed as soon as possible

           (b) May advert potential lawsuit by early corrective action

  3. Follow-up call initiated at preoperative visit

    a. Information provided to patient that call will be made

        i. Verify accurate telephone number

        ii. Where will the patient be staying

        iii. Any restraints requested by patient or family

           (a) Not to call at work

           (b) Not to divulge to family members who is calling

           (c) Best time to call

  4. Second postoperative call

    a. Made several weeks after surgery

    b. Pursue issues of infection control, long-term recovery issues

        i. Return to work

        ii. Level of activity

        iii. Personal expectations/actual experience

        iv. Complications and resolution

  5. Call used as quality-improvement tool

    a. Information gained studied and compiled to change practices if needed

    b. Data used to increase patient satisfaction

III. Alternatives to Home Care—Phase III Recovery Care

  A. Recovery center

    1. Offers skilled nursing on the level with a PACU Phase II unit, to patients when the patient or the family feels they cannot provide the care but acute nursing care is not required

a. May be adjacent to a freestanding ambulatory center

b. May be a hotel-like atmosphere with private rooms

c. Family members are allowed to stay with the patient

d. Hotel-like services are provided to the patient, including meals, TV, video, and stereo

2. Length of admission is up to 72 hours

a. Patients provide basic self-care needs

b. Pain management needs to be achieved within the 72 hours

c. Education is a focus to teach the proper skills for self-care at home

3. Procedures that may go to a recovery center may include but are not limited to:

a. Joint, tendon, and ligament reconstructions

b. Cholecystectomy

c. Hemorrhoidectomy

d. Mastectomy

e. Extensive plastic surgeries

f. Laparoscopic abdominal surgeries

4. Prototype of care developed by California legislature

a. Original project—12 facilities with up to 20 beds

b. Evaluated whether inpatient-type procedures could be performed more economically than hospitals without compromising care or safety

c. Projected saving of 30–60% over traditional hospital-based care

B. Hospital hotels

1. Bed-and-breakfast type facility within the hospital

a. Line drawn between guest and patient

b. Risk that patient and family equate level of care with that of the rest of the hospital

2. Utilization

a. Elderly

b. Patients who travel more than one hour to the hospital or center

C. Outpatient observation

1. Came into existence following Medicare DRG program which denied many admissions

2. Need for longer period of observation for some patients

3. Considered as a nonhospitalized patient for up to less than 24 hours

4. Fees prorated on length of stay, usually charging hourly rate

5. Also provides service to physician when patient needs additional observation before discharge

D. Freestanding medical motels

1. Nonmedical facility

2. Offers comfortable, inexpensive, convenient place to recuperate

3. Care given by family or friends

4. Transitional care may be provided by a home health nurse

5. More complex procedures may be done on an outpatient basis with follow-up by a home health nurse

6. Hotel staff only trained in cardiopulmonary resuscitation

IV. **The pediatric ambulatory patient**

A. Unique aspect of pediatric care is that the patient is a growing organism

1. Understanding of the growth and development patterns of the pediatric patient is essential

2. Normal physical and psychologic parameters must be understood and any deviation readily recognized

B. Postoperative home care starts with the preoperative visit
1. Patient and family are interviewed to gather data, educate, and to provide emotional support to the child and to the family
2. Education on the entire surgical experience is given
3. Care the parent will provide is given in detail
   a. Verbally discussed with parents or caregiver
   b. Procedure-specific handout
      i. Includes care points that need to be stressed
      ii. Includes complications to watch for
      iii. Includes telephone numbers to call (physician or hospital emergency department) to report untoward symptoms
4. Education and emotional support help to dispel the fear a parent may have in caring for the child at home
C. Common complications seen at home
1. Nausea and vomiting
   a. More common with tonsillectomy and adenoidectomy, strabismus surgery, and orchiopexy
   b. Twice as common in surgeries lasting over 20 minutes
   c. More common in children above three years of age
   d. Prevention during surgery with good fluid replacement and low dosage of droperidol
   e. Parents cautioned to provide adequate liquids and call if child cannot retain fluids for a period of time
2. Pain
3. Sleepiness, cough, sore throat, hoarseness, croup, and fever
D. Transportation home
1. Availability of responsible adult
2. Two adults ideal for infant or small child; one can tend to child during ride home
3. Child should adequately be restrained in appropriate car seat or seat belt; not held by adult
E. Home care
1. Follow-up phone call helpful the evening of surgery and within 24 hours
   a. Inquire of any complications
   b. Specific procedure-related questions are required
      i. Tonsillectomy—bleeding, nausea, vomiting, fluid intake
      ii. Hernia—nausea, vomiting, taut abdomen, unrelieved pain
      iii. Orthopedic—color, warmth, movement (of extremity if in cast)
2. In home nursing visit reserved for complicated, high-tech cases
3. Telephone support is usually sufficient
V. **The Geriatric Ambulatory Surgery Patient**
A. The geriatric population, 65 years and older, is the fastest growing age group in the United States
1. This age group will double its size between the years 1990 to 2030
2. The 100+ are the fastest growing group within the elderly population
B. The health-care industry will see major changes in the age group of patients that are being cared for:
1. By the year 2000 the rise of the geriatric patient in the hospital will rise from 34% in 1990 to 58%
2. 50% of persons 60 and older will require surgery before they die
C. The elderly patient is being treated with surgery more aggressively than in the past
1. Proper postoperative home care is one of the most important factors in geriatric ambulatory surgery

a. Evaluation of the home caregiver during the preoperative interview may include:
   i.   Reliability
   ii. Physical capability
   iii. Emotional maturity
b. Support services can be arranged in advance if needed:
   i.   Social worker
   ii. Home health care
   iii. Visiting nurse
   iv. Transportation

2. Risk of surgical intervention is reduced by careful preoperative evaluation, planning, and education
   a. Evaluation of psychosocial and education needs
      i.   Will alleviate many fears, risks, and complications
      ii. The patient may be concerned about a spouse for whom he/she is caring, a pet, or a parent
   b. The discharge plan
      i.   The discharge planner or case manager may be needed to help with the patient's concerns
      ii. Preoperative discharge planning can evaluate if the patient needs home nursing care postoperatively
   c. Family members should be included in the preoperative education session on how they can help and reinforce the postoperative care

3. Assessment of physiologic functioning and chronic illness is done to plan the care of the elderly patient through the entire surgical phase

4. Successful outcome of ambulatory surgery for the elderly depends on:
   a. Elective versus emergency surgery
   b. Optimum physical condition
   c. Thorough preoperative assessment
   d. Close intraoperative and postoperative monitoring
   e. Preventive measures to decrease any complications

D. Discharge instructions
   1. Education should be done in a non-hurried manner
      a. Needs extra time to assimilate information
      b. Quiet atmosphere can help patient focus attention on what is being presented
      c. Preoperative teaching can effectively be done in the home by home health nurses
         i.   Teaching done in the patient's home make the patient more receptive to the instruction
         ii. Familiarity to surroundings reinforces learning
   2. Instructions need to be written
      a. Large type may be needed
      b. Colored paper (yellow or tan) will make instructions easier to read
      c. Gives patient sense of control
         i.   Patient can refer to instructions that are easily understood
         ii. Self-esteem is reinforced as patient doesn't need to ask for help
   3. Instructions for hearing- or sight-impaired
      a. Special provisions may need to be made
      b. Braille standardized instructions for the sight-impaired or audio tapes
      c. Sign interpretation for the hearing-impaired

VI. Home Health Care Nursing
   A. Definition
      1. Provision of health care services specifically designed to meet the individual needs of the patient; services are provided in the patient's place of residence
         a. Promotes and maintains health
         b. Maximizes level of independence
         c. Emphasizes focus on wellness
         d. Services planned, coordinated, and made available through home health-care agencies
   B. Levels of care
      1. Concentrated or intensive services
         a. For those needing hospitalization
         b. Coordination of services under professional supervision allows the patient to be treated at home
      2. Intermediate services
         a. Convalescent/rehabilitation-type of care
         b. Less concentrated type of care provided
         c. Personal care
         d. Environmental supportive social services
      3. Basic or maintenance services
         a. Long-term care needs
         b. Prevents or postpones hospital care
         c. Personal and supportive environmental care
         d. Social services
         e. Condition stable—periodic monitoring only
   C. Role of the nurse in home health care—all encompassing
      1. To teach the family to care for the patient; including, but not limited to:
         a. Changes in patient condition—infections
         b. Medications—use, times to be given, and side effects
         c. Skin care—prevent skin breakdowns
         d. Nutrition—good nutrition program to promote healing of surgical wounds
         e. Elimination—changes that might occur in bowel movements from pain medications
         f. Mobilization and dressing the patient
         g. Wound dressing changes
         h. Safety of the patient
      2. Assessments
         a. Patient's physical assessment
         b. Assessment of the family and caregiver
            i. Family dynamics—possible or anticipated changes
            ii. Type of relationships in the family
            iii. Educational and cultural backgrounds
               (a) Education affects the patient's ability to read, listen, and follow directions
               (b) Attitude towards health and illness may be related to cultural background
         c. Assessment of the community in which the patient is a part
      3. Support
         a. Link to physician and health care services
            i. Physical and occupational therapies
            ii. Community resources
               (a) Meals on Wheels
               (b) Visitors

          (c) Senior centers
          (d) Home care social worker—can be link to community resources for the patient
       iii. Home health aide
          (a) Gives personal care to the patient
          (b) Reinforces care given by other health-care workers
          (c) Reports changes in patient condition to other health-care professionals
       iv. Arrange for equipment needed during convalescence
       v. Refer patient to organizations that can help with financial considerations if needed
          (a) Red Cross
          (b) American Cancer Society
          (c) Multiple Sclerosis Society
          (d) Muscular Dystrophy Association
          (e) St. Vincent de Paul Society
          (f) United Way
    b. Support of decisions made by family regarding patient
  4. Performance of specific skills in connection with the patient's condition
    a. Involvement of the family in these skills reinforces teaching and connection to the patient
D. Expands complexity of procedures performed under ambulatory surgery
  1. Procedures performed may include but are not limited to:
    a. Vaginal hysterectomy
    b. Mastectomy
    c. Anterior cruciate ligament repair
    d. Endoscopic abdominal surgery
       i. Salpingoopherectomy
       ii. Cholecystectomy
       iii. Appendectomy
       iv. Hysterectomy
       v. Nephrectomy
       vi. Nephrolithotomy
  2. Plan of care—outpatient vaginal hysterectomy
    a. Careful preoperative screening according to selected criteria
       i. Decision involves patient and family agreement
       ii. Requires active participation by family
    b. Detailed education on the surgical experience
    c. Postoperative care map is followed for Phase I and Phase II recovery
    d. Meets discharge criteria
       i. Hematocrit remains constant
       ii. Ambulates successfully
       iii. Voids
       iv. Tolerates clear liquid
    e. Average length of stay is 9.5 hours
    f. Transportation home
       i. Private transportation
       ii. Ambulance with a registered nurse
    g. Home health care follow-up
       i. Protocols differ per institution
          (a) Registered nurse remains in attendance for 48 hours
            (i) IV fluids, narcotics, IV antibiotics are available
          (b) Visit by home health nurse on post days one and two

      ii. Detailed postoperative instructions given

     iii. Role of nurse

        (a) Physical assessment

        (b) History since discharge—observing for possible complications

        (c) Blood drawn each day

        (d) Progress reported to physician or hospital-based protocol nurse

     iv. Surgeon maintains contact via telephone

      v. Extended follow-up

        (a) Physician office visit at 2 and 6 weeks

     vi. Outcome

        (a) Patient satisfaction expressed

        (b) Favorable outcome based on good education and support system

   3. Plan of Care—anterior cruciate ligament repair

     a. Protocol of care established between the physician's office, visiting nurse association, and the hospital

       i. Preoperative instructions and education received

        (a) Receive standard preoperative instructions from hospital admission nurse

        (b) Instructed by hospital physical therapist on postoperative exercises and use of continuous passive motion (CPM) machine

     ii. Home care follow-up

        (a) Visits day of surgery and first postoperative day

        (b) Administers IM injection of ketorolac each day

        (c) Assesses patient including neuroassessment of affected limb

        (d) Teaches/reinforces teaching on dressing care, exercises, CPM machine, self-assessment of involved leg, crutch walking

        (e) Physician visit 7–10 postoperative and then every 2 weeks for 3 months

VII. Summary

   A. The trend will increase to do surgery on an outpatient basis to keep hospital costs down

   B. The outcome for a successful experience depends on thorough and detailed education: preoperatively, during the facility stay, and postoperatively

   C. Home health resources are enabling major surgeries to be done on an outpatient basis

     1. Preoperative discharge planning

     2. Home health nursing

     3. Home health aides, physical therapist, occupational therapist

     4. Community resources can be utilized for equipment needs, meals, socialization, financial help

Bibliography

1. Allen, A. (1994). A model for rural health care. *J Post Anesth Nursing*, 9(2):120–122.
2. Allen, M., Knight, C., Falk, C., Strang, V. (1992). Effectiveness of a preoperative teaching programme for cataract patients. *J Adv Nursing*, (17)3:303–309.
3. Bailey, C. (1994). Education for home care providers. *J Obstetric, Gynecologic, and Neonatal Nursing*, 23(8): 724–729.
4. Bran, D.F., Spellman, J.R., Summitt, R.L. (1995). Outpatient vaginal hysterectomy as a new trend in gynecology. *AORN J*, 5(62):810–814.
5. Burden, N. (1993). *Ambulatory Surgical Nursing*. Philadelphia: Saunders.
6. Cruz, L. (1990). Ambulatory surgery—the next decade. *AORN J*, (51)1:241–247.
7. Dellasega, C., Burgunder, C. (1991). Perioperative nursing care for the elderly surgical patient. *Today's OR Nurse*, 13(6):12–17.
8. Drew, J. (1995). Testing the need for a follow-up visit after child day surgery. *Nursing Standards (AWH)*, 10(10):38–43.

9. Galazka, S.S. (1988). Preoperative evaluation of the elderly surgical patient. *J Family Practice, 27,* 622.

10. Ferguson, L.K., Kaplan, L. (1966). *Surgery of the Ambulatory Patient.* Philadelphia: Lippincott.

11. Fosko, S.W., Stecher, J.C. (1995). The role of home health nursing: A dermatologic case study. *Dermatology Nursing, 7*(3):185–187.

12. Fromm, C.G., Metzler, D.J. (1993). Preparing your older patient for surgery. *RN,* January: 38–43.

13. Jeffries, E. (1997). One-day mastectomy. *Home Healthcare Nurse, 15*(1):30–40.

14. Keating, H.J. (1987). Preoperative considerations in the geriatric patient. *Medical Clinics of North America,* (71):569.

15. Kendall, F. (1993). Documenting local anesthesia patient care. *AORN J, 58*(4):715–719.

16. Kenne, A. (1991). Perioperative assessment and nursing implications for the elderly. *Plastic Surgical Nursing, 11*(40):143–150.

17. Kirkpatrick, L., Kleinbeck, S.V.M. (1991). Surgery trends change nursing care: Operating room nurses share new procedures that will affect home healthcare. *Home Healthcare Nurse, 9*(6):13–20.

18. Kjernik, D.K., Weisensee, M.G. (1992). Empowering older people is a perioperative nursing challenge. *AORN J 55*(4):1086–1089.

19. Lea, S.G., Phippen, M. (1992). Client education in the ambulatory surgery setting. *Seminars in Perioperative Nursing, 1*(4):203–223.

20. Llewellyn, J.G. (1991). Short stay surgery—present practices, future trends. *AORN J, 53*(5):1179–1191.

21. Maligalig, R., Marina, L. (1994). Parents' perceptions of the stressors of pediatric ambulatory surgery. *J Post Anesth Nursing, 9*(5):278–282.

22. Marley, R.A., Moline, B.M. (1996). Patient discharge from the ambulatory setting. *J Post Anesth Nursing, 11*(1):39–49.

23. Meeker, M.H., Rothrock, J.C. (1995). *Alexander's Care of the Patient in Surgery.* St. Louis: Mosby.

24. Michel, L.L., Myrick, C. (1990). Current and future trends in ambulatory surgery and their impact on nursing practice. *J Post Anesth Nursing, 5*(5):347–349.

25. Neal, J.N. (1996). Outpatient ACL surgery: The role of the home health nurse. *Orthopaedic Nursing,* (15)4:9–13.

26. Orticio, L.P., Swan, J. (1992). Implementation of the postdischarge follow-up call in the patient care units. *Insight, 17*(2):15–9.

27. Redmond, M.C. (1993). Infection control monitoring in the ambulatory surgery unit. *J Post Anesth Nursing, 8*(1):28–34.

28. Redmond, M.C. (1994). Phase III recovery: Referral options in postoperative discharge planning. *J Post Anesth Nursing, 9*(6):353–356.

29. Redmond, M.C. (1995). Using home health agencies to meet patient needs in Phase III recovery. *J Post Anesth Nursing, 10*(1):21–26.

30. Richards, D.M., Irving, M.H. (1996). Cost utility analysis of home parenteral nutrition. *British J Surgery, 83*(9):1226.

31. Rivellini, D. (1993). Local and regional anesthesia. *Nursing Clinics of North America,* (28)3:547–572.

32. Rothman, N.L., Moriarty, L., et al. (1994). Establishing a home care protocol for early discharge of patients with hip and knee arthroplasties. *Home Healthcare Nurse, 12*(1):24–30.

33. Singer, H. (1993). Then and now: A historical development of ambulatory surgery. *J Post Anesth Nursing, 8*(4):276–279.

34. Singleton, R.J., Rudkin, G.E., et al. (1996). Laparoscopic cholecystectomy as a day surgery procedure. 24(2):231–236.

35. Smallwood, S.B. (1988). Preparing children for surgery through play. *AORN J,* (47)1:177.

36. Smeltzer, C.H., Flores, S.M. Preadmission discharge planning: Organization of a concept.

37. Spangenberg, A.B. (1994). Wound care: Complex care. *Nursing Times, 90*(7):74–78.

38. Stephenson, M.E. (1990). Discharge criteria in day surgery. *J Adv Nursing,* (15):601–613.

39. Stuart-Siddall, S. (1986). *Home Health Care Nursing: Administrative and Clinical Perspectives.* Rockville, MD: Aspen.

40. Summers, S., Ebbert, D.W. (1992). *Ambulatory Surgical Nursing: A Nursing Diagnosis Approach.* Philadelphia: Lippincott.

41. Suter-Gut, D., Metcalf, A.M., Donnelly, M.A., Smith, I.M. (1990). Post-discharge care planning and rehabilitation of the elderly surgical patient. *Clinics in Geriatric Medicine,* (6)3:543–556.

42. Thomas, J.S., Graff, B.M., et al. (1992). Home visiting for a posthysterectomy population. *Home Healthcare Nurse, 10*(3):47–52.

43. Weber, F. (1996). The challenge of changing healthcare systems. *Drugs,* (EC2)52(2):68–77.

44. Wetchler, B.V. (1991). *Anesthesia for Ambulatory Surgery, 2nd ed.* Philadelphia: Lippincott.

45. Whaley, L.F., Wong, D.J. (1991). *Nursing Care of Infants and Children, 4th ed.* St. Louis: Mosby.

46. Whedon, M.A., Sabin, P., et al. (1995). Practice corner: What do you do to expedite discharge after surgery? *Oncology Nursing Forum, 22*(1):147–150.

47. White, P.F. (1997). *Ambulatory Anesthesia and Surgery.* London: Saunders Company Limited.

48. Wolfson, J., Walker, G., Levin, P. (1993). Freestanding ambulatory surgery: Cost-containment winner? *Healthcare Financial Management, 47*(7):27.

49. Young, C.M. (1990). The postoperative follow-up phone call: An essential part of the ambulatory surgery nurse's job. *J Post Anesth Nursing,* (5)4:273–275.

REVIEW QUESTIONS

1. An ambulatory patient who is ready to be discharged home means that

   A. Patient is ready to assume all activities of daily living without additional aid
   B. Patient's condition is medically stable and that care at home can be provided by the patient with the aid of the family
   C. Patient will be able to go home but needs to have assistance from a professional caregiver
   D. Patient has no pain or nausea or vomiting

2. When the patient is ready for discharge

   A. The physician absolutely needs to see and evaluate the patient and write the discharge order
   B. The patient may be discharged by the RN in attendance when the patient meets the predetermined standardized discharge criteria
   C. Both the physician and anesthesiologist need to see the patient prior to discharge
   D. The nurse may discharge the patient when he/she is awake, taking fluids, free from pain, and wants to go home

3. The continuing plan of care contains the following facets of care except

   A. Discharge instructions are written and discussed with the patient and home caregiver
   B. The patient should not drive, make important decisions, or drink alcohol for 24 hours following discharge
   C. The patient should be able to do a return demonstration of a care skill before discharge
   D. The patient may return home alone with no care provider

4. The patient's home plan of care includes

   A. Written instructions on how to obtain emergency help if needed
   B. Telephone numbers of the patient's physician and hospital emergency care
   C. Assurance that the patient will have a responsible adult caregiver present for 24 hours
   D. All of the above

5. A follow-up phone call is done after the patient is discharged

   A. Within the first week after discharge
   B. To find out if the patient has any complaints about his/her care
   C. To inquire about the patient's condition and continuing recovery
   D. To find out if the patient drove him/herself home

6. The follow-up phone call accomplishes the following

   A. The patient's satisfaction with his/her care at the facility
   B. The patient's present status and compliance with discharge instructions
   C. To answer any questions the patient may have incurred since returning home
   D. Meets standards of accrediting agencies and community standards
   E. All of the above

7. Every patient may not feel comfortable going home due to various circumstances. An alternative method of care would be

   A. A hotel room near the hospital
   B. A recovery center that specializes in postoperative care
   C. Continuing care in the hospital up to a week postoperatively
   D. All of the above

8. Pediatric patients can be successfully cared for as ambulatory patients because

   A. Parents are usually competent in the care of their children
   B. The procedures performed on children are not serious and not life-threatening
   C. Most children are healthy and do not pose a problem with care
   D. Careful preoperative education will prepare the family or caregiver to provide the care the child needs

9. The following conditions make the geriatric patient a viable candidate for ambulatory surgery

   A. Extensive preoperative preparation and education
   B. Provision of a caregiver who the patient trusts and is familiar with
   C. Detailed discharge instructions are given to both the patient and the caregiver on admission and discharge
   D. Preventive measures are taken preoperatively to prevent untoward complications postoperatively
   E. All of the above

10. The goal of home health nursing is to

    A. Make sure the patient is compliant with his/her discharge instructions
    B. To allow the patient to be cared for at home with adequate support from health resources
    C. To avoid hospital admissions that cause a rise in health-care cost
    D. To give families a reprieve from providing care to their family member

11. The role of the home health nurse is

    A. To teach the families to care for the patient
    B. Assess the patient's postoperative condition
    C. To provide coordination of health and community services that are available to the patient and family
    D. All of the above

12. Surgeries that can safely be performed on an outpatient basis because of advanced technology and professional home health care are

    A. Vaginal hysterectomy
    B. Mastectomy
    C. Abdominal endoscopic surgeries
    D. Complex orthopedic procedures
    E. All of the above

13. Which of the following parameters is not a requirement for the care of major ambulatory surgical patients?

    A. Preoperative education
    B. Detailed plan of care
    C. Patient and family cooperation and willingness to participate
    D. Adequate insurance to afford home health services

ANSWERS TO QUESTIONS

1. B
2. B
3. D
4. D
5. C
6. E
7. B

8. D
9. E
10. B
11. D
12. E
13. D

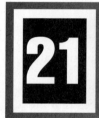

Transcultural Nursing

Christine Kelley
Elliot 1-Day Surgery Center
Manchester, New Hampshire

Objectives

1. Define transcultural nursing.
2. Describe nursing interventions for assessing culturally diverse patients.
3. Identify the three major sectors of health care.
4. Identify and describe the three world views of health and illness.
5. Compare and contrast the beliefs and values of African-Americans and African-Caribbean (Haitians).
6. State specific verbal and nonverbal communication techniques for at least two different cultures.

I. **Definitions**
   A. Culture
      1. Integrated system of learned values, beliefs, and practices
      2. Characteristic of a society
      3. Guides individual behavior
         a. Thoughts
         b. Feelings
         c. Actions
   B. Transcultural nursing
      1. Integrates the concept of culture into all aspects of nursing
      2. A humanistic and scientific area of formal study and practice (Leininger, 1991)
         a. Focuses on differences and similarities among cultures with respect to:
            i. Human care
            ii. Health (or well-being)
            iii. Illness
         b. Based on individual's:
            i. Cultural values
            ii. Beliefs
            iii. Practices
   C. Cultural competence (Luckmann, 1997)
      1. Knowing, utilizing, and appreciating the effects of culture in resolving individual, family, or community problems
      2. Requires awareness of own cultural values, beliefs, and practices
      3. Openness, understanding, acceptance of, and adjustment to cultural differences

II. **Culture**
  A. Values, norms, beliefs, and practices of a society
  B. Develops over time
  C. Learned responses, actions, words, and thoughts
  D. Passed down through generations
  E. Not genetic in nature
  F. Guides behavior
  G. Affects health-care practices

III. **The Transcultural Nursing Society**
  A. Founded in 1974
  B. Madeleine Leininger, founder
  C. Publications on transcultural nursing
  D. Annual transcultural nursing conferences
  E. Certification available

IV. **Major World Views of Health and Illness**
  A. Biomedical (scientific)
    1. Life regulated by biomedical and physical processes
    2. Health is absence of disease
    3. Illness is alteration in structure and function of body
    4. Treatment focuses on physical and chemical interventions
  B. Magicoreligious (supernatural)
    1. All that exists is dependent on supernatural forces
      a. Includes good and evil
    2. Health means person is blessed or favored by the supernatural
    3. The cause of disease is mystical
      a. Not based on scientific fact
      b. Foreign object or spirit enters the body
      c. Sign of punishment or possession by the supernatural
    4. Treatment aimed at removing foreign object or spirit
  C. Holistic
    1. Everything governed by laws of nature
    2. Health achieved by adapting to constantly changing environment
    3. Illness is imbalance or lack of harmony between forces
    4. Treatment aimed at restoring harmony or balance

V. **Major Sectors of Health Care**
  A. Types
    1. Popular
    2. Folk
    3. Professional
  B. Characteristics
    1. Each explains and treats illness differently
    2. Each defines who should be the health-care provider
    3. Each defines how the provider and patient should interact
    4. Sectors used individually, in combination, or simultaneously
  C. Popular sector
    1. Lay; nonprofessional, non-folk healer
      a. Define and treat illness
    2. Determine if additional care is needed (folk or professional)
    3. Activities
      a. Self care is administered using home remedies
      b. Consult with family, friends, clergy, neighbors, others who have had same condition
      c. Remedies include over-the-counter medications

        d. Care provided by:
           i.   Self
           ii. Family
           iii. Friends

D. Folk sector
  1. May be consulted when home remedies and self-care methods fail
  2. Ethnomedical and traditional
  3. Ethnomedical
     a. The study of non-Western, traditional, or folk medicine
     b. Encompasses cultural traditions, beliefs, and practices related to health and illness
     c. Not related to biomedical theory
  4. Characteristics
     a. Defines and removes supernatural causes
     b. Works to restore balance
     c. Strives to restore health and prevent illness
  5. Activities
     a. Holistic approach
     b. Treatment of illnesses due to:
        i.   Imbalances in individual, physical, social, and metaphysical environments
        ii. Supernatural forces
     c. Treatment of:
        i.   Culture-specific illnesses
        ii. Illnesses not controlled by home remedies or professional medicine
     d. Rituals
        i.   Incorporated to prevent illness, misfortune, and to enhance effects of biomedicine
  6. Acts as intermediary between popular and professional sectors
  7. May be the only sector consulted, depending on cause, signs, and symptoms
  8. Care provided by:
     a. Folk healers
        i.   Secular
        ii. Sacred
        iii. Combination of both

E. Professional sector
  1. Types
     a. Biomedicine—United States
     b. Traditional Chinese medicine—China
     c. Ayurvedic medicine—India
  2. Goal: to define, treat, and prevent disease and illness
  3. May be consulted when home remedies or folk sector treatments are ineffective
  4. Initially consulted if acute trauma, surgery, or restoration of body part necessary

F. Use of different sectors
  1. Folk sector
     a. New immigrants and refugees use as primary source
     b. Used by individuals from all socioeconomic groups
     c. Use dependent on cause of illness and availability of healers in other sectors

G. Nurse's role
  1. Understand why different sectors are used
     a. Enables nurse to better explain goals of nursing intervention and treatments

b. Ensure patient understands advantages and disadvantages and potential incompatibilities of treatments from multiple sectors

VI. **Traditional Healers**
 A. Description
  1. Not part of popular or professional health sector
  2. Specialize in forms of healing characteristic of ethnomedicine
  3. Deal with secular, sacred, or both
  4. Combine methods from both sacred and secular
 B. Secular
  1. Use organic and technical means to treat conditions due to natural causes
  2. Types of healers
   a. Herbalist
   b. Bone setters
   c. Granny midwives
   d. Tooth extractors
   e. Injectionists
 C. Sacred
  1. Use nonorganic methods to treat supernatural and natural causes
  2. Nonorganic
   a. Semimystical and religious practices
   b. Influence mind and faith of individual
   c. Examples:
    i. Chants
    ii. Prayers
    iii. Rituals
    iv. Amulets—object worn or cherished to ward off evil or attract good fortune
   d. Types of healers
    i. Sorcerers
    ii. Shamans
    iii. Spiritualists
    iv. Voodoo priests, priestesses
    v. Diviners
 D. Nurse's Role
  1. Determine if patient receiving treatment from traditional healer
  2. Inform patient if traditional treatments and biomedical treatments are incompatible (see Table 21–1)
  3. Consult with traditional healer, if necessary, to ensure all have understanding of same goal: assisting the patient to recovery
  4. Modify plan of care if no compromise is reached
VII. **Preoperative Interview/Nursing Assessment**
 A. Develop culture sensitivity
  1. Clarify own culture and value systems
   a. Reflect on actions, thoughts, communications, and beliefs of own culture
  2. Examine personal negative opinions of different cultures
  3. Increase awareness of other cultures through churches and schools
 B. Do not project own views on patients through:
  1. Verbal communication
  2. Nonverbal communications
   a. Facial expressions
   b. Gestures
   c. Posture

Table 21-1 • TRADITIONAL HEALERS, PREPARATION, AND AREA OF PRACTICE

HEALER	PREPARATION	PRACTICE
African-American (southern urban)		
Family members, especially grandmother	Word of mouth Practical experience	*Secular:* Common, everyday self-limiting illnesses that respond to home remedies Illness prevention
Wise woman ("old lady")	Practical experience of caring for and raising own children, grandchildren, and other kin Develops reputation among family, friends, and neighbors of being knowledgeable about home remedies for common illnesses No formal training	*Secular:* Treatment and prevention of common, everyday illnesses Advice about child care and child-rearing
Herbalist		*Secular:* Diagnose a variety of natural illnesses Dispense herbs to neutralize or eliminate harmful substances that impair the power of body to heal or protect itself
Spiritualist	No formal training Power may be present at birth (twins) or given by God later in life Usually associated with fundamentalist Christian religion (Holy Ghost, Pentecostal)	*Sacred:* Cure illnesses sent by God as punishment Cure ailments beyond the power of biomedical practitioners (e.g., arthritis, hypertension, diabetes mellitus) Power of God is present in the body of the spiritualist and transferred to the ill person through laying on of hands Draws on the faith of the individual *Sacred or Secular:* May combine laying on of hands with herbal therapy, massage, and life counseling
Root doctor (root worker, conjure man or woman, voodoo priest or priestess)	Apprenticeship May be born with magical powers	*Sacred or secular:* Serve as intermediary between supernatural and natural worlds Enact or remove spells Counteract or project against witchcraft or sorcery Combine magical powers with use of herbs Read omens and signs and prescribe therapy or preventive measures Counseling and magical powers with use of herbs

Group	Healer	Training	Function
African-Caribbean (Haitian)	Family members, primarily female	Word of mouth, generation to generation; Practical experience	*Secular:* Prevention and treatment of common, everyday illnesses
	Docteur feuilles, bocars, dokte fe (leaf doctors, herbalists)	Apprenticeship training; Hands-on experience; Learn "formulas" for healing	*Secular:* Treat patients with herbs, roots, medicinal plants, and rituals; Bone setting, burn treatments, and massage
	Droquistes	Apprenticeship	*Secular:* Make and sell potions to prevent or treat illnesses of natural causation
	Houngan (voodoo priest); Mambo (voodoo priestess)	Apprenticeship training in rituals; Knowledge of prayers and herbal remedies from elders; Long training in and study of mythology of spirits	*Sacred or secular:* Treatment of illnesses due to supernatural causation (angry voodoo spirits; dead ancestors; or magic, witchcraft, or sorcery); Treatment of illnesses that are long lasting or fail to respond to biomedicine
	Sages-femme, fam saj, matrone (lay midwife, wise woman)	Apprenticeship	*Secular:* Perform deliveries, prepartum and postpartum care, treats other "female" conditions related to reproduction; Uses herbs, massage, rituals, baths, and diet
	Piqurestes (injectionists)	Training in missions and other medical facilities; Word of mouth; Practical experience	*Secular:* Give injections, change dressings
Hispanic (Puerto Rican)	Family member, especially oldest female		*Secular:* Common everyday illnesses that respond to home remedies
	Curandero or cuandera	Apprenticeship; Gift from God	*Sacred or secular:* Knowledge of herbs, diet, massage, and ritual; Commune with supernatural; Conduct religious curing ceremonies
	Partera (lay midwife)	Apprenticeship training from older female relatives	*Secular:* Prepartum and postnatal care, herbal remedies, massage, treatment of natural illnesses affecting women
	Yerbero (herbalist)	No formal training	*Secular:* Preventative and curative care; Treats both ethnomedical and biomedical illnesses affecting women
	Santiguadore (sabador)	Apprenticeship	*Secular:* Massage and manipulation of body for illnesses affecting the musculoskeletal and gastrointestinal systems

Table continued on following page

Table 21–1 • **TRADITIONAL HEALERS, PREPARATION, AND AREA OF PRACTICE** *Continued*

HEALER	PREPARATION	PRACTICE
Spiritualist (espiritualista, brujera, santero)	May be born with gift to foretell future Perfect skills through apprenticeship	*Sacred:* Prevention and diagnosis of illness due to magic, witchcraft, or sorcery; uses amulets, prayers, and other artifacts Some limited curative functions
Moslem (Iranian) Family members, especially older women	Knowledge handed down generation to generation	*Secular:* Self-care measures such as bed rest, diet, herbs, home remedies, and childbirth assistance
Dais (traditional midwife)	Apprenticeship Older women who have raised their own families	*Secular:* Prepartum and postpartum care Childbirth Newborn care Herbal therapies Massage
Mullah (religious healer)	Religious training	*Sacred:* Prevention of illnesses via preparation of tawiz (amulet with verses from the Koran) Treat emotional problems, nervousness, excessive anxiety, and mental illness
Injectionists	Self-taught	*Secular:* Administer medications prescribed by physicians Purchase and prescribe injectable medications on their own
Hakimji (traditional healer)	Apprenticeship	*Sacred or secular:* Combine procedures and medicines from Urani and Greco-Arabic medical traditions
Bonesetters	Apprenticeship	*Secular:* Sets broken bones Treats sprains, strains, dislocations, and generalized body pains

Native American (Navajo Indian)			
Family members	Knowledge handed down from generation to generation	*Secular:* Common everyday illnesses of natural origin Prevention of illness Herbal remedies
Medicine man	Born with power to heal Acquire power to heal via vision or quest Apprenticeship with medicine man once power to heal is known	*Sacred:* Diagnose and treat supernatural or natural illness (meditation, trance state, divination, or star gazing) Use combination of herbs and curing ceremonies
Diagnostician	As per medicine man	*Sacred:* Diagnose underlying cause of illness via divination
Herbalists	Knowledge passed down generation to generation Apprenticeship	*Secular:* Diagnose and treat common illnesses of natural causation

From Luckmann, J. (ed.). (1997). *Saunders Manual of Nursing Care.* Philadelphia: Saunders, pp. 37–39.

    C. Observe client's family and support system

    D. Respect the patient

        1. All cultures are unique

        2. All individuals are unique

    E. Tips for effective communication

        1. Introduce yourself

           a. Exhibit confidence; avoid arrogance

           b. Shake hands if appropriate

           c. Explain reason for your presence

           d. Explain upcoming sequence of events (admission assessment, preop holding, intraoperative, postoperative)

        2. Avoid assuming where the patient comes from; the patient will tell you if he/she wants you to know

        3. Show respect, especially to males

           a. Males are often the decision maker

           b. If patient is child or woman, male may be the one making decisions regarding care and follow-up

        4. In some cultures it is customary for children to go everywhere with parents

           a. Poorer families may not have child-care options available to them

           b. Include children in perioperative experience

        5. Understand traditional health-related practices

           a. Do not show disapproval of them

           b. If practice is potentially harmful, inform patient

        6. Be cognizant of folk illnesses and remedies for the cultural population in your service area

        7. When possible, involve leaders of local groups

           a. Leader may have understanding of problem

           b. May be able to assist in offering acceptable interventions

           c. Ensure confidentiality is maintained

        8. Accept diversity as an asset, not a liability

VIII. Health Habits

    A. Western

        1. Care providers

           a. Physician is most common care provider

           b. Physician assistants

           c. Nurse practitioners

           d. Chiropractors

           e. Doctors of osteopathy

           f. Doctors of podiatry

        2. Causes for illness

           a. Genetic

        3. Toxins

           a. Cigarettes

           b. Asbestos

           c. Environmental

        4. Dietary

           a. Inappropriate diet

           b. Excessive fat intake

           c. Excessive alcohol intake

        5. Illness is treatable or curable

        6. Focus on prevention of illness

B. Non-Western (folk medicine)
   1. Care providers
      a. Indigenous healers
         i.   Surgeons
         ii. Spiritualists
         iii. Herbalists
   2. Causes for illness
      a. Evil spirits
      b. Witches
      c. Dysfunction within the harmony of the body

IX. **Cultural Beliefs of Asians (Chinese-Americans)**
  A. Basis for health–culture beliefs and practices is holistic
    1. Oneness of all things with nature, the universe, and the divine
  B. Health
    1. Results when body works in rhythmic and finely balanced manner
    2. Body adjusts to external environment
    3. Functions and emotions are in harmony
  C. Traditional Chinese medicine (TCM)
    1. System of preventive medicine
    2. Components
       a. Tao
          i.   Way of life, virtue, heaven, and death
          ii. Individuals should:
             (a) Flow with nature
             (b) Avoid excesses and extremes
             (c) Maintain a middle position
             (d) Practice moderation
       b. *Ch'i* (vitality)
          i.   "Universal energy"
          ii. Fundamental concept of entire system of TCM
          iii. Origin of all disease
          iv. Health is balance of harmony in the flow of *ch'i*; illness results from imbalance
       c. Yin and yang
          i.   Represents duality and unity of universe and Tao
          ii. Balanced of yin and yang
             (a) The negative and positive energy forces
             (b) Gift from prior generations
             (c) Harmony and balance of physical and spiritual with nature
       d. Law of five elements
          i.   Association between external physical worlds and internal milieu of body
          ii. Includes fire, earth, metal, water, and wood
       e. Meridians and pulses
          i.   Invisible systems or pathways that carry *ch'i* through the body
          ii. Regulate organs, blood flow, and connect internal and external organs
          iii. Pulses
             (a) Present in each organ
             (b) Pulse indicates status of organ
                (i) Balance
                (ii) Imbalance
             (c) No difference among pulses indicates perfect balance

      f. Causative factors of disease
        i. Internal
           (a) Excess or lack of emotion
           (b) Constitution
           (c) Anxiety
           (d) Irregularity of food and drink
        ii. External
           (a) Cold, heat, humidity, fire, dryness, dampness, and wind
        iii. Illness results from:
           (a) Excess or deficiency of internal or external causative factors
           (b) Interruption in flow of *ch'i*
           (c) Loss of *ch'i*
           (d) Imbalance of yin and yang

D. Illness
  1. Prevented by:
    a. Conforming with nature
    b. Wearing of jade charms to prevent harm
  2. Disruption of yin and yang energy forces caused by:
    a. Overexertion
    b. Lying or sitting for prolonged periods
  3. Treatment
    a. Herbs such as ginseng
    b. Acupuncture
    c. Curing methods
      i. Cold treatments
      ii. Hot treatments (moxibustion—application of heat to skin)
E. Grief handled stoically and internalized
F. Family
  1. Is valued
  2. Act as caregivers
  3. Respect and value elders
G. Language/communication
  1. Mandarin is official language
  2. Many dialects; not all are understood by other groups
  3. Silence is valued
  4. Do not verbalize disagreements
  5. Unacceptable to display affection to opposite sex in public
  6. Excessive eye contact may be interpreted as rude
H. Death
  1. Viewed as religious experience
I. Medical conditions linked to Asians
  1. Thalassemia
  2. Lactose intolerance
J. Medical care provided by healers
K. Nursing implications
  1. Expect use of multiple sectors; attempt to accommodate alternative therapies
  2. Patient will use self-care measures; support and encourage patient
  3. Incorporate family in planning care
  4. Patient tends to be submissive, quiet, and agreeable
    a. Ability to maintain harmonious relationship supersedes disagreement
    b. Impolite to disagree with authority figures
    c. Will say "yes" even when patient does not fully understand to prevent disruption in harmony

        d. Will not openly express pain

        e. Will not ask for assistance

    5. Do not draw large amounts of blood from patient

        a. Blood contains *ch'i*

        b. Vital energy for TCM

    6. Avoid lengthy conversations and questioning of patient

        a. May confuse patient or convey incompetence

        b. Combine health teaching with interactive techniques and demonstration

X. Cultural Beliefs of Hispanics (Puerto Rican-American)

  A. Basis for health–culture beliefs and practices is holistic

  B. Health

    1. Luck or gift from God

    2. Balance/harmony among mind, body, spirit, and nature

        a. Forces of "hot" and "cold," "wet" and "dry"

    3. Maintain equilibrium through

        a. Proper balanced diet

        b. Avoiding conflict

        c. Moderate lifestyle

        d. Sharing resources with others

        e. Honoring God

    4. Maintain health by:

        a. Praying to God

        b. Consumption of herbs and spices

        c. Wearing amulets

        d. Keeping religious materials in home

        e. Proper conduct

        f. Proper nutrition

  C. Illness

    1. Caused by God as punishment for misconduct

    2. Cause may be natural or supernatural

    3. Cause determined by:

        a. Previous social behavior

        b. Religious behavior

    4. Spiritism

        a. Supernatural illness

        b. Cause is external force

        c. Individual is "passive" instrument in treatment

        d. Failure of patient to respond to biomedical treatment may confirm presence of supernatural cause

  D. Family

    1. Respect for one another is important

    2. Plays key role in health care

    3. Strong sense of family, both nuclear and extended

        a. Needs of family supersede needs of individual

        b. Men are dominant providers, women are homemakers

        c. Female health consultant is oldest female in family

  E. Treatment

    1. Medical care provided by western and non-western (healers)

    2. Healer *(curandero)*

        a. Cures hot illness with cold medicine and vice versa

        b. Uses massage and cleanings

        c. May use herbs and spices for prevention and healing

3. *Brujo*
   a. Uses witchcraft for healing illnesses related to jealousy and envy
F. Medical conditions linked to Hispanics
   1. Diabetes mellitus
   2. Tuberculosis
G. Language/communication
   1. Primary language is Spanish
   2. Direct confrontation considered rude and disrespectful
H. Death
   1. Predominantly Catholic
   2. Believe in heaven and hell
   3. Administration of sacraments of the sick is important
I. Nursing implications
   1. Key cultural concepts
      a. Respect
         i.   Treat others and expect to be treated with dignity and respect
              (a) Professional attire
              (b) Correct tone of voice
              (c) Professional image
              (d) Providing proper explanations for treatments
              (e) Answering all questions completely
              (f) Allowing patient opportunity to express his/her feelings
         ii. *Personalismo:* treating each patient as an individual
              (a) Establish rapport with patient initially
              (b) Touch arm, shoulder, or back during interactions
              (c) Allow patient opportunity to express concerns
              (d) Take initiative to learn a few words in Spanish
   2. Expect full physical for any complaint or problem
   3. Very expressive, dramatic
      a. Cultural norm
   4. Difficult to express degree or location of pain
   5. Prefer Hispanic health-care professional
      a. Understand and respect traditional health-care beliefs
XI. **Cultural Beliefs of Native Americans (Navajo Indians)**
   A. Basis of traditional Navajo health–culture beliefs and practices is holistic
      1. Health achieved by living in harmony with universe
      2. Individuals have spiritual and physical dimensions
      3. Physical dimension
         a. Individuals treat bodies and nature with respect
      4. Spiritual dimension
         a. Individuals participate in development of own potential through will or volition
      5. World is governed by supernatural powers and holy people
         a. Failure to honor supernatural results in lack of harmony
         b. Harmony essential for good health
   B. Cultural traditions
      1. Emphasize cooperation rather than competitiveness
      2. Share and give to others
      3. Continue to develop self throughout lifetime
      4. Believe nature is more powerful than humans
      5. Respect elders
      6. Welfare and security of family more important than individual success
      7. Strive to live in balance with nature

C. Health
  1. Harmony within self and environment
  2. Ability to survive under difficult circumstances
D. Illness
  1. Caused by disharmony within self and environment
    a. Action of witches
    b. Disturbing physical world
    c. Angering the spirit world
    d. Failure to follow established rituals
    e. Not taking care of self
    f. Failure to observe moderation and balance in all things
    g. Being disrespectful
  2. Do not believe in infection, communicable agents, or physiologic processes
  3. Do not believe in germ theory
  4. Prevention by rituals
E. Healing
  1. Occurs when ill person becomes one with holy people
  2. Establishes harmony with universe
F. Treatment
  1. Biomedical and ethnomedical systems sought for treatment
  2. Medical care provided by Medicine Man
    a. Healing achieved only through ethnomedicine
    b. Healing cannot be separated from religion and individual spirituality
    c. Chanting used at traditional healing ceremonies
      i.   Used to diagnose and restore balance
  3. Nature is powerful force
  4. Medicine, rest, diet, isolation, and sweat baths
  5. Medications made of herbs and plants
  6. In order for medication to be effective, it must be administered according to proper ceremony
G. Family
  1. Should be included for nursing care
  2. Strong sense of community/extended family
H. Prevention of illness
  1. Wearing of amulets to ward off illness or witchcraft
  2. Amulets can be bags of herbs, fetishes, or other symbolic objects that are believed to have curative or protective powers
  3. Blessing occurs at important events
    a. Enhance good fortune, happiness, and health
I. Medical conditions associated with Native Americans
  1. Lactose intolerance
  2. Tuberculosis
J. Language/communication
  1. Navajo or English
  2. Silence shows respect
  3. Eye contact avoided
XII. **Cultural Beliefs of African-Americans**
  A. Basis of health–culture beliefs and practices is magicoreligious and holistic
    1. Perceptions about health and illness come from popular, ethnomedical, and biomedical health culture
    2. Little distinction between science and religion, or body and mind
    3. Good health equates to good fortune

        4. Illness viewed as misfortune
- B. Health
  1. Is synonymous with good luck
  2. Is harmony with nature
- C. Illness
  1. Causes
     a. Disharmony with nature
     b. Demons
     c. Personal tragedy
  2. Classified as natural and unnatural
  3. Natural illness caused by failure to follow three laws of nature (God's law)
     a. Humans are bound by same laws of nature
     b. Humans are to know, love, and serve God
     c. Humans are to love each other
  4. Unnatural illness caused by God withdrawing divine protection
     a. Makes person vulnerable to evil influences
     b. Devil is in control
     c. Evil influences not responsive to treatment
  5. Individuals vulnerable to illness
     a. Elderly
     b. Young
     c. Women
     d. Unborn fetus
- D. Treatment
  1. Medical care by both western and non-western
  2. Cannot be separated from religious beliefs and practices
  3. Occurs around practice of religious ceremonies
  4. Prevention by:
     a. Proper nutrition
     b. Adequate rest
     c. Taking care of relationship with God, nature, and others
- E. Family
  1. Strong family ties
  2. Extended family assists with health care
- F. Medical conditions linked to African-Americans
  1. Sickle cell anemia
  2. Hypertension

XIII. Cultural Beliefs of Haitian-Americans (Caribbean)
- A. Basis of health–culture beliefs is magicoreligious and holistic
  1. Believe in healing power of Christian God
  2. Believe in traditional folk religion such as voodoo
     a. Maintaining health and recovery from illness depends on faith
     b. Power of supernatural works in conjunction with traditional healers and biomedical health-care providers
     c. Usually seek biomedical care after appropriate rituals performed
- B. Health
  1. Ability to carry out activities of daily living
     a. Looks well
     b. Good appetite
     c. Shiny skin
     d. Bright eyes
     e. Good color
     f. Able to move about without pain

C. Illness
   1. Natural
      a. Dominant illnesses
   2. Supernatural
      a. Rare
      b. Suspected when:
         i.   Child becomes ill or dies
         ii. Home remedies, biomedicine, or treatments from secular healers do not work
         iii. Social conflict occurs prior to symptoms
         iv. Sudden onset
         v.   Illness becomes life-threatening
         vi. Other misfortunes occur at same time
         vii. Occurs after one has good fortune; caused by envy and anger of others
D. Family
   1. Rely on family, kin, and friends
   2. Usually use extended family
   3. Health care in home managed by grandmother, mother, or maternal aunt
   4. Older siblings care for younger siblings
E. Nursing implications
   1. Patient may regard questions with suspicion
      a. Keep questions to a minimum
      b. Explain reason for questions
      c. If health-care practitioner asks too many questions, may be viewed as lacking competence
   2. Oral medications not so effective as parenteral
   3. View vitamin injections as important for maintaining blood
   4. Explain reason for all blood tests; very concerned about status of their blood
   5. Commonly use purgatives with castor oil
      a. Assess for signs and symptoms of dehydration, especially in children
   6. Have difficulty expressing location of pain
      a. Have patient point to area
      b. Give opportunity for patient to describe pain
      c. Not accustomed to using pain rating scales to describe intensity

XIV. **Cultural Beliefs of White or Anglo-Americans**
   A. Basis of health–culture beliefs and practices is scientific
      1. Incorporate variety of self-care measures and home remedies
      2. Number of illness episodes brought to health-care practitioner are limited
      3. Faith in God
         a. Assists in protecting from illness
         b. Aids in recovery
         c. Assists in coping with illness
         d. May consider illness as punishment from God
      4. Supernatural causes
         a. Evil eye and curses
   B. Health
      1. Absence of illness
      2. Ability to function in acceptable manner
   C. Illness
      1. Interferes with ability to function in acceptable manner
      2. Experienced when:
         a. Pain occurs
         b. Changes in bodily feelings or functions occur

        3. Most illnesses due to natural causes
        4. Dominant theory is germ theory
    D. Prevention
        1. Diet and nutrition
        2. Taking vitamins, minerals, and tonics
        3. Exercising
        4. Maintaining normal bowel function
        5. Moderate lifestyle
        6. Adequate sleep and rest
    E. Family
        1. Structure usually nuclear family only
        2. Spouse generally main health consultant
        3. Mother or wife primary caregiver
            a. Diagnoses illness when it occurs
    F. Nursing implications
        1. Wide variation among groups
        2. Some groups have difficulty expressing signs and symptoms
        3. May not openly express pain
XV. **Aspects of Communication**
    A. Communication techniques
        1. Use open-ended questions
        2. Approach in nonthreatening manner
        3. Allow time for patient's responses
        4. Do not hurry through interview
        5. Use professional interpreters whenever possible; patient may be more willing to give important health history information through stranger than family member (especially information regarding sexual matters)
        6. Avoid use of medical terms; use language appropriate to patient's level of understanding
        7. Use language dictionary appropriate to culture
        8. Use pictures and gestures
        9. Speak slowly
    B. Culture specific—verbal
        1. Chinese-Americans
            a. Soft tone
            b. Slow speech with silence at times
            c. Silence is valued
        2. Hispanics
            a. Loud tone
            b. Rapid speech
        3. Native Americans
            a. Soft tone
            b. Slow speech with silence at times
        4. African-Americans
            a. Loud tone
            b. Rapid speech
    C. Culture specific—nonverbal
        1. Chinese-Americans
            a. Avoid eye contact
            b. Discomfort expressed privately
            c. Avoid excessive touch

2. Hispanics
   a. Maintain eye contact
   b. Discomfort expressed openly
   c. Tactile culture
3. Native Americans
   a. Respect indicated by avoiding eye contact
   b. Respect indicated by periods of silence
   c. Discomfort expressed privately
   d. Light touch or hand passing
4. Orthodox Jews
   a. Eye contact may have sexual connotation
   b. Older male to female other than wife
   c. Tactile culture
5. African-Americans
   a. Maintain eye contact (avoid prolonged eye contact)
   b. Open display of discomfort

XVI. Nutritional Concerns
A. Ethnic/religious food preferences
   1. Chinese-Americans
      a. Prefer rice with all meals
   2. Native Americans
      a. Usually consists of corn, beans, and squash
   3. African-Americans
      a. Prefer salted and spiced foods
      b. High intake of yellow and dark green leafy vegetables
   4. Hispanics
      a. Foods and illness have varying degrees of "hot" and "cold" (not related to temperature of food)
      b. Easier to digest hot foods—chili peppers, onions, garlic
      c. Cold foods include fresh vegetables, corn, beans, squash, tropical fruits
   5. Jehovah's Witnesses
      a. No food that blood is an additive, such as lunch meats
   6. Seventh-Day Adventists
      a. Avoid meat or foods with shells
      b. Avoid caffeine
      c. Vegetarian diet encouraged
      d. Protein deficiency may need to be considered
   7. Jews
      a. Consider pigs unholy or unclean
      b. Pork products not allowed
      c. Cannot mix meat with milk
      d. Kosher products
   8. Muslim
      a. No pork or food products made with pork
      b. No animal fat shortening
   9. Manner of preparation
      a. Identify any cultural preconditions
   10. Frequency
      a. Identify any cultural requisites
   11. Nursing implications
      a. Incorporate normal diet into postoperative plan of care
      b. Consult with nutritionist if areas of concern are identified

XVII. Spiritual/Religious Needs
A. Practices pertaining to health care
  1. Availability of spiritual resources
  2. Pray before meals
  3. Religious articles made available
B. Chinese
  1. Taoism
  2. Buddhism
  3. Islam
  4. Christianity
C. Hispanics
  1. Catholicism
D. Christian Science
  1. Prayer heals the body
  2. Children treated by Christian Science practitioners only
E. Jehovah's Witnesses
  1. Opposed to homologous blood transfusions
  2. May submit to autologous blood transfusions
  3. May refuse surgery if blood transfusion is required
  4. Do not partake in national holidays including Christmas
F. Seventh-Day Adventists
  1. Belief that their body is a temple of God
  2. Avoidance of meat, caffeine, drugs, tobacco, and alcohol
  3. May refuse foods with shells (lobster, crab)
G. Nursing implications
  1. Be cognizant of patient's religious needs
  2. Patient may request private time prior to procedure (preoperative holding)

XVIII. Perioperative Nursing Considerations
A. Preoperative teaching
  1. Be alert and sensitive to cultural differences
  2. Differences may:
    a. Dictate type of teaching method based on patient's learning style
    b. Show variation in patient's educational needs
    c. Cause variation in patient's response to teaching
    d. Cause variations in patient's discharge plan
B. Consent
  1. Decision for surgery may be made by head of family or group of elders in a religious community
  2. Decision-maker and patient must understand importance of surgery
  3. Ensure consent forms signed appropriately, according to facility policy
C. Body hair
  1. Shaving may violate some cultural beliefs and practices
    a. Sikh religion (East India): forbids shaving of hair
    b. Greece: manhood is linked to body hair
    c. Native Americans: body hair sign of health and strength
D. Removal of jewelry
  1. Some cultures view as religious articles
  2. Not permitted to be removed from body
    a. If site interferes with surgery, may consent to placement of article on another part of body
    b. May need to be secured (taped) on person prior to procedure
    c. Document presence of article in nursing record

  E. Pain
    1. Emphasize that it is acceptable to express pain
      a. Patient may not verbalize or may continue to deny pain
      b. Incorporate nonverbal patient reactions into nursing assessment of pain
      c. Medicate as necessary
    2. Cultural belief to express stoic attitude toward pain
      a. Patient may refuse pain medication
    3. Meditation
      a. Used by Eastern religions
      b. Relaxation techniques may be helpful in minimizing postoperative pain
  F. Postoperative dietary needs
    1. Incorporate cultural food practices into dietary teaching for the postoperative patient
  G. Geriatric considerations
    1. Nursing approach
      a. Elderly person is unique individual
      b. Avoid imposing own attitude and belief toward aging on the patient
XIX. **Loss of Privacy Throughout Perioperative Experience**
  A. History and physical
    1. Use of touch during assessment: respect individual's cultural practice
    2. Need to remove clothing: respect individual's cultural practice; accommodate patient's requests
    3. Communication with physician regarding "taboo" topics
      a. Incorporate cultural practices into plan of care if appropriate
  B. Exposure during perioperative experience
    1. Reinforce confidentiality; respect cultural practices; accommodate patient requests
    2. Keep personnel to a safe minimum
    3. Avoid overexposure
XX. **Personal Space**
  A. Determined by individual cultures
    1. Close personal space
      a. Chinese-Americans
      b. Hispanics
      c. Native Americans
      d. African-Americans
    2. Distant personal space
      a. Whites

Bibliography

1. Giger, J., Davidhizar, R. (1995). *Transcultural Nursing, Assessment & Intervention.*
2. Kozier, B., Erb, G., Blais, K., Wilkinson, J.M. (1995). *Fundamentals of Nursing,* 5th ed. Redwood City, CA: Addison-Wesley Nursing.
3. Leininger, M. (1991). Transcultural nursing: The study and practice field. *Imprint,* 38(2):55–66.
4. Luckmann, J. (ed). (1997). *Saunders Manual of Nursing Care.* Philadelphia: Saunders.
5. Smith, C., Maurer, F. (1995). *Community Health Nursing, Theory and Practice.* Philadelphia: Saunders.

REVIEW QUESTIONS

1. Culture
   (1) Is an integrated system of learned values, beliefs, and practices
   (2) Is a characteristic of a society
   (3) Encompasses genetic responses to illness
   (4) Is guided by an individual's thoughts, feelings, and actions

   A. 1, 2
   B. 1, 2, 3
   C. 1, 2, 4
   D. 2, 3, 4
   E. All of the above

2. Transcultural nursing focuses on differences and similarities among cultures with respect to
   (1) Human care
   (2) Health or well-being
   (3) Genetics
   (4) Illness

   A. 1, 2
   B. 1, 2, 4
   C. 2, 3, 4
   D. 1, 3, 4
   E. All of the above

3. Major world views of health and illness include all of the following except

   A. Folk
   B. Biomedical (scientific)
   C. Holistic
   D. Magicoreligious

4. Activities provided by care providers in the popular sector include all of the following except

   A. Self care administered using home remedies
   B. Over-the-counter medications
   C. Consultation with family, friends, clergy, neighbors, and others who have had the same disease
   D. Incorporating rituals to prevent illness and misfortune into treatments

5. Traditional healers of the secular type include all of the following except:

   A. Spiritualists
   B. Herbalists
   C. Bonesetters
   D. Injectionists
   E. Midwives

6. Hispanics believe that equilibrium is maintained through
   (1) Proper balanced diet
   (2) Avoiding conflict
   (3) Maintaining a moderate lifestyle
   (4) Sharing resources with others
   (5) Honoring God

   A. 1, 3, 5
   B. 2, 3, 5
   C. 1, 4, 5
   D. 1, 2, 4
   E. All of the above

7. Which ethnic group does not believe in illness being caused by infection, communicable agents, or physiologic processes?

   A. Hispanics
   B. African-Americans
   C. Native Americans
   D. African-Caribbean
   E. Asian, Chinese-Americans

8. Failure to follow the three laws of nature (God's law) is the belief of which ethnic group?

   A. Hispanics
   B. African-Americans
   C. Native Americans
   D. African-Caribbean
   E. Asian, Chinese-Americans

9. The most important reason for the use of professional interpreters during interactions with patients undergoing health-care interventions is because

A. They can interpret medical terminology
B. They are easily available in all health-care settings
C. The patient may be more at ease giving a stranger personal information rather than a close family member
D. Family members may not be truthful in their interpretation of information

10. Effective communication with culturally diverse populations requires health-care professionals to
   (1) Exhibit confidence
   (2) Show respect
   (3) Understand traditional health-related practices
   (4) Accept diversity as an asset, not a liability
   (5) Be cognizant of folk illnesses and remedies for the cultural population in the area served

A. 1, 2, 3
B. 2, 3, 5
C. 2, 3, 4, 5
D. 1, 2, 3, 5
E. All of the above

ANSWERS TO QUESTIONS

1. C
2. B
3. A
4. D
5. A

6. E
7. C
8. B
9. C
10. E

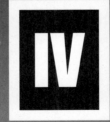

PART

IV

Anesthesia
Review

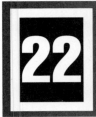

Anesthetic Agents for Ambulatory Surgery (Adults and Pediatrics)

Lois Schick
Exempla Healthcare, Saint Joseph Hospital
Denver, Colorado

I. Definitions

Consider anesthesia as a continuum from conscious state to an unconscious state.

A. Conscious state
   1. Patient remains conscious
   2. May have alteration of mood and/or relief of anxiety
   3. Some analgesia
   4. Protective reflexes remain intact
B. Conscious sedation or monitored anesthesia care (MAC)
   1. Minimally depressed level of consciousness
   2. Patient maintains patent airway independently and continuously
   3. Patient responds to verbal commands
   4. Patient does not lose consciousness
   5. When provided by anesthesiologist is known as monitored anesthesia care (MAC)
C. Deep sedation
   1. Patient may sleep but is arousable
   2. Partial or complete loss of protective reflexes
D. Unconsciousness
   1. Patient incapable of appropriate response to command
   2. Respiration is automatic and involuntary
   3. Breathing response to blood CO_2 levels
   4. Muscle tonus lost
   5. Diminished to absent reflexes depending on depth of anesthesia

1. List inhalation agents used by anesthesia.
2. Differentiate between depolarizing and nondepolarizing muscle relaxants.
3. Describe anesthetic options used today.
4. Identify reversal agents used for narcotics and benzodiazepines.
5. List contraindications for regional techniques.

413

E. General anesthesia
  1. Controlled state of unconsciousness
  2. Patient cannot be aroused
  3. Reversible state providing:
     a. Analgesia
     b. Sedation
     c. Appropriate muscle relaxation
     d. Appropriate control of autonomic nervous system
     e. Partial or complete loss of protective reflexes
F. Regional anesthesia
  1. Production of analgesia and anesthesia in a part of the body
  2. Types of blocks
     a. Topical: anesthetic agent applied to surface (skin, mucous membrane, urethra, nose, or pharynx)
     b. Infiltration: injection of local anesthetic into tissue to be cut
     c. Peripheral nerve blocks: injection of local anesthetic at a specific site to block conduction of impulses
        i.   Plexus block—cervical, brachial, lumbosacral, perivascular
        ii. Upper or lower peripheral nerve blocks—intercostal, elbow, wrist, ankle
        iii. Intravenous—bier
        iv. Sympathetic blocks—stellate ganglion, celiac plexus, lumbar paravertebral
     d. Conduction anesthesia
        i.   Depositing local anesthetic agent into nerve or nerves that supply a region of the body
        ii. Eliminates sensation or motor control or both
        iii. Types:
             (a) Spinal
                 (i) Administration of local anesthetic into the lumbar intrathecal space
                 (ii) Local anesthetic blocks conduction in the spinal nerve roots, dorsal root ganglia, and the periphery of spinal cord
             (b) Epidural
                 (i) Injecting the local anesthetic into the extradural space

II. Premedication
  A. Tranquilizers/benzodiazepines
    1. Agents
       a. Diazepam (Valium)
       b. Midazolam (Versed)
       c. Lorazepam (Ativan)
    2. Advantages
       a. Effective anxiolytic
       b. Amnesia
       c. Patient acceptance high
       d. Physiologic stress decreased
       e. Midazolam burns less on injection
    3. Disadvantages/risks
       a. Depression of central nervous system (CNS) with profound sedation
       b. Compromised respiratory function
       c. Diazepam burns on injection—potential phlebitis
       d. Prolonged sedation especially with diazepam
          i.   Elderly
          ii. Patients with severe liver dysfunction

B. Narcotics/opioids
  1. Action
    a. Blunt cardiovascular response to surgical stimulus
    b. Decrease requirement for inhalation agents
    c. Provides analgesia
  2. Agents
    a. Morphine sulfate
    b. Meperidine (Demerol)
    c. Fentanyl (Sublimaze)
      i.   Short-acting due to lipid solubility
      ii. No histamine release
    d. Alfentanil (Alfenta)
      i.   One-tenth as potent as fentanyl
      ii. One-third the duration of fentanyl
      iii. Rapid onset and brief duration
      iv. Patients may require longer-acting narcotics for pain relief
    e. Sufentanil (Sufenta)
      i.   Potency 5–7 times that of fentanyl
      ii. May see decreased respiratory drive or increased airway resistance
      iii. May see chest wall rigidity
    f. Remifentanil (Ultiva)
      i.   Extremely short-acting
      ii. Broken down by cholinesterases, therefore do not need to rely on liver
           for metabolism
      iii. Patients may require longer-acting narcotics for pain relief
  3. Disadvantages
    a. Nausea and vomiting due to direct stimulation of chemoreceptor trigger
       zone (CTZ)
    b. Narcotic depressants enhanced with:
      i.   Phenothiazines
      ii. Monoamine oxidase inhibitors (MOA)
      iii. Tricyclic antidepressants
    c. Respiratory depression varies according to:
      i.   Medication dose
      ii. Pre-existing pulmonary disease
      iii. Patient age
      iv. Other medications
C. Antiemetics (no antiemetic is completely effective in treating nausea and vomiting)
  1. Agents
    a. Ondansetron (Zofran)—serotonin receptor antagonist
      i.   Prevents nausea and vomiting without prolonged sedation
      ii. Does not affect respiratory function
      iii. Does not affect cardiovascular function
      iv. Metabolized by liver
    b. Droperidol (Inapsine)
      i.   Causes sedation—potentiates CNS depressants and narcotics
      ii. May be accompanied by dysphoria
      iii. May cause extrapyramidal effects
      iv. May cause hypotension
      v.   May cause vasodilatation
    c. Metoclopramide (Reglan)
      i.   Increases lower esophageal sphincter pressure
      ii. Speeds gastric emptying

        iii.   Prevents/alleviates nausea and vomiting
        iv.   May cause dysphoria or extrapyramidal reactions
        v.   Gastrokinetic action is contraindicated in bowel obstruction
    d. Hydroxyzine (Vistaril, Atarax)
        i.   Antihistamine
        ii.   Potentiates barbiturates, narcotics, and CNS depressants
    e. Prochlorperazine (Compazine)
        i.   Phenothiazine, antiemetic, antipsychotic
        ii.   Potentiates sedation
        iii.   Depresses cough reflex
    f. Promethazine (Phenergan)
        i.   Dopaminergic receptor antagonist
        ii.   Some histamine properties
    g. Ephedrine
        i.   Sympathomimetic vasoconstrictor
  2. Advantages
    a. Decreased aspiration potential in high-risk patients
        i.   Peptic ulcer disease
        ii.   Hiatal hernia
        iii.   Obesity
        iv.   History of emesis
        v.   Young females
    b. Avoid dangerous and unpleasant vomiting causing:
        i.   Bleeding
        ii.   Tearing or rupture
        iii.   Electrolyte imbalance
        iv.   Increased pain
    c. Prevents or diminishes nausea and vomiting following emetic-producing procedures
        i.   Laparoscopy
        ii.   Orchiopexy
        iii.   Strabismus
        iv.   Otologic procedures
        v.   Nasal/nasopharyngeal procedures
    d. Administer prior to predisposing factors
        i.   Use of narcotics
        ii.   Use of nitrous oxide
        iii.   Gastric distention
        iv.   Severe pain
        v.   Postural hypotension
        vi.   Hypoxia
D. Anticholinergics (no longer routinely administered preoperatively)
  1. Agents
    a. Atropine
    b. Glycopyrrolate (Robinul)
    c. Scopolamine
  2. Advantages
    a. Antisialagogue
        i.   Dries the mouth
        ii.   Given prior to airway manipulation
    b. Vagolytic
        i.   Bradycardia stimulus

   3. Disadvantages
      a. Dry mouth
      b. Sore throat
      c. CNS toxicity
         i.   Delirium
         ii. Restlessness
         iii. Confusion
      d. Augment tachycardia
      e. Augment dysrhythmias
      f. Avoid with glaucoma
         i.   Dilates pupils
         ii. Causes blurred vision
         iii. Causes photophobia
   E. Histamine blockers (H2 receptor blocking agent inhibit gastric acid secretion)
      1. Agents
         a. Cimetadine (Tagamet)
         b. Ranitidine (Zantac)
         c. Famotidine (Pepcid)
      2. Advantages
         a. Most effective when administered orally
            i.   One to one-and-a-half hours prior to induction
            ii. Morning of surgery
         b. Indicated for patients at risk for acid aspiration syndrome (AAS)
            i.   Obese patients
            ii. Pregnant patients
            iii. Patients with gastrointestinal disorders
      3. Disadvantages
         a. Cimetadine prolongs elimination of:
            i.   Theophyllin
            ii. Diazepam (Valium)
            iii. Propranolol (Inderal)
            iv. Lidocaine (Xylocaine)
            v.   Metronidazole (Flagyl)
            vi. Warfarin-type anticoagulants
         b. Doses in patients with renal failure require reduction by 50%
         c. May increase creatine (nitrogenous compound found mainly in muscle tissues)
   F. Gastrokinetic agents (stimulates gastric motility)
      1. Metoclopramide (Reglan)
         a. Increase gastric emptying
         b. Lower esophageal sphincter tone
         c. Relax pylorus and duodenum
         d. Antiemetic effect
      2. Cisapride (Propulsid)
         a. Treat gastroesophageal reflux
         b. Causes less sedation
         c. Reduces delay in gastric emptying
         d. Duration of action longer than metoclopramide
III. **Inhalation Agents**
   A. Indications
      1. Administered for maintenance of general anesthesia

2. Used for induction particularly in pediatric patients
3. Rapid induction
4. Insoluble agents provide rapid onset and rapid emergence

B. Nitrous Oxide
  1. Properties
    a. Light anesthetic
    b. Combined with other anesthetics to potentiate their action
    c. Insoluble
  2. Advantages
    a. Analgesic
    b. Amnesic
    c. Combines with other agents
    d. Rapidly absorbed through the lungs
    e. Excreted rapidly through the lungs with small amount through the skin
    f. Not thought to undergo biotransformation
  3. Disadvantages
    a. Increases pressure within air-containing spaces
    b. Can diffuse into endotracheal cuff markedly increasing cuff pressure
    c. Postoperative nausea and vomiting
    d. Rapid movement from blood to the alveoli, therefore results in potential for diffusion hypoxia
    e. Oxygen is indicated for 5–10 minutes after discontinuation to avoid diffusion hypoxia
    f. Mild respiratory and myocardial depressant

C. Halothane (Fluothane)
  1. Properties
    a. Nonflammable liquid
    b. Fruity, non-irritating odor
    c. Often combined with nitrous oxide
    d. Saturated hydrocarbon
    e. 60–80% eliminated by lungs unchanged; 20–40% metabolized by liver
  2. Advantages
    a. Favorite pediatric and pre-adolescent agent
      i.   Less noxious odor
      ii. Less irritating to airway
    b. Bronchodilator, therefore drug of choice in pre-existing airway pathology
      i.   Asthma
      ii. Smoking
      iii. COPD
  3. Disadvantages
    a. Untoward cardiovascular effects
      i.   Hypotension
      ii. Decreased cardiac output
      iii. Decreased heart rate
    b. Ventricular dysrhythmias
      i.   Avoid respiratory acidosis
      ii. Avoid hypoxia
      iii. Avoid light anesthesia
      iv. Avoid subcutaneous or parenteral epinephrine
    c. Postoperative shivering
    d. Depresses mucociliary function up to 6 hours

    e. Depresses pharyngeal reflex increasing chance of aspiration

    f. Avoid in patient with liver dysfunction

    g. Avoid use on patients undergoing repetitive procedures

    h. May trigger malignant hyperthermia

D. Enflurane (Ethrane)

  1. Properties

    a. Volatile liquid halogenated ether

    b. Potent evaporative vapors

    c. General anesthesia produced at low concentrations: 25%—minimal alveolar concentration (MAC)

    d. Absorbed by lungs: 80–95% excreted by lungs and 2–5% excreted by liver

  2. Advantages

    a. Vascular dilatation may be used to produce deliberate hypotension

    b. May cause less nausea and vomiting in PACU

    c. Produces dose-related muscle relaxation

    d. Potentiates effects of nondepolarizing muscle relaxants

    e. Suited for ambulatory surgery because of rapid recovery

  3. Disadvantages

    a. Lowers seizure threshold

    b. Moderately pungent

    c. May precipitate:

      i.   Hiccoughs

      ii. Laryngospasm

      iii. Breath holding

    d. Lipid soluble, therefore prolonged duration in obese patients

    e. Could cause profound cardiovascular depression

    f. May trigger malignant hyperthermia

E. Isoflurane (Forane)

  1. Properties

    a. Nonflammable

    b. Volatile pungent halogenated ether with ether-like odor

  2. Benefits

    a. Agent for those requiring stable cardiovascular effect

    b. Rapid recovery (absorption/excretion almost exclusively by lungs)

    c. Less nausea and vomiting than halothane

    d. Produces muscle relaxation

    e. Potentiates nondepolarizing muscle relaxants

    f. Successful ambulatory agent for both short and long procedures

    g. Low potential for toxicity

F. Desflurane (Suprane)

  1. Properties

    a. Potent nonflammable fluorinated ether

    b. Strong pungent odor

  2. Advantages

    a. Rapid induction

    b. Rapid recovery

    c. Minimal metabolism

    d. Elimination almost exclusively by the lungs

    e. Safe and effective for *maintenance* in children

  3. Disadvantages

    a. Strong vasodilator

    b. Dose-related respiratory depression

      c. Dose-related cardiovascular depression
      d. Greater airway irritant than isoflurane
      e. Requires expensive vaporizer
      f. May see:
         i.   Breath holding
         ii.   Apnea
         iii. Laryngospasm
      g. May trigger malignant hyperthermia
      h. Not recommended as *induction* agent in children

  G. Sevoflurane (Ultane)
    1. Properties
      a. Less soluble than desflurane
      b. Halogenated ether
    2. Advantages
      a. Rapid onset and rapid recovery
      b. Little pungency
      c. Produces minimal airway irritation allowing anesthesia induction with a mask
      d. Does not sensitize heart to catecholamines
      e. Strong vasodilator
      f. Does not depress kidney or liver functions
    3. Disadvantages
      a. Respiratory depressant
      b. Metabolites include fluoride and hexafluoropropanol which do not show evidence of toxicity
      c. May trigger malignant hyperthermia
      d. Expensive

IV. Intravenous Medications
  A. Barbiturates
    1. Thiopental (Sodium Pentothal)
      a. Properties
         i.   Produces unconsciousness in 30 seconds
         ii.   Elimination half-life is 10–12 hours
      b. Advantages
         i.   Rapid pleasant induction
         ii.   Used as sole anesthetic
            (a) Electroconvulsive therapy (ECT)
            (b) Cardioversion
      c. Disadvantages
         i.   No analgesia
         ii.   Cardiovascular impact
            (a) Decrease arterial blood pressure
            (b) Decrease cardiac output
            (c) Increase heart rate
            (d) Venous irritation
         iii. Respiratory impact
            (a) Decrease tidal volume
            (b) Apnea may occur
         iv. Garlic taste
         v.   Fatty tissue functions as reservoir with slow release in obese patients, therefore prolonged somnolence seen
         vi. Yawning, hiccoughing, and occasional laryngospasm

2. Methohexital (Brevital)
    a. Properties
        i.   Ultra short-acting barbiturate
        ii.   Rapid recovery (with 4–7 minutes)
    b. Advantages
        i.   Used in short procedures
           (a) ECT
           (b) Prior to blocks
               (i)   Retrobulbar or peribulbar
               (ii) Regional
               (iii) Local
           (c) Cystoscopy
           (d) Dental
        ii.   May be used rectally
           (a) Uncooperative patients
           (b) Young patients
        iii. Rapid psychomotor function recovery
    c. Disadvantages
        i.   Slower recovery of fine motor skills
        ii.   Burns on administration
        iii. Administer slowly
           (a) Tremors minimized
           (b) Muscle twitching minimized

B. Benzodiazepines
  1. Diazepam (Valium)
    a. Properties
        i.   Rapid onset of sedation (1–5 minutes)
        ii.   Duration 2–6 hours
        iii. Half-life 20–40 hours
        iv. Potent amnesic
        v.   Effective anxiolysis
        vi. Hepatic metabolism and renal excretion
    b. Advantages
        i.   Use alone or with opioids
        ii.   Anticonvulsant
        iii. Mild muscle relaxant
    c. Disadvantages
        i.   Not compatible with IV solutions or other medications
        ii.   High lipid solubility, therefore storage in fatty tissues
        iii. Burns on administration
        iv. Venous irritation and phlebitis
        v.   May cause respiratory depression
  2. Midazolam (Versed)
    a. Properties
        i.   Rapid onset of sedation (3–5 minutes)
        ii.   Short duration of action (2–6 hours)
        iii. Half-life 1.2–12.3 hours
        iv. Potent amnesic
        v.   Effective anxiolytic
        vi. Hepatic clearance ten times faster than Diazepam
    b. Advantages
        i.   Use alone or with opioids
        ii.   Provides sedation and tranquility

        iii.   Water soluble so does not burn on injection
        iv.   Patient acceptance high
    c. Disadvantages
        i.   Vital signs fluctuate
        ii.   Hypotension
        iii.   Hiccoughs
        iv.   Over sedation
        v.   Apnea
  3. Lorazepam (Ativan)
    a. Properties
        i.   5–10 times more potent than valium
        ii.   Onset 15–20 minutes
        iii.   Moderate duration of action (6–8 hours)
        iv.   Shorter elimination half-life (16 hours)
        v.   Renal and hepatic elimination
    b. Advantages
        i.   Anticonvulsant action
        ii.   Minimal cardiovascular effects
        iii.   Minimal sedation
        iv.   Good amnesia
    c. Disadvantages
        i.   Poor IV compatibility
        ii.   Slow onset and long duration
C. Nonbarbiturates/Hypnotics
  1. Propofol (Diprivan)
    a. Properties
        i.   Rapid distribution and elimination
        ii.   Onset 40–80 seconds
        iii.   Duration of action 10–20 minutes
        iv.   Twice as potent as Thiopental
        v.   Short elimination half-life (2–8 minutes)
    b. Advantages
        i.   Rapid recovery of consciousness
        ii.   Rapid return of psychomotor abilities
        iii.   Low incidence of nausea and vomiting
        iv.   Low doses may produce conscious sedation
    c. Disadvantages
        i.   Depressed myocardial contractility
        ii.   Venous irritation, so inject into large vein
        iii.   Depressed respiratory status
           (a) Depressed rate
           (b) Decreased tidal volume
           (c) Apnea within 30–90 seconds
        iv.   Delivered in intra-lipid emulsion
           (a) Watch for soy or egg allergy
           (b) No preservative—ampoule: use within 6 hours; vial: use within 12 hours
           (c) White milky fluid incompatible with other meds
        v.   Reduce doses with:
           (a) Other anesthetics
           (b) Elderly
           (c) Hemodynamically compromised
        vi.   Comparatively costly

2. Etomidate (Amidate)
   a. Properties
      i. Induction is rapid
      ii. Potent hypnotic
      iii. No analgesic properties
      iv. No histamine release
   b. Advantages
      i. Quick acting with little effect on cardiovascular system
      ii. Increases respiratory rate with decreased tidal volume
      iii. Useful for unstable patients
         (a) Hypovolemic patients
         (b) Excessive intraoperative blood-loss cases
      iv. Decreases cerebral blood flow and cerebral oxygenation
      v. Induction agent of choice for neurosurgical patients with increased intracranial pressure
   c. Disadvantages
      i. Myoclonia and dyskinesia
      ii. Nausea and vomiting postoperatively
      iii. Venous irritation
      iv. May suppress adrenal steroid synthesis up to 24 hours
D. Dissociative agent—ketamine hydrochloride (Ketalar)
   a. Properties
      i. Rapid-acting potent agent
      ii. Onset 1–2 minutes IV; 5 minutes IM
      iii. Duration of action 1–2 hours
      iv. May be used alone
      v. May be administered IV or IM
   b. Advantages
      i. Profound analgesia and anesthesia
      ii. Provides amnesia
      iii. Produces cardiovascular stimulation
         (a) Increases heart rate
         (b) Increases blood pressure
         (c) Increases cardiac output
      iv. Respiratory stimulant
      v. Airway reflexes maintained
      vi. Does not release histamine
   c. Disadvantages
      i. Emergence delirium
         (a) Confusion
         (b) Disorientation
         (c) Bad dreams
         (d) Hallucinations
      ii. Psychotic side effects treated with:
         (a) Midazolam
         (b) Diazepam
      iii. Increased nausea
      iv. Increased salivary and tracheobronchial secretions
E. Narcotics
   1. Agents
      a. Morphine sulfate
      b. Meperidine (Demerol)
      c. Fentanyl (Sublimaze)

       d. Alfentanil (Alfenta)

       e. Sufentanil (Sufenta)

       f. Remifentanil (Ultiva)

       g. Tramadol hydrochloride (Ultram)

       h. Synthetic agonist-antagonists

          i.   Nalbuphine (Nubain)

          ii.   Butorphanol (Stadol)

          iii. Buprenorphine (Buprenex)

          iv. Dezocine (Dalgan)

  2. Advantages

       a. Intraoperatively produces:

          i.   Mild amnesia

          ii.   Analgesia

          iii. Unconsciousness

          iv. Alter perception of pain

       b. Reduces minimal alveolar concentrations (MAC) of potent anesthetics

       c. Decreases incidence of dysrhythmias

       d. Provides cardiac stability

  3. Disadvantages

       a. Produces dose-related respiratory depression

       b. May cause nausea and vomiting due to direct effect on vomiting center in medulla

       c. Can prolong recovery

          i.   Patients with liver disease

          ii.   Elderly patients

          iii. Obese patients

          iv. Congestive heart failure (CHF) patients

       d. Urinary retention

       e. High doses may result in peripheral vasodilatation and bradycardia

       f. Depressant narcotic effects may be enhanced by:

          i.   Phenothiazines

          ii.   MAO inhibitors

          iii. Tricyclic antidepressants

F. Nonsteroidal antiinflammatory drugs—ketorolac tromethamine (Toradol)

  1. Properties

       a. Narcotic sparing effect

       b. No known effect on opiate receptor

       c. Peak analgesia 45–60 minutes

       d. Duration of action is 6–8 hours

       e. Potency 800 times greater than aspirin (ASA)

  2. Advantages

       a. Administer IM or IV

       b. Minimal nausea and vomiting

       c. Minimal, if any, respiratory depression

  3. Disadvantages

       a. Avoid in:

          i.   Coagulation disorders

          ii.   Anticoagulated patients

          iii. Aspirin-allergy/asthmatic patients

       b. Renal failure is associated with drug

       c. Can cause:

          i.   Peptic ulcer

  ii.   GI bleeding
  iii. GI perforation
  d. Contraindicated for:
  i.   Intrathecal or epidural administration because of preservative of alcohol
  ii.   Labor and delivery
  iii. Nursing mothers
G. Depolarizing muscle relaxants
  1. Succinylcholine (Anectine, Quelicin)
  a. Properties
  i.   Used for intubation and induction
  ii.   Mimic action of acetylcholine at postjunctional nicotinic cholinergic
        receptor located at neuromuscular junction
  iii. Is not pharmacologically reversed
  b. Advantages
  i.   Hydrolysis by plasma pseudocholinesterase
  ii.   Rapid induction (1 minute)
  iii. Rapid recovery (4–6 minutes)
  iv.   Used for endotracheal intubation particularly for rapid sequence
        induction
  v.   Used for short procedures requiring profound skeletal muscle relaxation
  c. Disadvantages
  i.   Contraindicated in pediatric patients except in emergencies
  ii.   Avoid in patients with decreased cholinesterase activity
  iii. Post usage complaints of muscle pain—myalgia
  iv.   Serum potassium increases, therefore use caution in patients with:
        (a) Burns
        (b) Hyperkalemia
        (c) Neuromuscular disorders
        (d) Trauma
        (e) Spinal cord trauma
  v.   Recovery may be prolonged with:
        (a) Atypical pseudocholinesterase (1:2,800 people)
        (b) Liver disease
        (c) Renal disease
        (d) Peripartum patients
        (e) Severe anemia
        (f) Malnutrition
        (g) Prolonged pyrexia
  vi.   Has caused rhabdomyolysis and cardiac arrest in children with
        undiagnosed myopathies
  vii. Increases:
        (a) Intraocular pressure
        (b) Intragastric pressure
        (c) Intracranial pressure
  viii. Triggers malignant hyperthermia
H. Nondepolarizing muscle relaxants
  1. Properties
  a. Act by competing with nicotinic cholinergic receptors in postjunctional
     membrane of neuromuscular junction
  b. Intermittent dosing in OR
  c. May be required for intubation

    d. Prolonged duration with:
       i.   Hypothermia
       ii. Acidosis
       iii. Inhalation agents
    e. Reversal agents include:
       i.   Anticholinesterases
       ii. Anticholinergics
2. Disadvantages
    a. Medications potentiate:
       i.   Halothane
       ii. Enflurane
       iii. Some antibiotics
            (a) Streptomycin
            (b) Clindamycin
            (c) Neomycin
            (d) Gentamicin
       iv. Local anesthetics
       v.   Furosemide (Lasix)
       vi. Quinidine
       vii. Calcium channel blockers
    b. Antagonism may be difficult in following situations:
       i.   Impaired renal and hepatic functions
       ii. Hypothermia
       iii. Hypokalemia
       iv. Respiratory acidosis
       v.   Metabolic alkalosis
    c. Magnesium decreases the nerve terminal by competing with calcium
    d. Medications that antagonize:
       i.   Phenytoin (Dilantin)
       ii. Theophylline (Aminophyllin)
       iii. Caffeine
       iv. Calcium
       v.   Steroids (chronic use)
3. Depolarizing neuromuscular blocking agents
    a. Long-acting
       i.   Pipecuronium bromide (Arduan)
            (a) Cardiovascular stability
            (b) No histamine release
            (c) Duration 60–120 minutes
            (d) Elimination 80–100% renal; 20–25% biliary
       ii. Pancuronium (Pavulon)
            (a) Useful for patients requiring complete muscle relaxation for
                mechanical ventilation
            (b) No histamine release
            (c) Contraindicated in:
                (i)   Chronic digitalis therapy
                (ii) Renal disease
                (iii) Coronary artery disease
                (iv) Myasthenia gravis
            (d) Elimination 60–80% renal; 15–40% hepatic; 5–10% biliary
            (e) Difficult to reverse in first 20–30 minutes after injection

    iii. Metocurine (Metubine)
        (a) Slight histamine release
        (b) Cardiovascular stability
        (c) Avoid in iodine-allergic patients
        (d) Elimination 80–100% renal
    iv. d-Tubocurarine (Curare)
        (a) Histamine release
           (i)   Hypotension
           (ii) Bronchospasm
           (iii) Increased secretions
        (b) May contain sulfite preservatives
        (c) Elimination 50% renal; 10–20% biliary; <1% hepatic
    v. Doxacurium (Nuromax)
        (a) Minimal to no histamine release
        (b) No vagolytic effects
        (c) Cardiovascular stability
        (d) Elimination 80–100% renal
 b. Intermediate acting
    i. Vecuronium (Norcuron)
        (a) No histamine release
        (b) Cardiovascular stability
        (c) Prolonged effect in severe hepatobiliary disease
        (d) Elimination 75% hepatobiliary; 25% renal
    ii. Atracurium besylate (Tracrium)
        (a) Slight histamine release
        (b) Cardiovascular stability
        (c) Does not depend on renal or hepatic elimination
        (d) Breaks down through Hoffman elimination and ester hydrolysis
    iii. Cistatracurium (Nimbex)
        (a) No histamine release
        (b) Cardiovascular stable
        (c) Excellent intubating conditions in 1.5–2 minutes
        (d) Duration 40–60 minutes (pediatric patients, 30 minutes)
        (e) Elimination by Hoffman elimination, minor renal and hepatic
    iv. Rocuronium (Zemuron)
        (a) Rapid to immediate onset
        (b) Increases pulmonary vascular resistance
        (c) Minimal cardiovascular effects
        (d) Onset 1–1.5 minutes
        (e) Duration 20–40 minutes
        (f) Elimination 50% biliary; 30% renal
 c. Short-acting
    i. Mivacurium (Mivacron)
        (a) Onset 1.5–3 minutes
        (b) Duration of action is 10–15 minutes
        (c) Recovery short and predictable
        (d) Minimal cardiovascular effects
        (e) Dose-related histamine release
        (f) Metabolized by hydrolysis in plasma
        (g) Elimination by plasmacholinesterase; <10% renal and biliary

I. Pediatric and geriatric considerations
   1. Pediatric
      a. Recover more quickly from muscle relaxants
      b. May need to use larger doses of nondepolarizing agents
   2. Geriatric
      a. Distribution affected by decreased lean body mass and increased body fat
      b. Takes longer time to maximal effect
      c. Recovery may be delayed due to slowed physiologic responses, disease states
J. Anticholinesterases (bind to enzyme acetylcholinesterase allowing acetylcholine to rebuild)
   1. Edrophonium (Tensilon)
      a. Advantages
         i.   Rapid onset
         ii.   Short activity
         iii. Minimal muscarinic effects
         iv. 75% renal excretion
      b. Disadvantages
         i.   Short action inadequate for profound blockade
         ii.   Bradycardia requiring atropine
         iii. Abdominal cramping
         iv. Nausea
   2. Neostigmine (Prostigmin)
      a. Advantages
         i.   Slightly slower action and duration
         ii.   Bradycardia has slower onset
            (a) Treated with glycopyrrolate (Robinul)
            (b) Treated with atropine
         iii. 50% renal excretion
         iv. May reverse Phase II block
      b. Disadvantages
         i.   Stimulation muscarinic receptors
            (a) Abdominal cramping
            (b) Nausea
            (c) Bradycardia
            (d) Miosis
            (e) Increased secretions
            (f) Bronchoconstriction
            (g) Hypotension
         ii.   Stimulation nicotinic receptors
            (a) Muscle cramps
            (b) Weakness
         iii. May cause dysrhythmias
   3. Pyridostigmine (Regonol, Mestinon)
      a. Advantages
         i.   Fewer muscarinic effects than neostigmine
         ii.   Onset 4–20 minutes
         iii. Duration 120–135 minutes
         iv. 75% renal excretion
      b. Disadvantages
         i.   Longer onset time
         ii.   Less potent

K. Anticholinergic agents
  1. Properties
    a. Minimizes side effects of anticholinesterases including:
       i.   Increasing heart rate
       ii. Decreasing intestinal tone
       iii. Decreasing oral secretions
    b. Block action of parasympathetic system
  2. Glycopyrrolate (Robinul)
    a. Lower incidence of dysrhythmias
    b. Slow change when increasing heart rate
    c. Does not cross blood brain barrier
    d. Devoid of sedative effects
  3. Atropine
    a. Rapid onset
    b. Tachydysrhythmias increase oxygen demand
    c. Drug crosses blood brain barrier resulting in:
       i.   Restlessness
       ii. Disorientation
       iii. Agitation
    d. Decreases salivary, bronchial, and gastric secretions
    e. Pupillary dilatation
V. Antagonists
  A. Physostigmine (Antilirum)
    1. Properties
      a. Anticholinesterase that crosses blood brain barrier
      b. Inhibits acetylcholinesterase
      c. Reverses central anticholinergic syndrome
      d. Nonspecific reversal of scopolamine, ketamine, benzodiazepines
    2. Advantages
      a. Increase level of consciousness
      b. Decrease disorientation
      c. Decrease agitation
    3. Disadvantages
      a. Bradycardia
      b. Hypotension
      c. Nausea and vomiting
  B. Naloxone (Narcan)
    1. Properties include being a specific antagonist
    2. Advantages
      a. Reverses respiratory depression
      b. Rapid results
      c. Lipid-soluble
    3. Disadvantages
      a. Short duration
         i.   Narcotic may outlast naloxone
         ii. May need to redose
         iii. Monitor patient
      b. Reverses analgesia
      c. May result in noncardiogenic pulmonary edema (NCPE)
         i.   Use with caution in patients with pre-existing cardiac disease
         ii. Use with caution in patients who receive potentially cardiotoxic drugs

    d. Sympathetic stimulation and catecholamine release
- i. Tachycardia
- ii. Hypertension
- iii. Increased peripheral vascular resistance
- iv. Ventricular dysrhythmias

C. Flumazenil (Romazicon)
1. Properties
    a. Specific benzodiazepine antagonist to reverse
- i. Anticonvulsant effect
- ii. Amnesia
- iii. Relaxant effect
- iv. Respiratory depression

    b. Does not reverse analgesic effect of narcotics on board
2. Disadvantages
    a. May cause slight agitation
    b. Benzodiazepine may outlast reversal
    c. Adverse effects include:
- i. Headache
- ii. Nausea and vomiting
- iii. Dizziness
- iv. Injection site pain
- v. Emotional lability

VI. Regional Anesthesia
Inducing loss of sensation in a specific region of the body

A. Sequence of neural blockade
1. Vasodilation and skin temperature elevation
2. Loss of pain and temperature sensation
3. Loss of proprioception
4. Loss of touch and pressure sensation
5. Motor paralysis

B. Spinal (subarachnoid block)
1. Local anesthetic injected into cerebrospinal fluid of second or lower lumbar vertebrae
2. The dura puncture and injection of local anesthetics are made below the spinal cord itself
3. The level of anesthesia depends on:
    a. Amount of local anesthetic
    b. Area of injection
    c. Patient position
4. Indications for use of spinal are procedures done on lower body and extremities

C. Level of blockade
1. Three types of blockade
    a. Sympathetic—nerves block first so one might see hypotension
    b. Sensory—sensation of dullness or lack of sensation
    c. Motor—result in loss of motor function
2. Sympathetic is two dermatones above sensory level
3. Motor is two dermatones below sensory level
4. Spinal blocks progress from sympathetic to sensory to motor
5. Spinal blocks regress from motor to sensory to sympathetic
6. Patients may be able to move extremities but not feel them

D. Contraindications for spinal
   1. Patient refusal
   2. Infection at puncture site
   3. Septicemia
   4. Hypovolemia
   5. CNS disease
   6. Vasomotor instability
   7. Coagulopathies
   8. Severe headache or backache
   9. Disease of spinal column
   10. Allergy to anesthetic medications

E. Complications of spinal
   1. PDPH (post dural puncture headache) secondary to loss of cerebrospinal fluid (CSF)—low incidence
   2. Urinary retention
   3. Bradycardia
   4. Respiratory depression
   5. Hypotension
   6. Nausea and vomiting
   7. Total spinal blockade—hypoventilation
   8. Infection
   9. Backache
   10. Allergy to medication
   11. Neurological sequelae
      a. Cauda equina syndrome
         i.   Compression of spinal nerve roots
         ii. Dull pain and anesthesia of buttocks, genitalia, and thigh
         iii. Impaired bladder and bowel function
      b. Peripheral neuropathy

F. Epidural
   1. Local anesthetic injected above the dura into the potential space called the epidural space
   2. The local anesthetic diffuses through the dura to produce analgesia and anesthesia
   3. Indications for epidural include:
      a. Procedure on abdomen
      b. Procedure on lower extremities
      c. Treatment of chronic pain
   4. Advantages of epidural
      a. Catheter placed so subsequent doses of medication may be given
      b. Narcotics can be used for postoperative pain management
   5. Complications of epidural block
      a. Unintentional arachnoid puncture, with or without headache (larger bore epidural needle may cause increase loss of CSF)
      b. Neurologic sequelae (epidural hematoma)
      c. Nausea and vomiting
      d. Backache
      e. Urinary retention
      f. Hypotension
      g. Infection
      h. Allergy to/seizure from medication

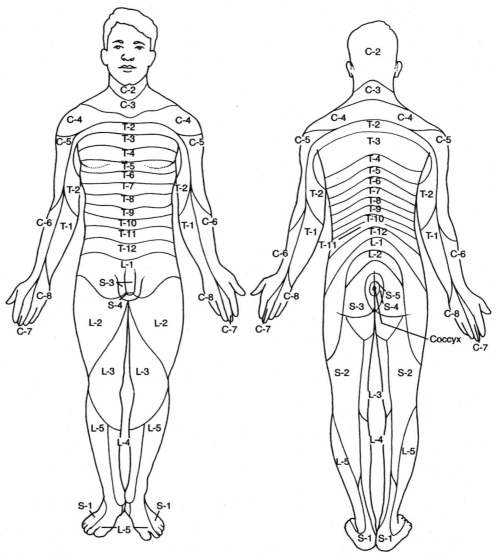

Figure 22–1. Dermatomes (cutaneous innervation of spinal nerves).   (From Ignatavicius, D., Workman, M.L., Mishler, M. [1995]. *Medical-Surgical Nursing,* 2nd ed. p. 1087. Philadelphia: Saunders.)

    6. Level of blockade for surgery types (see Figure 22–1)
      a. Rectal: S1-S5
      b. Foot: L2-L3
      c. Lower extremity: L1
      d. Hip, TURP, vagina, ovaries, testes, lower extremities: T 10
      e. Forceps delivery: T 10
      f. Upper abdominal: T 6 (xiphoid)
      g. Lower abdominal: T 4 (nipple)
      h. C-Section, tubal ligation: T 4
   G. Use of epinephrine with regional anesthesia
      1. Causes vasoconstriction
      2. Slows vascular absorption
      3. Prolongs effect

4. Epinephrine may cause:
   a. Anxiety
   b. Hypertension
   c. Tachycardia
   d. Dysrhythmias
H. Baricity of solution
   1. Cerebrospinal fluid (CSF) specific gravity ranges from 1.003–1.009
   2. Primary determinant of spinal level is the specific gravity of the local agent injected
      a. Hypobaric
         i.   Specific gravity less than normal (1.001–1.002) for CSF
         ii. Use distilled water as diluent
         iii. Used for perineal, rectal, and total hip arthroplasty procedures
      b. Isobaric
         i.   Normal CSF specific gravity is 1.003–1.009
         ii. Use CSF to dilute agent
         iii. Used when anesthesia required at specific level, i.e., lower extremity surgery, fractured hips
         iv. Not widely used
      c. Hyperbaric
         i.   Specific gravity greater than normal (1.023–1.035) for CSF
         ii. Use dextrose 10% as diluent
         iii. Solution settles to most dependent aspect of subarachnoid space
         iv. Most frequently used
   3. Dose requirement may be increased up to 40% in patients with high abdominal pressure
      a. Obese
      b. Pregnant
      c. Ascites
      d. Bowel obstruction
      e. Dose requirements probably secondary to decreased epidural and intrathecal space secondary to engorged venous structures
   4. Level of spinal determined by:
      a. Baricity of solution
      b. Position of patient at time of injection
      c. Dose and volume of medication injected
      d. Presence of vasoconstrictors
VII. **Local Agents and Their Use in Regional Techniques**
   A. General
      1. Levels of anesthesia are dependent upon:
         a. Dose of agent
         b. Rate of injection
         c. Specific gravity of fluid
         d. Position of the patient
      2. Rare allergic response may be due to preservative, not medication
      3. Toxicity is predictable and dose-related
         a. Metallic taste
         b. Ringing in ears
   B. Amino-esters
      1. Agents
         a. Cocaine
         b. Procaine (Novocain)

       c. Chloroprocaine (Nesacaine)

       d. Tetracaine (Pontocaine)

    2. Hydrolyzed in the plasma

    3. Poor penetrance

    4. Fair to poor stability

    5. Rare allergic response

  C. Amino-amides

    1. Agents

       a. Lidocaine (Xylocaine)

       b. Mepivacaine (Carbocaine)

       c. Prilocaine (Citanest)

       d. Bupivacaine (Marcaine)

       e. Etidocaine (Duranest)

       f. Ropivacaine (Naropin)

    2. Metabolized by liver

    3. Good penetrance

    4. Very stable

    5. Very rare allergic response

VIII. Specific Agents

  A. Cocaine

    1. Amino-ester

    2. Low potency

    3. Duration 10–55 minutes

    4. Used as topical typically for vasoconstriction of nasal mucosa

  B. Procaine

    1. Amino-ester

    2. Low potency

    3. Duration 30 minutes (short duration)

    4. If epinepherine added, duration 45 minutes or more

    5. Uses

       a. Local

       b. Peripheral nerve blocks

       c. Subarachnoid

  C. Chloroprocaine (Nesacaine)

    1. Low potency

    2. Short acting amino-ester

    3. Duration 30–60 minutes

    4. Uses

       a. Local

       b. Peripheral nerve blocks

       c. Epidural

  D. Tetracaine (Pontocaine)

    1. High potency amino-ester with long duration

    2. Duration 3–4 hours

    3. Duration when used with epinephrine is 5–7 hours

    4. Uses

       a. Topical

       b. Subarachnoid

  E. Lidocaine

    1. Intermediate amino-amide potency

    2. Duration 1–1.5 hours

    3. Duration 2–2.3 hours when used with epinepherine

    4. Uses
      a. Local
      b. Topical
      c. Peripheral nerve block
      d. Intravenous
      e. Epidural
      f. Subarachnoid

F. Mepivacaine (Carbocaine)
    1. Intermediate amino-amide potency
    2. Duration 1.5 hours
    3. Duration 2 hours when used with epinephrine
    4. Uses
      a. Local
      b. Peripheral nerve block
      c. Epidural

G. Prilocaine (Citanest)
    1. Intermediate potency amino-amide
    2. Duration 60 minutes
    3. Less vasodilatation than lidocaine
    4. Uses
      a. Local
      b. Peripheral nerve block
      c. Intravenous
      d. Epidural
      e. Subarachnoid

H. Bupivacaine (Marcaine, Sensorcaine)
    1. High potency amino-amide
    2. Long duration of action 3 to 10 hours
    3. Uses
      a. Local
      b. Peripheral nerve block
      c. Intravenous
      d. Epidural
      e. Subarachnoid

I. Etidocaine (Duranest)
    1. High potency amino-amide of long duration
    2. Duration 5–10 hours
    3. Need high concentration for adequate sensory block
    4. Uses
      a. Local
      b. Peripheral nerve block
      c. Epidural

J. Ropivacaine (Naropin)
    1. High potency amino-amide
    2. Similar to bupivacaine
    3. Produces less motor blockage than bupivacaine
    4. Duration as long as 12 hours
    5. Uses
      a. Epidural
      b. Safe for obstetric use

K. Eutetic mixture local anesthetic (EMLA)
    1. Topical preparation

2. Lidocaine 2.5% plus prilocaine 2.5%
3. Penetrates intact skin
4. Apply to skin under an occlusive dressing one hour prior to procedure
5. May apply to two sites so backup site available in case first venipuncture unsuccessful

IX. **Regional Anesthesia in Ambulatory Surgery Patients**
   A. Advantages
      1. Postoperative analgesia
      2. Alert patient
      3. Decreased nausea and vomiting
      4. Not as intense nursing care
      5. Shorter discharge time
   B. Disadvantages
      1. Longer preparation time
      2. Potential urinary retention
      3. Possible orthostatic hypotension
      4. Needle injections required
      5. Numb extremity

Bibliography

1. Barash, P., Cullen, B., Stoelting, R. (1991). *Handbook of Clinical Anesthesia*. Philadelphia: Lippincott.
2. Burden, N. (1993). *Ambulatory Surgery Nursing*. Philadelphia: Saunders.
3. DiPiro, J., Talbert, P., Hayes, P., Yee, G., Matzke, G., Posey, L.M., 1993. *Pharmacotherapy: A Pathophysiologic Approach*, 2nd ed. East Norwalk, CT: Appleton & Lange.
4. Drain, C., (1994). *The Post Anesthesia Care Unit*, 3rd ed. Philadelphia: Saunders.
5. Fetzer-Fowler, S. (1992). State of the art: Regional anesthesia using anesthetic admixtures. *J Post Anesth Nursing*, 7(4):229–237.
6. Kang, S., Rudrud, L., Nelson, W., Baier, D. (1994). Postanesthesia nursing care for ambulatory surgery patients: Post-spinal anesthesia. *J PeriAnesth Nursing*, 9(2):101–106.
7. Kirby, R., Gravenstein, N. (1994). *Clinical Anesthesia Practice*. Philadelphia: Saunders.
8. Litwack, K. (1995). *Post Anesthesia Care Nursing*, 2nd ed. St. Louis: Mosby.
9. Litwack, K. (1994). *Core Curriculum for Post Anesthesia Nursing Practice*, 3rd ed. Philadelphia: Saunders.
10. McGoldrick, K. (ed.), (1995). *Ambulatory Anesthesiology*. Baltimore: Williams & Wilkins.
11. Omoigui, S. (1992). *The Anesthesia Drug Handbook*. St. Louis: Mosby.
12. *PDR® Nurses Handbook for Certified Registered Nurse Anesthetists*. (1997). Montvale, NJ: Medical Economics.
13. Schweinefus, R., Schick, L. (1991). Succinylcholine: Good guy, bad guy. *J Post Anesth Nursing*, 6(6): 410–419.
14. Stein, R. H. (1995). The perioperative nurse's role in anesthesia management. *AORN J*, 62(5):794–804.
15. Twersky, R. S. (1995). *The Ambulatory Anesthesia Handbook*. St. Louis: Mosby.
16. Vender, J., Spiess, B. (1992). *Post Anesthesia Care*. Philadelphia: Saunders.
17. Walker, J. (1997). Neuromuscular relaxation and reversal: An update. *J PeriAnesth Nursing*, 12(4): 264–274.
18. White, P. (1997). *Ambulatory Anesthesia and Surgery*. Philadelphia: Saunders.
19. Wong, D. (1995). *Whaley & Wong's Nursing Care of Infants and Children*, 5th ed. St. Louis: Mosby.

REVIEW QUESTIONS

1. Which of the following medications is not reversed by using the drug flumazenil (Romazicon)?

   A. Morphine
   B. Lorazepam (Ativan)
   C. Diazepam (Valium)
   D. Midazolam (Versed)

2. An absolute contraindication to spinal anesthesia includes all of the following except

   A. Localized infection at site of injection
   B. Patient refusal
   C. Uncorrected coagulation defect
   D. Multiple sclerosis

3. Which of the following has the lowest baricity?

A. Lidocaine 5% in dextrose 7.5%
B. Equal volume of tetracaine 1% and water
C. Bupivacaine 0.75% in dextrose 7.5%
D. Equal volume of tetracaine and dextrose 10%

4. The addition of epinephrine to local anesthetic solutions provides all of the following except

A. Prolongation of duration of anesthesia
B. Minimization of peak blood levels
C. Reduced surgical bleeding
D. Decrease in blockade intensity

5. Which of the following does not increase the block of nondepolarizing muscle relaxants?

A. Lidocaine
B. Aminoglycide antibiotics
C. Halothane
D. Carbamazepine (Tegretol)

6. All of the following tend to cause pain on injection except

A. Diazepam
B. Propofol
C. Methohexital
D. Ketamine

7. Which of the following has the shortest recovery time after induction?

A. Propofol
B. Methohexital
C. Ketamine
D. Thiopental

8. The following decrease cerebral blood flow and intracranial pressure except

A. Thiopental
B. Propofol
C. Ketamine
D. Midazolam

9. Which of the following is associated with the highest incidence of nausea and vomiting?

A. Propofol
B. Midazolam
C. Ketamine
D. Etomidate

10. Which of the following is a long-acting local anesthetic?

A. Cocaine
B. Bupivicaine
C. Procaine
D. Lidocaine

11. Halothane is known to be a potent

A. Bronchodilator
B. Antihypertensive
C. Narcotic
D. Cardiac stimulant

12. All inhalation agents are known to be

A. Narcotics
B. Muscle stimulants
C. Respiratory depressants
D. Respiratory stimulants

ANSWERS TO QUESTIONS

1. A
2. D
3. B
4. D
5. D
6. D

7. A
8. C
9. C
10. B
11. A
12. C

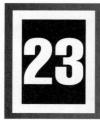

Malignant Hyperthermia

Lois Schick
Exempla Healthcare, Saint Joseph Hospital
Denver, Colorado

Objectives

1. Define malignant hyperthermia (MH).
2. Identify triggering agents of malignant hyperthermia.
3. State medication of choice to treat malignant hyperthermia.
4. Describe nursing interventions in PACU for patients in MH crisis.
5. Identify signs and symptoms of malignant hyperthermia.

I. Malignant Hyperthermia

An inherited muscle disorder that, when triggered by potent inhalation anesthetics and some other drugs, i.e., succinylcholine, may cause a life-threatening crisis.

  A. General
    1. Malignant hyperthermia (MH) is an inherited disorder of skeletal muscle
    2. Actual cause is not yet known with certainty
    3. Research points to a generalized derangement of processes that regulate muscle contractions; underlying pathology is consistent with a defect in the sarcoplasmic reticulum (area in muscle cells that stores calcium)
    4. An increased concentration of calcium in the muscle cell is found; high calcium levels cause the muscles to contract and become rigid, leading to greatly increased metabolism
    5. A hypermetabolic state results
    6. Heat production and muscle-cell breakdown occur from the hypermetabolic state
    7. Potentially lethal
    8. Incidence 1 in 5,000 to 1 in 65,000 anesthetic administrations
    9. Previous general anesthesia does not rule out MH susceptibility; 50% of patients with MH had previous surgery without a problem
  B. Demographics
    1. More common in children 1:10,000 as compared with adults 1:50,000, but may occur at any age (7 months to 87 years)

    2. Children under 15 represent 52% of MH cases
    3. Occurs in either sex but predominantly males (55.9%)
    4. Identified in every country
    5. MH susceptibility is inherited (autosomal dominant)
    6. All races are susceptible
    7. Relationship between MH and certain muscle diseases suggested
        a. Muscular dystrophy
        b. Central core disease
        c. Congenital myotonic dystrophy
        d. Physical characteristics associated but not proven
            i. Extraocular muscle defect (ptosis, strabismus)
            ii. Spinal deformity (scoliosis)
           iii. Congenital hernias
           iv. Clubfoot
C. Triggering agents
    1. All volatile inhalation agents
        a. Halothane
        b. Enflurane
        c. Isoflurane
        d. Sevoflurane
        e. Desflurane
    2. Muscle relaxant succinylcholine
D. Safe agents to use
    1. Barbiturates
    2. Local anesthetics
    3. Opioids
    4. Nitrous oxide
    5. Benzodiazepines
    6. Propofol
    7. Ketamine
    8. Etomidate
    9. All nondepolarizing muscle relaxants
E. Signs and symptoms
    1. Anesthetist will note an increase in end tidal carbon dioxide (ETCO$_2$)
    2. Tachycardia and dysrhythmias
    3. Tachypnea
    4. Generalized muscle rigidity
    5. Masseter (jaw) muscle rigidity (early sign)
    6. Hyperthermia (often late sign)
F. Biological signs include:
    1. Metabolic acidosis
    2. Respiratory acidosis
    3. Hyperkalemia
    4. Elevated blood creatinine kinase levels (CPK) with myoglobinuria (only 40% of MH patients have elevated CPK)
    5. Hypercalcemia
    6. Disseminated intravascular coagulopathy (DIC)
    7. Left ventricular failure (late sign)
G. After onset of MH, the attack is rapidly progressive
H. Establish MH emergency kit/cart/equipment
    1. Dantrolene with sterile preservative-free water to reconstitute
    2. Ice packs

3. Cold wound irrigation
4. Cold intravenous solutions—iced normal saline, not lactated ringers
5. Nasogastric tubes
6. Three-way irrigation Foley catheter
7. Syringes (blood gas syringes, 60 cc to reconstitute dantrolene, 5, 10, and 20 cc)
8. Lab tubes for electrolytes and coagulation studies
9. Urine specimen containers
10. Medications
   a. Sodium bicarbonate
   b. Mannitol
   c. Furosemide
   d. Lidocaine
   e. Procainamide
   f. Calcium chloride
   g. Regular insulin
   h. Dextrose 50%

II. Perioperative Management

A. Preoperative assessment
   1. Patient/family assessment
   2. Any unexpected deaths or complications after family member having anesthesia
   3. Any muscle disorder history
   4. Any dark-colored (cola-colored) urine after anesthesia
   5. Any history of unexplained fevers, muscle rigidity during surgery
B. Intraoperative
   1. Preparation of susceptible patients
      a. Hypothermia blanket on OR table
      b. Fully stocked malignant hyperthermia kit/cart with dantrolene
      c. Ice and cold intravenous irrigations
   2. Available emergency supplies and equipment
   3. Anesthesia provider should
      a. Avoid the use of MH-triggering anesthetics
      b. Be familiar with the signs and treatment of MH
      c. Continuously monitor the patient's carbon dioxide concentration ($ETCO_2$)
      d. Continuously monitor the patient's temperature
      e. Consider hyperkalemia as cause in the sudden cardiac arrest in a male child with normal oxygenation and must treat accordingly if hyperkalemia
         i. Treat with glucose and insulin
      f. Evaluate any unexpected hypercarbia, tachycardia, tachypnea, or dysrhythmia
      g. Have an MH kit or cart in the OR stocked with an adequate supply of dantrolene
C. Postoperative in PACU
   1. MH may present in PACU (usually within first hour postprocedure but may be up to 12 hours postoperative)
   2. Monitor for myoglobinuria
      a. Is clear urine prerequisite for discharge?
      b. Educate patient and family to observe for cola-colored urine
   3. Monitor temperature and electrocardiogram on patients
   4. Patients with intraoperative/postoperative episode will be admitted to ICU for 24–48 hours
   5. Provide education on MH for:
      a. Patient
      b. Family
      c. Other staff

D. Documentation should include:
1. Patient response
2. Interventions
3. Times
4. Personnel involved
5. Patient outcomes
6. Register MH episode with North American MH registry at 1-717-531-6936

III. **Treatment of MH**

A. Identify crisis
1. Recognize signs and symptoms (tachycardia, masseter muscle rigidity, dysrhythmias)
2. Summon help
3. Discontinue potent inhalation agents and succinylcholine
4. Hyperventilate patient with 100% oxygen (2–3 times normal minute ventilation)
5. Can use oxygen flow of 15–20 L/min to purge anesthesia machine of trace gases and change breathing circuit and gas hose while hyperventilating patient with ambu or change to new anesthesia machine

B. Treat patient
1. Administer dantrolene
   a. 2.5 mg/kg intravenously up to 10 mg/kg IV; in some instances may be as much as 20 mg/kg IV
   b. Fast-acting muscle relaxant
   c. Sufficient quantity needs to be available (36 vials)
   d. Crystalline powder is not easy to mix and must be diluted with 60 cc preservative-free sterile water
2. Treat dysrhythmias/cardiac arrest
   a. May use lidocaine for dysrhythmia or procainamide
   b. Do not use calcium channel blockers for dysrhythmias
   c. Avoid suppressing tachycardia with beta blockers until MH has been ruled out
3. Treat acidosis
   a. Hyperventilate patient
   b. Administer bicarbonate 1–2 mEq/kg
4. Treat hyperthermia
   a. Ice pack to body surfaces (head, neck axillae, groin)
   b. Lavage with ice solutions to:
      i. Nasogastric tube
      ii. Bladder
      iii. Wound
      iv. Rectum
   c. Cool patient to 38°C (if cool lower, may have problems)
   d. Monitor core temperature with esophageal, rectal, or tympanic probes
5. Monitor lab values for:
   a. Blood gases
   b. Electrolytes
   c. Coagulation
6. Monitor urine output
   a. Myoglobinuria common after MH
   b. May lead to renal failure
   c. Insure diuresis 2ml/kg/hr
7. Observe patient in ICU for 24–48 hours
   a. Recrudescence may occur within hours to days

  b. Monitor for renal failure
  c. Monitor for DIC
  d. Administer dantrolene for at least 48 hours post episode
8. Continue to monitor creatinine kinase
  a. Guide to status of muscle destruction
  b. CK's peak at 24 hours after muscle damage
9. Educate patient and family
  a. Refer to testing center (directory of centers may be obtained from MHAUS, address to follow)
    i. Notify family members of incident
    ii. To diagnose must test with caffeine–halothane contracture test from muscle obtained from a muscle biopsy; the testing must take place at a designated testing center
  b. Neurology workup may be indicated
10. Physical therapy in severe muscle destruction may be indicated
  a. Muscle pain may limit mobility
  b. Muscle pain may lead to contractures

IV. **Malignant Hyperthermia Association of United States (MHAUS)**
  A. Address:
  P.O. Box 1069
  32 S. Main Street
  Sherburne, New York: 13460
  1-607-674-7901
  Hotline: 1-800-98M-HAUS (1-800-986-4287)
  Internet: http://www.mhaus.org
  B. Brochures, posters, and educational information available, including videos on MH
  C. Newsletter, *The Communicator*, published quarterly with updated information

V. **Future Considerations**
  A. Develop inexpensive testing method to diagnose MH-susceptible patients
  B. Develop dantrolene solution requiring less difficulty to reconstitute
  C. Continue research about MH
  D. Continue education programs for the public and health-care providers

Bibliography

1. Aubert, M., Borsarelli J., Khambatta H.J., Kezak Ribkens G., (English Version): A. Wald. (ed.). (1993). *International Congress Malignant Hyperthermias.* Englewood, NJ: Normed Verlag.
2. Burden, N. (1993). *Ambulatory Surgery Nursing.* Philadelphia: Saunders.
3. Drain, C. (1994). *The Postanesthesia Care Unit*, 3rd ed. Philadelphia: Saunders.
4. Kirby, R., Gravenstein, N. (1994). *Clinical Anesthesia Practice.* Philadelphia: Saunders.
5. McGoldrick, K. (ed.). (1995). *Ambulatory Anesthesia: A Problem Oriented Approach.* Baltimore: Williams & Wilkins.
6. MHAUS. (August 1997). "What Is Malignant Hyperthermia?" "Managing MH, Drugs, Equipment & the Antidote Dantrolene Sodium," and "An Anesthesia Protocol." http://www.mhaus.org.
7. MHAUS. (1996). *Malignant Hyperthermia, a Concern for OR and PACU Nurses.* Sherburne, NY: MHAUS.
8. Quinn, D. (ed.). (1995). *Ambulatory Postanesthesia Nursing Outline: Content for Certification.* Thorofare, NJ: ASPAN.
9. Twersky, R. (1995). *The Ambulatory Anesthesia Handbook.* St. Louis: Mosby.
10. White, P. (1997). *Ambulatory Anesthesia and Surgery.* Philadelphia: Saunders.

REVIEW QUESTIONS

1. Patients with an increased risk for malignant hyperthermia can safely tolerate

   A. Depolarizing muscle relaxants
   B. Volatile halogenated hydrocarbons
   C. Prolonged physical stress
   D. Nondepolarizing muscle relaxation

2. Anesthesia drugs implicated as triggering an MH crisis include

   A. Barbiturates and benzodiazepines
   B. Inhalation agents and succinylcholine
   C. Benzodiazepines and narcotics
   D. Barbiturates and narcotics

3. Malignant hyperthermia has been defined as

   A. Syndrome triggered in susceptible individuals by using inhalation agents and succinylcholine
   B. Inherited disorder of skeletal muscle
   C. Common in children, treatable, but potentially lethal
   D. All of the above

4. Avoid suppressing tachycardia with which of the following until MH as been ruled out?

   A. Procainamide
   B. Lidocaine
   C. Beta blockers
   D. Digoxin

5. Treatment of choice for hyperkalemia in an MH crisis is

   A. Glucose and insulin
   B. Kayexalate
   C. 50% glucose
   D. Potassium chloride

6. According to MH literature, the recommended number of vials of dantrolene to be stocked in a facility are

   A. 6
   B. 18
   C. 36
   D. 72

7. The antidote recommended in an MH crisis is

   A. Sodium bicarbonate
   B. Furosemide
   C. Procanamide
   D. Dantrolene

8. Early signs and symptoms of MH include

   A. Pulmonary edema
   B. Seizure activity
   C. Muscle rigidity
   D. Cyanosis

9. The initial dantrolene doses usually start at

   A. 1 mg/kg
   B. 2.5 mg/kg
   C. 5 mg/kg
   D. 10 mg/kg

10. One would perform the following test to **confirm** the patient was MH susceptible.

   A. CPK
   B. ABGs
   C. Electrolytes
   D. Caffeine–halothane contracture test from muscle biopsy specimen

ANSWERS TO QUESTIONS

1. D
2. B
3. D
4. C
5. A

6. C
7. D
8. C
9. B
10. D

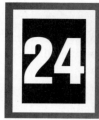

Pain Management

Lois Schick
Exempla Healthcare, Saint Joseph Hospital
Denver, Colorado

Objectives

1. Identify five factors that influence pain.
2. Differentiate between acute and chronic pain.
3. List the quantifiable aspects of pain.
4. Identify nonpharmacologic pain management techniques.
5. State regional techniques utilized to treat patients for pain.

I. Pain

"Unpleasant sensory and emotional experience associated with actual or potential tissue damage." (Salerno & Willens, 1996)

"Pain is whatever the experiencing person says it is, existing whenever the experiencing person says it does." (McCaffery & Beebe, 1989)

A. Goals for management of pain
   1. Reduce incidence and severity of patient's postoperative or posttraumatic pain
   2. Educate patients about the need to communicate unrelieved pain so they can receive prompt evaluation and effective treatment
   3. Enhance patient comfort and satisfaction
   4. Contribute to fewer postoperative complications and, in some cases, shorter stays after surgical procedures
B. Pain is determined and influenced by many factors
   1. Type of procedure performed
   2. Medical condition
   3. Developmental level
   4. Emotional and cognitive states
   5. Personal concerns
   6. Family issues and attitudes
   7. Culture
   8. Personality
   9. Age
   10. Experiences
   11. Personal bias
   12. Environment

C. Anatomy and physiology
   1. Nociception—transmission of noxious stimuli
   2. Pain—unpleasant sensory and emotional experience (person's perception of the event)
      a. Involves the body's peripheral and central nervous systems
         i. Receptors detect the noxious event
         ii. Pathways relay information to central processing system to trigger a response
   3. Response to tissue injury results in:
      a. Increased blood flow to area
      b. Tissue edema
      c. Sensitization to nociceptors
   4. Biochemical response to injury
   5. Release of neurotransmitters
      a. Histamine—located in tissue, platelet, basophils, mast cells
      b. Bradykinin—contained in plasma
         i. Released when clotting cascade is activated
         ii. Directly activates nociceptors
         iii. Causes vasodilatation
         iv. Increases vascular permeability
      c. Prostaglandin—located in tissue, biosynthesized in body from certain polyunsaturated fats
      d. Serotonin—located in tissues, mast cells, platelets
      e. Norepinephrine—located in dorsal horn
      f. Substance P—located at nerve terminal
         i. Peptide manufactured by cells in dorsal root ganglia
         ii. Involved in pain transmission
         iii. Causes blood vessels to release conduction chemicals: bradykinin, histamine, serotonin
D. Pain transmission is carried out through:
   1. Elaborate network of receptors
   2. Peripheral nerves
      a. Nerve endings found in skin, blood vessels, subcutaneous tissue, muscle fascia, periosteum, and visceral joints
   3. Spinal cord
      a. Spinothalmic tract
         i. Lateral—sharp localized pain
         ii. Ventral—aching, dull, nonlocalized pain
   4. Supraspinal pathways
E. Primary afferent fibers
   1. A-fibers that cause acute, prickling-type pain
      a. Alpha
      b. Beta
      c. Gamma
      d. Delta—provoke bright well-localized pain
   2. C-fibers that cause slower, burning sensations
      a. Small
      b. Slow
      c. Myelinated
   3. A and C-afferent fibers explain double pain
      a. A-fibers cause first perception of stinging
      b. C-fibers cause second burning pain

II. Theories of Pain
  A. Gate control theory—dorsal horns of spinal column serve as gates for controlling entry of pain signals
    1. Physiologic aspect of nociception
    2. Stimulation evokes nervous impulses that are transmitted to three spinal cord systems
      a. Substantia gelatinosa in dorsal horn
      b. Dorsal column fibers
      c. Central transmission cells
    3. Amount of activity in large diameter fibers inhibits transmission of pain, therefore "closing the gate"
    4. Amount of activity in smaller fibers results in transmission of pain, therefore "opening the gate"
  B. Opiate receptor theory
    1. Biochemical focus emphasizing descending system to inhibit nociception
    2. Enkephalins—in the head
    3. Endorphins—endogenous morphine
      a. Three distinct classes concentrated in descending inhibitory system
        i.   Enkephalins
        ii. Dynorphins
        iii. B-endorphins
    4. Opiate binding receptors
      a. Mu receptor
        i. Mediate supraspinal analgesia
        ii. Mediate spinal analgesia, bradycardia, respiratory depression
      b. Kappa—located in dorsal horn
      c. Delta—mediate analgesia through enkephalin substance
    5. Opiate receptors found in:
      a. Spinal and medullary dorsal horn
      b. Substantia nigra
      c. Periaqueductal gray
      d. Hypothalmus
      e. Amygdala

III. Pain Assessment and Reassessment
  A. Quantifiable aspects of pain
    1. Location—have patient point to exact location of pain
    2. Intensity—none to mild to excruciating
      a. Numeric scales
      b. Visual scales
    3. Timeliness—onset, duration, time intensity, pattern
    4. Quality—describe what pain is like
    5. Personal meaning
  B. Physiologic signs of pain (use as adjunct to verbal signs if patient can talk)
    1. Tachycardia
    2. Tachypnea
    3. Hypertension
  C. Behavioral observations (not a qualitative measure)
    1. Facial expressions—grimace, clinch teeth, tightly shut lips, tearing
    2. Vocalization—moan, groan, grunt, sigh, cry, scream
    3. Verbalization—pray, swear, count
    4. Body action—thrash, pound, bite, rock
    5. Behaviors—massaging, immobilization, apply pressure/hot/cold, positioning

    D. Cognitive statements
       1. Patient reports pain
       2. Patient reports estimation of intensity of pain
    E. Tools of pain assessment
       1. Numeric scales
       2. Visual analog scale
       3. Descriptive intensity scale
       4. Pain inventory (diary)
       5. Faces of pain scale
       6. Questionnaires related to pain
    F. Mismanagement of pain
       1. Inadequate knowledge by health-care professional
       2. Ineffective communication
       3. Poor assessment
       4. Concern about regulation of controlled substance
       5. Fear of addiction
       6. Concern with side effects
       7. Concern with patient becoming tolerant to medications
       8. Patient's reluctance to report pain
       9. Patient's reluctance to take pain medications
      10. Inadequate reimbursement
      11. Restrictive regulations
      12. Availability
IV. Preoperative Assessment
    A. Ensure patient understands procedure to be performed
    B. Discuss previous experience with pain, including drug preferences that work
    C. Provide information regarding pain management
       1. Pain is normal and can be affected by attitude
       2. Pain is amplified by muscle tension
       3. Relaxation may help alleviate pain
       4. Position changes prevents strain on injured part
    D. Develop with patient a plan for pain assessment
    E. Select a pain-assessment tool
       1. Visual analog scale
       2. Simple descriptive pain intensity scale
       3. Zero to ten numeric pain intensity scale
       4. Face rating scale
    F. Teach patient how to use selected pain-assessment tool
    G. Provide patient with education about pain control; include training in nonpharmacologic options such as relaxation and diversion
    H. Assess patient willingness to incorporate nonpharmacologic pain-control measures
    I. Emphasize the importance of a factual report of pain-avoiding stoicism or exaggeration
    J. Instruct patient it is more difficult to play "catch up" once pain is established
V. Intraoperative
    A. Anesthesia techniques used
       1. Local
       2. General anesthetics
       3. Regional
    B. Surgical procedure may include usage of local anesthetic infiltration or application to wound

C. Avoid pain extraneous to operative site, misalignment of body, positioning, pressure from equipment or personnel, and unnecessary manipulation of body tissue

VI. Postoperative
A. General
1. Assess patient perceptions in conjunction with behavioral and physiologic responses
2. Use patient self-report as an indication for medication
   a. Most reliable indicator of patient's pain
3. Assess and reassess pain frequently
4. If pain is poorly controlled, increase frequency of assessment and revise pain-management plan
5. Record pain intensity
6. Record response to pain intervention
7. Identify pharmacologic and nonpharmacologic interventions
8. Administer medications per physician orders and protocols using appropriate delivery system
   a. Monitor effectiveness at frequent intervals
   b. Record assessment data
   c. Intervene at onset of pain
9. Position for comfort
10. Encourage proper posture and alignment
11. Provide touch as appropriate
12. Provide supportive environment
13. Provide discharge instructions to patient
14. Provide referral or information on community services

VII. Acute versus Chronic Pain
A. Acute pain (brief duration that subsides as healing occurs, lasts for less than 6 months)
1. Characteristics of acute pain
   a. Associated with identifiable injury, disease, or procedure
   b. Accompanied by anxiety and sympathetic nervous system stimulation
   c. Less than six months in duration
   d. Subsides with healing
   e. Not associated with psychopathology
2. Prevention of pain is better than having to treat pain
3. Key to management of pain is a routine systematic assessment
4. Pharmacologic interventions
   a. Opioids
   b. Nonsteroidal antiinflammatory drugs (NSAIDs)
   c. Patient-controlled analgesia (PCA)
5. Nonpharmacologic interventions
   a. Supportive measures: bandages, splints
   b. TENS (transcutaneous electrical nerve stimulator)
   c. Acupuncture
   d. Cryoanalgesia
6. Psychologic interventions
   a. Distraction
   b. Relaxation methods
7. Music therapy
8. Hypnosis
9. Muscle relaxation

B. Chronic pain (prolonged 6 months and longer; recurrent, acute, ongoing)
1. Tend to show development of psychological factors
2. Pain is subjective experience
3. Examples of chronic pain:
   a. Low back pain
   b. Neck pain
   c. Peripheral neuropathy
   d. Post herpetic neuralgia
   e. Reflex sympathetic dystrophy
   f. Headache
4. Chronic pain interventions
   a. Pharmacologic
      i.   Tricyclic antidepressants
      ii. Anticonvulsants
      iii. Selective serotonin reuptake inhibitors (SSRI)
      iv. Opiates
   b. Nonpharmacologic
      i.   Distraction
      ii. Exercise
      iii. Heat and cold
      iv. Relaxation
      v.   TENS (transcutaneous electrical nerve stimulator)

VIII. Pharmacologic Interventions
A. Nonopioid analgesics
1. Acetaminophen—may be given preoperatively for preventative pain control
2. Aspirin (ASA) and salicylate salts
3. NSAIDs (nonsteroidal antiinflammatory agents)
   a. Ketorolac tromethemine (Toradol)
   b. Ibuprofen
   c. Naproxen (Naprasyn)
4. Three effects of NSAIDs
   a. Antiinflammatory
   b. Analgesic
   c. Antipyretic
5. Indications
   a. Mild to moderate pain of peripheral origin
   b. In conjunction with narcotics in severe acute pain
   c. Conditions associated with excessive prostaglandin at site of injury (postoperative pain)
   d. Patient's desire to avoid mind-altering drugs
6. Advantages
   a. No respiratory depression
   b. Little physical tolerance
7. Disadvantages
   a. Undesirable effects in some patients
      i.   GI disturbance
      ii. Allergic response
      iii. Increased bleeding time
      iv. Fluid retention
   b. Analgesic ceiling
   c. Organ damage with long-term use
8. Contraindications
   a. History of ulcers or GI problems

      b. Renal failure

      c. Allergy to NSAIDs

      d. Ketorolac tromethemine (Toradol)

         i.   Used for short-term management (up to 5 days)

         ii.   May not be used if patient allergic to ASA

         iii. Requires high doses for antiinflammatory effects

  B. Opioids

    1. Physiologic response

      a. Indications

         i.   Relieves moderate to severe pain

         ii.   Titration based on patient's analgesic response and side effects

      b. Opioids bind to opiate receptors (mu, kappa, delta)

      c. Agonists

         i.   Morphine ("gold" standard for opioids)

         ii.   Fentanyl (Sublimaze)

         iii. Remifentanil (Ultiva)

         iv. Codeine

         v.   Methadone (Dolophine)

         vi. Meperidine (Demerol)

         vii. Hydromorphone (Dilaudid)

         viii. Oxycodone (Percocet)

         ix. Propoxyphene (Darvocet-N, Darvon)

         x.   Tramadol hydrochloride (Ultram)

         xi. Hydrocodone (Vicodin)

      d. Partial or mixed agonist/antagonist

         i.   Pentazocine (Talwin)

         ii.   Butorphanol (Stadol)

         iii. Buprenorphine (Buprenex)

         iv. Nalbuphine (Nubain)

         v.   Dezocine (Dalgan)

      e. Agonist/antagonists may cause withdrawal symptoms in patients

IX. Nonpharmacologic Pain Management

  A. Indications

    1. Supplement and augment pharmacologic interventions

    2. Promote patient involvement in own care

  B. Advantages

    1. Any nurse is qualified to use effectively with some training

    2. Special equipment is not required

    3. Does not interfere with medical treatment

  C. Peripheral techniques

    1. Cryotherapy—application of cold to body surface

      a. Decreases release of pain-causing chemicals (kinins, serotonin, histamine)

      b. Decreases edema formation by decreasing lymph production and cell permeability

      c. Slows conduction velocity of small unmyelinated nerves

      d. Use for clinical situations including initial posttraumatic pain, swelling, and muscle spasm

      e. Contraindications

         i.   Patients with history of peripheral vascular disease

         ii.   Raynauds disease

         iii. Angina patients with intolerance to cold

      f. Techniques easily taught to patient and family

2. Massage—kneading, manipulation or application of pressure and friction to body
   a. Improves circulation
   b. May release body endorphins
   c. Decrease pain by soothing and relaxing patient
   d. Used to comfort and ease back discomfort
   e. Contraindications
      i.   Fractures
      ii. Phlebitis
      iii. Skin lesions
      iv. Lacerations
      v.   Area of recent injury or trauma
   f. Easily taught to patient and family
   g. Creates opportunity to spend time with patient
D. Acupuncture
   1. Requires special training and skill to perform
   2. Provides body a boost
   3. May release histamine at acupuncture site
   4. May stimulate reflex mechanism that closes off pain sensation and transmission
   5. Not readily accepted by Western medicine
E. Acupressure—involves applying finger pressure to points that correspond to many of the points of acupuncture
   1. Little known as to how accupressure exerts analgesic effect
   2. Can treat many pain complaints
   3. Contraindicated in pregnant patients
   4. Nurse can provide a safe, simple inexpensive, noninvasive treatment
   5. Requires little time to learn or perform
F. TENS (transcutaneous electrical nerve stimulator)—electroanalgesia
   1. May activate large diameter, A-beta fibers closing the gate to pain impulse from the periphery
   2. May activate deep fibers by releasing endorphin
   3. Clinical uses include:
      a. Acute postoperative pain
      b. Other acute pain
         i.   Labor pain
         ii. Angina
         iii. Trauma
         iv. Low back pain
         v.   Headaches
   4. Contraindications
      a. Contact dermatitis
      b. Early pregnancy
      c. Cardiac pacemakers
   5. Nurse's role
      a. Requires physician order
      b. Document TENS stimulus to include intensity, frequency, and pulse width
      c. Mixed reviews as to being a good adjunct to other pain-management modalities
      d. Turn output to lowest setting when putting in new batteries and then gradually increase to patient tolerance
G. Relaxation—state of relative freedom from anxiety and skeletal muscle tension
   1. Decreases oxygen consumption
   2. Decreased muscle tone

3. Decreases heart rate and respiratory rate
4. Reduces distressing thoughts and anxiety
5. Nurse's role includes:
    a. Deep breathing, exhaling, yawning
    b. Humor
    c. Jaw relaxation
    d. Simple touch, massage

H. Music therapy
    1. Use preoperatively and intraoperatively to decrease anxiety
    2. Use postoperatively to decrease pain
    3. Adjunct to conventional therapy
    4. Music must be patient's preference
    5. Earphones for private listening

I. Distraction
    1. May increase tolerance to pain
    2. Useful in any type of pain
    3. Must be consistent with patient's energy and ability to concentrate
    4. Stimulates other major sensory modalities including:
        a. Hearing
        b. Vision
        c. Touch
        d. Movement

J. Imagery—development of an image on which to concentrate
    1. May be used to alter perception of pain
    2. Used to reduce fear and anxiety related to pain
    3. Nurses assist patient to convert pain to nonpain
    4. Use pain scales to assess

X. **Regional Techniques**
    A. Nerve blocks done for following purposes:
        1. Diagnostic
            a. Determine anatomic source of pain
            b. Differentiate central from peripheral pain
        2. Prognostic—predicts effects of other therapies
        3. Prophylactic—prevent chronic pain syndrome
        4. Therapeutic—provide anesthesia and postoperative analgesia
    B. Anesthesia agents (see Chapter 22 for more information)
        1. Two types of local anesthesia agents
            a. Esters
                i.   Hydrolyzed in plasma
                ii. Procaine, cocaine, chloroprocaine, tetracaine
            b. Amides
                i.   Metabolized by liver
                ii. Lidocaine, mepivacaine, bupivacaine, etidocaine
            c. Action of local anesthetics depends on:
                i.   Lipid solubility
                ii. Protein binding
                iii. Dissociation constant
        2. Neurolytic drugs
            a. Used to permanently destroy peripheral nerve pathways
            b. Indications
                i.   Ischemic vascular conditions
                ii. Advanced incurable cancer
                iii. Sympathetic dystrophy

3. Corticosteroids
   a. Used for reducing inflammation
   b. Relief of neuralgia pain associated with back pain
4. Alpha adrenergic drug
   a. Clonidine (Duroclon) approved in United States
   b. Epidural use for treating chronic pain

C. Peripheral nerve blocks
   1. Cranial nerve blocks
      a. Diagnose and treat pain syndromes associated with cancer
   2. Stellate ganglion blocks
      a. Used for causalgia, reflex sympathetic dystrophy, peripheral neuropathies, Raynauds syndrome, herpes zoster (shingles)
      b. Used for management of pain in:
         i.   Upper limbs
         ii. Neck
         iii. Thoracic viscera
      c. Successful block shows signs of:
         i.   Horner's syndrome
              (a) Ptosis of eyelid on blocked side
              (b) Miosis
              (c) Enophthalmos
              (d) Diminished sweating
              (e) Flushing of the face
         ii. Sensation of lump in throat with slight difficulty swallowing
         iii. Hoarseness
         iv. Nasal congestion
         v.   Warmth
         vi. Vasodilatation of arm on blocked side
      d. Complications
         i.   Pneumothorax
         ii. Hematoma
         iii. Hemoptysis
         iv. Seizure
         v.   Potential CSF injection
   3. Brachial plexus blocks
      a. Surgery
      b. Postoperative pain relief
      c. Chronic pain of upper extremities
      d. Four approaches
         i.   Interscalene
         ii. Supraclavicular
         iii. Infraclavicular
         iv. Axillary
   4. Peripheral nerve block of extremities
      a. Lumbosacral plexus which is made up of the following:
         i.   Sciatic nerve
         ii. Femoral nerve
         iii. Obturator
         iv. Lateral femoral cutaneous
   5. Sympathetic nerve blocks
      a. Block somatic nerve
      b. Intravenous regional infiltration
      c. Intraspinal block

6. Sympathetic blockade of lumbar chain
   a. Indication
      i.   Causalgia
      ii.   Reflex sympathetic dystrophy
      iii. Post amputation syndrome
      iv.   Peripheral vascular disease
   b. Signs of successful block
      i.   Increased skin temperature
      ii.   Flushing of blocked side
   c. Complications
      i.   Puncture of kidney
      ii.   Hematuria
      iii. Hypotension
      iv.   Abdominal pain
      v.   Persistent weakness in legs
D. Central nerve blocks
   1. Epidural
      a. Local anesthetic acts directly on nerve root after diffusing across dura
      b. Then it produces a paravertebral block
   2. Caudal epidural analgesia
      a. Good analgesia in pediatric population
      b. Pain control for circumcision, hypospadius, hernia, ureteral reimplant
      c. Dural puncture rarely a problem
      d. Larger volumes of local anesthetic agents are generally required compared
         with an epidural or lumbar puncture
   3. Subarachnoid (spinal)
      a. Local injection into cerebral spinal fluid
      b. Acts on superficial layers of spinal cord
      c. Spinals done for pain relief result in accompanying sympathetic blockade
   4. Complications associated with epidural and subarachnoid
      a. Neurologic changes
      b. Hypotension
      c. Headache
      d. Backache
      e. Hematoma
      f. Infection
      g. Respiratory depression especially from high central nerve block
   5. Epidural narcotics
      a. To control moderate to severe pain
      b. May be continuous or bolus
      c. Narcotics frequently used
         i.   Fentanyl
         ii.   Sufentanil (Sufenta)
         iii. Duramorph
         iv.   Dilaudid
      d. Complications
         i.   Sedation
         ii.   Pruritus
         iii. Nausea and vomiting
         iv.   Urinary retention
         v.   Respiratory depression

6. Interpleural regional analgesia—epidural catheter placed percutaneously in interpleural space
    a. Indications
        i.   Pain management after unilateral incision of chest
        ii. Pain management after unilateral incision of abdomen
    b. Contraindications
        i.   Pulmonary disease
        ii. Sepsis
        iii. Local infection
        iv. Coagulation abnormalities
    c. Complications
        i.   Pneumothorax
        ii. Local analgesia toxicity
        iii. Pleural effusions
        iv. Horner's syndrome—flushing, ptosis, hoarseness, difficult swallowing, decreased sweating
        v.   Phrenic nerve block

XI. Special Considerations
A. Pediatric patients
   1. Treat anticipated procedure-related pain prophylactically
   2. Ensure competence of individual performing procedure and the timeliness of the procedure—delays can escalate pain and anxiety
   3. Provide adequate unhurried preparation of the patient/family/responsible adult
   4. Be attentive to environmental stimuli and manner in which child is handled
   5. Allow parents to be with the child; the parents' presence may be a great source of comfort to the child
   6. Tailor treatment options, both pharmacologic and nonpharmacologic, to the child's and family's needs and preferences, to the procedure, and to the perioperative experience
   7. If possible, administer pharmacologic agents by a route that is not painful
   8. Dovetail pharmacologic and nonpharmacologic options to complement one another
   9. Provide monitoring and resuscitative equipment if medications are used for sedation
   10. Manage pre-existing pain optimally before beginning the procedure
   11. Historically, studies show undertreatment of infants and children
       a. Causes for undertreatment include:
           i.   Fear of addiction
           ii. Fear of respiratory depression
           iii. Lack of recognition/denial of pediatric pain
       b. A child's response to pain is related to developmental age and body image
   12. After the procedure, review with the child and family their experiences and perceptions about the effectiveness of pain-management strategies
B. Elderly patients
   1. General
       a. Suffer acute and chronic painful diseases
       b. Have multiple diseases
       c. Take numerous medications
       d. Metabolize medications less efficiently

2. Pain assessment may present unique problems as the elderly report pain differently due to the following changes associated with aging
   a. Physiologic
      i. Changes in drug absorption, distribution, metabolism, and excretion
      ii. Hepatic changes affect drug metabolism prolonging half-life and reducing total plasma clearance
   b. Psychologic
      i. Mental status may contribute to altered perceptions of pain experience
      ii. Patients with impaired cognition may be less able to report pain
   c. Cultural
      i. Assess patient's needs, ways, and customs as thoroughly and sensitively as possible
      ii. Establish a relationship by listening, showing respect, and allowing the patient to help formulate and choose treatment options
3. Elderly people are at risk for under- and overtreatment of pain
4. Attention should be directed to musculoskeletal, neurologic, and vascular systems as major sources of pain in the elderly
5. Attitudes of health-care professionals, the lay public, and the patients themselves may impede appropriate care because acute and chronic pain are often considered a part of normal aging
6. The widespread belief that aging results in increased pain thresholds may be a myth

Bibliography

1. *Acute Pain Management in Adults: Operative Procedures.* (1992). Quick Reference Guide for Clinicians. AHCPR Pub. No. 920019. Rockville, MD: Agency for Health Care Policy and Research, Public Health Service, U.S. Department of Health and Human Services.
2. *Acute Pain Management in Infants, Children, and Adolescents: Operative and Medical Procedures.* (1992). Quick Reference Guide for Clinicians. AHCPR Pub. No. 920019. Rockville, MD: Agency for Health Care Policy and Research, Public Health Service, U.S. Department of Health and Human Services.
3. *Acute Pain Management: Operative or Medical Procedures and Trauma.* (1992). Quick Reference Guide for Clinicians. AHCPR Pub. No. 920019. Rockville, MD: Agency for Health Care Policy and Research, Public Health Service, U.S. Department of Health and Human Services.
4. Carpenter, Randall. (1995). Does outcome change with pain management? In Barash, P.C., ed., *Refresher Courses in Anesthesiology.* Philadelphia: Lippincott. Chapter 3.
5. DiPiro, J.T., Talbert, R., Hayes, P.E., Yee, G.C., Matzke, G.R., Posey, L.M., ed. (1993). *Pharmacotherapy: A Pathophysiologic Approach,* 2nd ed. Norwalk, CT: Appleton-Lange.
6. Drain, C. (1994). *The Post Anesthesia Care Unit,* 3rd ed. Philadelphia: Saunders.
7. Litwack, K. (1995). *Post Anesthesia Care Nursing,* 2nd ed. St. Louis: Mosby.
8. Lefkowitz, M. (1994). Chronic Pain. In Barash, P.C. ed., *Refresher Courses in Anesthesiology.* Philadelphia: Lippincott. Chapter 14.
9. *Management of Cancer Pain: Adults.* (1994). Quick Reference Guide for Clinicians. Number 9. AHCPR Pub. No. 920019. Rockville, MD: Agency for Health Care Policy and Research, Public Health Service, U.S. Department of Health and Human Services.
10. McCaffery, M., Beebe, A. (1989). *Pain: Clinical Manual for Nursing Practice.* St. Louis: Mosby.
11. McGoldrick, K., ed. (1995). *Ambulatory Anesthesia.* Baltimore: Williams & Wilkins.
12. Meeker, M.H., Rothrock, J. (1995). *Alexander's Care of the Patient in Surgery,* 10th ed. St. Louis: Mosby.
13. Salerno, E., Willens, J.S. (1996). *Pain Management Handbook.* St. Louis: Mosby.

REVIEW QUESTIONS

1. In the PACU, the single most reliable indicator of a patient's pain is

   A. Change in behavior
   B. Crying
   C. Change in cardiovascular system
   D. Patient report of pain

2. The advantages of nonpharmacologic pain management include

   A. Any nurse is qualified to use it effectively with some training
   B. Specialized equipment is not required
   C. It does not interfere with medical treatment
   D. All of the above

3. Quantifiable aspects of pain include

   A. Location
   B. Intensity
   C. Timeliness
   D. Quality
   E. All of the above

4. Physiologic signs of pain include all of the following except

   A. Tachycardia
   B. Tachypnea
   C. Hypertension
   D. Hypoxia

5. Acute pain is defined as lasting

   A. Less than 6 months
   B. Less than 6 hours
   C. Less than 2 days
   D. Less than 1 year

6. Nonsteroidal antiinflammatory drug effects include all of the following except

   A. Antiinflammatory
   B. Analgesia
   C. Antipyretic
   D. Narcotic antagonist

7. Contraindications to nonpharmacologic pain management with cryotherapy include

   A. Patients with history of peripheral vascular disease
   B. Raynauds disease
   C. Angina patients with intolerance to cold
   D. All of the above

8. Opiate receptors primarily affected by morphine sulfate are

   A. Mu
   B. Alpha
   C. Beta
   D. Sigma

9. Contraindications to transcutaneous electrical nerve stimulator (TENS) include

   A. Contact dermatitis
   B. Early pregnancy
   C. Cardiac pacemakers
   D. All of the above

10. A successful stellate ganglion block will be evident by the evidence of occurrence of

   A. Horner's syndrome
   B. Cardiac dysrhythmias
   C. Hypotension
   D. Hypertension

ANSWERS TO QUESTIONS

1. D
2. D
3. E
4. D
5. A

6. D
7. D
8. A
9. D
10. A

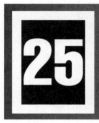

Anesthetic Complications

Lois Schick
Exempla Healthcare, Saint Joseph Hospital
Denver, Colorado

I. Nausea and Vomiting

Most common complication in inpatient and outpatient population.

    A. Emesis—retching is controlled by vomiting center in medulla; vomiting center receives input from:
        1. Cerebral cortex (olfactory, visual, emotional stimuli)
        2. GI tract
        3. Vestibular system
        4. Chemoreceptor trigger zone (CTZ)
    B. Risk factors for developing postoperative nausea and vomiting (PONV)
        1. Predisposing factors
            a. Female patient
            b. Motion sickness
            c. Vestibular problems
            d. Morbid obesity
            e. Early pregnancy
        2. Increased gastric volume
            a. Delayed gastric emptying
            b. Excessive anxiety
            c. Solid food ingestion
        3. Anesthetic agents
            a. Inhalation agents
                i.   Nitrous oxide
                ii. Volatile agents
            b. Intravenous agents
                i.   Ketamine
                ii. Etomidate
                iii. Analgesics including opioids

Objectives

1. Identify most common complications in inpatient and outpatient population.
2. List five examples of respiratory complications.
3. Identify three etiologies of delayed arousal.
4. State seven causes of emergence delirium.
5. Describe signs and symptoms seen when succinylcholine is administered to a patient with a pseudocholinesterase deficiency.

4. Surgical procedures
   a. Laparoscopy
   b. Strabismus
   c. Tonsillectomy and adenoidectomy
   d. Middle ear procedures
   e. Orchiopexy
5. Postoperative factors
   a. Severe pain
   b. Hypotension
   c. Dehydration

C. Interventions
1. Most effective treatment is prevention
   a. Assess for risk factors
   b. Hydrate adequately
   c. Avoid brisk head movement
   d. Administer pain medication
   e. Encourage deep breathing
   f. Avoid gastric distention
   g. Position appropriately—patient comfort
   h. Provide mouth care
2. Nasogastric tube
3. Limit movement immediately postoperative
4. Medicate patient
   a. Anticholinergics
      i. Atropine
      ii. Scopolamine
   b. Phenothiazines
      i. Prochlorperazine (Compazine)
      ii. Chlorpromazine (Thorazine)
   c. Antihistamines
      i. Promethazine (Phenergan)
      ii. Hydroxyzine (Vistaril, Atarax)
      iii. Diphenhydramine (Benadryl)
   d. Butyrophenones
      i. Droperidol (Inapsine)
      ii. Haloperidol (Haldol)
   e. Benzamide
      i. Metoclopramide (Reglan)
   f. Serotonin
      i. Ondansetron (Zofran)
      ii. Granisetron—for chemotherapy induced N and V
      iii. Dolasetron—currently under study in United States
      iv. Tropisetron—long acting; used in Europe and used with patient-controlled morphine drips
   g. Other
      i. Ephedrine

II. **Respiratory Complications**
A. Airway obstruction
1. Causes
   a. Soft tissue obstruction
   b. Tongue displacement (most common)
   c. Airway edema

        d. Foreign body

        e. Laryngospasm

    2. Signs and symptoms

        a. Snoring

        b. Flaring of nostrils

        c. Retraction

        d. Asynchronous movement of chest and abdomen

        e. Increased accessory muscle usage

        f. Increased pulse

        g. Decreased oxygen saturation

        h. Decreased breath sounds

    3. Interventions

        a. Chin support/jaw thrust

        b. Positive pressure with mask/ambu

        c. Artificial airways

           i.   Oral

           ii. Nasal

           iii. Endotracheal tube

B. Hypoventilation (desaturation most frequent event)

    1. Factors associated with hypoventilation

        a. Greater than 60 years of age

        b. Obese patients

        c. Longer operations

        d. High-dose muscle relaxant use

        e. High-dose opioid use

        f. Male

    2. Causes

        a. Airway obstruction

        b. Residual effects of medications

           i.   Anesthetic agents

           ii. Muscle relaxants

           iii. Analgesics

        c. Splinting

    3. Signs and symptoms

        a. Lethargy

        b. Confusion

        c. Restlessness

        d. Anxiety

        e. Dysrhythmias

        f. Cyanosis

        g. Decreased SpO_2

        h. Increased PCO_2

    4. Interventions

        a. Stir-up regimen

        b. Ventilatory assistance

        c. Oxygen

        d. Elevating head of bed

        e. Reversal of sedatives, narcotics, muscle relaxants

C. Laryngospasm

    1. Causes

        a. Asthma history

        b. Irritable airway

      c. Smoking
      d. Chronic obstructive pulmonary disease
      e. Endotracheal tube usage
      f. Anesthetic agents
      g. Vocal cord irritation
          i. Secretions
          ii. Blood
          iii. Vomitus
  2. Signs and symptoms
      a. Dyspnea
      b. Hypoxia
      c. Hypoventilation
      d. Crowing sounds
      e. Hypercarbia
  3. Interventions
      a. Hyperextend head
      b. Elevate head of bed
      c. Medications
          i. Oxygen
          ii. Racemic epinephrine
          iii. Decadron
          iv. Lidocaine
          v. Atropine
          vi. Muscle relaxants
      d. Intubation
      e. Positive pressure ventilation
D. Bronchospasm
  1. Causes
      a. Light anesthesia
      b. Residual effect of muscle relaxants
      c. Irritable tracheobronchial tree
      d. Mechanical factors
  2. Signs and symptoms
      a. Wheezing
      b. Shallow noisy respiration
      c. Chest retractions
      d. Dyspnea
      e. Tachypnea
      f. Decreased SpO_2
  3. Interventions
      a. Remove irritant
      b. Increase oxygen
      c. Administer muscle relaxants
      d. Deepen anesthesia
      e. Administer medications
          i. Lidocaine
          ii. Glycopyrollate
          iii. Hydrocortisone
          iv. Inhaled sympathomimetic bronchodilator aerosol (Albuterol)
          v. Theophylline
          vi. Terbutaline
          vii. Epinephrine

E. Noncardiogenic pulmonary edema
  1. Causes
     a. Pulmonary aspiration
     b. Allergic reactions
     c. Upper airway obstruction
     d. Rapid naloxone administration
     e. Sepsis
  2. Signs and Symptoms
     a. Tachypnea with respiratory distress
     b. Shortness of breath
     c. Rales
     d. Rhonchi
     e. Pink frothy sputum
     f. Pulmonary infiltrates
  3. Interventions
     a. Oxygen
     b. Pulmonary toilet
     c. Maintain unobstructed airway
     d. Diuretics
     e. Fluid restriction
     f. Morphine sulfate
     g. Mechanical ventilation
F. Aspiration—rare event related to anesthesia
  1. Factors related to aspiration pneumonitis
     a. Increased gastric residual volume
     b. Decreased gastric pH
     c. Presence of particulate matter in stomach
     d. Difficulty in protecting airway
  2. Higher risk populations for aspiration include:
     a. Morbid obesity
     b. Diabetics
     c. Surgical factors
        i.   Upper abdomen surgery
        ii. Straining on ETT (endotracheal tube)
  3. Types of aspiration
     a. Large particle
     b. Clear acidic fluid
     c. Clear nonacidic fluid
     d. Food stuff or small particle
     e. Contaminated material
  4. Sign and symptoms
     a. Tachypnea
     b. Tachycardia
     c. Hypoxia
     d. Chest infiltrate
     e. Wheezing
     f. Coughing—dyspnea
     g. Apnea
     h. Hypotension
     i. Bradycardia
  5. Interventions
     a. Position on side with head turned
     b. Bronch if large particles

       c. Oxygen
       d. Ventilate if needed
       e. Inotropic medications
       f. Antiemetics
  G. Pulmonary embolism
    1. Precipitating factors
       a. Venous stasis
       b. Hypercoagulability
       c. Vascular wall damage
    2. Signs and symptoms
       a. Hypoxia
       b. Restlessness
       c. Headache
       d. Apprehension
       e. Delirium
       f. Splinting
       g. Retractions
       h. Peripheral edema
       i. Distended neck veins
       j. Pleuritic pain
    3. Diagnosis
       a. Chest X-ray—nonspecific
       b. ECG—usually normal
       c. ABG—show hypoxemia and hypocapnia
       d. Lung scan—shows obstructed flow, perfusion defect
    4. Interventions
       a. Oxygen
       b. Bedrest
       c. Heparinization
       d. Narcotics
       e. Vasopressors
       f. Fluids
       g. Elastic hose
       h. Leg exercises

III. Cardiovascular Complications
  A. Dysrhythmia (see Chapter 11)
  B. Hypotension—25–30% decrease in systolic blood pressure from resting baseline value
    1. Causes
       a. Anesthesia—vasodilating effect
       b. Regional anesthesia—sympathetic block
       c. Hypovolemia
       d. Cardiac dysrhythmias
       e. Hypoxia
       f. Myocardial infarction
       g. Hypoglycemia
    2. Interventions
       a. Treat underlying cause
       b. Fluid challenge
       c. Elevate legs
       d. Oxygen
       e. Pressor drugs

C. Hypertension—pressures exceeding 140/90 mm Hg
  1. Causes
     a. Pain
     b. Hypoxemia
     c. Hypercarbia
     d. Fluid overload
     e. Delirium
     f. Distended bladder
     g. Shivering
     h. Hypothermia—vasoconstriction
     i. Improper sized BP cuff (too small)
     j. Poorly controlled hypertension
  2. Interventions
     a. Treat underlying cause first
     b. Analgesic administration
     c. Vasodilators
     d. Ganglionic blockers
     e. Calcium channel blockers
     f. Diuretics
D. Acute myocardial infarction
  1. Patients at risk
     a. Pre-existing coronary artery disease
     b. Diabetics
     c. Obesity
     d. Debilitated state
  2. Signs and symptoms
     a. Midsternal chest pressure with or without radiation to neck
     b. Jaw pain
     c. Left arm pain
     d. Diaphoresis
     e. Nausea
     f. Dyspnea
     g. Orthopnea
     h. Bradycardia
     i. Tachycardia
     j. Hypotension
  3. Interventions
     a. Relieve chest pain
     b. Decrease workload of heart
     c. Maintain stable cardiac rhythm
     d. Detect and treat complications

IV. **Delayed Arousal**
  A. Etiology
     1. Prolonged action of anesthesia medications
     2. Metabolic causes
     3. Neurologic causes
  B. Anesthesia causes
     1. Residual anesthesia
     2. Hyperventilation due to high concentration of inhaled agents
     3. Narcotics may contribute to hypercarbia and sedation
     4. Hypothermia

C. Metabolic causes
  1. Hepatic dysfunction
  2. Renal disease
  3. Electrolyte imbalance
     a. Hypocalcemia
     b. Dilutional hyponatremia
     c. High magnesium levels, especially eclamptic patients
  4. Diabetic ketoacidosis
  5. Thyroid dysfunction
  6. Malignant hyperthermia
D. Neurologic causes
  1. Ischemia
  2. Cardiovascular accident
  3. Intracranial hemorrhage
  4. Air emboli
  5. Uncontrolled hypotension
  6. Embolism
  7. Mass lesions
  8. Seizure disorders
E. Interventions
  1. Assess oxygenation needs
  2. Ensure adequate oxygen exchange
  3. May need to reverse narcotics and benzodiazepines
  4. Warm patient if cold
  5. Treat electrolyte imbalance appropriately
  6. Identify causes to treat specifically

V. Emergence Delirium—Agitation/Dysphoria

Common in children as well as healthy patients

A. Causes
  1. Anesthetic agents
     a. Ketamine
     b. Atropine
     c. Lidocaine
     d. Droperidol
     e. Scopolamine
     f. Residual neuromuscular blockers
     g. Residual inhalation agents
  2. Pain
  3. Urinary bladder distension
  4. Anxiety
  5. Substance abuse including alcohol withdrawal
  6. Hypoxia
  7. Hypercarbia
  8. Metabolic/endocrine problems
  9. Hypoglycemia
  10. Hyponatremia
  11. Hyper/hypothyroidism
  12. Hypoadrenalism
  13. Cerebral hypoxia
     a. Systemic

  b. Hypotension
  c. Severe anemia
 14. Sepsis
B. Signs and symptoms
 1. Responsive or unresponsive agitation
 2. Crying
 3. Tachycardia
 4. Verbalizations
 5. Unable to follow commands
 6. Low saturation levels
 7. Restlessness
 8. Disorientation
 9. Irrational talking, screaming, shouting
 10. Confusion
C. Interventions
 1. Treat underlying cause
 2. Oxygen if indicated
 3. Narcotics or sedation if needed
 4. May need to reverse narcotics or benzodiazepines
 5. Provide quiet environment
 6. Speak softly and directly to patient
 7. Maintain safety

VI. Hypothermia

A. Causes
 1. Anesthesia
 2. Surgery
 3. Cold OR
B. Mechanisms of heat loss
 1. Radiation—heat transfer between two surfaces of different temperatures
 2. Convection—heat loss at a surface caused by fluid flowing across at a lower temperature
 3. Conduction—heat transfer due to a temperature difference between two objects in contact
 4. Evaporation—insensible water loss from skin, the respiratory tract, open incisions, and wet drapes
C. Potential complications from hypothermia
 1. Wound infection
 2. Cardiac disturbances
 3. Altered medication effect
 4. Coagulopathy
 5. Shivering
 6. Increased oxygen consumption
 7. Delayed emergency from anesthesia
D. Interventions
 1. Warmed cotton blankets
 2. Thermal drapes
 3. Fluid warmers
 4. Heat-moisture exchangers
 5. Heated humidifiers
 6. Warm ORs
 7. Infrared lights
 8. Forced-air therapy

VII. Pseudocholinesterase Deficiency

Atypical pseudocholinesterase unable to break down succinylcholine; pseudocholinesterase breaks down succinylcholine within 3–5 minutes normally.

- A. Causes
  - 1. Genetic
    - a. Affects 1 in 2,500–2,800 people
  - 2. Prolonged duration of action of succinylcholine in patients with abnormal or low levels of plasmacholinesterase
    - a. Patients with liver disease
    - b. Patients with severe anemia
    - c. Patients with malnutrition
    - d. Pregnant patients
    - e. Dialysis patients
    - f. Acidosis
    - g. Medications
      - i. Antibiotics
      - ii. Local anesthetics
      - iii. Beta blockers
      - iv. Diuretics
      - v. Magnesium
      - vi. Cytotoxic drugs
- B. Signs and symptoms
  - 1. Apnea
  - 2. Lack of muscle control—"floppy fish"
- C. Interventions
  - 1. Ventilate until efficient respirations obtained
  - 2. Offer psychological support
  - 3. May need to administer sedative
  - 4. Educate family and patient of not receiving succinylcholine in the future
  - 5. Laboratory studies may be indicated (dibucaine levels)

VIII. Shivering

Heat production by muscular contractions.

- A. Causes
  - 1. Intraoperative hypothermia
  - 2. General anesthesia
  - 3. Regional anesthesia
- B. Implications of hypothermia and shivering
  - 1. Increased oxygen consumption up to 400–500%
  - 2. Cardiac dysrhythmias
  - 3. Decreased level of consciousness
  - 4. Decreased metabolism parenteral medications
  - 5. Delayed excretion sedatives, narcotics, muscle relaxants
- C. Signs and symptoms
  - 1. Postoperative shivering
  - 2. Difficult to deliver care
  - 3. Interference with monitoring
  - 4. Increased risk of trauma
  - 5. Elicit marked increase in cardiac output and minute ventilation
  - 6. Tonic and clonic activity

   D. Interventions
     1. Supplemental oxygen
     2. Maintain core temperature
     3. Warm ambient air
     4. Warm intravenous fluids
     5. Warm irrigation fluids
     6. Passive assistance with radiant lighting
     7. Blankets
     8. May try medications
        a. Morphine
        b. Meperidine
        c. Droperidol
        d. Chloropramazine
        e. Clonidine
 IX. **High/Total Spinal**
   A. Causes
     1. Overdose local anesthetic
     2. Incorrect patient position
     3. Rapid injection
     4. Variations in spinal pressures
   B. Interventions
     1. Immediate recognition
     2. Intubate and ventilate
     3. Increase intravenous fluids
     4. Trendelenburg—constant monitoring
     5. Emotional support
  X. **Toxicity of Local Anesthetic**
   A. Systemic Effects
     1. CNS
        a. Tinnitus
        b. Light headedness
        c. Confusion
        d. Circumoral numbness
        e. Tonic–clonic convulsions
        f. Generalized CNS depression
        g. Unconsciousness
     2. Cardiovascular
        a. Hypertension
        b. Tachycardia
        c. Myocardial depression
        d. Peripheral vasodilatation
        e. Sinus bradycardia
        f. Ventricular dysrhythmias
        g. Circulatory collapse
   B. Treatment
     1. Postpone surgery
     2. Maintain patent airway
     3. Symptomatic treatment
     4. Observe for delayed toxicity
     5. Epinephrine reduces risk of toxicity

XI. Allergic Reactions

Occur approximately once every 10,000 anesthetics. Vast majority of intravenous-induced allergic reactions occur within 3 minutes of administration.

- A. Causes
    1. Drug sensitivity
    2. Allergy, i.e., latex, foods, chemicals, materials
- B. Signs and symptoms
    1. Conjunctivitis
    2. Urticaria
    3. Angioedema
    4. Gastrointestinal disturbances
    5. Laryngeal edema
    6. Bronchospasm
    7. Hypotension
    8. Dysrhythmias
    9. Cardiac arrest
    10. Coma
- C. Treatment
    1. Maintain patent airway
    2. Adrenergic agonists (epinephrine)
    3. Methylxanthines (Aminophyllin)
    4. Anticholinergics (Atropine, Glycopyrollate, Scopolamine)
    5. Antihistamines (Benadryl)
    6. Corticosteroids
    7. Volume expanders
    8. Hemodynamic monitoring

Bibliography

1. Barash, P., Cullen, B., Stoelting, R. (1991). *Handbook of Clinical Anesthesia.* Philadelphia: Lippincott.
2. Burden, N. (1993). *Ambulatory Surgery Nursing.* Philadelphia: Saunders.
3. DiPiro, J., Talbert, R., Hayes, P., Yee, G., Matzke, G., Posey, L.M. (1993). *Pharmacotherapy: A Pathophysiologic Approach,* 2nd ed. East Norwalk, CT.: Appleton & Lange.
4. Drain, C. (1994). *The Post Anesthesia Care Unit,* 3rd ed. Philadelphia: Saunders.
5. Fetzer-Fowler, S. (1992). State of the art: Regional anesthesia using anesthetic admixtures. *J Post Anesth Nursing,* 7(4):229–237.
6. Kang, S., Rudrud, L., Nelson, W., Baier, D. (1994). Postanesthesia nursing care for ambulatory surgery patients: Post-spinal anesthesia. *J PeriAnesth Nursing,* 9(2):101–106.
7. Kirby, R., Gravenstein, N. (1994). *Clinical Anesthesia Practice.* Philadelphia: Saunders.
8. Litwack, K. (1995). *Post Anesthesia Care Nursing,* 2nd ed. St. Louis: Mosby.
9. Litwack, K. (1994). *Core Curriculum for Post Anesthesia Nursing Practice,* 3rd ed. Philadelphia: Saunders.
10. McGoldrick, K. (ed.) (1995). *Ambulatory Anesthesiology.* Baltimore: Williams & Wilkins.
11. Omoigui, S. (1992). *The Anesthesia Drug Handbook.* St. Louis: Mosby.
12. *PDR® Nurses Handbook for Certified Registered Nurse Anesthetists.* (1997). Montvale, NJ: Medical Economics.
13. Schweinefus, R., Schick, L. (1991). Succinylcholine: Good Guy, Bad Guy. *Post Anesth Nursing,* 6(6): 410–419.
14. Silverman, D., Connelly, N.R. (1995). *Review of Clinical Anesthesia.* Philadelphia: Lippincott.
15. Stein, R. H. (1995). The perioperative nurse's role in anesthesia management. *AORN J,* 62(5):794–804.
16. Twersky, R.S. (1995). *The Ambulatory Anesthesia Handbook.* St. Louis: Mosby.
17. Vender, J., Spiess, B. (1992). *Post Anesthesia Care.* Philadelphia: Saunders.
18. Walker, J. (1997). Neuromuscular relaxation and reversal: An update. *J PeriAnesth Nursing,* 12(4): 264–274.
19. White, P. (1997). *Ambulatory Anesthesia and Surgery.* Philadelphia: Saunders.
20. Wong, D. (1995). *Whaley & Wong's Nursing Care of Infants and Children,* 5th ed. St. Louis: Mosby.

REVIEW QUESTIONS

1. Predisposing risk factors for developing postoperative nausea and vomiting include the following except

   A. Morbid obesity
   B. Vestibular problems
   C. Early pregnancy
   D. Male patients

2. The most common cause of upper airway obstruction is

   A. Tongue
   B. Laryngospasm
   C. Patient position
   D. Incorrectly placed endotracheal tube

3. An effective way to prevent hypoventilation in a young healthy PACU patient is

   A. Stir-up regimen
   B. Provide humidified oxygen
   C. Administer naloxone
   D. Flush residual anesthesia with IV solution

4. Rapid administration of naloxone in an anesthetized patient may result in

   A. More sedate patient
   B. Bradycardia
   C. Noncardiogenic pulmonary edema
   D. Pain-free patient

5. One of the most common causes of hypotension in the PACU is

   A. Unreplaced volume loss
   B. Myocardial dysfunction
   C. Dysrhythmias
   D. Medication intolerance

6. Frequent causes of hypertension in the PACU include

   A. Pain
   B. Distended bladder
   C. Too-small blood pressure cuff
   D. All of the above

7. A common cause of delayed awakening in patients emerging from anesthesia is

   A. Barbiturate premedication
   B. Hypoxic injury
   C. Residual inhaled or injected anesthetic agents
   D. Hyperthermia

8. Causes for emergence delirium in the PACU include

   A. Hypoxia
   B. Anesthetic agents
   C. Cerebral hypoxia
   D. All of the above

9. A prolonged duration of action of succinylcholine in patients with abnormal or low levels of plasmacholinesterase is seen in

   A. Pregnant patients
   B. Patients with severe anemia
   C. Patients with liver disease
   D. All of the above

10. Shivering can increase oxygen consumption by

    A. 50%
    B. 100%
    C. 200%
    D. 400%

ANSWERS TO QUESTIONS

1. D
2. A
3. A
4. C
5. A

6. D
7. C
8. D
9. D
10. D

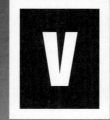

P A R T

V

General and
Abdominal-
Thoracic
Surgeries

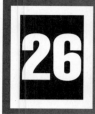

General Surgery

Lonnie Lane
Columbia Physicians Daysurgery Center
Dallas, Texas

I. **Anatomy and Physiology**
   A. Breast
      1. Mammary glands (bilateral)
      2. Lie on pectoralis major fascia of the anterior chest wall
      3. Surrounded by layers of fat encased in envelope of skin
      4. Weight
         a. Non-lactating breast: 150 to 250 grams
         b. Lactating breast: 400–500 grams
      5. Muscle
         a. Fixed to overlying skin and underlying pectoral fascia with fibrous bands (Cooper's ligaments)
      6. Lobes
         a. 12 to 20 lobes subdivided into lobules, composed of acini
         b. Arranged in a spiral fashion around the nipple
         c. Each lobe is drained by a duct, 12 to 20, which open on nipple
      7. Nipple
         a. Center of fully developed breast in adult women
         b. Located in 4th intercostal space
         c. Bundles of smooth muscle fibers have erectile properties
         d. Pigmented areola (that surrounds the nipple) diameter 1.5 to 2.5 cm
         e. 15 to 20 lactiferous ducts arranged radially under areola

Objectives

Study of the information represented by this outline will enable the learner to:
1. State the classification and pathophysiology of benign disorders of the breast.
2. State factors that may be associated with cholelithiasis.
3. State the classifications of hemorrhoids according to the degree of involvement.
4. Identify the differences between an open-approach and a laparoscopic-approach herniorrhaphy.
5. Develop a patient teaching plan for the patient having partial, subtotal, or total thyroidectomy.
6. State the rationale for observations necessary in PACU care of the general surgery patient.

      f. Areolar epithelium contains small hairs and glands
         i. Sebaceous glands (Montgomery's glands)
        ii. Sweat glands
      iii. Accessory mammary glands

8. Blood supply
    a. Artery
        i. Internal mammary
       ii. Lateral branches of anterior aortic intercostal arteries
    b. Veins
        i. Main veins follow the arterial pattern
       ii. Superficial veins frequently become dilated during pregnancy
      iii. Superficial veins often dilate over area which contains disease

9. Lymph drainage system
    a. Generally follows course of blood vessels
    b. Drain into axillary nodes (approximately 53) and into internal mammary nodes (few in number)

10. Nerve supply
    a. Anterior cutaneous branches of upper intercostal nerves
    b. 3rd and 4th branches of cervical plexus
    c. Lateral cutaneous branches of intercostal nerves

11. Pathophysiology
    a. Affected by three types of physiological changes
        i. Those related to growth and development
       ii. Those related to menstrual cycle
      iii. Those related to pregnancy and lactation
    b. Description of benign tumors of breast
        i. Fibrocystic disease
           (a) Accounts for over 45% of all biopsied female breast lesions
       ii. Adenofibroses
           (a) Disease of the youth, mean age 21
      iii. Papilloma (intraductal papillomas)
           (a) Growing in the terminal portions of a duct or throughout the duct system of a sector (multiple)
      iv. Duct ectasia (comedomastitis)
           (a) Disease of the ducts in the subareolar zone
           (b) Disease of the aging breast, most common in or near menopause
           (c) No demonstrated association with carcinoma
    c. Classification of malignant tumors of the breast
        i. Early: solitary, unilateral, hard, painless, solid, irregular, poorly outlined, non-mobile lump usually located in the upper, outer quadrant of the breast, and opaque to translumination
       ii. Moderately advanced locally: axillary nodes, nipple retraction or elevation, skin dimpling, nipple discharge
      iii. Far advanced locally: supraclavicular nodes, fixation of axillary nodes, fixation of tumor to chest wall, edema (peau d'orange or redness over more than a third of the breast), edema of the arm, ulceration of the skin, satellite nodules
      iv. Distant metastasis: inoperable, partial, osseous or visceral

B. Gallbladder

Refer to Figure 26–1

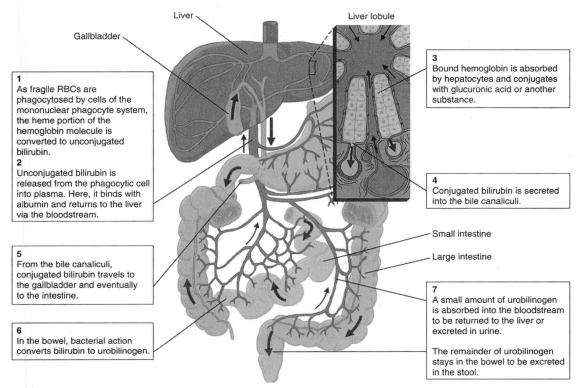

Liver

Gallblader

Liver lobule

1
As fragile RBCs are phagocytosed by cells of the mononuclear phagocyte system, the heme portion of the hemoglobin molecule is converted to unconjugated bilirubin.

2
Unconjugated bilirubin is released from the phagocytic cell into plasma. Here, it binds with albumin and returns to the liver via the bloodstream.

3
Bound hemoglobin is absorbed by hepatocytes and conjugates with glucuronic acid or another substance.

4
Conjugated bilirubin is secreted into the bile canaliculi.

Small intestine

Large intestine

5
From the bile canaliculi, conjugated bilirubin travels to the gallbladder and eventually to the intestine.

6
In the bowel, bacterial action converts bilirubin to urobilinogen.

7
A small amount of urobilinogen is absorbed into the bloodstream to be returned to the liver or excreted in urine.

The remainder of urobilinogen stays in the bowel to be excreted in the stool.

Figure 26–1. Bile formation, metabolism, and excretion. *Inset* shows bile formation in the liver lobule. *Thin arrows* indicate the direction of blood flow; *fat arrows* indicate the direction of digestive system flow. (From Black, J.M, Matassarin-Jacobs, E. [1997]. *Medical Surgical Nursing*, 5th ed. [p. 1839]. Philadelphia: Saunders.)

1. Location
   a. Lies in sulcus on undersurface of right lobe of liver
   b. Terminates in cystic duct
   c. Provides a channel for flow of bile to gallbladder, where bile becomes highly concentrated during storage period
2. Bile
   a. Consists chiefly of water, salts of bile acids, pigments, inorganic salts, cholesterol, and phospholipids
3. Bile movement
   a. Presence of certain food stuffs—particularly fat in duodenum—causes release of hormone cholecystokinin–pancreozymin, which then reaches the gallbladder via blood and brings on contraction
   b. As sphincter of Oddi in ampulla of Vater relaxes, bile pours forth, flowing into the duodenum to aid in digestion
4. Blood supply
   a. From cystic artery, a branch of the hepatic artery
5. Pathophysiology
   a. Gallstones (cholelithiasis)
      i. Formation results from changes in bile components or bile stasis, which may be associated with such factors as:
         (a) Infection
         (b) Cirrhosis
         (c) Pancreatitis
         (d) Celiac disease

          (e) Diabetes mellitus

          (f) Pregnancy

          (g) Oral contraceptives

     ii.   Acute cholecystitis

        (a) May be calculous (with gallstones) or acalculous (without gallstones) and can result from:

          (i)   Obstruction of cystic duct with an impacted gallstone (90% to 95% of cases)

          (ii) Tissue damage due to trauma, massive burns, or surgery

          (iii) Gram-negative septicemia

          (iv) Multiple blood transfusions

          (v) Prolonged fasting

          (vi) Hypertension

          (vii) Overuse of narcotic analgesics

        (b) Calculi usually form from solid constituents of bile

          (i)   Cholesterol gallstones

            a) Most common type

            b) Thought to form in supersaturated bile

          (ii) Pigment gallstones

            a) Formed mainly of unconjugated pigments in bile precipitate

          (iii) Mixed types

            a) Characteristics of cholesterol and pigment stones

        (c) Most patients have smaller pool of bile acids in general and often less chenodeoxycholic acid in particular

C. Hemorrhoids

   1. Masses of vascular tissue found in anal canal

     a. Internal hemorrhoids

       i.   Found above pectinate line

       ii. Arise from superior hemorrhoidal venous plexus

       iii. Covered with mucosa

     b. External hemorrhoids

       i.   Found below pectinate line

       ii. Arise from inferior hemorrhoid venous plexus

       iii. Covered by anoderm and perianal skin

     c. Patient may have combination of internal and external hemorrhoids

     d. Classification according to degree of involvement

       i.   1st degree: project slightly into the anal canal

       ii. 2nd degree: prolapse with defecation and reduce spontaneously

       iii. 3rd degree: prolapse with defecation and reduce manually

       iv. 4th degree: irreducible

   2. Pathophysiology

     a. Bleeding can be severe enough to cause iron-deficiency anemia

     b. Strangulation: prolapse hemorrhoid in which blood supply is cut off by the anal sphincter

     c. Thrombosis: clotting of blood within hemorrhoid

D. Anal Fissure

   1. Small tear in lining of anus

   2. Tear resembles a slit-like crack and may extend from anal verge to pectinate line

   3. Usually caused by trauma from passing large, hard stools

   4. Loss of elasticity of anal canal may predispose due to:

     a. Laxative abuse

     b. Scarring from anal surgery

      c. Chronic diarrhea disease

      d. Frequent anal intercourse

E. Anorectal fistula

    1. Hollow, fibrous tunnel or tract with two openings

    2. Primary, or internal, opening usually at a crypt near the pectinate line

    3. Infection in crypt progresses to form abscess that drains (spontaneously or with surgical drainage), and tract is preserved as abscess heals

    4. Associated with:

      a. Traumatic injury

      b. Crohn's disease

      c. Cancer

      d. Radiation therapy

    5. May have single or multiple fistulas

F. Pilonidal disease

    1. Occurs in midline of upper portion of gluteal fold

    2. Sinus channel develops; lined with epithelium and hair

    3. Occurs during embryonic development when small amount of endothelial tissue is included beneath skin

    4. Rarely becomes symptomatic until adulthood

G. Hernia

Refer to Figure 26–2

    1. Sac lined by peritoneum that protrudes through defect in layers of abdominal wall

    2. May be acquired or congenital

    3. Weak places or intervals in abdominal aponeurosis

      a. Inguinal canals

      b. Femoral rings

      c. Umbilicus

    4. Contributing factors

      a. Age

      b. Sex

      c. Previous surgery

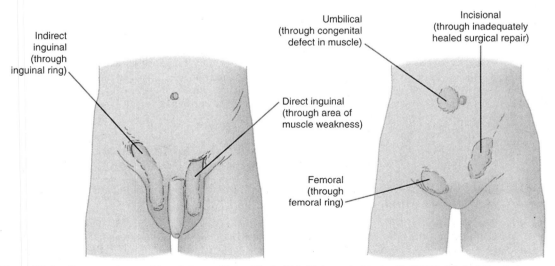

Figure 26–2. Common types of herniation. (From Black, J.M, Matassarin-Jacobs, E. [1997]. *Medical Surgical Nursing*, 5th ed. [p. 1817]. Philadelphia: Saunders.)

      d. Obesity
      e. Nutritional status
      f. Pulmonary and cardiac disease
      g. Loss of skin turgor
         i. Aging
        ii. Chronic debilitating diseases
   5. Pathophysiology
      a. Internal hernias
         i. Congenital
        ii. Associated with failure of intestine to rotate in usual sequence in fetus
      b. External hernias:
         i. Inguinal hernia
            (a) Most common
            (b) Indirect: herniation protrudes through inguinal ring and follows round ligament or spermatic cord
            (c) Direct: herniation goes through posterior inguinal wall
        ii. Femoral
            (a) More frequent in women
            (b) Protrusion through femoral ring into femoral canal
            (c) Seen as bulge below inguinal ligament
            (d) Can strangulate easily
        iii. Ventral
            (a) Associated with muscle weakness from abdominal incisions
            (b) Spontaneous occurring
               (i) Epigastric
                  a) Protrusions of fat through defects in abdominal wall
                  b) Between xiphoid process and the umbilicus
              (ii) Umbilicus
                  a) More common in children
                  b) Frequently disappears spontaneously by two years
                  c) Adult
                     (1) Acquired
                     (2) More common in women
                     (3) Increased abdominal pressure
                     (4) Obese persons
                     (5) Multiparity
            (c) Postoperative
               (i) Incisional
                  a) Muscle weakness from previous surgeries
                  b) Poor nutritional state
                  c) Faulty surgical technique
                  d) Obese associated with ascites
                  e) Those who have had wound infection
                  f) Wounds healed by secondary intention
H. Thyroid
   1. Butterfly-shaped gland composed of two lobes positioned on either side of trachea and joined by isthmus
      a. Isthmus situated near base of neck
      b. Upper pole of gland beneath upper end of sternothyroid muscle
      c. Lower pole extends to sixth tracheal ring
      d. Posterior surface of isthmus adherent to anterior surface of tracheal ring
      e. Enclosed by pretracheal fascia

2. Blood supply
   a. External carotid arteries via superior thyroid artery and subclavian artery via inferior thyroid arteries
   b. Drained by three pairs of veins that extend from a plexus formed on surface of gland and on front of trachea
   c. Capillaries form a dense plexus in connective tissue around follicles
3. Nerve supply
   a. Superior laryngeal nerve lies bilateral in proximity to superior thyroid artery
   b. Recurrent laryngeal nerve that supplies vocal cord ascends from mediastinum and in close association with tracheoesophageal sulcus and interior thyroid artery
   c. Sympathetic and parasympathetic nerves enter gland, probably exerting influence primarily on blood supply
4. Physiology
   a. In response to thyroid-stimulating hormone (TSH, released by pituitary in response to thyrotropin-releasing hormone)
   b. Produces thyroxine (T_4) and triiodothyronine (T_3) each day
      i. T_3 has short half life
      ii. T_4 has half life of 5 to 7 days
      iii. Peripheral tissue converts T_4 to T_3
      iv. T_3 considered as true tissue thyroid hormone, whereas T_4 considered a plasma pro-hormone
      v. Control of hormones exists in hypothalamus and pituitary on negative-feedback cycle
5. Pathophysiology
   a. Multinodular toxic diffuse enlargement, Graves' disease
   b. Adenomas
   c. Malignancy
   d. Thyroiditis
      i. Viral, autoimmune, or unknown etiology
      ii. Immunoglobulins found in serum of hyperthyroid patients mimic thyrotropin (also called thyroid-stimulating hormone, or TSH)

I. Parathyroid

Refer to Figure 26–3

1. Consists of four small masses of tissue lying behind or, rarely, within thyroid gland, inside pretracheal fascia
   a. Upper pair lie behind superior pole of thyroid
   b. Lower pair lie near pole of thyroid
2. Aberrant nodules of parathyroid tissue may be found outside pretracheal fascia as low as superior mediastinum, especially within thymus
3. Glands are brownish
4. Normally measure 3 to 4 mm in diameter
5. Blood supply
   a. Derived from superior and inferior thyroid arteries
6. Physiology
   a. Parathyroid hormone (PTH) regulates and maintains metabolism and hemostasis of blood calcium concentration
   b. Refer to Figure 26–4: Regulation of parathyroid hormone secretion
7. Pathophysiology
   a. Primary hyperparathyroidism characterized by hypercalcemia and hyperphosphatemia

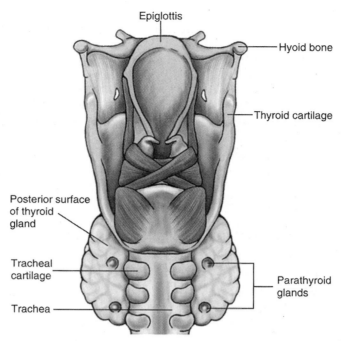

Figure 26–3. The parathyroid glands are positioned on the posterior surface of the thyroid gland. Although the parathyroids may be located anywhere on the posterior surface of the thyroid, one parathyroid gland is usually located in the upper half and one in the lower half of each thyroid lobe.   (From Monahan, F.D., Neighbors, M. [1998]. *Medical Surgical Nursing,* 2nd ed. [p. 1212]. Philadelphia: Saunders.)

    b. Disturbances in calcium and phosphate result in major kidney and bone lesions

    c. Secondary hyperparathyroidism results from parathyroid hyperplasia, producing decreased serum calcium levels

    d. Bone lesions are primary outcomes

    e. Overactivity of one or more parathyroid glands

    f. Excessive secretion of PTH

    g. Imbalance in calcium and phosphate metabolism; increased 10.5 ml/dL (normal 9–10.6 ml/dL)

II. Assessment

  A. General

    1. Testing requirements are individualized according to institutional policy

    2. Laboratory tests

      a. Basic hematology and electrolyte studies

      b. Urinalysis

    3. Radiologic examinations

      a. Chest x-ray film

    4. General history and physical

    5. Electrocardiogram (ECG) with follow-up evaluation as dictated by medical history and/or physical findings

    6. Psychological assessment

  B. Breast

    1. Clinical manifestations

      a. Benign breast tumors may include:

        i.   Breast pain and tenderness

        ii.   Change in mass size (larger and smaller) with menstrual cycle

        iii.   Palpable masses: firm, round, and freely movable

   b. Conditions affecting the nipple include:
       i.   Bloody nipple discharge (intraductal papilloma)
       ii. Eczematous or ulcerated nipple (Paget's disease)
       iii. Usually minimal pain
   c. Breast cancer may include:
       i.   A nontender lump, usually in an upper, outer quadrant
       ii. Pain (late)
       iii. Axillary lymphadenopathy (late)
       iv. Fixed, nodular breast mass (late)
2. Diagnostic studies
   a. Monthly breast self-examination
   b. Annual breast examination by physician
   c. Annual or other periodic mammography for asymptomatic women 50 years of
       age and older
   d. Annual or periodic mammography for women 40 years of age and older and:
       i.   Familial history of breast cancer
       ii.   Early menarche
       iii. Late menopause
       iv.   Multiparous or birth of first child after 34 years of age
       v.   High-fat diet
       vi.   Oral contraceptive use
       vii. Radiation exposure
       viii. Presence of other cancer

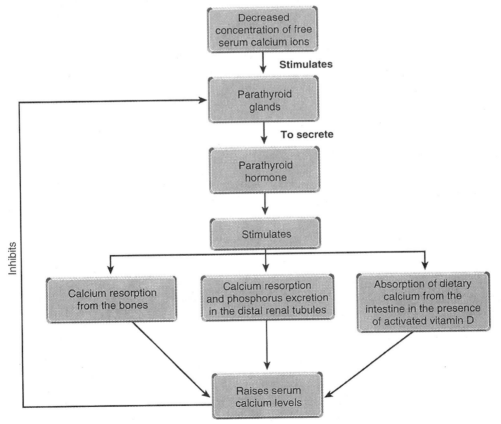

Figure 26–4. Regulation of parathyroid hormone secretion by negative feedback control.   (From Monahan, F.D., Neighbors, M. [1998]. *Medical Surgical Nursing,* 2nd ed. [p. 1213]. Philadelphia: Saunders.)

3. Laboratory studies
   a. Estrogen receptor protein
   b. Carcinoembryonic antigen (CEA)
   c. Gross cystic disease protein
   d. Liver function studies
4. Scans
   a. Bone scanning
   b. Brain or computed tomography (CT) scan
   c. Chest roentgenogram
   d. Ultrasonography
   e. Thermography
C. Laparoscopic cholecystectomy
   1. Clinical manifestations
      a. Episodic, cramping pain in right upper abdomen quadrant or epigastrium, possibly radiating to the back near right scapular tip (biliary colic)
      b. Nausea and/or vomiting
      c. Fat intolerance
      d. Fever and leukocytosis
      e. Signs and symptoms of jaundice
      f. Heart burn
      g. Flatulence
   2. Laboratory studies
      a. Serum enzyme levels
      b. Serum markers (e.g., carcinoembryonic antigen [CEA])
      c. Bilirubin studies, liver function tests, alkaline phosphate
   3. Radiographic studies
      a. Flat plate of abdomen
      b. Ultrasonography
      c. Gallbladder series (oral cholecystogram)
      d. Cholangiogram (intravenous)
      e. Upper gastrointestinal series
D. Hemorrhoidectomy
   1. Clinical manifestations
      a. Digital rectal exam
         i. Tone of internal sphincter; usually increased in young men with hemorrhoids; may be low in older men and women
      b. Anoscopy
         i. Visualization of hemorrhoids as instrument is removed
         ii. Sigmoidoscopy
         iii. Barium enema
            (a) To rule out carcinoma and inflammatory disease
            (b) Particularly important in patient over 40 years of age
E. Anal fissure
   1. Clinical manifestations
      a. Digital rectal examination:
         i. Induration
         ii. Tenderness
         iii. Sphincter spasm
         iv. Hypertrophied and papillae
      b. Anoscopy (proctoscopy)
         i. Visualization of anorectal fissure; a superficial tear that bleeds easily and has a reddish base

2. Differential diagnosis
    a. If fissure is not found in midline, rule out:
        i. Inflammatory disease
        ii. Bowel disease
        iii. Carcinoma
        iv. Tuberculosis
        v. Syphilis
        vi. Herpes or other venereal disease

F. Anal fistula
  1. Clinical manifestations
    a. Digital rectal examination
        i. Palpate tract direction internally
    b. Anoscopy (proctoscopy)
        i. May reveal the primary opening in a cyst
    c. Sigmoidoscopy
        i. Used to rule out other sources of fistula formation
    d. Fistulography
        i. Used if tract is of questionable origin
        ii. Rules out colonic, small bowel, and urethral fistulas

G. Pilonidal disease
  1. Clinical manifestations
    a. Perineal area
        i. Hairy dimple in gluteal fold
        ii. Open, draining lesion in sacral region with hair protruding from sinus opening

H. Herniorrhaphy
  1. Clinical manifestations
    a. Physical examination of abdomen
        i. Examine supine and sitting
        ii. Can often see hernia "bulge" or protrude as person changes position, coughs, or when children cry or laugh
        iii. Palpate weakened muscle area
        iv. Abdominal distention, nausea, and vomiting may be early signs of intestinal obstruction
        v. Pain of increasing severity, fever, tachycardia, and abdominal rigidity are signs of strangulation

I. Thyroid (hyperthyroidism)
  1. Clinical manifestations
    a. Nervousness, irritability, hyperactivity, emotional lability, and decreased attention span
    b. Weakness, easy fatigability, exercise intolerance
    c. Heat intolerance
    d. Weight change (loss or gain), increased appetite
    e. Insomnia, interrupted sleep
    f. Frequent stools, diarrhea
    g. Menstrual irregularities, decreased libido
    h. Warm, sweaty, flushed skin with a velvety-smooth texture, spider telangiectasis
    i. Tremor, hyperkinesia, hyperreflexia
    j. Exophthalmos, retracted eyelids, staring gaze
    k. Hair loss
    l. Goiter
    m. Bruits over thyroid gland
    n. Elevated systolic blood pressure, widened pulse pressure, S3 heart sound

2. Diagnostic laboratory testing
   a. Thyrotropin-releasing hormone (TRH) stimulation test
      i. Little or no response of TSH to TRH stimulation
   b. Serum T_4 and T_3
   c. Serum free T_4 and T_3
      i. Increased
   d. Radioactive T_3 uptake (RT_3U)
      i. High
   e. Radioactive iodine uptake (RAIU)
      i. High in Graves' disease and toxic nodular goiter
      ii. Low in thyroiditis and thyrotoxicosis
   f. TSH
      i. Suppressed and does not respond to TRH
   g. Thyroid-stimulating immunoglobulins (TSI)
      i. Present in Graves' disease
J. Parathyroid
   1. Clinical manifestations
      a. Fatigue, muscular weakness, listlessness
      b. Height loss and frequent fractures
      c. Renal calculi
      d. Anorexia, nausea, abdominal discomfort
      e. Memory impairment
      f. Polyuria, polydipsia
      g. Back and joint pain
      h. Hypertension
   2. Diagnostic laboratory testing
      a. Serum calcium levels
         i. Greater than 5.3 mEq/L in adults
         ii. Greater than 6.0 mEq/L in children
      b. Serum PO4
         i. Less than 1.8 mEq/L
      c. Urinary calcium levels
         i. Less than 25 mEq/L
      d. Urinary PO4
         i. Greater than 25 mEq/L
      e. Creatine clearance
         i. Decreased
      f. Hydroxyproline
         i. Increased
      g. Urinary cAMP
         i. Increased

III. Operative Procedures
A. Breast

Refer to Figure 26–5

1. Needle biopsy
   a. Vim–Silverman or disposable cutting-type needle is introduced and advanced into breast mass to entrap a core or plug of tissue
   b. The needle is withdrawn and tissue specimen sent for diagnostic examination
   c. Definitive surgical treatment should never be performed without a formal biopsy

2. Incisional biopsy
   a. A portion of mass is surgically excised using a curved incisional line
   b. Tissue is sent for pathological examination
3. Excisional biopsy
   a. Entire tumor mass is surgically excised from adjacent tissue
   b. Specimen sent for examination as with incisional biopsy
   c. The biopsy procedure has little risk and is usually done under local anesthesia
   d. The short delay between biopsy and further treatment does not adversely affect survival
4. Incision and drainage for abscess
   a. Incision of an inflamed and suppurative area of the breast is performed for drainage of abscess
   b. Abscesses occur most frequently as result of infections in a lactating breast
   c. Chronic abscesses are rare
   d. Free drainage is required with association of abscess around nipple or in breast tissue
5. Partial mastectomy (lumpectomy, tylectomy, segmental resection, quadrant resection, wedge resection)
   a. Removal of tumor mass with at least one inch of surrounding tissue
   b. Combined with axillary node dissection and irradiation in stages I and II breast cancer appears to provide results equal to a more radical procedure
6. Subcutaneous mastectomy
   a. Removal of all breast tissue with overlying skin and nipple left intact
   b. Recommended for patients who:
      i. Have central tumors of noninvasive origin
      ii. Chronic cystic mastitis
      iii. Hyperplastic duct changes
      iv. Multiple fibroadenomas
      v. Have undergone number of previous biopsies
   c. Prosthesis may be inserted at time of mastectomy or at a later date
7. Simple mastectomy
   a. Removal of entire involved breast without lymph node dissection
   b. Performed to remove extensive benign disease, if malignancy is believed to be confined only to breast tissue, or as a palliative measure to remove an ulcerated advanced malignancy
B. Gallbladder
   1. Laparoscopic cholecystectomy: removal of the gallbladder laparoscopically
   2. Purpose: treatment of diseases involving the gallbladder, such as acute or chronic inflammation (cholecystitis) or stones (cholelithiasis)
C. Hemorrhoids
   1. Hemorrhoidectomy: excision and ligation of dilated veins in anal region
   2. Purpose: to relieve discomfort and control bleeding
D. Anal fissure
   1. Anal fissurectomy: involves dilatation of anal sphincter and removal of lesion
   2. Purpose: to relieve discomfort
E. Anal fistula
   1. Anal fistulotomy or fisulectomy: fistula incised and drained or excised and packed to heal by granulation
   2. Purpose: to treat, either by incision or excision, fistulous tracts in anal canal
F. Pilonidal cyst
   1. Pilonidal cystectomy: removal of cyst with sinus tract, removing necrotic tissue, debris, hair; wound may be packed open, closed, or closed with tissue flaps

Surgical Interventions for Breast Cancer

Procedure	Description	Diagram
Lumpectomy or tylectomy	Removal of the breast tumor and small amounts of surrounding tissue	
Partial mastectomy or segmental resection	Removal of the tumor plus approximately 2 to 3 cm of surrounding tissue	
Quadrantectomy	Removal of a quadrant of the breast with the tumor, and fascia covering the greater pectoral muscle.	
Local regional treatment	Removal of the tumor with the surrounding tissue and axillary lymph nodes	

Figure 26–5.   (From Monahan, F.D., Neighbors, M. [1998]. *Medical Surgical Nursing,* 2nd ed. [pp. 1861–1862]. Philadelphia: Saunders.)

Surgical Interventions for Breast Cancer *(Continued)*

Procedure	Description	Diagram
Total mastectomy	Removal of the entire breast, with the pectoral muscles and axillary lymph nodes left intact	
Modified radical mastectomy	Removal of the entire breast, skin, and axillary lymph nodes. The pectoral muscles are left intact.	

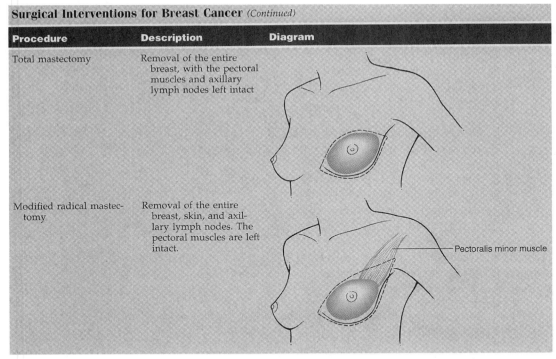

Pectoralis minor muscle

Figure 26–5. *Continued.*

2. Purpose: to prevent recurrence of infection and abscess formation in pilonidal sinus
G. Hernia
   1. Open approaches: herniorrhaphy—surgical repair of hernia; hernioplasty—reinforcement of weakened area with wire, fascia, or mesh
   2. Laparoscopic approach
      a. Advantages
         i. Requires less oral analgesics
         ii. Recovery period shorter
         iii. Lower wound infection rate
         iv. Tension-free application of mesh
         v. Bilateral herniorrhaphy can be performed using same port sites
      b. Disadvantages
         i. Longer surgical time
         ii. Increased general anesthesia exposure time
         iii. Increase cost
   3. Purpose: to reduce or repair hernia; may be inguinal, femoral, ventral, umbilical, or incisional in origin
H. Thyroid
   1. Types of procedures
      a. Subtotal thyroid lobectomy: unilateral or bilateral excision of portion of lobe(s)
      b. Thyroid lobectomy: removal of one lobe
      c. Total thyroidectomy: removal of entire gland
   2. Purpose
      a. Graves' disease is associated with diffuse, bilateral enlargement
      b. Hashimoto's thyroiditis, thought to be an autoimmune disease, nontender enlargement occurs

     c. Surgery is performed to relieve trachea obstruction

     d. Nontoxic nodular goiter does not produce an excess of hormones and is noninflammatory in character

     e. Surgery may be indicated to relieve tracheal or esophageal obstruction or rule out a malignant nodule

I. Parathyroid

  1. Types

     a. Total parathyroidectomy: removal of all glands

     b. Partial parathyroidectomy: removal of up to 3½ to 4 glands, leaving metal clips in place to identify remaining glandular tissue

  2. Purpose

     a. Presence of adenomas (hypersecreting neoplasms)

     b. Hyperplasia

     c. Carcinomas require surgical excision

     d. Resection of lymphatic is essential

     e. Inability to locate glands

     f. Underlying medical conditions such as renal failure or severe cardiac disorders

     g. Hypercalcemia from nonparathyroid etiology

IV. Postanesthesia Priorities: Phase I

  A. General immediate postanesthesia care

    1. Initial assessment: refer to Chapter 8 for general assessment information

  B. Breast surgery

    1. Monitor and document drainage output

    2. Monitor competency of drainage hemovac, grenade drain, or other low-suction system

    3. Monitor dressing for hemorrhage or oozing

    4. Assess comfort level

      a. Pain may increase anxiety and feeling of powerlessness

      b. If severe, may limit chest expansion

      c. If pain medication given, assess for relief

    5. Position in bed

      a. Usually supine

      b. Affected arm may be elevated on pillow to decrease swelling and enhance circulation

    6. Psychological support

      a. Respond appropriately to questions and responses that may be verbalized

      b. Privacy should always be respected

    7. Complications

      a. Drain becomes unattached or occluded

      b. Hematoma

      c. Hemorrhage or shock

      d. Wound infection

      e. Electrolyte and fluid imbalances

  C. Laparoscopic cholecystectomy

    1. Assess nasogastric tube for proper placement; if ordered, discontinue

    2. Monitor intake and output every hour

      a. Assess bladder for distention if no indwelling catheter in place

        i. Bladder distention is common postoperatively

      b. Assess indwelling catheter

        i. Note color of urine

        ii. Discontinue indwelling catheter if ordered

      c. Assess comfort level
          i. Location of discomfort (i.e., at incision site or in shoulders, chest, neck)
          ii. Position patient for comfort
          iii. Administer prescribed medications
          iv. Evaluate pain relief
      d. Complications
          i. Atelectasis and respiratory problems
          ii. Bladder distention
          iii. Hemorrhage or shock
          iv. Wound infection
          v. Dehiscence or evisceration
          vi. Hiccups
          vii. Pneumoperitoneum
          viii. Electrolyte and fluid imbalance

D. Hemorrhoidectomy
  1. Observe perianal area for signs of bleeding
  2. Assess amount, character, and threshold for pain or discomfort
    a. Position patient in most comfortable position
    b. Provide analgesics as ordered
  3. Monitor patient for hypotension secondary to vasodilation of pelvic blood vessels
  4. Complications
    a. Atelectasis and respiratory problems
    b. Bladder distention
    c. Hemorrhage or shock
    d. Uncontrolled pain threshold
    e. Electrolyte and fluid imbalance
    f. Constipation

E. Anal fissurectomy
  1. Observe perianal area for signs of bleeding
  2. Assess amount, character, and threshold of pain or discomfort
    a. Position patient in most comfortable position
    b. Provide analgesics as ordered
  3. Monitor patient for hypotension secondary to vasodilation of pelvic blood vessels
  4. Complications
    a. Bladder distention
    b. External fistulas
    c. Hemorrhage or shock
    d. Wound infection
    e. Electrolyte and fluid imbalance

F. Anal fistulectomy
  1. Observe perianal area for signs of bleeding
  2. Assess amount, character, and threshold for pain or discomfort
    a. Position patient in most comfortable position
    b. Provide analgesics as ordered
  3. Monitor patient for hypotension secondary to vasodilation of pelvic blood vessels
  4. Complications
    a. Bladder distention
    b. External fistulas
    c. Hemorrhage or shock
    d. Wound infection
    e. Electrolyte and fluid imbalance

G. Pilonidal cystectomy
    1. Observe gluteal fold area for signs of bleeding
    2. Assess amount, character, and threshold for pain or discomfort
       a. Position patient in most comfortable position
       b. Provide analgesics as ordered
    3. Monitor patient for hypotension secondary to vasodilation of pelvic vessels
    4. Complications
       a. Wound infection
       b. Uncontrollable pain threshold
       c. Bladder distention
       d. Hemorrhage or shock
       e. External fistulas
       f. Electrolyte and fluid imbalance

H. Herniorrhaphy
    1. Open approach
       a. Use ice packs for scrotal edema per physician's order
       b. Assess for bladder distention
       c. Encourage patient to cough by splinting the incision with hands or pillows
    2. Laparoscopic approach
       a. Monitor for hematoma formation
          i. Bowel perforation caused by blind sticks from Veress needles
          ii. Perforation of epigastric vessels
          iii. Perforation or damage of ilioinguinal vessels
       b. Monitor for scrotal edema and ecchymosis
       c. Monitor for sensory/motor alterations
          i. Damage of ilioinguinal nerves during manipulation and dissection of different anatomical structures
       d. Assess bladder distention
          i. Perforation of urinary bladder during dissection
       e. Assess abdominal girth, hardness, or tenderness
    3. Complications
       a. Pneumoperitoneum
       b. Atelectasis and respiratory problems
       c. Bladder distention
       d. Paralytic ileus
       e. Hemorrhage or shock
       f. Wound infection
       g. Dehiscence or evisceration
       h. Electrolyte and fluid imbalances
       i. Pulmonary embolus

I. Thyroidectomy
    1. Focus assessment on surgical site
       a. Assess neck dressing for hemorrhaging
       b. Assess and document presence of drain/drainage
       c. Assess neck for swelling
          i. Nerve damage, have patient say "e"
          ii. Obstructed airway
          iii. Vascularity of neck
       d. Uncommon postoperative problems
          i. Hypothyroidism
          ii. Thyroid storm
    2. Instruct patient in importance of remaining silent to rest vocal cords
    3. Instruct patient to remain calm and prevent neck thrashing

J. Parathyroidectomy
  1. Focus assessment on surgical site
     a. Assess neck dressing for hemorrhaging
     b. Assess and document presence of drain/drainage
     c. Assess neck for swelling
        i.   Nerve damage, have patient say "e"
        ii. Obstructed airway
        iii. Vascularity of neck
  2. Instruct patient to remain calm and prevent neck thrashing
  3. Complications
     a. Tetany
     b. Hyperparathyroid crisis

V. **Postanesthesia Priorities: Phase II**
  A. General patient care
     1. PACU Phase II admission assessment: refer to Chapter 8 for general assessment information
  B. Breast surgery
     1. Assess dressing/bra firmness
     2. Assess security of drain
     3. Reassure emotional feelings
     4. Key educational components
        a. Emphasize the need for safety precautions, including need for firm-fitting bra for support
        b. Stress the need for adequate nutrition
        c. Provide information about resources and support systems such as "Reach to Recovery" program of the American Cancer Society
     5. Provide adequate written and verbal instructions and ensure patient/family understanding
  C. Laparoscopic cholecystectomy
     1. Assess dressings
     2. Assess abdominal girth
     3. Key educational components
        a. Instruct patient and family on routine care following major abdominal surgery
           i.   Ambulate at regular times
           ii. Rest frequently
           iii. Slowly increase activity as tolerated
           iv. Keep incisions dry
           v.   Report any signs of redness, pain, or drainage from incisions
           vi. Avoid heavy lifting for at least one week (check with surgeon)
           vii. Splint abdomen when coughing
        b. Identify importance of follow-up care with surgeon
        c. Instruct patient and family regarding pneumoperitoneum (retained CO_2 under diaphragm via phrenic nerve)
        d. Stress need for adequate nutritional intake; low- to moderate-fat diet
     4. Provide adequate written and verbal instructions and ensure patient/family understanding
  D. Hemorrhoidectomy
     1. Assess dressing or packing
     2. Assess level of pain
     3. Assess adequate intake and output

    4. Key educational components
      a. Instruct in management and prevention of constipation with diet, fluids, and physical activity
      b. Patient needs to respond to urge to defecate, to avoid straining, and to administer stool softener as needed
      c. Emphasize the need for warm sitz baths and compresses
    5. Provide adequate written and verbal instructions and ensure patient/family understanding

  E. Anal fissurectomy
    1. Assess dressing and/or packing
    2. Assess pain control
    3. Assess adequate intake and output
    4. Key educational components
      a. Emphasize importance of keeping postoperative site clean and free of stool by use of sitz bath and careful cleansing
      b. Instruct patient and family of possibility of hypotension secondary to vasodilation of pelvic blood vessels during sitz bath
      c. Provide patient and/or family with information on natural methods of relieving or preventing constipation (i.e., diet high in bulk and fiber, increased fluid intake, avoidance of harsh laxatives and constipating medications such as codeine)
    5. Provide adequate written and verbal instructions and ensure patient/family understanding

  F. Anal fistulectomy
    1. Assess dressing and/or packing
    2. Assess pain control
    3. Assess adequate intake and output
    4. Key educational components
      a. Instruct in wound irrigation, shaving of perianal area, and application of wound dressing
      b. Sitz bath can be used to cleanse wound but does not replace irrigation procedure
      c. Instruct in use of mirror to inspect area and look for redness or firm reddened areas of increased itching and tenderness
      d. Provide patient and/or family with information on natural methods of relieving or preventing constipation (i.e., diet high in bulk and fiber, increased fluid intake, avoidance of harsh laxatives and constipating medications such as codeine)
    5. Provide adequate written and verbal instructions and ensure patient/family understanding

  G. Pilonidal cystectomy
    1. Assess dressing and/or packing
    2. Assess pain control
    3. Assess adequate intake and output
    4. Key educational components
      a. Instruct patient and/or family in dressing change as needed
      b. Instruct in importance of keeping wound free of fecal and urinary contamination
      c. Instruct in cleansing wound as needed
      d. Instruct in proper use of sitz bath
      e. Instruct patient and family of possibility of hypotension secondary to vasodilation of pelvic blood vessels during sitz bath

    f.   Instruct in pain control measures

    g.   Provide patient and/or family with information on natural methods of relieving or preventing constipation (i.e., diet high in bulk and fiber, increased fluid intake, avoidance of harsh laxatives and constipating medications such as codeine)

  5. Provide adequate written and verbal instructions and ensure patient/family understanding

H. Herniorrhaphy

  1. Assess adequate intake and output

  2. Assess pain control

  3. Assess dressing for hemorrhage

  4. Assess patient's ability to ambulate

  5. Key educational components

    a. Open approach

      i.   Instruct patient regarding application of ice packs to incisional area

      ii. Instruct patient to avoid heavy lifting until follow-up appointment with surgeon

      iii. If patient is discharged with a binder, provide correct instruction regarding application

      iv. Instruct in application of scrotal support if ordered

      v.   Instruct in proper maintenance of incisional area

      vi. Instruct in identification of possible infection (i.e., redness, fever, tenderness, drainage from incision)

    b. Laparoscopic approach

      i.   Instruct patient and family regarding pneumoperitoneum (retained CO_2 under diaphragm via phrenic nerve)

  6. Provide written and verbal instruction and ensure patient/family understanding

I. Thyroidectomy

  1. Assess airway, symmetry of neck, swelling of neck

  2. Assess dressing for hemorrhaging

  3. Assess patency of drain(s)

  4. Assess complaints of numbness and tingling of lips, fingers, and toes

  5. Assess adequate intake and output

  6. Key educational components

    a. Instruct patient in signs and symptoms of hyperthyroidism, hypothyroidism, and hypocalcemia

    b. Instruct in surgical site care

      i.   Report to surgeon any signs of redness, swelling, drainage, fever, and/or incisional pain

    c. Teach patient to support head and neck with folded towel during mobility

    d. Establish alternate means of communication (pencil and pad)

    e. Identify with patient importance of follow-up care

  7. Provide written and verbal instructions and ensure patient/family understanding

J. Parathyroidectomy

  1. Assess for adequate intake and output

  2. Assess neurologic sequelae

    a. Hyperthermia

    b. Increased intracranial pressure

    c. Cerebrospinal fluid leakage

    d. Convulsions

  3. Assess dressing and drain(s)

> **BOX 26–1. Key Educational Patient Outcomes**
>
> - The patient who has undergone a hernia repair is able to verbalize the importance of monitoring the surgical site for signs and symptoms of infection and understands the importance of reporting any signs and symptoms to the physician immediately
> - The patient who has undergone a mastectomy can verbalize the importance of wearing a firm support bra, the steps to empty the drainage system, and measures for pain control
> - The patient who has undergone a thyroidectomy can verbalize the signs and symptoms of hyperthyroidism, hypothyroidism, and hypocalcemia and can identify the steps to take if the signs and symptoms appear
> - The patient who has undergone a rectal procedure is able to verbalize the proper procedure for a sitz bath and the importance of keeping the area clean and dry

    4. Key educational components
      a. Teach signs and symptoms of hypocalcemia
        i.   Paresthesia
        ii. Muscle cramps in extremities
        iii. Tingling in fingers and around mouth
      b. Instruct patient in care of incision
      c. Teach body mechanics and importance of mobility, especially for patients with irreversible skeletal impairment
      d. Instruct patient regarding dietary supplements containing calcium and their use in treatment of hypocalcemia
      e. Instruct patient regarding calcium replacement medication
      f. Instruct in importance of monitoring weight
    5. Provide written and verbal instructions and ensure patient/family understanding

VI. Postanesthesia Care: Phase III
  A. General
    1. Reinforce instructions regarding care for operative site(s) and dressing care
    2. Emphasize importance of continued pain management
    3. Instruct patient to continue to monitor for nausea, vomiting, and dizziness
    4. Instruct patient to continue to monitor nutritional and elimination status
    5. Teach patient to monitor for fever
    6. Emphasize importance of need for follow-up care with surgeon
    7. Emphasize importance of establishing contact should an emergency occur
      a. Provide with emergency contact numbers
        i.   Surgeon
        ii. Anesthesia
        iii. Hospital
        iv. Surgery Center

BIBLIOGRAPHY

1. Atkinson, L.J., Kohn, M.L. (1986). *Introduction to Operating Room Technique*, 6th ed. New York: McGraw-Hill.
2. Black, J.M., Matassarin-Jacobs, E. (Eds). (1997). *Medical Surgical Nursing*, 5th ed. Philadelphia: W. B. Saunders.
3. Braasch, J.W., et al. (Eds). (1991). Laparoscopic cholecystectomy. *Atlas of Abdominal Surgery*. Philadelphia: W. B. Saunders.
4. Burden, N. (1993). *Ambulatory Surgical Nursing*. Philadelphia: W. B. Saunders.
5. Collins, L.G. (1996). Laparoscopic extraperitoneal herniorrhaphy. *AORN Journal*, 63(6):1089–1098.
6. Darzi, A., et al. (1994). Laparoscopic herniorrhaphy. Initial experience in 126 patients. *Journal of Laparoendoscopic Surgery*, 4:179–183.
7. Donohue, J.H., Farnell, M.B. et al. (1992). Laparoscopic cholecystectomy: Early Mayo Clinic experience. *Mayo Clinical Procedures*, 67:449–455.
8. Eubanks, S., Newman, L., Lucas, G. (1993). Reduction of HIV transmission during laparoscopic procedures. *Surgical Laparoscopy & Endoscopy*, 3:2–5.

9. Felix, E.L., Michas, C., McKnight, R.L. (1994). Laparoscopic repair of recurrent groin hernias. *Surgical Laparoscopy & Endoscopy*, 4:200–204.

10. Ferrara-Love, R. (1997). Laparoscopic surgery. *Nursing Clinics of North America*, 32(2):429–440.

11. Forrest, D.M. (1993). Practical points in the postoperative management of a laparoscopic inguinal herniorrhaphy patient. *JoPAN*, 8(4):280–285.

12. Ganong, W. (1991). *Review of Medical Physiology*, 15th ed. Norwalk, CT: Appleton & Lange.

13. Gonzalez-Cortes, S.B., Preuniar, C.E. (1994). Laparoscopic inguinal herniorrhaphy. *AORN J*, 60(3): 419–436.

14. Hargrove-Huttel, R.A. (1996). *Lippincott's Review Series: Medical–Surgical Nursing*, 2nd ed. Philadelphia: Lippincott.

15. Jacob, S.W., Francone, C.A., Lossow, W.S. (1982). *Structure and Function in Man*, 5th ed. Philadelphia: W. B. Saunders.

16. Keating, J.P., Morgan, A. (1993). Femoral nerve palsy following laparoscopic inguinal herniorrhaphy. *Journal of Laparoendoscopic Surgery*, 3:557–559.

17. Kleinbeck, S.A., Hoffart, N. (1994). Outpatient recovery after laparoscopic cholecystectomy. *AORN J*, 60(3):394–402.

18. Lichtenstein, I.L., Shulman, A.G., Amid, P.K. (1992). The editors comment. *Laparoscopy in Focus*, 1(1):8–9.

19. Litwack, K. (Ed.). (1995). *Core Curriculum for Post Anesthesia Nursing Practice*, 3rd ed. Philadelphia: W. B. Saunders.

20. Litwack-Saleh, K. (1992). Practical points in the care of the patient post-thyroid surgery. *JoPAN*, 7(6): 404–406.

21. Mayo Clinic. (1993). Laparoscopic herniorrhaphy: Goal in reduction of postoperative pain and duration of convalescence. *Mayo Clinical Update*, 9:1–3.

22. McKernan, J.B. (1991). Laparoscopic cholecystectomy. *The American Surgeon*, 57(5):309–312.

23. McKernan, J.B., Laws, H.L. (1992). Laparoscopic peritoneal prosthetic repair of inguinal hernias. *Surgical Rounds*, 7:597–610.

24. Meeker, M.H., Rothrock, J.C. (Eds). (1995). *Alexanders Care of the Patient in Surgery*, 10th ed. St. Louis: Mosby.

25. Monahan, F.D., Neighbors, M. (Eds). (1998). *Medical Surgical Nursing: Foundations for Clinical Practice*, 2nd ed. Philadelphia: W. B. Saunders.

26. Morris, P.B. et al. (1992). Outpatient CO_2 laser cholecystectomy: Laser techniques, patient outcomes, cost containment. *AORN J*, 55:984–992.

27. Peters, J.H., Ellison, E.C. et al. (1991). Safety and efficacy of laparoscopic cholecystectomy: A prospective analysis of 100 initial patients. *Ann Surg*, 213(1):3–12.

28. Reddick, E., Olsen, D. (1991). *Laparoscopy for the General Surgeon*. Tuttlingen, Germany: Karl Storz GmbH & Co.

29. Salky, B. (1990). *Laparoscopy for Surgeons*. New York: Igaku-Shoin.

30. Saltzstein, E.C. et al. (1992). Outpatient open cholecystectomy. *Surgery, Gynecology & Obstetrics*, 174: 173–175.

31. Spaw, A.T., Ennis, B.W., Spaw, L.P. (1991). Laparoscopic hernia repair: The anatomic basis. *Journal of Laparoendoscopic Surgery*, 1:269–276.

32. Steckler, R.M. (1986). Outpatient thyroidectomy: A feasibility study. *The American Journal of Nursing*, 152:417–419.

33. Stillman, A. (1993). Laparoscopic cholecystectomy. *AORN J*, 57(2):429–436.

34. Toy, F.K., Smoot, R.T. (1991). Toy–Smoot laparoscopic hernioplasty. *Surgical Laparoscopy & Endoscopy*, 1:151–155.

35. Ulrich, S.P., Canale, S.W., Wendell, S.A. (1995). *Nursing Care Planning Guides: A Nursing Diagnosis Approach*, 2nd ed. Philadelphia: W. B. Saunders.

36. William, K.W., Kosik, M.L., Doolas, A. (1994). A prospective comparison of transabdominal preperitoneal laparoscopic hernia repair versus traditional open hernia in a university setting. *Surgical Laparoscopy & Endoscopy*, 4:247–253.

37. Zucker, K.A. (1990). Laproscopically guided cholecystectomy. *Problems in General Surgery*, Special issue, 7(5):175–184.

REVIEW QUESTIONS

1. All of the following are contributing factors to hernia formation except:

   A. Previous surgery
   B. High-fat diet
   C. Age
   D. Obesity

2. Nursing interventions for the patient who has undergone laparoscopic cholecystectomy include:

   A. Maintaining patency of tubes and drains
   B. Monitoring fluid status
   C. Maintaining oxygenation
   D. All of the above

3. Which of the following laboratory reports will the PACU nurse be primarily concerned with in a patient following a total thyroidectomy?

   A. ABGs
   B. CBC
   C. Calcium level
   D. Potassium level

4. Thyroid storm is characterized by:

   A. Hypocalcemia with acute symptoms
   B. Bradycardia, hypotension, hypoxemia
   C. Fever, diaphoresis, severe neck pain
   D. Hypertension, tachycardia, heat intolerance

5. Complications that may occur following pilonidal cystectomy include all of the following except:

   A. Hypotension
   B. Reoccurrence
   C. Pneumoperitoneum
   D. Constipation

6. A ventral hernia may be classified as which of the following?

   A. Indirect inguinal, femoral, epigastric
   B. Hiatal, incisional, epigastric
   C. Epigastric, umbilicus, incisional
   D. External direct, inguinal, umbilicus

7. Which of the following physiological changes have an affect on the breast?

   A. Those related to growth and development
   B. Those related to the menstrual cycle
   C. Those related to pregnancy and lactation
   D. All of the above

8. Acute cholecystitis can result from:

   A. Tissue damage due to trauma, massive burns, or surgery
   B. Multiple blood transfusions
   C. Prolonged fasting
   D. All of the above

9. Congenital hernias

   A. Are external
   B. Are associated with failure of the intestine to rotate in usual sequence in the fetus
   C. Are most common
   D. All of the above

10. Clinical manifestations of hyperthyroidism include all of the following except:

    A. High energy
    B. Hyperactivity, irritability
    C. Insomnia, interrupted sleep
    D. Heat intolerance

ANSWERS TO QUESTIONS

1. B
2. D
3. C
4. A
5. C

6. C
7. D
8. D
9. B
10. A

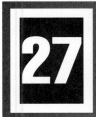

Laparoscopic and Minimally Invasive Surgery

Gayle Miller
St. Luke's Hospital
Jacksonville, Florida
Christine Kelley
Elliot 1-Day Surgery Center
Manchester, New Hampshire

NOTE: This chapter is not intended to discuss details of pre- and postprocedure care of the patient undergoing minimally invasive procedures. Refer to other sections of this book for details. The goal here is to familiarize the perianesthesia nurse with the technology involved in minimally invasive and techno-logic procedures that are seen in ambulatory surgery. Providing information on these issues will help the perianesthesia nurse gain new perspective on what the patient will experience. This information should help in patient education preoperatively, and enable the nurse to better understand complications to be alert for postoperatively.

I. **Trends**
   A. Trend over recent years has been toward more surgical procedures done on an outpatient basis
      1. Trend has been influenced by several factors
         a. New or improved, short-acting pharmaceutical agents and anesthesia techniques
            i. Allow rapid recovery
         b. Technologic advances such as laparoscopic equipment and techniques
         c. Lasers and other modalities
         d. The push by third-party payers for health-care dollar efficiencies
         e. The desire of the health-care consumer for procedures that decrease postoperative pain and/or recuperation time
            i. Hastens return to routine activities

Objectives

1. Discuss the historical trends of minimally invasive surgery.
2. Describe the types of minimally invasive procedures seen in ambulatory surgery.
3. Discuss the preoperative needs of the minimally invasive surgery candidate.
4. Describe the techniques involved in minimally invasive procedures.
5. Discuss risks and complica-tions related to laparoscopic procedures.
6. Describe the use of lasers in ambulatory surgery.
7. Discuss safety measures required for laser procedures.
8. Discuss the management issues related to the use of technology in surgery.

II. Trends in Technology
A. Historical overview of laparoscopy
1. Minimally invasive techniques began as early as the tenth century
2. Arabian physician used reflected light to examine the cervix
3. The bladder and nasal passages examined in this way
4. Early problems
   a. Lack of adequate illumination
   b. Burns from light sources
5. An Italian physician, Philip Bozzini, developed a "light guide" in 1806
   a. Device used a candle for illumination
6. In 1853 Frenchman Desmoreaux presented to the Academy of Paris a device that utilized an alcohol lamp and wick
7. In the 1860s, a German dentist developed a means of illumination that used a platinum wire heated by electrical current
   a. Method used water for cooling
   b. Not sufficient to avoid burns
   c. Edison's invention of the incandescent bulb in 1880 eliminated the need for the water-cooling apparatus
B. Early diagnostic procedures
1. In 1901 Kelling introduced cystoscope into abdomen of dog to insufflate and inspect the internal organs
2. First performed on human in 1910 by Jacobaeus
   a. Simple syringe used to instill air into abdomen for insufflation
   b. Air of concern because of risk of air embolus
3. In the 1940s, Goetz and Veress introduced needles for safely introducing gas into the abdomen
   a. Initially utilized oxygen
   b. Oxygen discontinued as introduction of electrocautery presented an increased fire hazard in oxygen-rich environment
4. In 1944 Pilmer employed Trendelenburg positioning to get air into the abdominal cavity following the introduction of a needle in the cul-de-sac
5. Pilmer stressed the importance of monitoring intraabdominal pressure
6. Device for automatically insufflating introduced by Semm in 1964
7. In 1966, a physicist named Hopkins, who along with Kapany developed fiberoptics in 1952, introduced a rod–lens system that greatly improved image brightness and clarity
8. Fiberoptic light sources introduced in the 1960s
   a. Eliminated the problem of bowel burns from incandescent light
   b. Problem of bowel burns from unipolar coagulation decreased, but not eliminated with the introduction of bipolar devices
   c. Visualization initially limited to one person through a cumbersome system of articulated mirrors
9. In 1986, computer chips and TV camera attached to laparoscope revolutionized minimally invasive surgery
10. Laparoscopic techniques in gynecology became widespread in 1960s and 1970s
11. 500,000 procedures performed by 1973 when the First International Congress of Gynecological Laparoscopy was held
12. 1987—first laparoscopic removal of a gallbladder by Mouret of France
13. 1988 and 1989 in the United States, McKernan, Saye, and Reddick started the revolution in cholecystectomy
    a. Within 3 years the procedure nearly replaced traditional open cholecystectomy

      b. Laparoscopic cholecystectomy described as catalyst in growth of minimally invasive general surgery

III. Minimally Invasive Surgery
  A. Arthroscopy
     1. Introduction of arthroscopic techniques eliminated need for arthrotomy in many orthopedic procedures
     2. Diagnostic arthroscopy may precede an arthrotomy
     3. Assists surgeon to determine any needed modifications to the surgical plan
     4. Advantages of arthroscopy to the patient include:
       a. Decreased infections
       b. Shortened rehabilitation time
       c. Minimal hospital stay
       d. Smaller incisions
       e. No disruption of extensor mechanisms
       f. Decreased postoperative pain
     5. Preoperative preparation
       a. Important for patient to abstain from aspirin products or other drugs that can affect clotting
       b. If the surgeon plans to inject local anesthetic into the joint, the patient should be advised that the lack of discomfort is temporary and does not preclude the observation of activity restrictions
  B. Types of arthroscopies
     1. Knee
       a. Diagnostic arthroscopy
          i.   With or without subsequent arthrotomy
       b. Meniscus repair
       c. Anterior cruciate ligament (ACL) repair
       d. Posterior cruciate ligament repair
     2. Shoulder
       a. Diagnostic arthroscopy
          i.   With or without subsequent arthrotomy
       b. Removal of loose bodies
       c. Lysis of adhesions
       d. Biopsy of the synovium
       e. Bursectomy
       f. Rotator cuff tear repair
       g. Glenoid labrum tear repair
       h. Biceps tendon repair
       i. Relief of impingement syndrome
     3. Elbow
       a. Diagnostic arthroscopy
          i.   With or without subsequent arthrotomy
       b. Removal of loose bodies
       c. Debridement
       d. Partial synovectomy
       e. Lysis of adhesions
       f. Fracture evaluation
     4. Ankle
       a. Diagnostic arthroscopy
          i.   With or without subsequent arthrotomy
       b. Removal of loose bodies
       c. Ligament reconstruction
       d. Biopsy

C. Knee arthroscopy
   1. Intraoperative procedure
      a. Leg is placed in a limb holder about 4 inches above patella
      b. Tourniquet may be placed on leg and may or may not be inflated
      c. Leg prepared
      d. Portal sites are identified and marked prior to the insertion of a Veress needle or another type of irrigation cannula into the suprapatellar pouch
      e. Joint is distended with fluid (e.g., lactated ringers)
      f. Sharp trocar with scope sheath is inserted through stab wound
      g. Joint is entered with blunt trocar
      h. Arthroscope is inserted through sheath
      i. Drainage tube, light source cord, and video camera are attached
      j. Second stab incision made to insert instruments through
      k. Arthroscopy pump regulates the flow of fluid in and out of joint and controls pressure within
      l. When procedure completed joint is thoroughly irrigated
      m. Portal sites are closed by suture
      n. Local anesthetic with epinephrine may be instilled into the joint to decrease postoperative pain and bleeding
      o. Dressing applied
      p. Splint applied if ordered
   2. Equipment issues
      a. Arthroscope and light cord should not be sterilized in steam autoclave (unless arthroscope and light cord are newer models and manufacturer recommends steam sterilization)
         i. Results in damage to arthroscopes and the lens cement
         ii. Equipment can be sterilized in an ethylene oxide sterilizer
         iii. Can be disinfected by soaking in glutaraldehyde
            (a) Minimum of 20 minutes is current recommendation for disinfection
            (b) Items must be soaked for 12 hours for sterilization
            (c) Rinse items thoroughly with sterile water prior to use to remove disinfectant
            (d) Fiberoptic cables should never be kinked or twisted
               (i) Can cause damage to the fibers
               (ii) Prevents transmission of light
            (e) Steris or other sterilization techniques may be appropriate, depending on manufacturer recommendations
D. Cystoscopy
   1. Examination of the urinary bladder
      a. One of the earliest minimally invasive procedures in history
      b. Modern urological practice encompasses many commonly done outpatient procedures
   2. Procedures
      a. Bladder fulguration
      b. Bladder biopsy
      c. Cystoscopy
      d. Fulguration of bladder neck
      e. Ureteroscopy
      f. Stent insertion or removal
      g. Ureteral catheterization and pyelography
      h. Transurethral uretopyleoscopy

3. Equipment
   a. Can be done with either a rigid or flexible cystoscope
   b. Flexible scope
      i. Useful in a patient with obstructive disease due to prostatic hyperplasia
      ii. For patients with limited mobility who cannot be placed in lithotomy position
4. Intraoperative procedure
   a. Can be done under local, IV sedation, or general anesthesia
   b. Diagnostic and therapeutic modalities utilized in conjunction with cystourethroscopy include:
      i. Ultrasound
      ii. Fluoroscopy
      iii. Laser
      iv. Lithotripsy

E. Laparoscopy
   1. History
      a. Expanding development of laparoscopic procedures major reason for growth in outpatient surgery
      b. Gynecologists utilized early laparoscopic techniques
      c. Initially for diagnosis
      d. Later for tubal sterilization and ovarian biopsy
      e. General surgeons continuing to find more applications for laparoscopic procedures to replace or supplement traditional open techniques
   2. Care of equipment and instrumentation
      a. Requires specialized equipment
      b. Staff need to be familiar with the use and care of all equipment and instrumentation
      c. Improper handling can cause damage
         i. May result in inadequate support for the surgeon
         ii. Potential of injury to patient
         iii. Considerable expense for the institution
      d. AORN published recommended practices related to the use and care of endoscopic equipment
         i. Includes:
            (a) Inspection
            (b) Handling
            (c) Cleaning
            (d) Decontamination
            (e) Sterilization
            (f) Documentation
         ii. Education
            (a) Equipment should not be sterilized in a steam autoclave unless approved by the manufacturer
               (i) Results in damage to scopes and the lens cement
            (b) The equipment can be sterilized in an ethylene oxide sterilizer
            (c) Can be soaked in a liquid disinfectant such as glutaraldehyde
            (d) Newer sterilization modalities using chemical processes are being adapted for use with endoscopic equipment
   3. Equipment—basic items needed for laparoscopy (disposable or reusable)
      a. Veress needle or other pneumo peritoneal needle
         i. Used to penetrate and insufflate the abdomen
         ii. Has a spring-loaded inner blunt tip and sharp outer tip

          iii. When penetrating the abdomen, the blunt tip retracts
          iv. Exposes the sharp beveled sheath
          v. Blunt tip advances to protect underlying tissues
          vi. Insufflation tubing is attached at hub of needle

    b. Insufflator
          i. Device delivers gas through filtered sterile tubing at a controlled rate
          ii. Monitors intraabdominal pressure
          iii. Carbon dioxide gas is provided in tanks

    c. Trocar and cannula
          i. Two components
             (a) Outer sheath
             (b) Sharp inner obturator
          ii. Technique
             (a) Sharp obturator penetrates abdomen after insufflation **or**
             (b) Cannula is inserted using open laparoscopy technique
          iii. Surgical procedure performed through several cannulae
          iv. Trocar valve attached to insufflation tubing to maintain pneumo-peritoneum
          v. Second valve prevents loss of pneumoperitoneum when no instruments in place
          vi. Cannulae come in different sizes to adapt to laparoscope and instruments

    d. Laparoscope
          i. Consists of lenses and channels for fiberoptics and viewing
          ii. Laparoscope may be used with video camera
          iii. 5- or 10-mm laparoscope used
          iv. Laparoscope available in 0-, 5-, 30-, and 45-degree angles
             (a) The 0-degree laparoscope views straight out
             (b) Others provide angled views to look over and around intraabdominal tissue

4. Intraoperative procedure
    a. The laparoscope can be maintained in position by an assistant or a mechanical scope holder attached to OR table
    b. Surgeon is working in two dimensions
    c. Maintenance of scope position is important for orientation
    d. Light source
          i. High-intensity light sources
             (a) Xenon, mercury, or halogen vapor bulbs provide illumination
             (b) Illumination channeled through fiberoptic cables to laparoscope
             (c) Light is controlled so image is not washed out
    e. Camera and video
          i. Microchip technology enables image to be real-time video imaging
             (a) Earlier technology allowed only surgeon direct visualization of operative field, unless there was a teaching port on the scope
          ii. Camera is attached to laparoscope
          iii. Images transmitted via cable through camera box
          iv. Changed into video image and displayed on monitor
          v. A VCR can be utilized to provide documentation of the procedure
    f. Instruments
          i. Disposable instruments
          ii. Reusable instruments
          iii. Insulated for use with electrosurgical devices

g. Instrument classification
  i. Grasping
  ii. Retracting
  iii. Cutting
F. Endoscopic/Laparoscopy Techniques
  1. Insufflation
    a. Prior to insufflation, test pressure/flow shut-off mechanism
    b. Insufflator turned on to a flow of >6 L/minute
    c. Pressure should register zero
    d. Rate is then lowered to 1 L/min and tubing is kinked
    e. Pressure should rise to 30 mm Hg
    f. Flow of CO_2 should stop
    g. Test blunt retractable tip of the Veress needle prior to use
  2. Procedure—Laparoscopy
    a. Patient placed in head-down position
    b. Puncture site dependent upon previous surgical history
    c. If no previous surgery
      i. Site is at superior or inferior border of the umbilical ring
      ii. Or directly through umbilicus for abdominal, gynecological, or obese patients
    d. After stabilizing umbilicus, small stab incision is made
    e. Needle is passed by shaft
    f. Surgeon should feel change in resistance as:
      i. The needle passes through fascia
      ii. And again through peritoneum
    g. A 10 cc syringe with 5 cc of NS is used
      i. To aspirate and check for blood or bowel contents
      ii. To instill saline and ascertain there is easy flow
    h. Veress needle is stabilized
      i. Insufflator tubing is attached
      ii. CO_2 flow is initiated
    i. Pressure in abdomen at start of insufflation should be less than 10 mm Hg
      i. 15 mm Hg should not be exceeded
      ii. High pressures or pressures reached quickly may indicate incorrect needle placement
        (a) Could be resting on omentum, adhesion, bowel, etc.
        (b) Correct by:
          (i) Rotating the needle
          (ii) Withdraw and attempt again
    j. Surgeon must be sure of placement before continuing to insufflate
    k. Surgeon will watch abdomen for symmetrical expansion
    l. Loss of dullness with percussion over the liver will be noted
    m. Insufflate until maximum of 15 mm Hg and/or 3 to 6 liters of CO_2 are instilled
      i. Percussion is reminiscent of a ripe watermelon
    n. Alternate method of insufflation is to insert Veress needle through posterior fornix or transuterine in female patients
  3. Laparoscopy options
    a. The surgeon may choose to insert a trochar prior to insufflation
      i. Accomplished by making a 1 cm incision through skin and down to fascia
      ii. Grasp and raise abdominal wall manually prior to inserting trochar
      iii. Same loss of resistance is noted as in previously described technique

b. Open cannula or Hasson technique
    i.   A 2- to 3-cm incision is made through skin
    ii.   Subcutaneous tissues are dissected with scissors
    iii.   Fascia is identified and incised
    iv.   Peritoneum is grasped with hemostats and incised
    v.   Surgeon manually inspects to confirm entry into abdominal cavity and determine presence of adhesions
    vi.   Cannula (which has a conical sleeve) is passed through opening and secured in place by sutures that have been placed at fascial incision
    vii.   Abdominal cavity is then insufflated
    viii.   Pneumoperitoneum can be achieved as rapidly if not more so than the Veress needle technique
    ix.   Method is considered safer to use on patients who have had previous surgeries

4. Electrocautery
  a. Electrosurgical unit (ESU) (commonly called the bovie)
  b. Device has been adapted for use in laparoscopic procedures
  c. ESU generates high-frequency current
    i.   Used either in monopolar or bipolar mode
    ii.   Used to either coagulate or cut in monopolar
  d. Must be inspected carefully before each use for breaks or defects in insulation
  e. To prevent electrical injury to the skin:
    i.   Ground pad must be placed on the patient for monopolar use
    ii.   Pad placement
        (a) On the same side or as close to the surgical site as possible
        (b) Over a muscle mass if possible
        (c) Avoid placement over:
            (i)   Bony prominence
            (ii)   Metal implant areas
            (iii)   Hairy areas
            (iv)   Pooling of prep solution in the area of the pad
  f. Electrosurgery is not without its risks
    i.   Leakage current can pass through a break in insulation
    ii.   Occurs through phenomenon known as capacitance to instruments or tissues
    iii.   The risk of capacitive coupling decreased by using all metal or all plastic cannulae and skin anchors
    iv.   Hybrid systems with metal cannula and plastic anchors should be avoided
    v.   Laparoscopic procedures may have limited view
        (a) Injuries can go undetected
        (b) Disastrous effects such as bowel perforation and peritonitis may result

5. Laser
  a. Laser used to cut and coagulate (discussed in-depth later in this chapter)

6. Staples and clips
  a. Surgical clips and staples have long been used in open procedures
  b. Adapted for use in laparoscopy
  c. Made of titanium
    i.   Used to ligate vessels

      ii.   Used to close abdominal structures with lumens such as bowel, bladder, or ureter

      iii. Used to reapproximate tissue

   d. Two forms of clips: occlusive and tacking

      i.   Come in single or multiload applier

      ii.   Sizes vary from 2.5 to 4.8 mm

      iii. Lengths of 3 or 6 cm

   e. Staples are pushed into tissue and closed; tissue between is cut

   f. Devices save time in surgery

   g. Less difficult than laparoscopic knot tying

   h. Disposable and reusable varieties available

IV. Preoperative Issues

A. Patient selection

  1. Not all patients are appropriate candidates for laparoscopic procedures

  2. Proper screening must be done preoperatively

  3. Contraindications

   a. Relative contradictions

      i.   Prior abdominal/pelvic surgery

      ii.   Previous peritonitis or pelvic fibrosis

      iii. Obesity

      iv. Unreducible abdominal or inguinal hernia

      v.   Diaphragmatic hernia

      vi. Umbilical abnormality

      vii. Abdominal/iliac aneurysm

      viii. Severe pulmonary disease

      ix. Bowel obstruction

      x.   Intolerance to positioning

      xi. Pregnancy

   b. Absolute contraindications

      i.   Generalized peritonitis

      ii.   Hypovolemic shock

      iii. Large pelvic or abdominal mass

      iv. Severe cardiac decompensation

      v.   Uncorrected coagulopathy

      vi. Inability to tolerate laparotomy

      vii. Inexperienced surgeon

B. Patient education

  1. Preoperatively about the usual preparatory activities

  2. Methods of education vary

   a. Based on patient's ability and readiness to learn

  3. Patients having laparoscopic surgery tend to minimize seriousness of procedure

  4. Need to be prepared for the procedure

   a. Potential complications

   b. Aftercare needed

V. Intraoperative Issues

A. Room layout for laparoscopic procedures

  1. Requires a significant amount of high-technology equipment

  2. Equipment must be organized in efficient and accessible arrangement

  3. Provide visualization for both primary surgeon and assistant; video monitors may be positioned on either side of the patient or at foot of bed

B. Insufflation equipment, electrosurgical unit or laser must be easily accessible and observable by surgical team

C. Anesthetic considerations
  1. Laparoscopic surgery patients at greater risk of regurgitation and aspiration of stomach contents
  2. Precautionary measures may include
     a. Strict NPO status for at least 8 hours preoperatively
     b. Water bolus 2 to 3 hours preoperatively (bolus may stimulate gastric peristalsis and emptying)
     c. Administration of metoclopramide (Reglan) or an H2 blocker such as cimetidine or ranitidine
  3. Anesthetic techniques
     a. May use local anesthetics for brief, simple procedures (e.g., gynecological cases)
        i. Technique involves injecting local anesthetic with epinephrine (to potentiate duration) at each trochar site
        ii. Abdominal organs are sprayed with an anesthetic solution prior to being manipulated
     b. Monitored anesthesia care (MAC) can be used in conjunction with a local anesthetic technique
     c. Advantages of these techniques consists of:
        i. Avoidance of general anesthesia risks
        ii. Less postoperative nausea and vomiting
        iii. Rapid postoperative recovery
     d. Disadvantages include
        i. Intraoperative anxiety
        ii. Respiratory compromise
        iii. Shoulder and abdominal pain from insufflation
  4. Epidural anesthesia not often used
     a. Is a viable alternative to avoid risks of general anesthetic
  5. General anesthesia most common technique for laparoscopy
     a. Endotracheal intubation decreases risk of regurgitation and aspiration
     b. Allows control of ventilation to compensate for compromised intraoperative pulmonary status
     c. Anesthetist must monitor patient closely with pulse oximetry and capnography
  6. Anesthetic goals
     a. Keep $ETCO_2$ less than 40 mm Hg
     b. Keep SpO_2 at or above 93%
  7. Anesthesia research studies
     a. Compare inhalation general anesthesia to total intravenous anesthesia
        i. Patients with IV agents had faster recovery and less postoperative nausea and vomiting
  8. Physiological effects of laparoscopy on the respiratory, cardiovascular, and gastrointestinal systems
     a. Cardiovascular effects caused by the pneumoperitoneum created by insufflation with CO_2
        i. Increased pressure in abdominal cavity
           (a) Causes circulatory impairment by decreasing venous return
           (b) Decrease CVP which is managed with fluids
           (c) Can lead to acute pulmonary edema in patients with cardiac compromise
        ii. CO_2 is absorbed from abdomen into circulation
           (a) Leads to hypercarbia and dysrhythmias
           (b) Anesthetist must increase tidal volume to compensate

        iii. Increased tidal volume
            (a) Results in increased wedge pressures
            (b) Decreases stroke volume
            (c) Decreases cardiac output
        iv. Cardiovascular collapse can occur from:
            (a) CO_2 embolus
            (b) Vagal effects
            (c) Manipulation of abdominal organs
   b. The pulmonary system effects include:
        i.   Atelectasis
        ii. Decreased functional residual capacity
        iii. High peak airway pressures
   c. Gastrointestinal effects are stated above and can be minimized by:
        i.   Decompression of stomach with nasogastric or orogastric tube
            (a) Decreases risk of injury to organs during trocar placement
   d. Effect of pneumoperitoneum on kidneys
        i.   Renal cortical perfusion diminished with pressure of 15 mm Hg
            (a) Results in oliguria
        ii. Perfusion rapidly restored when pressure released
        iii. Urinary output may not promptly return
        iv. May be due to abdominal compartment syndrome
            (a) Studied in patients with ascites
            (b) Affects ADH and aldosterone
 9. Significant effects caused by pneumoperitoneum have led to alternative methods of laparoscopic surgery being developed and studied
   a. Devices that elevate peritoneum by means of slings, wires, T-, L-, or fan-shaped devices
        i.   Utilized to facilitate visualization of abdomen without risks of pneumoperitoneum
        ii. Devices require additional puncture sites for retractors
        iii. Enable use of ordinary surgical instruments instead of laparoscopic
        iv. Entire procedure for cholecystectomy becomes less time consuming in patients with inflamed gallbladder

D. Complications
   1. Abdominal trauma most likely to occur during insertion of Veress needle or trocar placement
   2. Minor vascular injury controlled with pressure
   3. Major vascular injury requires clips, suturing, or open vascular repair
   4. Injury to the bowel can be caused by:
      a. Veress needle
      b. Trocar
      c. Various instruments
      d. Electrosurgical unit
      e. Laser
   5. Puncture injuries usually seen at time of occurrence
   6. Thermal injuries may not be apparent
      a. Abdominal pain, nausea, and fever 2 or 3 days postoperatively may indicate thermal injury
   7. Injury to the bladder uncommon if the bladder is emptied at beginning of procedure
   8. Bladder injury can occur (particularly with gynecological procedures)
      a. Ureters can be damaged by puncture, laser, or electrocautery

9. Complications related to pneumoperitoneum include:
   a. Pneumothorax and pneumomediastinum
      i.   Identify by chest X-ray
      ii. Treatment
           (a) Decompress pneumoperitoneum
           (b) Terminate procedure
           (c) Reverse muscle relaxants
           (d) Ventilate with oxygen
   b. Subcutaneous emphysema
      i.   Causes
           (a) Improper positioning of Veress needle
           (b) May occur in conjunction with pneumothorax, pneumomediastinum, or both
           (c) Weak areas in diaphragm allow carbon dioxide to leak through and enter mediastinum
      ii. Diagnosis
           (a) Increase in end-tidal CO_2
               (i) Cannot be lowered by increasing tidal volume or increasing rate of ventilation
      iii. Symptoms
           (a) Crepitus noted upon palpation of head and neck
           (b) May also include facial and conjunctival subcutaneous emphysema
   c. Gastric reflux
      i.   Risk
           (a) Increased with history of:
               (i)   Obesity
               (ii) Hiatal hernia
               (iii) Gastric outlet obstruction
      ii. Cause
           (a) Increased abdominal pressure associated with pneumoperitoneum
      iii. Treatment
           (a) Nasogastric or orogastric tube insertion
           (b) Decompress stomach
               (i)   Decreases risk of visceral puncture
               (ii) Improves visualization
               (iii) Decreases risk of aspiration
               (iv) Decreases incidence of postoperative nausea and vomiting
           (c) Pharmacological interventions
               (i)   Administer metoclopramide 10 mg preoperatively to promote gastric emptying
               (ii) Administer metoclopramide at the end of surgical procedure to decrease potential for nausea and vomiting
   d. Carbon dioxide embolus
      i.   Cause
           (a) Large amounts of CO_2 enter central venous circulation through opening in venous channels
      ii. Signs and symptoms
           (a) Sudden decrease in blood pressure
           (b) Cardiac dysrhythmias
           (c) Hear murmur
           (d) Cyanosis
           (e) Pulmonary edema
           (f) Increase in end-tidal CO_2

        iii. Increased incidence with high intraabdominal insufflation

        iv. Treatment

            (a) Deflate peritoneum immediately

            (b) Place patient in left lateral decubitus position

            (c) Head positioned below the level of the right atrium

            (d) Establish IV access to central circulation to aspirate gas from the heart

    e. Cardiovascular collapse

        i. Possible causes include:

            (a) Hemorrhage

            (b) Pulmonary embolus

            (c) Myocardial infarction

10. Abdominal wall hematoma
11. In laparoscopic cholecystectomy bile duct can be damaged by:
    a. Electrocautery
    b. Clips
    c. During cholangiography

VI. Lasers in Surgery

A. Laser basics
   1. Laser is an acronym for **l**ight **a**mplification by **s**timulated **e**mission of **r**adiation
   2. Theory on which laser based is stimulated emission
   3. Formulated by Albert Einstein in 1917
   4. Light is electromagnetic energy released as photons
   5. Visible light only part of the optical spectrum
       a. Optical spectrum part of larger electromagnetic spectrum
   6. All types of radiation are considered radiation
       a. Radiation in laser technology is not the ionizing radiation of X-rays
   7. Nonionizing radiation of lasers has no biological effects or health hazards
   8. Ordinary light travels in waves that have four characteristic properties
       a. Wavelength
       b. Amplitude
       c. Velocity
       d. Frequency
   9. Three characteristics that differentiate laser light from ordinary light
       a. Monochromatic
       b. Collimated
       c. Coherent
   10. Monochromatic laser light is all one color
   11. Ordinary light is polychromatic
   12. Collimated light waves are parallel to each other
       a. Do not diverge as they travel
   13. Ordinary light spreads out as it travels
   14. Property of collimation reduces loss of power
       a. Allows for focusing with precision
   15. Laser light is coherent
       a. Waves travel in phase and in one direction
   16. Ordinary light waves are choppy and travel in many directions
   17. General components of a laser
       a. Energy source
       b. Active medium
       c. Resonant cavity

18. The active medium may be:
    a. Solid
    b. Liquid
    c. Gas
19. The energy source can be:
    a. Electrical current
    b. High-powered lamp
    c. Chemical reaction
20. Light beam passes through active medium
21. Photons stimulate other photons
22. Energy is continually built up
23. Collimation could occur as process occurs in a long tube
24. Short cylinder with mirrors at either end is used to reflect light back and forth and create laser beam
25. The space between mirrors is resonant cavity
26. One of the mirrors is only partially silvered
    a. Allows light to leave cavity as a collimated beam
    b. Beam can be pulsed or continuous
27. A laser delivery system can utilize:
    a. Fibers
    b. Articulated arm
    c. Fixed optics
28. The delivery system can be connected to an operating microscope or used through an endoscope

B. Laser–tissue interaction
   1. Laser energy has four effects on tissue
      a. Reflection
      b. Scattering
      c. Transmission
      d. Absorption
   2. Reflection can be a positive property
      a. Mirrors utilized to get laser beam into hard-to-reach area
      b. Reflection can be a hazard if beam is reflected inadvertently off an instrument
         i. Special instruments are required for use in laser procedures
            (a) Ebonized instruments
            (b) Nonreflecting instruments
   3. Laser beams can scatter
      a. In tissues
      b. Back up endoscope causing damage to optics
   4. Some wavelengths are transmitted through tissue with little effect
      a. Argon going through the eye to retina
      b. Nd:YAG through fluid to the bladder wall
   5. Absorption of a laser beam is dependent on:
      a. Wavelength
      b. Tissue characteristics
         i. Color
         ii. Consistency
         iii. Water content
   6. The argon and Nd:YAG beams are absorbed by tissue with high melanin and hemoglobin content

7. Color is irrelevant to the CO_2 laser absorption
   a. Primarily affects water molecules in tissue
   b. Cellular water is heated, steams, and bursts the cell membrane
   c. Effects vary with temperature to which tissue is heated
   d. Reactions vary from:
      i. No visible tissue change at 37 to 60°C
      ii. To vaporization, carbonization, and a smoke plume at 100°C
      iii. Temperatures between these temperatures cause:
         (a) Blanching
         (b) Gray color
         (c) Puckering
         (d) Resultant coagulation
         (e) Protein denaturization
         (f) Drying of tissues
C. Laser types
   1. Categorized by the active medium utilized
      a. Solid-state lasers utilize a crystal such as:
         i. Ruby
         ii. yttrium–aluminum–garnet (YAG)
         iii. yttrium–lithium–fluoride (YLF)
         iv. yttrium–aluminum–oxide (YALO) lasers
      b. Gas lasers include:
         i. Helium–neon
         ii. CO_2
         iii. Argon
      c. Dye lasers have limited applications
         i. Require use of toxic dyes
      d. Semiconductor diode lasers have been used
         i. In consumer products and fiberoptic communication systems
         ii. For medical use in ophthalmology and endoscopic application
      e. Experimental lasers include:
         i. Metal vapor lasers
         ii. Free-electron lasers
   2. Ruby laser
      a. First successful medical laser
      b. Has been replaced by newer technology
      c. Still used for such applications as removing tattoos
   3. Nd:YAG solid-state laser
      a. YAG is a garnet crystal of aluminum and yttrium oxides
      b. Minimal portion of yttrium atoms replaced with neodymium, creating the Nd:YAG
      c. Resultant crystal can be used in continuous wave or pulsed laser applications
         i. Wavelength is 1064 nm
         ii. Creates an invisible beam that penetrates tissue deeply
         iii. If wavelength is halved by combining with certain other crystals to create second harmonic generation, beam becomes visible and penetration is less deep
   4. The KTP (potassium–triphosphate) YAG produces a green beam
   5. Other combinations of YAG-pulsed lasers
      a. Alexandrite
      b. Holmium
      c. Erbium

6. CO_2 gas laser
   a. Operates at a 10,500 nm wavelength
   b. Utilizes low wattage
   c. Requires an articulating arm system
   d. Reflecting mirrors as opposed to fiberoptics because it is absorbed by glass
   e. H_2O molecules absorb energy superficially, creating a water vapor
   f. Very effective for cutting
7. Excimer laser
   a. Used primarily in ophthalmology
   b. Argon–fluoride laser
   c. Has short wavelength photons
   d. Has photoablative qualities leaving a smooth surface
8. Dye lasers
   a. Limited applications
      i. Photodynamic therapy
9. Diode laser
   a. Medical use currently limited to ophthalmic photocoagulation
   b. May have more applications in the future (such as for pain management)
D. Laser safety
   1. Use of lasers and/or recommend safe practice governed by:
      a. Regulatory agencies
      b. Industry
      c. Professional organizations
   2. Lasers are considered a class III medical device
      a. Subject to the jurisdiction of the FDA
   3. The U.S. Department of Health and Human Services and The American National Standards Institute (ANSI) subdivide lasers into four classes
      a. Most lasers used in medicine considered class IV
   4. The Occupational Safety and Health Administration (OSHA)
      a. Does not have any specific standards related to lasers
      b. Has jurisdiction under general safety clauses
      c. Expects laser users to provide a safe laser program and follow the general guidelines of ANSI
      d. If a person were to be injured in the use of a laser, OSHA could inspect facility
   5. The National Institute for Occupational Safety and Health (NIOSH)
      a. Conducts research utilized by OSHA in making regulations
      b. Has determined that plume formed during laser procedures is potentially harmful
   6. The Center for Devices and Radiological Health (CDRH)
      a. The FDA regulatory agency responsible for:
         i. Laser manufacturing standards
         ii. Approval of investigational permits for new laser technologies
   7. The Safe Medical Device Act of 1990
      a. Mandates reporting
         i. Serious injury or illness related to the use of lasers
         ii. Malfunctions that may occur
   8. Not all states regulate lasers
      a. States that regulate include:
         i. Florida
         ii. Texas
         iii. Arizona

        iv. Alaska

        v. New York

        vi. California

        vii. Georgia

        viii. Illinois

        ix. Massachusetts

        x. Oregon

        xi. Virginia

        xii. Vermont

    b. Regulations include:

        i. Issues related to registration of laser devices

        ii. Training requirements

        iii. Laser safety officer responsibilities

        iv. Safety rules

9. American National Standards Institute (ANSI), a nongovernmental organization of laser experts
   a. Establish standards and recommendations for the safe use of lasers (since 1973)
   b. Guidelines are the gold standard for laser safety
   c. Include definition of:
       i. Classes of lasers
       ii. Hazards of lasers
       iii. Control measures
       iv. Medical surveillance

10. The Joint Commission for Accreditation of Healthcare Organizations (JCAHO)
    a. Does not specifically deal with laser safety
    b. Considers lasers as they would any other medical equipment
        i. Staff must be properly trained in the use of equipment
        ii. Competency maintained
        iii. Equipment managed appropriately
        iv. Safe practices in place

11. Laser safety program
    a. Laser safety committee
        i. Structure of a laser safety program in a facility varies
        ii. Factors influencing structure include:
            (a) Size of the facility
            (b) Number of laser devices
            (c) Procedures
        iii. Laser safety could be under the jurisdiction of an OR committee
            (a) Could be a subset of the safety committee
        iv. Committee membership varies
            (a) May include the laser safety officer (LSO)
            (b) Risk management
            (c) Administration representatives
            (d) Physician users of laser technology
            (e) OR director
        v. Committee guides and oversees use of lasers in facility
            (a) Oversees issues such as education of users
            (b) Makes recommendations to credentialing body on practitioners requesting laser privileges
            (c) Monitors laser usage

     vi. Laser safety officer
- (a) Laser safety officer (LSO) plays a key part
  - (i) Role is recommended by ANSI
  - (ii) Required by some states
  - (iii) Must be knowledgeable in the safe use of lasers
  - (iv) Responsible for imparting knowledge to all parties involved with use of laser
  - (v) Oversees direct use of lasers
  - (vi) Must be educated in all aspects of laser safety and applicable regulations
  - (vii) Monitors and enforces all related safety practices in compliance with regulatory guidelines and institutional policies

     vii. Staff education
- (a) All persons involved in use of laser
  - (i) Must receive education and training prior to involvement
  - (ii) Basic laser safety training program includes:
    - a) Information about laser biophysics
    - b) Laser equipment
    - c) Laser–tissue interaction
    - d) Safety procedures
    - e) Clinical applications
  - (iii) Knowledge and skills are verified and updated
    - a) Ensure staff competency
    - b) Measurements of competency developed and facilitated by LSO

     viii. Physician credentialing
- (a) Must demonstrate knowledge and skill prior to independent practice
- (b) Education of physicians can occur in:
  - (i) Residency
  - (ii) Fellowship programs
  - (iii) Postgraduate courses offered by various sources related to laser usage
- (c) Credentialing requirements are dictated by the bylaws of institution
- (d) Credentialing varies between settings—requirements may include:
  - (i) Proof of both didactic and hands-on training
  - (ii) Proctoring by a physician staff member currently credentialed to perform specific laser procedures
  - (iii) Scope and currency of experience is considered for renewal application
- (e) Laser safety committee may serve to review and make recommendations in matters of physician credentialing and recredentialing

     ix. Protective measures
- (a) Eye safety
  - (i) Eyes are very susceptible to damage from laser radiation
  - (ii) CO_2 laser and the Holmium laser can cause scleral and corneal damage because their wavelength is absorbed by these tissues
  - (iii) Argon and Nd:YAG can cause damage to retina by passing through cornea and being focused by the lens
  - (iv) Damage to retina can be acute or develop slowly with continual exposure
  - (v) Early damage may go unnoticed

(vi) Damage may be caused by direct or reflected beam

(vii) Amount of risk to personnel is calculated based on concepts of:

    a) Maximum permissible exposure (MPE)

    b) Nominal hazard zone (NHZ)

(viii) Anyone entering OR where laser is in use is considered at risk for eye damage

(ix) To decrease risk of eye damage, protective eyewear *must* be worn

(x) The patient's eyes must also be protected:

    a) Eyewear

    b) Moist gauze pads

(xi) Different lasers require different eyewear

    a) Optical densities appropriate for filtering specific wavelengths

    b) Applicable wavelength should be clearly marked on eyewear

    c) Care must be taken to prevent damage to protective lenses

    d) Scratches compromise protective filtering capacity

    e) Filtering devices are available for operative microscopes and endoscopes

    f) Nonreflective instruments must be utilized to prevent reflection of laser beam causing eye or skin injury

    g) Eye examinations to establish an ocular history baseline recommended for personnel routinely involved with laser use

    h) Examinations should be done following any ophthalmic laser-exposure incidents

        (1) Some states may require exposures to be reported

x. Environmental controls

(a) Alert personnel

    (i) Identify laser-use areas

    (ii) ANSI standards recommend signs with a specific laser safety symbol

    (iii) Limit traffic in laser-use areas

    (iv) Specific eye protection with proper wavelength must be worn by personnel in room where laser is used

    (v) Extra goggles should be available outside the room

    (vi) Glass windows in room must be covered to prevent unintentional laser beams affecting persons outside the room

    (vii) Laser key must be available only to authorized personnel—not left with laser

(b) Fire safety measures

    (i) Laser always presents a risk of fire

    (ii) Education important for those involved in laser usage

    (iii) Ignition could occur with:

        a) Surgical drapes

        b) Anesthesia tubing

        c) Surgical sponges

    (iv) Contributions to flammability:

        a) Oxygen

        b) Anesthetic gases

        c) Vapors from alcohol-based prep solutions

      (v)   Special drapes and endotracheal tubes can be utilized
      (vi)   Sponges should be kept wet
      (vii) Oxygen concentrations kept low
      (viii) Prep solutions patted dry to prevent pooling
      (ix)   Foot pedal with which the surgeon activates laser beam must be placed such that it is not accidentally engaged

    (c) Laser plume
      (i)   Smoke produced by use of laser is known as plume
      (ii)   May contain particles of tissue, toxins, and steam
      (iii)   Studies done about the content of the plume and the risks it poses to caregivers
         a) Plume can be irritating, causing burning, watery eyes
         b) May contain viable cells that transmit disease such as human papilloma virus (HPV), since laser is a common treatment for genital warts
      (iv)   Smoke evacuators
         a) Filters the high efficiency particulate air (HEPA)
         b) Removes smoke and particles; high-filtration masks filter plume not captured by the smoke evacuator

VII. Other Technologies

1. Ultrasound
  a. Sound waves are mechanical energy
    i.   Waves at frequencies above the audible range are defined as ultrasonic
    ii. At lower frequencies ultrasonic waves have no tissue effect
      (a) Commonly employed for diagnostic purposes
  b. Newer devices adapt external modality to laparoscopic applications
  c. At higher frequencies ultrasound is utilized in two different devices
    i.   The cavitational ultrasonic aspirator
    ii. The ultrasonically activated scalpel
  d. The aspirator is utilized in neurosurgical and other procedures
    i.   It fragments and aspirates tumor cells
  e. Scalpel (also known as the harmonic scalpel) is utilized primarily in gynecology or general surgery
    i.   Used in either open or laparoscopic procedures
    ii. Employs either multiuse or disposable instruments such as:
      (a) Hooks
      (b) Coagulators
      (c) Shears
      (d) Can cut and coagulate
    iii. May use at times in place of lasers
    iv. May use at times in place of electrosurgical unit
    v.   Also used in place of endoscopic stapling devices used in laparoscopic procedures (such as laparoscopic assisted vaginal hysterectomy)
    vi. No electric current transmitted to patient
    vii. Eliminates risk of burns to patient
    viii. Little risk of inadvertent damage to adjacent tissues
    ix. Does not create smoke like electrosurgical unit or laser
    x.   Eliminates risk of plume for surgical team
    xi. Affords clear visualization during laparoscopic procedures
2. Intraoperative cholangiography
  a. ERCP (endoscopic retrograde cholangiopancreatography) or intraoperative cholangiography during laparoscopic cholecystectomy
    i.   Done to visualize and remove stones in biliary tract

ii.   Various catheters, baskets, dilators, balloons, etc. are utilized in dealing with cholelithiasis
iii. For cholangiography contrast medium is injected to visualize biliary tree
iv.   Flat plate x-ray or real time c-arm fluoroscopy is utilized
   (a) Real time is preferable
   (b) No need to wait for films to be developed and read
  b.   Laparoscopic transcystic common duct exploration
    i.   If stones are found via cholangiography
     (a) A flexible choledochoscope used to explore common bile duct
       (i)   To retrieve stones
     (b) Duct is dilated using a balloon dilator
       (i)   A series of sequential bougie type dilators may be used
       (ii) Balloon type less likely to injure duct
       (iii) Must be passed over a wire using fluoroscopy
     (c) Stones are retrieved via a choledochoscope, using a basket snare
3. Robotics
  a.   Not common in the ambulatory setting
  b.   Technology introduced for clinical use in the 1980s
  c.   Robot is a combination of mechanical manipulators and a computer
  d.   Computer controls complex movements of joints and arms of manipulators
  e.   Robotic applications in minimally invasive procedures have been trialed
  f.   Manipulation of laparoscope has been trialed
    i.   Difficult to maintain proper alignment of the camera throughout procedure
    ii. Surgeon relies on stability of image to maintain orientation to anatomical structures
  g.   Mechanical scope holders available
    i.   Surgeon must interrupt his/her activities and readjust as needed
  h.   The AESOP (Automated endoscopic system for optimal positioning) is approved by FDA
    i.   Used successfully for this purpose
    ii. Device is anchored to OR table
    iii. Controlled by surgeon with foot pedal
    iv. Camera does not move unless surgeon commands it to
     (a) Picture remains stable and upright
    v.   Device can take over role of assistant who is holding camera
    vi. Allows personnel to concentrate on other patient-care activities
  i.   Studies using robot for urological procedures proved the device successful

VIII. Management Issues
A. Risk management
  1. Advances from technology impacts ambulatory procedures
  2. Advances are not without risk and cost
  3. Should include proper training and credentialing of both personnel and physicians
  4. Competence of staff in performance of procedures should be assessed annually
  5. Competence of staff in use of equipment should be assessed annually
  6. Maintenance of equipment and instrumentation is essential
  7. Staff caring for patients postprocedure must be aware of signs of complications both in the immediate postoperative period as well as after the patient goes home
  8. Patients and/or caregivers must be instructed to recognize complications should they occur

9. Prompt intervention can make a critical difference in patient outcome should problems arise
10. Patients must be carefully instructed and advised of risks prior to surgery

B. Resource management
   1. Revenues from third-party payers is shrinking
   2. Managed care has become more prevalent
   3. Competition for contracts is intense
   4. The challenge is to provide high quality in most cost-effective means possible
   5. Surgical services obvious area where costs need to be addressed
      a. All persons involved in care of patients must be cost conscious
      b. Managers look at ways to control costs through:
         i. Staffing
         ii. Changing skill mix
         iii. Adding new types of multiskilled worker
         iv. Supplies used intraoperatively for minimally invasive procedures
         v. Fluency in budgeting methods
         vi. Maintenance of a close working relationship with materials management to facilitate purchasing
      c. Strategies to decrease cost
         i. Examine inventory for opportunities to consolidate and streamline inventory
         ii. Standardize wherever possible
         iii. When using disposables:
            (a) Keep items available—do not open until needed
         iv. Return to reusable products rather than disposable
            (a) Reusables are much improved over their original versions
            (b) Disposable trocars, clips, staplers, and instruments account for much of the cost in the OR
               (i) Disposables eliminated the need to reprocess and maintain items
                  a) Surgeon always had the assurance of a sharp sterile item to use
            (c) When considering a return to reusables, contemplate:
               (i) Capital investment
               (ii) Cost of repair and processing
               (iii) Quality of product
         v. Resposable items
            (a) Resposable instrument is partially reusable and partially disposable
            (b) Sharp part of the instruments are disposable
            (c) Eliminates concern of dull trocars
            (d) Eliminates need to periodically sharpen instruments
            (e) Resposable items available:
               (i) Trocars
               (ii) Clip appliers
               (iii) Staplers
               (iv) Scissors

Bibliography

1. Abbott, P. (1997). The best of both worlds—resposables. *Today's Surgical Nurse,* 19(2):35–38.
2. Allen, J.M., Phippen, M.L. (1994). Providing instruments, equipment and supplies. In Phippen, M.L., Wells, M.P. eds., *Perioperative Nursing Practice* (pages 183–197). Philadelphia: Saunders.
3. Amaral, J.F. (1994). Ultrasonic dissection. *Endoscopic Surgery and Allied Technologies,* 2(3/4):181–184.

4. Ball, K. (1995). *Lasers: The Perioperative Challenge*. St. Louis: Mosby.

5. Beadle, E. (1993). Complications of laparoscopy. In Graber, J.N., Schultz, L.S., Pietrafitter, J.J., Hickok, D.F., eds. *Laparoscopic Abdominal Surgery* (pages 75–82). New York: McGraw-Hill.

6. Berci, G. (1994). *History of Endoscopic Examination of the Foregut. Minimally Invasive Surgery of the Foregut.* St. Louis: Quality Medical Publishing.

7. Codeddu, J.A., Stoinovici, D., Kavoussi, L.R. (1997). Robotics in urologic surgery. *Urology*, 49(4):501–506.

8. Filipi, C.J., Fitzgibbons, R.J., Salerno, G. (1991). Historical review: Diagnostic laparoscopy to laparoscopic cholecystectomy and beyond. In Zucker, K.A. ed., *Surgical Laparoscopy* (pages 3–20). St. Louis: Quality Medical Publishing.

9. Goldstein, D.S., Chadhoke, P.S., Kavoussi, L.R., Odem, R.R. (1994). Laparoscopic equipment. In Soper, N.J., Odem, R.R., Clayman, R.V., McDougall, E.M., eds., *Essentials of Laparoscopy* (pages 104–147). St. Louis: Quality Medical Publishing.

10. Graus, C., Cedron, M. (1994). Urological surgery. In Phippen, M.L., Wells, M.P., eds., *Perioperative Nursing Practice* (pages 571–625). Philadelphia: Saunders.

11. Hill, D.L. (1993). The basics of laparoscopy. In Graber, J.N., Schultz, L.S., Pietrafitter, J.J., Hickok, D.F., eds., *Laparoscopic Abdominal Surgery* (pages 7–29). New York: McGraw-Hill.

12. Kalman, B.J. (1994). Orthopedic surgery. In Phippen, M.L., Wells, M.P., eds., *Perioperative Nursing Practice* (pages 571–625). Philadelphia: Saunders.

13. Kavoussi, L.R., Soper, N.J. (1994). Establishing the pneumoperitoneum. In Soper, N.J., Odem, R.R., Clayman, R.V., McDougall, E.M., eds., *Essentials of Laparoscopy* (pages 104–147). St. Louis: Quality Medical Publishing.

14. McDougall, E.M., Clayman, R.V., Soper, N.J. (1994). Laparoscopic clips and staples. In Soper, N.J., Odem, R.R., Clayman, R.V., McDougall, E.M., eds., *Essentials of Laparoscopy* (pages 184–203). St. Louis: Quality Medical Publishing.

15. Monk, T.G., Weldon, B.C. (1994). Anesthetic considerations for laparoscopic surgery. In Soper N.J., Odem, R.R., Clayman, R.V., McDougall, E.M., eds., *Essentials of Laparoscopy* (pages 24–33). St. Louis: Quality Medical Publishing.

16. Newman, L., Luke, J.P., Ruben, D., Eubanks, S. (1993). Laparoscopic herniorrhaphy without peritoneum. *Surgical Laparoscopy & Endoscopy*, 3(3):213–215.

17. Ordica, R.C., Das, S. (1994). History of laparoscopy. In Das, S., Crawford, D., eds., *Urological Laparoscopy* (pages 3–11). Philadelphia: Saunders.

18. Partin, A.W., Adams, J.B., Moore, R.G., Kavoussi, L.R. (1995). Complete roboti-assisted urological surgery: A preliminary report. *J American College of Surgeons*, 181:552–557.

19. *Recommended Practices for Use and Care of Endoscopes.* (1997). AORN Standards and Recommended Practices. Denver, CO: Association of Operating Room Nurses.

20. *Risk Analysis: Laparoscopic Electrosurgery.* (1995). ECRI Hospital Risk Control Bulletin.

21. Robotic arm returns direct scope control to surgeon. (1994). *Minimally Invasive Surgical Nursing*, 8(3):87–88.

22. Rohlf, S. (1995). Electrosurgical safety considerations for minimally invasive surgery. *Minimally Invasive Surgical Nursing*, 9(1):26–29.

23. See, W.A., Soper, N.J. (1994). Selection and preparation of the patient for laparoscopic surgery. In Soper, N.J., Odem, R.R., Clayman, R.V., McDougall, E.M., eds., *Essentials of Laparoscopy* (pages 1–10). St. Louis: Quality Medical Publishing.

24. Sliney, D.H., Trokel, S.L. (1993). *Medical Lasers and Their Safe Use.* New York: Springer-Verlag.

25. The risks of laparoscopic electrosurgery. (1995). *Health Devices*, 24(1):20.

REVIEW QUESTIONS

1. The gas used to establish pneumoperitoneum in laparoscopic surgery is

   A. Oxygen
   B. Argon
   C. Carbon dioxide
   D. Nitrous oxide

2. Relative contraindications to laparoscopic procedures are

   A. Uncorrected coagulopathy and previous abdominal surgery
   B. Pregnancy and adhesions
   C. Peritonitis and inguinal hernia
   D. Bowel obstruction and hypovolemic shock

3. A complication of laparoscopic surgery that may be evidenced several days postoperatively is

   A. Perforation of blood vessels
   B. Electrosurgical trauma to bowel
   C. Referred shoulder pain
   D. Subcutaneous emphysema

4. Subcutaneous emphysema is a complication of laparoscopic procedures related to

   A. Extraperitoneal insufflation
   B. Open laparoscopy
   C. Low insufflation pressures
   D. Veress needle injury

5. The structure frequently injured during laparoscopic procedures is the

   A. Colon
   B. Bladder
   C. Liver
   D. Small bowel

6. Elevated central venous pressure and potential pulmonary atelectasis may be seen in the patient undergoing laparoscopy due to

   A. Decreased functional residual capacity
   B. Decreased peak airway pressures
   C. Decreased intrathoracic pressure
   D. Decreased arterial carbon dioxide tension

7. Sympathetic vasoconstriction results in

   A. Increased total peripheral resistance
   B. Hypercarbia
   C. Increased intraabdominal pressure
   D. Decreased mean arterial pressure

8. The device used to access the abdominal cavity during laparoscopic procedures is the

   A. Veress
   B. Laparoscope
   C. Trochar
   D. Insufflator

9. Laser safety procedures include

   A. Universal laser goggles and nonreflective instrumentation
   B. Dry field and dual pedal activators
   C. Wavelength-specific goggles and window coverings
   D. Warning signage and reflective instrumentation

10. The organization that establishes standards for the safe use of lasers is

   A. OSHA
   B. ANSI
   C. AORN
   D. JCAHO

ANSWERS TO QUESTIONS

1. C
2. B
3. B
4. A
5. D

6. A
7. A
8. C
9. C
10. B

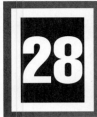

Cardiovascular Surgery

Beverly George-Gay
Medical College of Georgia
Augusta, Georgia
Vallire D. Hooper
Medical College of Georgia
Augusta, Georgia

1. Describe the effects of anesthesia on the basic functional properties of cardiac muscle.
2. Describe three factors regulating arterial and/or venous blood flow.
3. List five findings of a preoperative assessment that may be indicative of cardiac or peripheral vascular disease.
4. List three goals of anesthesia during cardiac or peripheral vascular procedures.
5. Identify at least one preoperative, intraoperative, and postoperative specific concern for each procedure discussed in this chapter.

I. Cardiac Anatomy and Physiology

A. Structure and function (See Figure 28–1)

B. Conduction system (See Figure 28–2)
1. Sino-atrial (AV) node: pacemaker of the heart
2. Internodal tracts/Bachman's Bundle
   a. Electrical pathways in atria
   b. Conducts impulse through atria and to the atrio-ventricular (AV) node
3. AV node: impulse briefly delayed
4. Ventricular conduction
   a. Bundle of His
   b. Left and right bundle branches
      i. Deliver impulse to the Purkinje fibers
      ii. Fibers carry impulse to the ventricular muscle

C. Cardiac cycle
1. Systole
   a. Ventricular contraction
      i. Occurs when ventricular pressure exceeds vascular pressure
      ii. Pulmonic and aortic valves open; tricuspid and mitral valves close
   b. Blood is ejected into the vasculature
2. Diastole
   a. Ventricular relaxation
      i. Ventricular pressure is less than vascular pressure

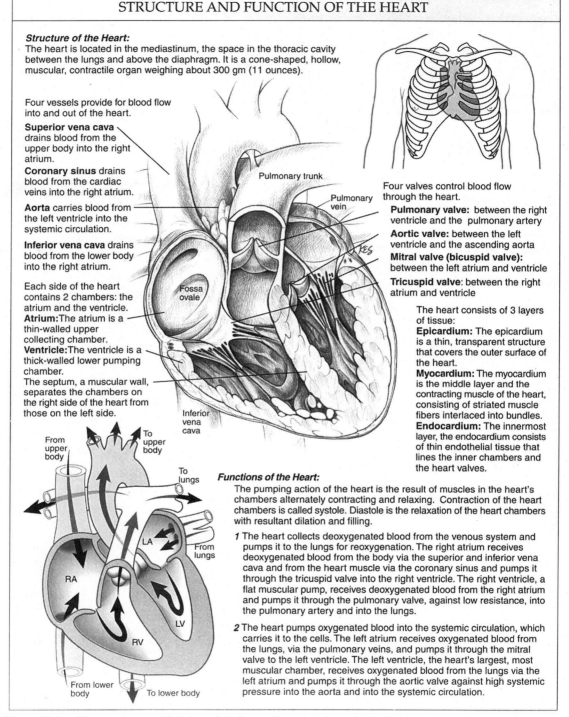

STRUCTURE AND FUNCTION OF THE HEART

Structure of the Heart:
The heart is located in the mediastinum, the space in the thoracic cavity between the lungs and above the diaphragm. It is a cone-shaped, hollow, muscular, contractile organ weighing about 300 gm (11 ounces).

Four vessels provide for blood flow into and out of the heart.
Superior vena cava drains blood from the upper body into the right atrium.
Coronary sinus drains blood from the cardiac veins into the right atrium.

Aorta carries blood from the left ventricle into the systemic circulation.

Inferior vena cava drains blood from the lower body into the right atrium.

Each side of the heart contains 2 chambers: the atrium and the ventricle.
Atrium: The atrium is a thin-walled upper collecting chamber.
Ventricle: The ventricle is a thick-walled lower pumping chamber.
The septum, a muscular wall, separates the chambers on the right side of the heart from those on the left side.

Pulmonary trunk

Pulmonary vein

Fossa ovale

Inferior vena cava

From upper body

To upper body

To lungs

From lungs

LA

RA

LV

RV

From lower body

To lower body

Four valves control blood flow through the heart.
Pulmonary valve: between the right ventricle and the pulmonary artery
Aortic valve: between the left ventricle and the ascending aorta
Mitral valve (bicuspid valve): between the left atrium and ventricle
Tricuspid valve: between the right atrium and ventricle

The heart consists of 3 layers of tissue:
Epicardium: The epicardium is a thin, transparent structure that covers the outer surface of the heart.
Myocardium: The myocardium is the middle layer and the contracting muscle of the heart, consisting of striated muscle fibers interlaced into bundles.
Endocardium: The innermost layer, the endocardium consists of thin endothelial tissue that lines the inner chambers and the heart valves.

Functions of the Heart:
The pumping action of the heart is the result of muscles in the heart's chambers alternately contracting and relaxing. Contraction of the heart chambers is called systole. Diastole is the relaxation of the heart chambers with resultant dilation and filling.

1 The heart collects deoxygenated blood from the venous system and pumps it to the lungs for reoxygenation. The right atrium receives deoxygenated blood from the body via the superior and inferior vena cava and from the heart muscle via the coronary sinus and pumps it through the tricuspid valve into the right ventricle. The right ventricle, a flat muscular pump, receives deoxygenated blood from the right atrium and pumps it through the pulmonary valve, against low resistance, into the pulmonary artery and into the lungs.

2 The heart pumps oxygenated blood into the systemic circulation, which carries it to the cells. The left atrium receives oxygenated blood from the lungs, via the pulmonary veins, and pumps it through the mitral valve to the left ventricle. The left ventricle, the heart's largest, most muscular chamber, receives oxygenated blood from the lungs via the left atrium and pumps it through the aortic valve against high systemic pressure into the aorta and into the systemic circulation.

Figure 28–1.   The structure and function of the heart. (From Luecke, L.E., Mancini, M.E., [1997]. Caring for people with cardiovascular disorders. In Luckman, J. ed. *Saunders Manual of Nursing Care,* [page 982]. Philadelphia: Saunders.)

  ii. Mitral valves open: ventricles fill passively

  iii. Pulmonic and aortic valves shut

 b. Provides for myocardial perfusion and ventricular filling

D. Functional properties of cardiac muscle

 1. Excitability: ability of a nerve to produce an action potential

 2. Automaticity: spontaneous depolarization and generation of an action potential

 3. Conductivity: ability to conduct electricity

 4. Refractoriness: resistance to stimulation while heart is still contracting from an earlier stimulus

 5. Contractility: ability to shorten when stimulated

 6. Extensibility: ability to stretch when heart fills with blood during diastole

 7. Rhythmicity

  a. Ability to function with a definite rhythm

  b. Stimulation–transmission–contraction–relaxation

 8. Irritability: ability to be stimulated

E. Effects of anesthesia on the heart

 1. Tachy and brady dysrhythmias

 2. Decreased contractility and cardiac output

II. **Vascular Structure and Function**

A. Structure (See Figure 28–3)

B. Function

 1. Arteries

  a. Transport oxygenated blood from the heart to the tissues

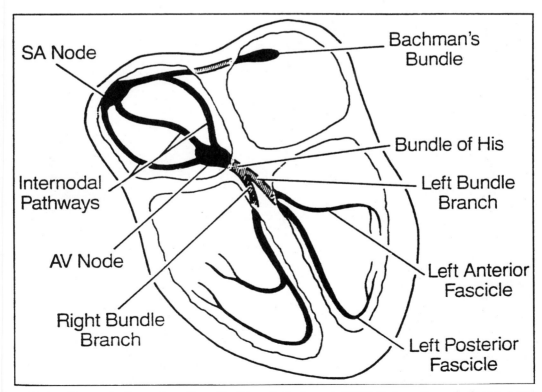

Figure 28–2. The conduction system. (From Van Riper, S., Luciano, A. [1994]. Basic cardiac arrhythmias: A review for postanesthesia care unit nurses. *JOPAN*, 9[1]:3.)

    b. Exception: pulmonary artery transports deoxygenated blood from the right ventricle to the lungs

  2. Capillaries: allow for the exchange of nutrients and wastes between the blood and cells

  3. Veins

    a. Transport deoxygenated blood from the tissues to the right side of the heart

    b. Exception: pulmonary vein transports oxygenated blood from the lungs to the left atrium

    c. Approximately 75% of total blood volume is found in the venous system at any given time

    d. Venous return is controlled by several factors

      i. Valves (See Figure 28–4)

        (a) Prevent backflow of blood, allowing flow to occur only in the direction toward the heart

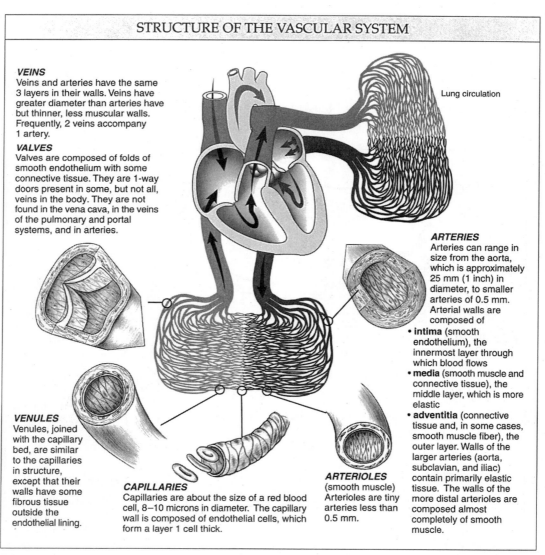

STRUCTURE OF THE VASCULAR SYSTEM

VEINS
Veins and arteries have the same 3 layers in their walls. Veins have greater diameter than arteries have but thinner, less muscular walls. Frequently, 2 veins accompany 1 artery.

VALVES
Valves are composed of folds of smooth endothelium with some connective tissue. They are 1-way doors present in some, but not all, veins in the body. They are not found in the vena cava, in the veins of the pulmonary and portal systems, and in arteries.

Lung circulation

ARTERIES
Arteries can range in size from the aorta, which is approximately 25 mm (1 inch) in diameter, to smaller arteries of 0.5 mm. Arterial walls are composed of

• **intima** (smooth endothelium), the innermost layer through which blood flows
• **media** (smooth muscle and connective tissue), the middle layer, which is more elastic
• **adventitia** (connective tissue and, in some cases, smooth muscle fiber), the outer layer. Walls of the larger arteries (aorta, subclavian, and iliac) contain primarily elastic tissue. The walls of the more distal arterioles are composed almost completely of smooth muscle.

VENULES
Venules, joined with the capillary bed, are similar to the capillaries in structure, except that their walls have some fibrous tissue outside the endothelial lining.

CAPILLARIES
Capillaries are about the size of a red blood cell, 8–10 microns in diameter. The capillary wall is composed of endothelial cells, which form a layer 1 cell thick.

ARTERIOLES
(smooth muscle) Arterioles are tiny arteries less than 0.5 mm.

Figure 28–3. Structure of the vascular system. (From Turner, J. [1997]. Caring for people with peripheral vascular and lymphatic disorders. In Luckman, J., ed. *Saunders Manual of Nursing Care,* [page 1092]. Philadelphia: Saunders.)

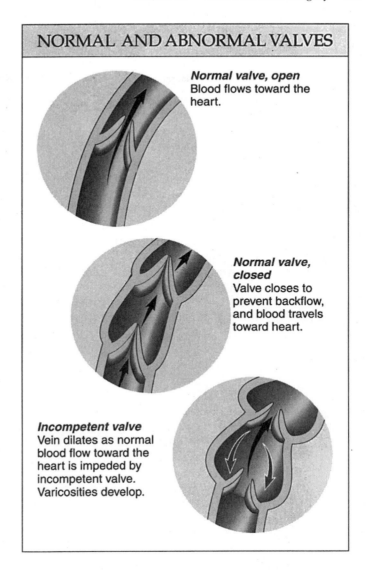

NORMAL AND ABNORMAL VALVES

Normal valve, open
Blood flows toward the heart.

Normal valve, closed
Valve closes to prevent backflow, and blood travels toward heart.

Incompetent valve
Vein dilates as normal blood flow toward the heart is impeded by incompetent valve. Varicosities develop.

Figure 28–4. Normal and abnormal valves. (From Turner, J. [1997]. Caring for people with peripheral vascular and lymphatic disorders. In Luckman, J., ed. *Saunders Manual of Nursing Care,* [page 1093]. Philadelphia: Saunders.)

       (b) Become incompetent when vein walls have been overstretched by excessive venous pressure
    ii. Venous elasticity
       (a) Venous walls are less elastic than arterial walls, thus allowing distention or pooling to occur.
       (b) This is known as *Venous capacitance*
    iii. Intrathoracic pressure
       (a) Negative intrathoracic pressure enhances flow into the heart by decreasing resistance
       (b) Positive intrathoracic pressure reduces flow into the heart by increasing resistance
  4. Arteriovenous anastomoses: channels where arterioles and venules connect without capillaries
C. Control of blood flow
  1. Neural control

a. Baroreceptors and chemoreceptors (stretch receptors) on the aortic arch, internal carotid sinus, and in the right atrium
   i.   Sense changes in blood flow
   ii. Send messages to the vasomotor center in the medulla
   iii. Stimulate the sympathetic nervous system (SNS) or parasympathetic nervous system to respond
      (a) Low flow:
         (i) Epinephrine and norepinephrine are released
         (ii) Cause vasoconstriction, increased heart rate, and contractility
      (b) High flow:
         (i) Acetylcholine released
         (ii) Causes vasodilation
2. Humoral control
   a. Also stimulated by the SNS in reaction to changes in blood flow, as well as other substances in the body
      i.   Low-flow states:
         (a) Adrenocorticotropic hormone (ACTH) released
            (i) Water reabsorption in renal tubules
            (ii) Increases intravascular volume
         (b) Renin–angiotensin–aldosterone system stimulated
            (i) Marked constriction of peripheral arteries
            (ii) Retention of sodium and water
      ii. High-flow states:
         (a) Bradykinin
            (i) Plasma protein
            (ii) Potent vasodilator
         (b) Histamine
            (i) Vasodilator
            (ii) Released following mast cell injury
3. Local control: autoregulation
   a. Blood vessels' ability to respond to tissue needs by dilating or constricting
   b. Utilized mainly by arterioles due to:
      i.   Decreased oxygen availability
      ii. Increased metabolic demand at the tissue level
III. **Assessment and Management**
   A. Preoperative
      1. Baseline preoperative assessment
      2. Cardiac-focused assessment
         a. Chest pain
            i.   Stable
            ii. Unstable
         b. Dyspnea
         c. Paroxysmal nocturnal dyspnea
         d. Syncope
         e. Unexplained weakness or fatigue
         f. Weight loss or gain
         g. Dependent edema
         h. Orthopnea
         i. Coughing at night
         j. Coughing up blood
         k. Rapid heartbeat or palpitations
         l. Need to urinate frequently at night time
         m. Intermittent claudication

3. Peripheral vascular focused assessment
   a. Skin
      i. Turgor
      ii. Edema
      iii. Compare temperature at different sites
      iv. Inspect for lesions or ulcerations
      v. Determine history of slow wound healing
      vi. Inspect for varicose veins: visibly engorged, palpable subcutaneous veins
      vii. Differentiate between venous and arterial insufficiency
         (a) Arterial insufficiency
            (i) Loss of hair
            (ii) Pallor
            (iii) Translucent, waxy appearance of skin
         (b) Venous insufficiency
            (i) Skin thickened
            (ii) Reddish-brown pigmentation
            (iii) Ulceration
   b. Vasculature/circulation
      i. Arterial
         (a) Capillary refill
            (i) Brisk: <3 seconds
            (ii) Sluggish: >3 seconds
         (b) Bruits
            (i) Low-pitched blowing sound due to turbulent flow
            (ii) Indicative of atherosclerosis
            (iii) Assess with bell of stethoscope
               a) Assess at carotid and femoral arteries
               b) Assess abdominal aorta
         (c) Determine strength of peripheral pulses
            (i) Absent: 0
            (ii) Diminished: +1
            (iii) Normal, easily palpated: +2
            (iv) Increased, strong: +3
            (v) Bounding: +4
         (d) Neurovascular assessment: Five P's indicative of arterial insufficiency
            (i) Pain
            (ii) Pulselessness
            (iii) Pallor
            (iv) Paresthesia
            (v) Paralysis
         (e) Ankle–brachial index (ABI)
            (i) Inexpensive, noninvasive, bedside assessment of arterial perfusion (atherosclerosis)
            (ii) Procedure
               a) Obtain the brachial blood pressure in both arms (use the higher systolic pressure for the calculation)
               b) Obtain the ankle blood pressure in the questionable extremity
               c) Divide the systolic ankle pressure by the systolic brachial pressure
               d) >.95 normal perfusion
               e) <.90 early asymptomatic disease, difficulty with wound healing, increased risk for cardiovascular event, i.e., MI or death

        f) <.60 wound probably will not heal, more advanced atheroma, greater risk for CV event or death

        g) >1.2 indicative of venous disease

  ii. Venous

    (a) Superficial thrombophlebitis: subcutaneous cords with overlying erythema

    (b) Deep vein thrombosis (DVT)

      (i) Silent at onset

      (ii) Shooting pain at moment of embolism, with numbness and weakness

      (iii) Followed by signs of ischemia

      (iv) Homan's sign

        a) Positive: pain in popliteal fossa and upper posterior calf on dorsiflexion of foot

        b) Helpful but not specific for DVT

4. Pre-existing disease states

  a. Arteriosclerotic heart disease

  b. Diabetes

  c. Hypertension

  d. Chronic obstructive pulmonary disease (COPD)

  e. Previous myocardial infarction (MI)

5. Specific allergies

  a. Shellfish

  b. Iodine

  c. Contrast media

6. Cardiac auscultation

  a. Normal heart sounds

    i. S_1 (first heart sound)

      (a) Represents closure of tricuspid and mitral atrioventricular (AV) valves

      (b) Occurs at the end of atrial contraction and with the onset of ventricular contraction

      (c) Loudest at the apex

      (d) Slightly longer and lower pitch than S_2

      (e) Occurs as the ventricles contract; almost synchronous with the carotid pulse

    ii. S_2 (second heart sound)

      (a) Caused by closure of the pulmonic and aortic valves at the end of ventricular contraction

      (b) Signals the beginning of diastole

      (c) Loudest at the base

      (d) Higher pitch than S_1, so is louder and transmits better

    iii. Split heart sounds

      (a) Split S_1: occurs if AV valves do not close at precisely the same time

      (b) Split S_2: occurs if semilunar valves do not close simultaneously

      (c) Normal occurrence; does not require treatment or monitoring

  b. Extra heart sounds

    i. S_3 (ventricular gallop)

      (a) Immediately follows S_2

        (i) Sounds like "lub-dup-a" or "Ken-tuc-ky"

        (ii) Dull and low-pitched

        (iii) Best heard at the apex with the bell of the stethoscope and the patient in the left lateral position

(b) Occurs when the AV valves open and atrial blood rushes into the ventricles
(c) Usually indicates decreased compliance of the ventricles commonly associated with heart failure
(d) May also indicate mitral or tricuspid AV valve incompetence
ii. S$_4$ (atrial gallop)
(a) Immediately precedes S$_1$
(i) Sounds like "da-lub-dup" or "Ten-nes-see"
(ii) Very low pitch
(iii) Best heard at the apex with the bell of the stethoscope
(b) Produced by atrial contraction when the ventricle is resistant to filling
(c) Heard in patients with:
(i) Increased resistance to ventricular filling as seen in hypertension and mitral stenosis
(ii) Increased stroke volume as seen with severe anemia and hyperthyroidism
(iii) Delayed conduction between the atria and ventricles
c. Murmurs
i. Caused by increased turbulence or blood flow through the heart
ii. Causes
(a) Valves will not open properly (stenosis)
(b) Valves will not close properly
(i) Incompetent
(ii) Insufficient
(iii) Regurgitant
(c) Presence of a congenital defect between chambers
(d) Dilated heart chamber
(e) Other
(i) Increased blood flow
(ii) Decreased blood viscosity
iii. Murmur description should include:
(a) Primary location related to valve where best auscultated
(b) Area of radiation or site of maximum intensity
(c) Timing as related to cardiac cycle
(d) Pitch
(e) Configuration or shape as determined by intensity over time
(f) Quality
(i) Blowing
(ii) Rumbling
(iii) Musical
(iv) Harsh
(g) Intensity
(i) Grade I: very faint, heard only after a period of intent listening
(ii) Grade II: quiet and faint, but heard immediately upon placing the stethoscope on the chest
(iii) Grade III: moderately intense
(iv) Grade IV: loud, associated with a thrill
(v) Grade V: very loud, can be heard with the stethoscope partially off the chest wall
(vi) Grade VI: very loud, can be heard with the entire chest piece just removed from the chest wall

      d. Pericardial friction rub

          i. Occurs if the pericardium becomes inflamed

          ii. Is a scratchy "to-and-fro"; should be heard with each heart beat

          iii. Best auscultated with patient sitting upright and leaning forward

   7. Laboratory studies

      a. Arterial blood gases as indicated

      b. Cardiac enzymes

          i. Creatine phosphokinase (CPK)

          ii. Lactate dehydrogenase (LDH)

          iii. Troponin I/Troponin Y

            (a) Detectable within 1 hour of myocardial cell injury

            (b) Peak elevation with 4 to 6 hours of MI

            (c) Remains elevated for up to 8 days

            (d) Useful in early detection of AMI, silent MI, microinfarctions, chest pain not accompanied by typical EKG changes

      c. Electrolytes critical to cardiac function (potassium, sodium, magnesium, calcium)

      d. Coagulation profile (PT/PTT/INR)

   8. Noninvasive diagnostic studies

      a. Chest X-ray

      b. Electrocardiogram (EKG)

          i. 12-lead EKG

          ii. Determines or detects:

            (a) Disturbances of rate, rhythm, or conduction

            (b) Ischemia or infarction

            (c) Electrolyte abnormalities

            (d) Anatomic orientation of heart

            (e) Chamber enlargement

            (f) Drug toxicity

      c. Echocardiography

          i. Ultrasonic exam

          ii. Detects abnormalities of anatomy and/or motion

      d. Radionuclide scans

          i. Perfusion imaging: evaluates myocardial blood flow

          ii. Infarction scintigraphy: detects injured or necrotic myocardium

      e. Exercise electrocardiography (stress testing)

   9. Invasive diagnostic studies

      a. Cardiac catheterization

      b. Ventriculography

      c. Pulmonary angiography

      d. Aortography

  10. Medications

      a. Types

      b. Dosages

      c. Consult with anesthesia or surgeon as to necessity of taking cardiac/antihypertensive medications the morning of surgery

      d. If unable to obtain consult, have patient bring medications with him/her the morning of surgery

  11. Determination of cardiac risk

      a. Goldman's Multifactorial Cardiac Risk Index (See Tables 28–1 and 28–2)

      b. Detsky's Multifactorial Index (See Tables 28–3 and 28–4)

Table 28–1 • GOLDMAN'S MULTIFACTORIAL CARDIAC RISK INDEX

		POINTS
History	Myocardial infarction within 6 mo	10
	Age over 70 y	5
Physical examination	S3 gallop or jugular venous distention	11
	Important aortic stenosis	3
Electrocardiogram	Rhythm other than sinus or sinus plus APBs* on last preoperative electrocardiogram	7
	More than 5 premature ventricular beats per minute at any time preoperatively	7
Poor general medical status	Pa_{O_2} <60 mm Hg, Pa_{CO_2} >50 mm Hg, K^+ <3.0 mEq $\cdot$ L^{-1}, HCO_3^- <20 mEq $\cdot$ L^{-1}, BUN >50 mg $\cdot$ dL^{-1} (18 mmol $\cdot$ L^{-1}), Creatinine >3 mg $\cdot$ dL^{-1} (260 mmol $\cdot$ L^{-1}), abnormal SGOT, signs of chronic liver disease, patient bedridden from noncardiac causes	3
Intraperitoneal, intrathoracic, or aortic surgery		3
Emergency operation		4
	Total:	53

*APB = atrial premature beat.

(From Goldman, L., Caldera, D, Nussbaum S.R., et al. [1977]. Multifactorial index of cardiac risk in non-cardiac surgical procedures. *N Engl J Med*, 197:848, by permission of the New England Journal of Medicine.)

B. Intraoperative/intraprocedural concerns
  1. Goals of anesthesia or sedation
     a. Maintain myocardial oxygen supply
     b. Keep oxygen demand as low as possible
     c. Maintain vital signs at, or near stable preoperative values
  2. Anesthesia choice based on procedure and cardiac stability
  3. Monitor for dysrhythmias; treat by ACLS protocol when indicated
  4. Monitor, control, and/or replace blood loss as indicated
  5. Monitor anticoagulation therapy and values as indicated
C. Postanesthesia Phase I
  1. Routine admission assessment and management
     a. Monitor vital signs per protocol
     b. Offer support and comfort
     c. Provide analgesics as indicated and ordered
     d. Administer antiemetics as indicated and ordered
     e. Ensure safe environment

Table 28–2 • PREDICTION OF PERIOPERATIVE CARDIAC COMPLICATIONS BY POINTS IN THE GOLDMAN INDEX

	POINT TOTAL	CARDIAC DEATH (%)	OTHER LIFE-THREATENING COMPLICATIONS* (%)
Class I	0–5	0.2	0.7
Class II	6–12	2.0	5.0
Class III	13–25	2.0	11.0
Class IV	≥26	56.0	22.0

*Nonfatal MI, CHF, and ventricular tachycardia.

(From Goldman, L., Caldera, D, Nussbaum S.R., et al. [1977]. Multifactorial index of cardiac risk in non-cardiac surgical procedures. *N Engl J Med*, 197:848, by permission of the New England Journal of Medicine.)

Table 28–3 • DETSKY'S MULTIFACTORIAL INDEX

Coronary artery disease	MI within 6 mo	10
	MI more than 6 mo previously	5
	Canadian Cardiovascular Society Angina:	
	Class III	10
	Class IV	20
Alveolar pulmonary edema	Within 1 wk	10
	Ever	5
Valvular disease	Suspected critical aortic stenosis	20
Arrhythmias	Rhythm other than sinus or sinus plus APBs on last preoperative electrocardiogram; more than 5 premature ventricular contractions at any time prior to surgery	5
Poor general medical status		5
Age over 70 y		5
Emergency operation		10

(From Detsky, A.S., Abrams, H.B., McLaughlin, J.R., et al. [1986]. Predicting cardiac complications in patients undergoing non-cardiac surgery. *J Gen Intern Med*, 1:213.)

2. ECG monitor
3. Assess heart sounds
4. Inspect and maintain pressure to procedure puncture sites
5. Assess peripheral pulses when appropriate
6. Neurovascular checks when appropriate
7. Procedure specific assessment
8. Monitor for other potential complications
   a. Bleeding
   b. Allergic reaction to dyes
   c. Pneumothorax
   d. Embolism
   e. Hematoma
   f. Septicemia
9. Monitor for venous access device displacement, damage, and destruction
   a. Facial edema
   b. Distention of thoracic and neck veins
   c. Swelling, redness, tenderness
   d. Leakage of fluid

Table 28–4 • LIKELIHOOD RATIOS OF PERIOPERATIVE CARDIAC COMPLICATIONS* BY POINTS IN THE DETSKY INDEX

CLASS (POINTS)	MAJOR SURGERY	MINOR SURGERY	ALL SURGERY
I (0–15)	0.42	0.39	0.43
II (15–30)	3.58	2.75	3.38
III (>30)	14.93	12.20	10.60

*Defined as MI pulmonary edema, ventricular tachycardia, or fibrillation, new or worsening CHF, and coronary insufficiency.

(From Detsky, A.S., Abrams, H.B., McLaughlin, J.R., et al. [1986]. Predicting cardiac complications in patients undergoing non-cardiac surgery. *J Gen Intern Med*, 1:213.)

      e. Inability to draw or infuse blood
      f. Bulging catheter
  D. Postanesthesia Phase II
      1. Routine assessment, management, and instruction
          a. Review/reinforce postprocedure routine
          b. Avoid tight-fitting clothing
          c. Resume preoperative medications
          d. Reinforce need for activity restrictions postprocedure
          e. Reinforce specific physician instructions
          f. Postoperative follow-up
              i.   Reinforce instructions and restrictions for home care
              ii. Emphasize need for long-term follow-up and care as indicated
              iii. Refer to home health care agency for follow-up as indicated
      2. Continue to monitor operative/puncture site
      3. Continue neurovascular/pulse checks
      4. Discharge teaching
          a. Instruct on signs and symptoms to report to physician
              i.   Increased temperature
              ii. Swelling, redness of involved limb
              iii. Involved limb assessment
                   (a) Numbness
                   (b) Acute pain
                   (c) Coldness
              iv. Bleeding from operative/puncture site
          b. Teach signs and symptoms of hemorrhage
          c. Instruct on management of postoperative bleeding
          d. Reinforce need for activity restrictions postprocedure
          e. Instruct on avoidance of situations causing blood pooling or interruption of
              blood flow
              i.   Crossing legs
              ii. Smoking
              iii. Sitting or standing for extended periods
          f. Teach pulse taking if indicated
          g. Teach shunt care if indicated
          h. Instruct on evaluation of thrill or bruit as indicated
          i. Explain aseptic technique
          j. Teach catheter care as indicated
  E. Postanesthesia Phase III
      1. Designed for the patient requiring extended care and/or monitoring for a period
          greater than 24 hours
      2. Utilization will increase as routine ICU procedures (carotid endarterectomy,
          laparoscopic heart surgery, angioplasty, etc.) become more popular and require
          shorter hospital stays
IV. **Operative procedures**
  A. AV shunt placement/revision
      1. Purpose: provide a permanent, internal vascular access for prolonged or long-term
          dialysis
      2. Description
          a. Surgically constructs an arteriovenous (AV) fistula
          b. Brings arterial blood flow pressure into the vein that will be used for dialysis
              i.   Significantly increases rate of venous flow to greater than 200 ml/min.
              ii. Allows for completion of dialysis in a reasonable length of time (3–4 hours)

  c. Minimum mortality rates

  d. Technical failure rate of 10 to 15%

 3. Preoperative care

  a. Physical assessment issues

   i. Respiratory

    (a) Common coexisting disease processes

     (i) Pneumonia

     (ii) Pulmonary edema

     (iii) Uremic pleuritis

    (b) Assess for:

     (i) Shortness of breath (SOB)

     (ii) Orthopnea

     (iii) Paroxysmal nocturnal dyspnea (PND)

   ii. Gastrointestinal (GI)

    (a) Common coexisting disease processes

     (i) Delayed gastric emptying

     (ii) GI bleeding

    (b) Assess for:

     (i) Regurgitation

     (ii) Nausea and vomiting (N/V)

     (iii) Early satiety

   iii. Hematology

    (a) Common coexisting disease processes

     (i) Anemia

     (ii) Bleeding diathesis

    (b) Assess for:

     (i) SOB

     (ii) Bruising

   iv. Genitourinary/endocrine (GU/ENDO)

    (a) Common coexisting disease processes

     (i) Oliguria/anuria

     (ii) Uremia

     (iii) Electrolyte/acid-base imbalance

     (iv) Diabetes

    (b) Assess for:

     (i) Weight (baseline and high)

     (ii) Hiccoughs

     (iii) Anorexia

     (iv) N/V

     (v) Diarrhea

     (vi) Diabetes

   v. Central nervous system (CNS)

    (a) Common coexisting disease processes

     (i) Encephalopathy

     (ii) Seizures

     (iii) Neuropathy

    (b) Perform musculoskeletal assessment

  b. Recommended diagnostic studies

   i. Chest X-ray (CXR)

   ii. Platelet count

   iii. Creatinine

   iv. BUN

      v.   HCO$_3$

      vi. Blood glucose

  c. Determine nondominant arm

      i.   Shunt should be easily accessible

      ii. Should be placed on nondominant arm when possible

         (a) Allows for easy self-cannulation for home dialysis patients

         (b) Allows for increased patient ease with performance of daily activities

4. Intraoperative concerns

  a. Types of internal vascular accesses

      i.   Internal AV fistula

         (a) Creation of an actual fistula

         (b) Not available for immediate use

            (i)   Wound healing must occur and edema subside

            (ii)   Usually not accessible for weeks to months after surgery

      ii. Internal graft AV fistula

         (a) Straight or looped natural or synthetic graft

         (b) Placed in arm or thigh

         (c) Preferred for obese individuals

      iii. Internal AV graft with external access device

         (a) External access port is attached to AV graft

         (b) Alleviates need for repeated needle insertions

  b. Common graft locations

      i.   Wrist

         (a) "Snuff-box" fistula

         (b) Antebrachium–cephalic vein to radial artery

      ii. Forearm: radial, ulnar, or brachial artery to antecubital or brachial vein

      iii. Upper arm: brachial artery above elbow to basilic or axillary vein

  c. Anesthesia techniques

      i.   MAC

      ii. Regional

      iii. General

  d. Other

      i.   Estimated blood loss (EBL): 25 to 100 cc

      ii. Length of case: 1 to 2 hours

5. Postanesthesia priorities: Phase I PACU

  a. Avoid venipuncture, BP measurements, injections in surgical arm

  b. Assess for graft/shunt patency

      i.   Gently palpate for thrill

      ii. Auscultate for bruit

  c. Elevate surgical arm to decrease swelling

  d. Avoid circumferential dressings, arm bands, to surgical arm

  e. Maintain adequate hydration

      i.   Maintains blood pressure

      ii. Protects patency of graft

  f. Assess for bleeding, apply pressure dressing for profuse bleeding

  g. Monitor for complications

      i.   Thrombosis

      ii. Infection

      iii. Aneurysm

      iv. Steal syndrome

         (a) Ischemic pain related to vascular insufficiency due to fistula formation

(b) Assess for:
  (i)   Diminished pulses
  (ii) Pallor
  (iii) Pain distal to graft site
(c) Surgical revision or additional procedures required when this syndrome occurs
  h. Report any suspected or actual complications to physician
6. Postanesthesia priorities: Phase II
  a. MAC/regional patients may be admitted directly to Phase II
  b. Continue Phase I level of care
  c. Pain management
    i.   Oral analgesia usually effective
    ii. Average discharge pain score: 1 to 2 (0 to 10 scale)
  d. Discharge teaching
    i.   Keep operative arm elevated for several days
    ii.   Avoid any venipuncture, BP measurements, injections in operative arm
    iii. Avoid wearing constrictive clothing, wristbands on operative site
    iv.   Instruct patient how to palpate for a thrill
    v.   Instruct patient in assessment for and management of possible complications
      (a) Infection very common
      (b) Synthetic grafts most susceptible to infection
7. Postanesthesia priorities: Phase III
  a. Autogenous fistulas must adequately heal before being used for dialysis
    i.   Blood flow increases with time
    ii.   Venous wall must adequately thicken to prevent tears and infiltration during dialysis
    iii. Maturation time varies from 3 to 6 weeks
    iv.   Fistula should not be used for 3 weeks to avoid aneurysm formation
  b. Teach importance to rotate injection sites when puncturing for dialysis
    i.   Prevents aneurysm formation
    ii.   Prevents shredding and eventual breakdown of shunt material
  c. Instruct patient that AV hemodialysis accesses have finite lifespan; replacements and revisions are common
  d. Support patient on waiting list for renal transplantation
    i.   Optimal therapy for end stage renal disease (ESRD)
    ii.   Waiting time varies considerably
B. Arteriography
  1. Purpose
    a. Commonly performed prior to any vascular surgery
    b. Aids in determination of surgical treatment options
    c. Provides morphologic visualization of arterial lumen
    d. Used to depict location, size, and/or condition of suspected stenosis, occlusion, aneurysm, or AV fistula
    e. Also allows visualization of collateral, proximal, and distal arterial circulation
  2. Description
    a. Performed in special procedures or radiology under sterile conditions
    b. Catheter is inserted percutaneously into an artery
    c. Radiopaque contrast medium is introduced
    d. Serial X-rays made of the movement of the dye
  3. Preoperative care
    a. Assessment issues
      i.   Pulses distal to catheter insertion site should be assessed and marked

      ii. History of allergy to shellfish, iodine, or contrast medium

     iii. Use of anticoagulants, over-the-counter (OTC) agents such as aspirin, NSAIDs

     iv. History of any renal disease

      v. Thorough assessment of involved body system

     vi. Rule out possibility of pregnancy when appropriate

  b. Recommended diagnostic studies

       i. PT/PTT/INR

      ii. BUN

     iii. Creatinine

     iv. H & H

      v. Beta HCG (when appropriate)

  c. Other nursing care

       i. Shave and prep catheter insertion site

      ii. Obtain IV access

     iii. Premedication

         (a) Benzodiazepine by oral or IV route most popular

         (b) Narcotic occasionally included

         (c) Usually given 30 to 60 minutes before procedure

4. Intraoperative care

  a. Anesthesia techniques

       i. Usually accomplished with injection of local anesthesia at catheter insertion site

      ii. Sedative agents may be indicated for extremely anxious patient

  b. Nursing care

       i. Provide reassurance and explanation throughout case

      ii. Patient may experience warmth, flushing, or burning sensation with dye injection

     iii. Monitor patient vital signs and ECG

     iv. Administer sedation when indicated and monitor appropriately

      v. Monitor injection site for irritation and thrombosis

     vi. Monitor for allergic reaction to dye

         (a) Skin rash

         (b) Itching

         (c) Bronchospasm

         (d) Anaphylaxis

         (e) Convulsions

         (f) Cardiac arrest

    vii. Discontinue catheter once procedure completed

         (a) Maintain pressure at catheter insertion site until all bleeding has stopped (length of time dependent on size of catheter and artery used)

         (b) Monitor insertion site for formation of hematoma

         (c) Apply pressure dressing to site

         (d) Assess distal pulses

5. Postanesthesia priorities: Phase I and Phase II

  a. Often admitted directly to Phase II

  b. Establish baseline assessment and vital signs

  c. Neurovascular checks distal to insertion site

  d. Observe catheter site for bleeding, hematoma

  e. Monitor closely for overt signs of bleeding

       i. Sensorium change

          ii. Increased restlessness

         iii. Drop in blood pressure

         iv. Increased heart rate

          v. Decreased peripheral pulses

    f. Maintain bed rest for 4 to 8 hours

          i. Extremity should be kept straight

         ii. Head of bed elevated no more than 30 degrees

         iii. Provide pain relief as needed

         iv. Assist with position changes to relieve back discomfort

          v. Teach patient to apply pressure at insertion site when coughing, sneezing, changing position, etc.

         vi. Instruct patient to notify nurse for any sensations of warmth or redness at the insertion site

    g. Monitor closely for allergic reaction

    h. Hydrate with IV and oral fluids to clear radiopaque dye

    i. Closely monitor intake and output (I&O)

    j. Discharge teaching

          i. Instruct patient in signs and symptoms of hemorrhage and hematoma formation

         ii. Encourage increased fluid intake

         iii. Encourage bed rest with as little ambulation as possible for 12 to 24 hours

         iv. Avoid stairs for 12 to 24 hours

          v. Instruct patient to continue holding pressure to site when ambulating, coughing, sneezing, etc.

         vi. Instruct caregiver in hemorrhage/hematoma management

            (a) Call emergency medical services

            (b) Have patient lie flat and still

            (c) Hold pressure over puncture site

  6. Phase III recovery

    a. Must have a caregiver capable of holding pressure with patient for the first 24 hours

    b. Must have immediate access to phone to call for help if needed

    c. Return to work/normal activities

          i. Dependent on type of work/activities

         ii. At the more strenuous the work/activities, the slower the return

C. Cardiac catheterization

  1. Purpose

    a. Confirms and evaluates lesions of the heart muscle and coronary vasculature

    b. Assesses left ventricular function

    c. Diagnoses CAD, cardiac status prior to heart surgery

    d. Measures pressures within the chambers of the heart, CO, and blood gases

  2. Description

    a. Right-sided catheterization

          i. The catheter is inserted into the femoral or brachial vein and advanced under fluoroscopy through the right atrium, right ventricle to the pulmonary artery

    b. Left-sided catheterization

          i. The catheter is placed into the femoral or brachial artery and advanced under fluoroscopy through the aorta into the left atrium and ventricle

            (a) Angiography: visualization of coronary circulation

               (i) The catheter is further advanced to the proximal end of the coronary arteries

            (ii)   Dye is injected and its progression through the coronary circulation is visualized and radiographed

         (b) Percutaneous transluminal coronary angioplasty (PTCA): treatment option for atherosclerosis of the coronary arteries

            (i)   A double lumen catheter with a distensible balloon is advanced into the affected coronary artery

            (ii)   The balloon is inflated to compress the atheroma

            (iii) If unsuccessful, coronary artery bypass grafting is recommended

3. Preoperative care (See Arteriography)
   a. May start aspirin 2 to 3 days prior to procedure
   b. Shave both groins
   c. Assess, mark, and document bilateral femoral, posterior tibial, and dorsalis pedis pulses
   d. Thorough respiratory and cardiac assessment
   e. Coagulation studies

4. Intraoperative Care (See Arteriography)
   a. Monitor multichannel ECG
   b. Heparinized saline is administered after cannulation to prevent thrombosis
   c. Patient may experience palpitations
   d. Injection of the contrast medium may cause a metallic taste in the mouth
   e. Tell the patient to report chest pain, headache, dyspnea, lightheadedness, nausea, itching

5. Postanesthesia priorities: Phase I and Phase II
   a. See Arteriography
   b. Manual pressure is applied for no less than 15 minutes
   c. Continue multichannel ECG monitoring for 12 to 24 hours
      i.   Assess for cardiac ischemia/injury
      ii. Rate changes
   d. Instruct patient to report any chest pain/discomfort
   e. Protamine sulfate may be administered to reverse the heparin

6. Phase III recovery
   a. See Arteriography
   b. Instruct patient to seek medical attention for any chest pain, discomfort, shortness of breath, lightheadedness, or dizziness
   c. Encourage cardiac rehab when indicated

D. Venography
   1. Purpose
      a. Most accurate way to diagnose deep vein thrombosis, determining location and severity
      b. Also used to determine competency of valves
   2. Description
      a. Performed in a special procedures area or radiology under sterile conditions
      b. Catheter is inserted percutaneously into an artery
      c. Contrast medium injected into vein previously emptied by gravity
      d. Injection followed by X-ray visualization of the area of suspected injury
      e. Carries high risk of complications; other noninvasive techniques typically utilized prior to this procedure
   3. Preoperative care
      a. See Arteriography
      b. Clear liquids occasionally allowed prior to the exam

    4. Intraoperative care
      a. Have patient flex feet and toes at end of procedure
      b. See Arteriography for rest of care
    5. Postanesthesia priorities: Phase I and Phase II
      a. Often admitted directly to Phase II
      b. Monitor for and instruct patient in signs and symptoms of postvenography syndrome
        i. Delayed calf discomfort
        ii. Subclinical or frank postvenographic deep vein thrombosis
        iii. Lower leg will be hot, red, and swollen
      c. See Arteriography
    6. Phase III recovery (See Arteriography)
  E. Carotid endarterectomy
    1. Purpose: to restore cerebral circulation
    2. Description
      a. For patients who have experienced retinal ischemic neurological deficits, transient ischemic attacks (TIA), or stroke
      b. Involves surgical removal of plaque from carotid artery by endarterectomy with or without a vein patch graft
      c. Plaque may also be removed intravascularly by a mechanical device
      d. Stroke risk
        i. Asymptomatic patients: 1 to 2%
        ii. Patient experiencing TIAs: 6 to 10%
        iii. Stroke risk greatly increases in asymptomatic patients with stenosis of >75%
      e. Perioperative mortality: 0-2.6%
        i. Highest from cardiac events
        ii. Followed by cerebrovascular events
      f. Perioperative risk of permanent neurological damage: 0 to 6.3%
    3. Preoperative care
      a. Physical assessment issues
        i. Thorough cardiovascular assessment
        ii. Respiratory
          (a) Often smokers with COPD
          (b) Assess for:
            (i) Cough
            (ii) Auscultate lung fields
        iii. Endocrine
          (a) Often coexists with diabetes mellitus
          (b) Assess for:
            (i) Ketoacidosis
            (ii) Diet/insulin control
        iv. CNS
          (a) May be symptomatic or asymptomatic
          (b) Assess for:
            (i) TIAs
            (ii) Ringing in ears
            (iii) Dizziness
            (iv) Changes in vision
            (v) Weakness
            (vi) Slurred speech
            (vii) Paralysis

   b. Recommended diagnostic studies
       i. ECG
       ii. Chest X-ray
       iii. Blood chemistry
       iv. Ultrasound scanning
       v. As needed:
           (a) EEG
           (b) Angiography
           (c) Stress test
           (d) Echocardiogram
           (e) CAT scan
4. Intraoperative care
   a. Rapid discharge protocol most effective when cases are done early in the morning
   b. Blood loss generally minimal and of little concern
   c. Anesthesia technique
       i. General
       ii. Regional
           (a) Becoming more popular with short-stay patients
           (b) Techniques include local, superficial infiltration with or without deep cervical plexus block
           (c) Nursing implications
               (i)   Constantly reassure patient
               (ii) Maintain constant vigilance in neurovascular assessment
               (iii) Avoid oversedation
5. Postanesthesia priorities: Phase I PACU
   a. Usually monitored in Phase I for a minimum of 2 hours when scheduled for rapid discharge
   b. Assessment/management includes:
       i. Position supine with HOB elevated 25 to 30 degrees
       ii. Level of consciousness
       iii. Neurological assessment
       iv. Bleeding or hematoma formation at incision site
       v. Meticulous blood pressure control
   c. Any alterations from baseline requires immediate attention and intervention
6. Postanesthesia priorities: Phase II
   a. Vital signs and neurological assessment every 2 hours or less for first 24 hours
   b. No invasive monitoring required
   c. IV fluids at maintenance volumes for first 24 hours postoperatively
   d. Hypotension treated with IV fluids
   e. Hypertension treated with sublingual nifedipine or intramuscular hydralazine
   f. Encouraged to eat and walk on day of surgery
7. Phase III recovery
   a. Expect 24- to 48-hour stay in acute care, Phase II-type environment
   b. Discharge teaching
       i. Rest for first week after surgery
       ii. Avoid strenuous activities
       iii. Resume preoperative medications, particularly antihypertensives as ordered
       iv. Majority receive postoperative aspirin or antiplatelet therapy
       v. Schedule follow-up appointment in 4 to 6 weeks

F. Vein ligation and stripping
  1. Purpose: surgical treatment for primary varicose veins, primarily for cosmetic purposes, but maybe for fatigue or pain that occurs upon standing
    a. Varicose veins: longitudinal enlargement of lower extremity veins due to loss of valvular competence; may be primary or secondary
      i. Primary varicose veins are an isolated condition due to weak thin-walled veins of the lower extremities
      ii. Secondary varicose veins are the result of an underlying condition such as deep vein thrombosis (DVT)
    b. Varicose veins affect:
      i. 15–20% of the adult population, with a familial tendency
      ii. Female-to-male ratio is 5:1, partly due to volume expansion and hormonal changes of pregnancy
  2. Description (See Figure 28–5): usually done bilaterally
    a. Individual varices are excised through small transverse incisions directly over the marked skin first
    b. The saphenous vein is ligated through incisions in the ankle above the malleolus and the upper thigh
    c. The saphenous vein is then removed with an internal vein stripper which is inserted through a small incision in the upper thigh
    d. A compressive dressing applied from the ankle upwards to reduce the risk of subcutaneous bleeding and hematoma
  3. Preoperative care
    a. Thorough vascular assessment

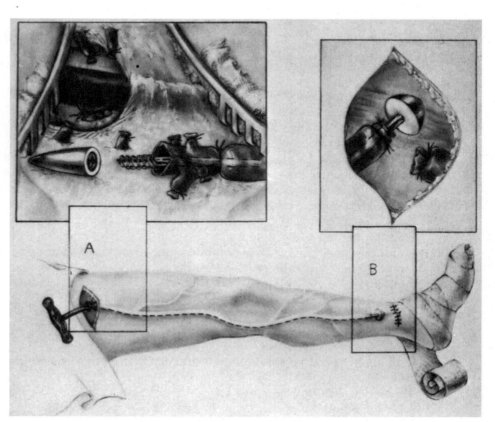

Figure 28–5. Vein ligation and stripping. (From Schenk, W.G. [1987]. Surgical disorders of the veins. In Sabiston, D.C., ed. *Sabiston's Essentials of Surgery,* [page 940]. Philadelphia: Saunders.)

   b. Mark posterior tibialis and dorsalis pedal pulses with indelible ink
   c. Assess whether primary or secondary; secondary must be distinguished as prognosis and treatment are related to the underlying condition, i.e., DVT
   d. Assess bleeding history: monitor PT, PTT, and INR if indicated
   e. Assist in locating and marking the varicosities with indelible ink while the patient is standing
   f. Prep the groin and affected lower extremities circumferentially
4. Routine intraoperative care
5. Postanesthesia priorities: Phase I
   a. Assess neurovascular status of affected extremity
   b. Assess for bleeding
   c. Elevate involved extremities without flexing the groin or knee
   d. Document the approximate number of incisions and their locations
   e. Offer oral analgesic
6. Postanesthesia priorities: Phase II
   a. Keep leg elevated first 24 hours with bathroom privileges
   b. Notify the physician of bleeding (rare), change in color, temperature or feelings of the involved extremity
   c. Isometric leg exercises while sitting or lying
   d. Ambulate several minutes per hour after the first 24 hours, gradually increasing daily
   e. Compressive dressing can be removed 48 to 72 hours after surgery with application of antiembolic hose
7. Phase III recovery
   a. Antiembolic hose should be worn for 8 to 12 weeks
   b. Instruct patient to report signs of DVT
   c. Instruct patient in prevention of recurrence
      i.   Maintain appropriate body weight
      ii.   Avoid prolonged standing and heavy lifting
      iii. Use comfortable support hose
      iv.   Avoid knee-length stockings
      v.   Increase muscular activity such as walking
      vi.   Elevate legs whenever possible
G. Transvascular endomyocardial biopsy
   1. Purpose
      a. Most often used to evaluate the histology of a heart graft postcardiac transplantation; identifies rejection in the early, more treatable stages
      b. Diagnose conditions including cancers of the heart, myocarditis, and cardiomyopathies
      c. Relatively safe: less invasive than percutaneous needle biopsy and open thoracotomy
   2. Description
      a. A #8 French Introducer is placed percutaneously into the superior vena cava; the right internal jugular or femoral vein may be used
      b. Biopsy forceps (Bioptome) are threaded through the introducer to the right ventricle (similar to the placement of a pulmonary artery catheter)
      c. Samples are taken from the wall of the right ventricle, usually three to five samples
      d. Forceps are removed and hemodynamic measurements are obtained
      e. The introducer may be left in place if needed, otherwise it is removed
   3. Preoperative care
      a. Thorough cardiovascular and pulmonary assessment

      b. Major contraindication for biopsy includes history of:
         i. Bleeding disorders
         ii. Left ventricular thrombus
      c. The cardiac transplant patient requires prophylactic antibiotic therapy due to his/her immunosuppressive drug regimen

    4. Intraoperative care
      a. Local anesthetic is used
      b. Strict sterile procedure is maintained to prevent infection
      c. Multichannel cardiac monitoring must be maintained
      d. Observe for atrial fibrillation, ventricular dysrhythmias, pneumothorax
      e. Apply pressure to the site at the end of the procedure

    5. Postanesthesia priorities: Phase I and Phase II
      a. Frequently admitted directly to Phase II
      b. Jugular approach
         i. Assess access site for bleeding
         ii. Keep HOB elevated 30 degrees
         iii. May discharge after 1 hour
      c. Femoral approach
         i. Assess access site for bleeding
         ii. Keep supine with HOB elevated no greater than 30 degrees for 1 hour
         iii. Assess distal pulses
         iv. Ambulate after 2 hours
         v. May discharge if no bleeding at this time

    6. Phase III recovery
      a. May return to work
      b. Avoid strenuous activity for 1 week
      c. Resume transplant precautions and previous medications

H. Temporal artery biopsy
    1. Purpose: for diagnosis of temporal arteritis (TA)
      a. A vasculitis of the temporal artery of unknown etiology
      b. Diagnosis is confirmed when significant inflammation of the vessel intima and the presence of giant cells are found (also known as giant cell arteritis)
      c. Occurrence
         i. Primarily seen in patients greater than 50 years of age
         ii. Incidence significantly increases after age 80
      d. Manifested by severe unilateral headache, pain on mastication, and ocular symptoms including sudden loss of vision if left untreated
      e. Nonspecific findings include fever, weight loss, and malaise

    2. Description
      a. Excisional biopsy
      b. A generous piece of the temporal artery is necessary (4–5 cm long) due to the patchy nature of the disorder
      c. If one side is negative and the patient is symptomatic, the other side should be biopsied, again due to the patchy nature of the disorder

    3. Preoperative care
      a. Assess the temporal artery for induration, tenderness, and bruits (see Figure 28–6)
      b. Obtain thorough history associated with findings as listed above

    4. Intraoperative care
      a. Local anesthesia
      b. No special precautions

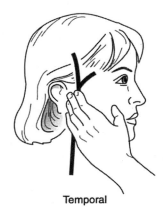

Temporal

Figure 28–6.   Temporal artery palpation. (From Keene, A. [1997]. Performing the basic physical assessment. In Luckman, J., ed. *Saunders Manual of Nursing Care*, [page 112]. Philadelphia: Saunders.)

    5. Postanesthesia priorities: Phase II
      a. Usually direct admission to Phase II
      b. Keep HOB elevated to reduce the risk of bleeding
      c. Monitor site for bleeding; apply direct pressure if bleeding occurs
      d. May be discharged in 1 to 2 hours
    6. Postanesthesia care: Phase III
      a. Follow-up with physician as to biopsy results
      b. Follow treatment plan based on biopsy results
  I. Vascular access device insertion
    1. Purpose
      a. Long-term intravascular access
      b. Avoid repeated venous puncture
      c. Administration of chemotherapeutic drugs
      d. Minimize the risk of drug extravasation
      e. Access for hemodialysis and repeated blood sampling
    2. Description
      a. Tunneled catheters (Hickman catheter, Groshong catheter, Raaf cath)
        i. The catheter is tunneled through the subcutaneous tissue, then inserted into a central vein
        ii. The tunneling reduces the risk of bacterial invasion directly into the central circulation
        iii. External site care required with routine flushing
      b. Implantable ports (Port-O-Cath, Infuse-A-Port, Life Port)
        i. Catheter and access port are implanted under the skin
        ii. Require needle puncture to access the port
        iii. No site care required when not in use
    3. Preoperative care
      a. Careful vascular assessment
      b. Assess patient ability to care for access device
    4. Intraoperative care
      a. General anesthesia is avoided
      b. Sedation may be utilized but not required
    5. Postanesthesia priorities: Phase II
      a. Usually admitted directly to Phase II
      b. Repeat vascular assessment and compare with preoperative assessment; report significant changes
      c. Monitor insertion site for bleeding or hematoma

      d. Monitor for signs of embolic event
        i. Changes in sensorium
        ii. SOB
        iii. Chest pain
      e. Assess external ports for patency
        i. Aspirate and flush with heparinized saline especially after each blood draw and medication administration
        ii. If clotted, streptokinase or other thrombolytic agent may be used by appropriately credentialed registered nurse

6. Phase III recovery
    a. Patient teaching
      i. Immediately report bleeding or swelling at site
      ii. Aseptic technique, good handwashing
      iii. Standard precautions
      iv. Report signs of infection such as foul-smelling drainage and erythema at site, fever, chills, malaise
      v. Report signs of embolic event
    b. Follow treatment and activity recommendation as indicated for disease process

J. Cardiac pacemaker insertion and battery change
  1. Purpose
    a. Permanent pacing is required for patients with symptomatic bradycardia of any type, usually second- or third-degree heart block or sinus node dysfunction
    b. Less commonly for tachycardias, such as atrial flutter, not responsive to medication
  2. Description
    a. An alternate, temporary pacemaker must be available and checked prior to the procedure
    b. The skin is prepped and the incision is made
    c. The pacing leads can be attached to the temporary pacer while the batteries are changed for battery change only
    d. The system is tested prior to closure
  3. Preoperative care
    a. Detailed cardiac history, reason for pacemaker
    b. Type of pacemaker and functional state
    c. Place on multi-channel cardiac monitoring
    d. Check serum potassium; level may affect pacing threshold
      i. Low potassium: loss of pacemaker capture
      ii. High potassium: ventricular tachycardia
  4. Intraoperative care
    a. Anesthesia requirements
      i. Local anesthesia with or without sedation for transvenous approach
      ii. General anesthesia for epicardial placement
    b. Maintain close cardiac monitoring
    c. Have atropine and isoproterenol available
  5. Postanesthesia priorities: Phase II
    a. Continue cardiac monitoring to assess pacemaker function as dislodgement of the leads is a postop consideration
    b. Assess pacemaker function
    c. Common pacemaker malfunctions
      i. Failure to sense

> BOX 28–1.   **Key Educational Patient Outcomes**
>
> - The patient who has undergone an AV shunt placement/revision is able to verbalize monitoring techniques to ensure patency of the site and signs and symptoms of infection
> - The patient and/or caregiver of the patient who has undergone arteriography will be able to recognize signs and symptoms of bleeding/hematoma and be able to manage appropriate interventions (pressure to site, obtaining emergency medical assistance, etc.)
> - The patient who has undergone a vein ligation and stripping will verbalize appropriate activity levels for home care (rest with leg elevated, increase ambulation slowly each day, etc.)
> - The patient who has had a vascular access device inserted will verbalize appropriate aseptic techniques for maintaining catheter

      ii. Failure to pace

      iii. Failure to capture

   d. Monitor site for bleeding

6. Phase III recovery

   a. Patient teaching: reinforce pacemaker precautions

      i. Proper technique for pulse taking

      ii. Avoid high-voltage areas, magnetic fields, radiation, microwaves, antitheft devices in stores

      iii. Avoid tight-fitting clothing

      iv. Avoid extreme arm movements

   b. Discharge

      i. Initial pacemaker placement

         (a) 24-hour telemetry and monitoring

         (b) Should ambulate before monitoring is discontinued

      ii. Battery-change patient may be discharged once ambulating without dizziness

Bibliography

1. Ahrens, T.S., Martin, N.K., Powers, C., et al. (1998). Angina pectoris and myocardial infarction. In Ahrens, T.S., Prentice, D., eds. *Critical Care Certification: Preparation, Review, and Practice Exams,* 4th ed. (page 63). Stamford, CT: Appleton & Lange.

2. Billingham, M.E. (1990). Endomyocardial biopsy diagnosis of acute rejection in cardiac allografts. *Prog Cardivas Dis,* 33(1):11–18.

3. Burden, N. (1998). The surgical specialties—part 2: Gynecologic and obstetric, urologic, orthopedic and podiatric, general, and cardiovascular surgical procedures. In Burden, N., ed. *Ambulatory Surgical Nursing,* (page 502). Philadelphia: Saunders.

4. Burrell, L.O., Streit, L.A. (1997). Cardiac arrhythmias. In Burrell, L.O., Gerlach, M.J.M., Pless, B.S., eds. *Adult Nursing: Acute and Community Care,* 2nd ed. (p. 375). Stamford, CT: Appleton & Lange.

5. Chernecky, C.C., Berger, B.J. (1997). *Laboratory Tests and Diagnostic Procedures,* 2nd ed. Philadelphia: Saunders.

6. Cunningham, A.J. (1997). AV graft for hemodialysis. In Roizen, M.F., Fleisher, L.A. eds. *Essence of Anesthesia Practice* (page 348). Philadelphia: Saunders.

7. Daily, K.A. (1994). Post anesthesia care of the vascular surgical patient. In Drain, C.B. ed. *The Post Anesthesia Care Unit: A Critical Care Approach to Post Anesthesia Nursing,* 3rd ed. (page 387). Philadelphia: WB Saunders.

8. DeAngelis, R. (1991). The cardiovascular system. In Alspach, J.G., ed. *Core Curriculum for Critical Care Nursing,* 4th ed. (page 132). Philadelphia: Saunders.

9. Detsky, A.S., Abrams, H.B., McLaughlin, J.R., et al. (1986). Predicting cardiac complications in patients undergoing non-cardiac surgery. *J Gen Intern Med,* 1:213.

10. Drain, C.B. (1994). Cardiovascular system anatomy and physiology. In Drain, C.B., ed. *The Post Anesthesia Care Unit: A Critical Care Approach to Post Anesthesia Nursing,* 3rd ed. (page 82). Philadelphia: Saunders.

11. Goldman, L., Caldera, D., Nussbaum, S.R., et al. (1977). Multifactorial index of cardiac risk in noncardiac surgical procedures. *N Engl J Med,* 197:848.

12. Gray, M., Rayome, R.G. (1997). Caring for people with urinary system disorders. In Luckman, J., ed. *Saunders Manual of Nursing Care,* (page 1173). Philadelphia: Saunders.

13. Guyton, A.C. (1991). *Textbook of Medical Physiology,* 8th ed. Philadelphia: Saunders.

14. Harbaugh, K.S., Harbaugh, R.E. (1995). Early discharge after carotid endarterectomy. *Neurosurgery,* 37:219.

15. Hicks, F.D. (1995). The cardiac surgical patient. In Litwack, K., ed. *Core Curriculum for Post Anesthesia Nursing Practice,* 3rd ed. (page 243). Philadelphia: Saunders.

16. Kaufman, J.L., Frank, D., Rhee, S.W., et al. (1996). Feasibility and safety of 1-day postoperative hospitalization for carotid endarterectomy. *Arch Surg,* 131:751.

17. Keeler, K.D. (1994). Post anesthesia care of the cardiac surgical patient. In Drain, C.B., ed. *The Post Anesthesia Care Unit: A Critical Care Approach to Post Anesthesia Nursing,* 3rd ed. (page 368). Philadelphia: Saunders.

18. Keene, A. (1997). Performing the basic physical assessment. In Luckman, J., ed. *Saunders Manual of Nursing Care,* (page 112). Philadelphia: Saunders.

19. Kennedy, M.M. (1998). Patient Assessment: Cardiovascular system cardiac history and physical examination. In Hudak, C.M., Gallo, B.M., Morton, P.G., eds. *Critical Care Nursing, A Holistic Approach,* (page 198). Philadelphia: Lippincott.

20. Korchek, N., Burrell, L.O. (1997). Nursing assessment and common cardiac interventions. In Burrell, L.O., Gerlach, M.J.M., Pless, B.S., eds. *Adult Nursing: Acute and Community Care,* 2nd ed. (page 353). Stamford, CT: Appleton & Lange.

21. Kristt, A.M. (1995). The peripheral vascular surgical patient. In Litwack, K. ed. *Core Curriculum for Post Anesthesia Nursing Practice,* 3rd ed. (page 279). Philadelphia: Saunders.

22. Limacher, M.C., Robbins, W.C. (1994). Cardiology consultation. In Kirby, R.R., Gravenstein, N., eds. *Clinical Anesthesia Practice,* (page 125). Philadelphia: Saunders.

23. Luecke, L.E., Mancini, M.E. (1997). Caring for people with cardiovascular disorders. In Luckman, J., ed. *Saunders Manual of Nursing Care,* (page 981). Philadelphia: Saunders.

24. Luna, G., Adye, B. (1994). Cost-effective carotid endarterectomy. *Am J Surg,* 169:516.

25. McDermott, M.M., et al. (1994). The prognostic value of ankle brachial index. *J Gen Intern Med,* 9:445–449.

26. Phillips, R.E., Feeney, M.K. (1990). *The Cardiac Rhythms: A Systematic Approach to Interpretation,* 3rd ed. Philadelphia: Saunders.

27. Pless, B.S. (1997). Nursing assessment and common vascular interventions. In Burrell, L.O., Gerlach, M.J.M., Pless, B.S., eds. (1997). *Adult Nursing: Acute and Community Care,* 2nd ed. (page 477). Stamford, CT: Appleton & Lange.

28. Quinn, D. (1994). *Ambulatory Post Anesthesia Nursing Outline: Content for Certification.* Thorofare, NJ: American Society of PeriAnesthesia Nurses.

29. Schenk, W.G. (1987). Surgical disorders of the veins. In Sabiston, D.C., ed. *Sabiston's Essentials of Surgery,* (page 933). Philadelphia: Saunders.

30. Shpritz, D.W. (1995). The neurological patient. In Litwack, K., ed. *Core Curriculum for Post Anesthesia Nursing Practice,* 3rd ed. (page 332). Philadelphia: Saunders.

31. Solymoss, B.C., Bourassa, M.G., Wesolowska, E. (1997). The role of cardiac troponin T and other new biochemical markers in evaluation and risk stratification of patients with acute chest pain syndromes. *Clin Cardiol,* 20(11):934.

32. Stark, J.L. (1991). The renal system. In Alspach, J.G., ed. *Core Curriculum for Critical Care Nursing,* 4th ed. (page 472). Philadelphia: Saunders.

33. Thompson, D., Farris, L. (1997). Coronary heart disease. In Burrell, L.O., Gerlach, M.J.M., Pless, B.S., eds. *Adult Nursing: Acute and Community Care,* 2nd ed. (page 425). Stamford, CT: Appleton & Lange.

34. Trankina, M.F. (1997). Pacemakers. In Roizen, M.F., Fleisher, L.A., eds. *Essence of Anesthesia Practice,* (page 239). Philadelphia: Saunders.

35. Turner, J. (1997). Caring for people with peripheral vascular and lymphatic disorders. In Luckman, J., ed. *Saunders Manual of Nursing Care,* (page 1091). Philadelphia: Saunders.

36. Van Riper, S., Luciano, A. (1994). Basic cardiac arrhythmias: A review for postanesthesia care unit nurses. *JOPAN,* 9(1):2.

37. Wiederhold, R. (1988). *Electrocardiography: The Monitoring Lead.* Philadelphia: Saunders.

38. Wilke, H.J., Ellis, J.E., McKinsey, J.F. (1996). Carotid endarterectomy: Perioperative anesthetic considerations. *J Cardio Vas Anes,* 10:928.

39. Youngberg, J.A. (1997). Carotid endarterectomy. In Roizen, M.F., Fleisher, L.A., eds. *Essence of Anesthesia Practice,* (page 363). Philadelphia: Saunders.

REVIEW QUESTIONS

1. The ability of the heart to resist stimulation while still contracting from an earlier stimulus is called

   A. Excitability
   B. Refractoriness
   C. Rhythmicity
   D. Conductiveness

2. All of the following indicate arterial insufficiency except

   A. Loss of hair
   B. Pallor
   C. Translucent, waxy appearance of skin
   D. Reddish-brown pigmentation

3. The laboratory study most useful in the early detection of a MI is

   A. Creatine phosphokinase
   B. Lactate dehydrogenase
   C. Troponin I
   D. Urokinase

4. Which of the following is not a goal of anesthesia during cardiac and peripheral vascular procedures ?

   A. Maintain myocardial oxygen supply
   B. Increase coronary artery fill time
   C. Reduce oxygen demand
   D. Maintain stable vital signs

5. A follow-up phone assessment to a post AV graft placement patient reveals complaints of diminished pulses, pain distal to the graft site, and complaints of pallor in the surgical arm. You suspect

   A. Steal syndrome
   B. Thrombosis formation
   C. Infection
   D. Carpal tunnel syndrome

6. A patient begins complaining of warmth and a flushing sensation during dye injection during a cardiac catheterization. Your best action would be to

   A. Assess the patient for allergies to shellfish
   B. Administer 100 mg of lidocaine
   C. Notify the physician and immediately halt the procedure
   D. Reassure the patient that this is a normal sensation

7. Signs and symptoms of post-venography syndrome include all of the following except

   A. Diminished pulses
   B. Positive Homan's sign
   C. Delayed calf discomfort
   D. Redness and swelling of the lower extremity

8. Discharge teaching for the carotid endarterectomy patient should include all of the following except

   A. Rest for the first week after surgery
   B. Avoid strenuous activities after surgery
   C. Continue to take antihypertensive medications
   D. Discontinue all preoperative aspirin therapy

9. Discharge teaching for the vein ligation and stripping patient should include all of the following except

   A. Keep leg elevated for the first 24 hours
   B. Bed rest with bathroom privileges only for the first 24 hours
   C. Advance activity as tolerated after 24 hours
   D. Remove compressive dressing after 72 hours

10. Which of the following is true about implantable vascular ports?

   A. Requires needle puncture to access
   B. They are tunneled through subcutaneous tissue
   C. External site care is required
   D. They must be flushed routinely

ANSWERS TO QUESTIONS

1. B
2. D
3. C
4. B
5. A

6. D
7. A
8. D
9. C
10. A

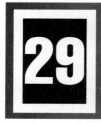

Gynecologic and Reproductive Surgery

Denise O'Brien
University of Michigan Health System
Ann Arbor, Michigan

I. **Anatomy and Physiology**
   A. External genitalia collectively known as vulva (see Figure 29–1)
      1. Mons: rounded fleshy prominence over the symphysis pubis
      2. Labia
         a. Majora: larger outer skin folds surrounding the vaginal orifice
         b. Minora: inner folds surrounding the vaginal orifice
      3. Clitoris: small projection of erectile tissue located at the upper ends of the labia minora
      4. Hymen: thin membrane partially covering the vaginal orifice
      5. Vestibule: space between the labia minora into which the urethra and vagina open
      6. Skene's ducts: paraurethral ducts that drain a group of urethral glands into the vestibule
      7. Bartholin's glands: two small mucoid-secreting glands on either side of the vaginal orifice
      8. Urinary meatus: opening of urethra, located between clitoris and vaginal orifice
      9. Perineum: between the vulva and anus
   B. Internal genital structures (see Figure 29–2)
      1. Vagina
         a. Canal, extending from vulva to cervix uteri, between the bladder and rectum
         b. Lined with mucous membrane; muscles and fibrous tissue form the walls
         c. Coital organ, passage for menstrual discharge, functions as the birth canal

1. Describe anatomy and physiology of female reproductive organs and structures pertinent to the ambulatory surgery patient undergoing gynecologic/reproductive procedures.
2. Identify assessment parameters for patients undergoing gynecologic/reproductive operative procedures.
3. Define nursing care priorities in each postanesthesia phase.
4. Describe patient education following gynecologic/reproductive procedures related to diet, pain management, wound care, activity, and follow-up.

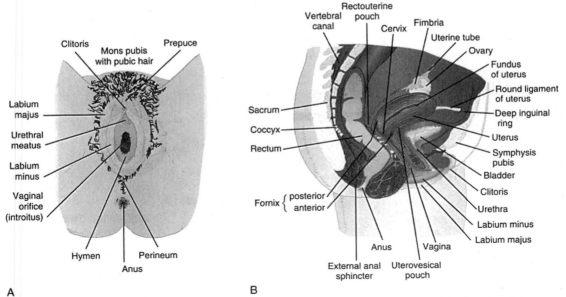

Figure 29–1. *A*, Anatomic landmarks of external female genitalia. *B*, Midsagittal section of the female pelvis. (From Black, J.M., Matassarin-Jacobs, E. [1997]. *Medical-Surgical Nursing, Clinical Management for Continuity of Care*, 5th ed. Philadelphia: Saunders.)

2. Uterus
   a. Hollow muscular organ, normally pear-sized; muscular walls, lined with mucous membrane
   b. Consists of:
      i. Fundus (dome): upper part
      ii. Corpus (body): middle part
      iii. Cervix (neck): lower, narrow part of uterus, extending into vagina
   c. Myometrium: muscular substance of uterus

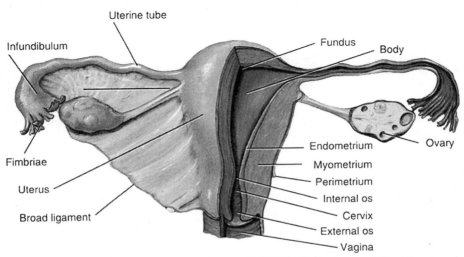

Figure 29–2. Uterus and uterine tubes. (From Applegate, E.J. [1995]. *The Anatomy and Physiology Learning System.* Philadelphia: Saunders.)

      d. Endometrium: inner lining composed of mucous membrane

      e. Functions:

         i. Contain products of conception until time of delivery

        ii. Lining shed (menstruation) in monthly cycle in the absence of fertilization and implantation of embryo

  3. Fallopian tube

      a. One of two tubes, attached on each side of uterus, extending to ovary

      b. Conveys ova to uterus, spermatozoa in opposite direction

      c. Fertilization usually occurs in the tube

  4. Ovary

      a. Paired oval organs one on either side of uterus

      b. Attached to the posterior surface of the broad ligament

      c. Functions:

         i. Production of ovum

        ii. Hormone production: estrogen, progesterone

  5. Ligaments

      a. Broad

      b. Round

      c. Cardinal

      d. Uterosacral

  6. Arteries

      a. Internal iliac

      b. Hypogastric

      c. Pudendal

      d. Uterine artery: superior, inferior

  7. Nerves

      a. Femoral

      b. Sciatic

      c. Pudendal

C. Associated structures

  1. Bladder, ureters, urethra

  2. Sigmoid colon

  3. Muscles: levator ani

  4. Lymph nodes

II. Assessment Parameters Specific to Procedures

A. Examination

  1. Pelvic

      a. Inspection of external genitalia

      b. Speculum exam of vagina and cervix

      c. Palpation of any visible abnormalities to determine consistency, mobility, and relation to adjacent structures

      d. Papanicoulaou's test (Pap smear): for detection and diagnosis of malignant and premalignant conditions of the vagina, cervix, endometrium

  2. Bimanual: the abdominal hand presses the pelvic organs to be palpated toward the intravaginal hand

  3. Menstrual history

      a. Onset of menses, length of cycles, regularity of cycles

      b. Duration, amount, and content of flow

      c. Date of last menstrual period

      d. Contraceptive use/absence

4. Gravidity
   a. Number of pregnancies
   b. Number of deliveries, terminations (spontaneous, elective)
5. Virilizing features: hair growth, irregular absent periods
6. Emotional state
   a. Psychosocial: family/partner support or lack of support
   b. Infertility
      i. May be associated with specific psychological problems, ranging from anxiety/stress disorders to compulsive/obsessive neurosis
      ii. Need sympathetic and understanding approach
   c. Loss of desired pregnancy
   d. Surgically-induced hormonal changes
   e. Concerns or fears for invasion of privacy
7. Other assessment factors
   a. Neurovascular assessment of lower extremities
   b. Test results: clotting times, Rh factor, pregnancy
   c. Physical limitations relating to:
      i. Arthritis
      ii. Musculoskeletal disorders
      iii. Implanted joints
   d. Resulting in potential alteration of anesthetic choice or positioning of patient (e.g., lithotomy)
   e. Allergies to dyes (injected during procedure)
B. Increased risk associated with history or need to alter perioperative management
   1. Deep vein thrombosis (DVT)
   2. Obesity
   3. Tobacco use
   4. Pregnancy
   5. Chronic pain
      a. Pain tolerance alterations
      b. Chronic analgesic use may alter postoperative analgesic management
   6. Developmentally challenged
      a. Potential behavioral problems (combative, disruptive, abusive)
      b. Legal authorization appropriately obtained before treatment commences
C. Determine the educational needs of patient, caregiver
   1. Analgesia, preoperative anxiety
   2. Projected effect (if any) on sexual activity, fertility
   3. Discharge planning
      a. Comfortable loose clothing to wear home, especially following laparoscopy
      b. Supply of dressings or supplies needed (perineal pads, tampons)
      c. Possible need for catheters and drains
      d. Caregiver available for first 24 hours postoperatively
D. Nursing diagnoses include:
   1. Risk for injury
   2. Anxiety
   3. Fear related to loss of control and unpredictable outcome
   4. Pain/discomfort
   5. Knowledge deficit
   6. Risk for infection
   7. Grieving related to loss of pregnancy
   8. Altered sexual patterns

III. Operative Procedures

Common operative procedures and techniques are included. The reader is referred to a comprehensive text on gynecologic and reproductive surgery for additional procedures and techniques.

    A. Cervical conization/colposcopy: removal of a cone of cervical tissue (partial excision) for diagnosis or treatment of cervical infection or carcinoma in situ

    B. Dilatation and curettage (D & C)
       1. Stretching the cervix beyond normal dimensions
       2. Removal of growths/other materials from the uterine cavity with a curet (spoon-shaped sharp-edged instrument)

    C. Dilatation and evacuation (D & E)
       1. Stretching the cervix beyond normal dimensions
       2. Removing the contents of the uterus by curettage, suction

    D. Excision/drainage of Bartholin cyst: removal by cutting or systematic withdrawal of fluids/discharges

    E. Endometrial ablation
       1. For treatment of abnormal uterine bleeding
       2. Nd:YAG laser with a hysteroscope or roller ball electrode with a modified resectoscope most commonly used

    F. Excision external lesion: removal of lesions (warts, papilloma, malignant growths) by cutting, laser, electrocautery methods

    G. Fertility procedures
       1. Cerclage: encircling an incompetent cervix uteri with a ring or loop (or a stitch into the cervix) to preserve uterine contents
       2. In vitro fertilization (IVF)
          a. Using transvaginal ultrasound-guided follicle aspiration, healthy mature oocytes are retrieved
          b. Oocytes and sperm are mixed
          c. The resultant embryo is transferred to the uterine fundus after two days
       3. Transcervical balloon tuboplasty
          a. Performed under fluoroscopy, sonography, or via hysteroscopy to open obstructed fallopian tubes
          b. A catheter is passed through the cervix and, after injecting dye to detect obstruction, the balloon attached to the catheter is inflated inside the fallopian tube to dilate the interior of the tube until recanalization is achieved
       4. Tubal ligation
          a. Obliteration of the fallopian tubes to cause infertility (sterilization)
          b. Rings, clips, ligation (ties), cauterization commonly used
       5. Gamete intrafallopian transfer (GIFT)
          a. Follicle stimulation and oocyte retrieval same as for IVF
          b. Gametes (oocytes and sperm) replaced through the distal fallopian tube, via laparoscopy or sonographically guided tubal cannulation
       6. Zygote intrafallopian transfer (ZIFT)—also known as tubal embryo transfer (TET)
          a. Follicle stimulation and oocyte retrieval same as for IVF
          b. Zygote replaced through the distal fallopian tube, via laparoscopy or sonographically guided tubal cannulation

    H. Hymenectomy: surgical excision of hymen membrane to enlarge the vaginal orifice

    I. Hymenotomy: surgical incision of the hymen membrane to open the vaginal orifice

    J. Hysteroscopy
       1. Inspection of the interior of the uterus with an endoscope, using either a liquid or gaseous distending medium

2. To examine the endometrium, secure specimens for biopsy, remove foreign bodies (e.g., IUD), remove cervical polyps, intrauterine adhesions or submucous fibroids, ablation, diagnose uterine abnormalities

K. Laparoscopy
1. Examination of the interior of the abdomen (abdominal and pelvic organs) by means of a lighted endoscope (laparoscope) through a small incision in the abdominal wall
2. Pneumoperitoneum is created using CO_2 to enhance visualization by lifting the abdominal wall
3. Diagnostic or therapeutic procedures may be performed (biopsies, removal of adhesions, sterilization, laser treatment of endometriosis)

L. Loop electrosurgical excision procedure (LEEP) of the cervix
1. Removes intact tissue
   a. Allows entire specimen to be sectioned for diagnosis
   b. Advantage over CO_2 laser for diagnostic excision, small biopsies, or ablations of human papillomavirus (HPV)-related lesions of anogenital tract
2. Primarily used for cervical lesions, but may also be used for external warts, or flat lesions of the vagina, vulva, or anus

M. Metroplasty
1. Repair septate uterus
2. Reconstructive surgery on the uterus

N. Minilaparotomy: surgical approach through small transperitoneal abdominal incision

O. Myomectomy
1. Surgical removal of a myoma (leiomyoma)—"fibroids"
2. May be accomplished laparoscopically or hysteroscopically, preserving uterine integrity/fertility

P. Oophorectomy: removal of an ovary or ovaries

Q. Ovarian cystectomy: excision of ovarian cyst, leaving functioning ovary

R. Salpingectomy: removal of fallopian tube

S. Salpingostomy: surgical restoration of the patency of the fallopian tube

T. Vaginal hysterectomy
1. Excision of the uterus through the vagina
2. May require 23-hour stay (extended recovery) following procedure

IV. **Intraoperative Priorities**
A. Anesthesia choice
1. General
   a. ETT, LMA, or mask depending on operative procedure, patient needs/physical habitus
   b. Use of total intravenous technique (propofol and an opioid analgesic) can reduce the incidence of postoperative nausea and vomiting (PONV)
2. Regional: spinal or epidural
3. Monitored anesthesia care (MAC)
4. Conscious sedation with local anesthesia
5. Local anesthesia used alone for minor or office procedures
   a. Paracervical block
   b. Pudendal block
6. Considerations unique to laparoscopic procedures
   a. Pulmonary and cardiovascular changes
      i. Pneumoperitoneum creates increased intraabdominal pressures
      ii. Pulmonary inspiratory pressure increases, compliance decreases, atelectasis develops, and functional residual capacity decreases

   b. CO_2 absorption from peritoneal cavity into the blood can cause hypercarbia and respiratory acidosis
   c. Trendelenberg positioning can lead to increased mean arterial pressure, pulmonary artery pressure, aortic compression, and systemic vascular resistance accompanied by a drop in cardiac output
   d. Marked hemodynamic changes may be brought about by a significant release of catecholamines, prostaglandins, and vasopressin during the procedure
   e. Stretching of the peritoneum and manipulation of viscera can lead to bradycardia which responds to atropine
   f. Pulmonary aspiration is a risk with abdominal insufflation
   7. Considerations unique to hysteroscopic procedures
   a. Fluid (saline, glycine, dextran) used as distending media
      i. Absorption and resultant circulatory overload
      ii. Dilution can lead to hyponatremia, hypoproteinemia, TUR syndrome (glycine)
      iii. DIC (dextran)
      iv. Anaphylaxis (dextran)
   b. Carbon dioxide used as distending medium
      i. Abdominal distention from leak via fallopian tubes
      ii. CO_2 absorption leading to acidosis, arrhythmias
      iii. CO_2 embolism
   c. Careful attention should be paid to amount of fluid instilled and removed; excessive administration can lead to the above complications
B. Intraoperative concerns
   1. Lithotomy position
   a. Elevate and lower legs together to avoid strain of back and leg muscles
   b. Avoid any abnormal movement of the knee or pressure on the knee
   c. Avoid extreme flexion of hips or popliteal pressure
   d. Pad lumbar region to prevent pressure
   e. After positioning assess neuromuscular status and reposition if compromised
   2. Arms and hands are safely positioned and shoulders are padded during Trendelenberg position
   3. Fingers need protection from impingement, especially when positioning and at end of procedure when repositioning for transfer
   4. Maintain patient's dignity
   5. Skin integrity can be compromised if iodine-based prep solutions are allowed to pool under the patient; can lead to burns of the skin
C. Procedural techniques

Special cautions and care are required with each technique. Refer to equipment training and maintenance literature for specific information on precautions, hazards, and safe use of the equipment in the OR environment.

   1. Microsurgical
   2. Endoscopic
   a. Laparoscope
      i. Usually use CO_2 gas as insufflating medium for creation of pneumoperitoneum
      ii. Gasless: uses a mechanical lift method
   b. Hysteroscope
      i. Rigid scope most commonly used
      ii. Flexible scopes available, not widely used

3. Laser, cautery, cryotherapy
4. Transvaginal ultrasonography
5. Transvaginal fluoroscopy: used infrequently due to risk of radiation exposure to reproductive organs

D. Intraoperative complications
   1. Gas embolism
   2. Fluid overload, dilutional hyponatremia
   3. Hemorrhage
   4. Perforation of hollow organs or vessels
   5. Thermal injuries
   6. Aspiration

V. Postanesthesia Priorities

A. Phase I
   1. Airway
      a. Spontaneous, unassisted breathing
      b. Adjunct or endotracheal tube in place
      c. Observe for respiratory complications
         i. Risk for pulmonary edema following hysteroscopy if excessive irrigant/distending media used
         ii. If intubated, assess location of tube by auscultating chest (dislocation of tube can occur from pneumoperitoneum)
   2. Hemodynamic stability
      a. Vital signs stable, consistent with baseline
      b. Observe for cardiovascular complications
         i. Hypotension
         ii. Hypertension, arrhythmias
   3. Bleeding
      a. Vaginal
         i. Cervical
         ii. Uterine
            (a) Assess uterine firmness following D & E
               (i) Oxytocin may be needed in advanced pregnancy termination
               (ii) Rh factor identified for Rh-negative patients to receive Rh immune globulin injection
            (b) Observe for passage of clots
      b. Incisional
         i. Oozing or frank bleeding
         ii. Hematoma beneath incision
      c. Internal
         i. Perforation of organ or vessel
         ii. Operative hemostasis not achieved or oozing
   4. Report from anesthesia/surgeon/perioperative nurse
      a. Positioning of patient intraoperatively
      b. Estimated blood loss
      c. Complications: perforation, burn, excessive fluid administration
   5. Discomfort
      a. Incisional
      b. Cramping
      c. Significant pain following procedure suspect perforation, hematoma formation, intraabdominal trauma
      d. Shoulder pain common following laparoscopy; referred pain due to diaphragmatic irritation from residual CO_2 in abdomen

    e. Cervical and intrauterine manipulation may result in prostaglandin release which can result in continued postoperative pain

    f. Peritoneal surface inflammation following laparoscopy may be caused by the formation of carbonic acid (reaction between CO_2 and interperitoneal fluid) and persist for 2 to 3 days postoperatively

    g. Nonsteroidal antiinflammatory drugs (NSAIDs) effective in managing postlaparoscopic pain

6. Dressing/drains

    a. Abdominal incisions

      i. Adhesive bandages or no dressing over trocar insertion sites following laparoscopic procedures

      ii. Gauze and tape dressing over longer incisions

    b. Perineal pad in place following cervical, uterine procedures

      i. Assess on arrival and regularly for type and amount of bleeding

      ii. Notify surgeon of bleeding saturating more than a pad an hour

    c. Vaginal packing: removable, absorbable, hemostatic material

      i. Observe minimal perineal bleeding

      ii. Patient may have urge to defecate from pressure of packing

    d. Drains in place after Bartholin cyst incision/drainage or marsupilization

7. Edema

    a. May observe subcutaneous edema from laparoscopic CO_2 insufflation

    b. External vulvar lesions: swelling may be reduced with application of ice or cold therapy

8. Fluids/nutrition

    a. Do not force fluids especially when nausea/vomiting present

    b. Causes of nausea and vomiting

      i. Narcotic analgesics, neuromuscular reversal (neostigmine and pyridostigmine have been associated with increased PONV)

      ii. Pain also major cause of nausea after gynecologic surgery

      iii. Starvation leading to weakness, low blood sugar levels

      iv. Controversy exists regarding effect of menstrual cycle and timing of operative procedure on PONV

    c. Hydrate with IV fluids (replacement and maintenance)

      i. Usual lactated ringers (Hartmann's) or dextrose-containing solutions

      ii. Long laparoscopic procedures with dry insufflating gases may increase patient's fluid-replacement needs

    d. When nausea/vomiting are present:

      i. Administer antiemetics as ordered; determine if antiemetic prophylaxis given

      ii. Commonly use droperidol, prochlorperazine, metoclopramide, ondansetron (See Chapters 8 and 22 for discussion on antiemetics)

    e. Hysteroscopy: fluid overload may be result of significant absorption of irrigant through tissue and blood vessels; may lead to pulmonary edema

      i. Monitor respiratory status

      ii. Check serum electrolytes

      iii. Diuretics and IV fluid restriction may be needed

9. Postlithotomy/postlaparoscopy neurovascular checks

    a. Sciatic nerve damage

    b. Pain, numbness, tingling of extremities should be reported

10. Urinary distention

    a. Risk following gynecologic procedures which either result in edema surrounding the urethra or injury to urethra and related structures (e.g., vaginal hysterectomy)

  b. Overdistention can cause temporary paralysis of the destrusor muscle, taking several days to resolve

  c. May require indwelling catheter or intermittent catheterization

 11. Emotional support needed; may express anger, fear, depression

  a. Adolescent/young adults embarrassed

  b. Pregnancy loss

  c. Negative findings/outcomes

 12. Nursing diagnoses

  a. Risk for urinary retention

  b. Fluid volume deficit

  c. Risk for altered body temperature: hypothermia

  d. Risk for altered respiratory function

  e. Risk for infection

  f. Pain/discomfort

B. Phase II

 1. Operative site

  a. Observe for bleeding, superficial hematoma formation around trocar insertion sites

  b. Change or reinforce dressing as necessary

  c. Monitor perineal pad drainage every hour and when patient ambulates first time

   i. Note amount and type of drainage

   ii. Notify surgeon of significant bleeding or passage of clots, excessive cramping

 2. Discomfort

  a. Gently palpate abdomen

   i. Expect soft, slightly tender to touch, slightly distended

   ii. Notify surgeon of excessive tenderness, firmness, swelling or suspected hematoma formation

  b. Oral analgesic medications initiated in preparation for discharge home

   i. May have started in PACU Phase I

   ii. Combination of opioid and NSAID can provide effective analgesia following gynecologic procedures

   iii. Determine effectiveness of medication before patient discharged home on same analgesic(s)

   iv. Patient with history of chronic pain or analgesia use may require greater support and alteration of usual pain-management protocols

   v. If ineffective may need prescription changed or other follow-up

  c. Comfort measures

   i. Positioning and repositioning to relieve or diminish discomfort

   ii. Back rub or massage may be comforting

   iii. Continue ice therapy as ordered

   iv. Promote relaxation techniques

 3. Urinary retention

  a. Assess bladder status

  b. Avoid overdistention

  c. Determine adequate fluid replacement

  d. May need intermittent catheterization until able to void

 4. Fluids/nutrition

  a. Avoid forced fluid intake if nausea and/or vomiting present

  b. Dry crackers may help ease nausea

  c. Maintain intravenous fluids to ensure adequate hydration

5. Education
   a. Includes patient/family/responsible adult
   b. Instructions
      i. Infections—signs and symptoms
      ii. Persistent pain or bleeding
      iii. Be alert for complications
      iv. Pain-relief alternatives

C. Phase III
   1. Nutrition/diet
      a. Eat lightly following the procedure
      b. If foods don't sound good, avoid and continue to drink fluids
      c. Usually can begin regular diet after 24 hours, if not earlier
      d. Encourage fluid intake especially during hot weather
      e. Avoid constipation through increased dietary fiber, bulking agents
   2. Nausea/vomiting
      a. Prepare patient and family/partner for possibility of nausea and vomiting
      b. Caution patient/family/partner to call surgeon/facility if nausea and/or vomiting persists for >6 hours
   3. Pain
      a. Oral analgesics
         i. Suggest contacting surgeon if pain is not relieved by prescribed analgesics, intolerable, or increasing
         ii. Unrelieved or increasing pain may indicate infection, peritonitis, perforation, hematoma
      b. Postoperative deep vein thrombosis can develop following hysterectomy or lengthy lithotomy procedures
         i. Lower extremity pain, edema, erythema, and prominent vascular pattern of the superficial veins may indicate deep vein thrombosis
         ii. Pleuritic chest pain, hemoptysis, shortness of breath, tachycardia, and tachypnea may be diagnostic of pulmonary embolism
         iii. Patient should call surgeon immediately and proceed to the nearest medical facility for diagnosis and treatment
      c. Alternatives
         i. Intermittent ice for external lesions to help reduce swelling, hematoma development, and pain
         ii. Sitz baths for easing discomfort of external lesions
         iii. Explore with patient/family/partner other potential pain-management techniques
   4. Medications: instruct on administration and how to apply
      a. Antibiotics
      b. Analgesics
      c. Vaginal applications
      d. Topical sprays/creams
   5. Wound care
      a. Instruct the patient to wash hands before and after changing pads, dressings, applying medications
      b. Perineal care
         i. Change pads every 4 hours or as needed
         ii. Note drainage: type, amount, and color
         iii. Gently wash the perineum with mild soap and warm water, rinse, and pat dry
         iv. Sitz baths or perineal wash as prescribed

   c. Incisional care
      i.   Keep wound clean and dry for minimum of 24 to 48 hours
      ii. May be instructed to remove dressing after 24 to 48 hours
      iii. Observe incision for signs of infection: redness, swelling, drainage
      iv. Replace original dressing with fresh gauze or adhesive bandage as needed
           or as ordered
      v.   Report signs and symptoms of infection to surgeon/nurse practitioner
   d. Vaginal bleeding
      i.   Heavier than a menstrual period must be reported to surgeon
      ii. Seven to 10 days after cone biopsy/cervical conization bleeding may
           increase
6. Urinary care
   a. Indwelling catheter (e.g., Foley) left in for continued urinary drainage
   b. Wash carefully around the urinary meatus with gentle soap and warm water
      and pat dry
   c. Keep drainage bag below level of bladder to prevent backflow
   d. Remove at home if ordered by surgeon (send with 10 cc syringe and
      instructions on how to aspirate balloon and pull catheter) or arrange return
      appointment for catheter removal
7. Activity
   a. Rest
      i.   Limit activity until pain and nausea/dizziness subside
      ii. While taking opioid analgesics, avoid operating machinery, automobiles,
           using sharp or potentially injurious articles, or drinking alcohol
   b. Exercise
      i.   For first 24 hours exercise is discouraged
      ii. Defer vigorous activity, heavy lifting
           (a) Restrict until surgeon allows; may be up to 4 weeks after surgery
           (b) Aerobic activity may increase heart rate and blood pressure leading to
               increased bleeding
   c. Sexual activity
      i.   Depending on location of incision, operative procedure
      ii. May be advised to avoid douching and coitus for up to 6 weeks
8. Follow-up care
   a. Arrange for return visit with surgeon in specified time interval
   b. Return to work dependent on procedure, patient work: usually next day for
      minor procedures; following hysterectomy: return in 1 to 2 weeks or when
      capable
   c. Home visit by a registered nurse may be arranged by the surgeon following
      certain procedures
   d. Fever: contact surgeon if temperature over 100.4°F (38°C) or as ordered by
      surgeon; check temperature every 4 hours for 2 days following procedures such
      as hysterectomy, twice a day following laparoscopic procedures (risk for
      development of peritonitis)
   e. Keep surgeon's/surgery facility's telephone number available when questions
      or concerns arise
VI. **Future Considerations in Gynecologic and Reproductive Surgery**
   A. Continued improvement in operative techniques and instrumentation
      1. Procedures only performed on an inpatient basis may move to the ambulatory
         surgery setting
      2. Size of endoscopic instrumentation expected to continue to decrease, resulting in:
         a. Decreased anesthetic needs

BOX 29–1.   **Key Patient Educational Outcomes**

Phase I
- Patient will express feelings of lessened anxiety
- Patient will describe minimal to tolerable pain
- Patient will request analgesic to manage pain

Phase II
- Patient tolerating discomfort following administration of oral analgesics
- Patient and family/partner describe wound care following instruction
- Patient progressing to upright position with minimal orthostatic effects: dizziness, lightheadedness, nausea

Phase III
- Patient and family/partner describe follow-up required
- Patient and family/partner identify risks associated with operative procedure: infection, hemorrhage, pain, vomiting
- Patient and family/partner describe wound observation and hand washing, and how to change dressing/pads, cleanse wounds, and expected drainage
- Patient and family/partner describe at-home activity, restrictions, diet, and pain management
- Patient and family/partner demonstrate knowledge of medications (analgesics, antibiotics, antiemetics, etc.) by describing purpose and administration of each medication prescribed
- Patient and family/partner express understanding of necessity to report uncontrolled bleeding or pain

---

        b. Enhanced postoperative recovery with:
           i. Decreased pain
          ii. Shorter length of stay
  B. Laparoscopic procedures will continue to expand to encompass a greater number of procedures
     1. Surgeons increase their skills
     2. Use of continually refined and improved equipment
  C. Home care services
     1. Provided by registered nurses
     2. Provide follow-up care on same day or day following surgery
     3. Increase type of procedures that can be performed on an outpatient basis
  D. Physician's office
     1. Increase in procedures being performed in office
     2. Require minimal anesthesia and recovery time
     3. May give rise to new kind of perianesthesia nursing role

Bibliography

1. Azziz, R., Murphy, A.A. (1997). *Practical Manual of Operative Laparoscopy and Hysteroscopy,* 2nd ed. New York: Springer-Verlag.
2. Black, J.M., Matassarin-Jacobs, E. (1997). *Medical-Surgical Nursing, Clinical Management for Continuity of Care,* 5th ed. Philadelphia: Saunders.
3. Carpenito, L.J. (1997). *Handbook of Nursing Diagnosis,* 7th ed. Philadelphia: Lippincott.
4. Darney, P.D., Horbach, N.S., Korn, A.P. (1996). *Protocols for Office Gynecologic Surgery.* Cambridge MA: Blackwell Science.
5. *Dorland's Illustrated Medical Dictionary,* 28th ed. (1994). Philadelphia: Saunders.
6. Evans, M.I., Johnson, M.P., Moghissi, K.S. (1997). *Invasive Outpatient Procedures in Reproductive Medicine.* Philadelphia: Lippincott-Raven.
7. Gershenson, D.M., DeCherney, A.H., Curry, S.L. (1993). *Operative Gynecology.* Philadelphia: Saunders.
8. Goldstone, J.C., Pollard, B.J. (1996). *Handbook of Clinical Anesthesia.* New York: Churchill Livingstone.

9. Mann, W.J., Stovall, T.G. (1996). *Gynecologic Surgery.* New York: Churchill Livingstone.

10. *Miller-Keane Encyclopedia & Dictionary of Medicine, Nursing, & Allied Health,* 6th ed. (1997). Philadelphia: Saunders.

11. Penfield, A.J. (1997). *Outpatient Gynecologic Surgery.* Baltimore: Williams & Wilkins.

12. Rock, J.A., Thompson, J.D. (1997). *TeLinde's Operative Gynecology,* 8th ed. Philadelphia: Lippincott-Raven.

13. Thompson, J.M., McFarland, G.K., Hirsch, J.E., Tucker, S.M. (1997). *Mosby's Clinical Nursing,* 4th ed. St. Louis: Mosby-Year Book.

14. Twersky, R.S. (1995). *The Ambulatory Anesthesia Handbook.* St. Louis: Mosby-Year Book.

15. White, P. (1997). *Ambulatory Anesthesia & Surgery.* Philadelphia: Saunders.

REVIEW QUESTIONS

1. One cause of postoperative nausea and vomiting following gynecologic procedures is

   A. Drinking juice
   B. Pain
   C. Positioning
   D. Bleeding

2. The patient and her partner arrive in the unit preoperatively. The patient appears agitated, demanding to see her surgeon immediately, and refusing to have her IV started. You will approach this infertility patient

   A. Brusquely, telling her everything's going to be fine and she shouldn't worry so much
   B. Asking her to calm down because you have to start her IV now and then you'll call her surgeon
   C. Demanding to know if she forgot to take her sedatives today
   D. Calmly, reassuring her and her partner that you will call her surgeon and then you'll be back to talk to her about what is planned

3. Prostaglandin release follows which of the following manipulations and can result in continued postoperative pain?

   A. Cervical and intrauterine
   B. Peritoneal and urethral
   C. Bladder
   D. Intestinal

4. The loop electrosurgical excision procedure (LEEP) offers advantages over CO_2 laser excision because

   A. Tissue is vaporized, reducing the cost of pathology examination
   B. It requires less complicated equipment and no laser technologist is needed
   C. It removes intact tissue which allows entire specimen to be sectioned for diagnosis
   D. It's less dangerous for the patient and surgeon

5. Cervical conization removes

   A. A cone of cervical tissue for diagnosis and treatment
   B. The entire cervical os for treatment of carcinoma in situ
   C. A layer of cervical tissue for microscopic examination
   D. One-third of the uterus

6. Stretching of the peritoneum and manipulation of viscera can lead to

   A. Tachycardia
   B. Bradycardia unresponsive to treatment
   C. Sinus arrest
   D. Bradycardia that responds to atropine

7. Shoulder pain following laparoscopy may be temporarily relieved by

A. Standing
B. Semi-Fowler's position
C. Flat or Trendelenberg position
D. Side-lying position

8. Hysteroscopy requires uterine distention for optimum diagnostic benefit. Distention can be accomplished using

A. O_2 or dextran
B. CO_2 or fluids (saline, glycine, dextran)
C. N_2O or fluids (saline, glycine, dextran)
D. Dextran or glycine

9. Ms. Smith calls 2 days after her laparoscopic tubal ligation complaining of persistent abdominal pain. She states she is afebrile, voiding without difficulty but her abdomen is tender and sore. You suspect

A. Peritonitis from thermal injury
B. Bladder perforation
C. Retroperitoneal hematoma
D. Peritoneal irritation from the CO_2 insufflation

10. Mrs. Jones underwent a vaginal hysterectomy today. During the postoperative instruction review with Mrs. Jones and her partner, she asks when she can resume intercourse. According to her surgeon's instructions, she may resume intercourse and douching

A. In 48 hours
B. In 4 weeks
C. When the bleeding stops
D. In 1 week

ANSWERS TO QUESTIONS

1. B
2. D
3. A
4. C
5. A
6. D
7. C
8. B
9. D
10. B

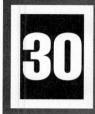

Urologic Surgery

Gayle Miller
St. Luke's Hospital
Jacksonville, Florida

Objectives

1. Discuss indications for common urologic surgical procedures.
2. Describe complications of cystoscopic procedures.
3. List appropriate nursing interventions following scrotal procedures.
4. Describe the anatomy and physiology of the genitourinary system.
5. Describe assessment parameters pertinent to care of the genitourinary surgical patient.

I. **Anatomy and Physiology**
   A. Kidney
      1. Description (see Figure 30–1)
         a. Pair of structures
         b. Lie in retroperitoneal space adjacent to T12 to L2 or L3 levels of spinal column
         c. Right kidney located slightly lower than left due to presence of liver
         d. Concave surface of kidney (hilum) lies near spine
         e. Convex surface of kidney is distal to concave surface
         f. Convex portion (renal hilum) is point where renal pelvis, renal artery, renal vein, nerves, and lymphatic system enter and exit the parenchyma
      2. Covering of kidneys
         a. Enclosed in thin, fibrous renal capsule
         b. Supported by layers of perineal fat
         c. Covers all of kidney except hilum
      3. Average size (adult)
         a. 12 to 14 cm (4¾ to 5½ inches) in length
         b. 5 to 7 cm (2 to 2¾ inches) in width
         c. 3 cm (1¼ inches) in thickness
      4. Average weight (adult): 150 g (5 oz.)
      5. Parenchyma
         a. Functional tissue of kidney
            i. Consists of cortex and medulla
            ii. Medulla
               (a) Pale cone-shaped pyramids
               (b) Base of pyramid faces concave surface of kidney

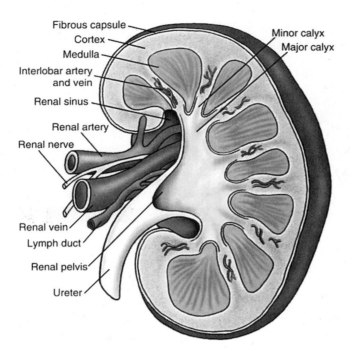

Fibrous capsule
Cortex
Medulla
Interlobar artery and vein
Renal sinus
Renal artery
Renal nerve
Renal vein
Lymph duct
Renal pelvis
Ureter
Minor calyx
Major calyx

Figure 30–1. The kidney. (From Monahan, F.D., Neighbors, M. [1998]. *Medical Surgical Nursing Foundations for Clinical Practice*, 2nd ed. Philadelphia: Saunders, p. 1330.)

(c) Apex faces hilum or pelvis of kidney
(d) Each kidney contains 8 to 18 pyramids
(e) Pyramids drain into 4 to 13 minor calices
(f) Minor calices drain into two or three major calices
(g) Major calices open directly into pelvis
(h) Major calices come together at center of medulla to form renal pelvis
iii. Cortex
(a) Extends inward between two pyramids; forms renal columns
(b) Contains nephrons
iv. Renal pelvis
(a) Cone-shaped structure that extends from center of medulla
(b) Exits kidney through hilum
(c) Curves downward to form ureter
(d) Holds approximately 5 to 7 ml (approximately ¼ oz.) of urine
6. Nephron
a. The functional unit of the kidney
b. Each kidney contains more than a million nephrons
c. One kidney can provide adequate renal function for body if other kidney becomes nonfunctional
d. Nephron contains glomerulus, Bowman's capsule, proximal tubule, loop of Henle, distal tubule, and collecting ducts
7. Glomerulus
a. A segment of the proximal nephron
b. Consists of a tuft of capillaries
c. Blood enters glomerulus via afferent arterioles
d. Blood exits glomerulus via efferent arterioles
e. Glomerulus is enclosed in Bowman's capsule
f. The glomerulus is the site of filtration of blood for selective excretion or reabsorption by kidneys

8. Bowman's capsule
   a. Membrane that surrounds the glomerulus
   b. Beginning of tubular system of nephron
9. Tubular system consists of:
   a. Proximal convoluted tubule
      i. Proximal convoluted tubule—site where about 65% of the glomerular filtrate is reabsorbed
   b. Loop of Henle
      i. Site of active reabsorption of sodium, potassium, chloride ions
   c. Distal convoluted tubule
      i. Site for reabsorption of water in the presence of antidiuretic hormone (ADH)
      ii. Terminates in one of many collecting ducts that pass through calices
      iii. Empties into renal pelvis
10. Blood supply
    a. Renal artery
       i. Receives 25% of cardiac output
       ii. Renal artery arises from abdominal aorta
       iii. Branches in to right and left renal artery
       iv. Enters kidney at renal hilum
       v. Bifurcates into superior and inferior branches
       vi. Subdivides into lobular vessels and glomerular capillaries
    b. Renal veins
       i. Empty into inferior vena cava
11. Nerve supply
    a. Sympathetic and parasympathetic innervation
    b. Supplied by splanchnic nerves
12. Function of kidney and urinary system (see Figure 30–2)
    a. Maintain internal homeostasis
       i. Accomplished by:
          (a) Glomerular filtration
          (b) Tubular reabsorption and secretion
          (c) Excretion
    b. Excreting the end products of metabolism
    c. Controlling the concentration of constituents of body fluids to maintain homeostasis
       i. Regulates fluid and electrolyte balance
    d. Provides long-term regulation of acid-base balance
    e. Assists with calcium metabolism and regulation of blood pressure
    f. Regulates production of red blood cells
    g. Renal function
       i. Kidney filters approximately 180 liters of plasma in 25 hours
       ii. 1 liter becomes urine; 179 liters are reabsorbed
       iii. Process can be affected by composition, pressure, and volume of blood flowing through kidney

B. Ureters
   1. Description
      a. Paired cylindrical fibromuscular tubes
      b. Transport urine from renal pelvis to bladder
   2. Average size
      a. 30 to 33 cm (12 to 13 inches) in length
      b. Diameter varies from 1 mm to 1 cm (approximately ¹⁄₂₅ to ³⁄₈ inches)

3. Mucosal fold prevents backflow (reflux) of urine from ureters to kidney
4. Function
   a. Carry urine from renal pelvis to urinary bladder
   b. Accomplished through peristaltic contractions of smooth muscle fibers of middle layer of ureters
C. Bladder
   1. Description
      a. Hollow muscular organ
      b. Serves as a reservoir for urine
   2. Average capacity
      a. 350 to 450 ml (12 to 15 oz.)
   3. Position
      a. Male: between rectum and pubis when empty
      b. Female: in front of vagina and uterus
      c. When distended, projects well into abdomen
         i. Can be easily palpated
   4. Openings
      a. Three orifices on floor of bladder
         i. Anterior orifice for urethra
         ii. Posterior portion (two) for two ureters
   5. Bladder composition
      a. Inner lining (mucosal layer) composed of transitional epithelium
      b. Submucosal layer made up of elastic and connective tissue
      c. Muscular layer and detrusor muscle outside of submucosal layer
   6. Bladder neck
      a. Thickening formed by the interlaced fibers of the muscular layer of bladder

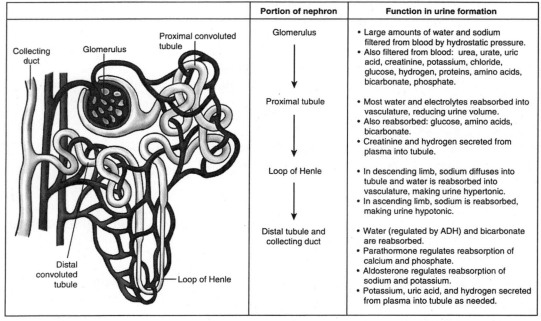

Portion of nephron	Function in urine formation
Glomerulus	• Large amounts of water and sodium filtered from blood by hydrostatic pressure. • Also filtered from blood: urea, urate, uric acid, creatinine, potassium, chloride, glucose, hydrogen, proteins, amino acids, bicarbonate, phosphate.
Proximal tubule	• Most water and electrolytes reabsorbed into vasculature, reducing urine volume. • Also reabsorbed: glucose, amino acids, bicarbonate. • Creatinine and hydrogen secreted from plasma into tubule.
Loop of Henle	• In descending limb, sodium diffuses into tubule and water is reabsorbed into vasculature, making urine hypertonic. • In ascending limb, sodium is reabsorbed, making urine hypotonic.
Distal tubule and collecting duct	• Water (regulated by ADH) and bicarbonate are reabsorbed. • Parathormone regulates reabsorption of calcium and phosphate. • Aldosterone regulates reabsorption of sodium and potassium. • Potassium, uric acid, and hydrogen secreted from plasma into tubule as needed.

Figure 30–2. Normal physiologic function of the nephron in urine formation. ADH, antidiuretic hormone. (From Monahan, F.D., Neighbors, M. [1998]. *Medical Surgical Nursing Foundations for Clinical Practice,* 2nd ed. Philadelphia: Saunders, p. 1332.)

7. Micturition (voiding)
   a. Highly coordinated process
   b. Two phases
      i. Urine storage
      ii. Bladder emptying
   c. Both phases controlled and coordinated by sympathetic, parasympathetic, and central nervous systems
8. Urine storage
   a. Filling phase
      i. Increase in volume of urine in bladder causes slow rise in pressure in bladder (intravesical pressure)
      ii. Stretch receptors in bladder wall convey afferent impulses through pelvic nerve to spinal cord
      iii. Results in stimulation of sympathetic efferent nerves
      iv. Impulses conveyed back to bladder and urethra via hypogastric nerves
      v. Results in activation of internal sphincter to maintain continence
      vi. Allows for complete bladder filling
      vii. When bladder sufficiently distended, nerve impulses transmitted to brain
         (a) Brain stem responsible for micturition
   b. Emptying stage
      i. To initiate voiding
         (a) Efferent pelvic nerve stimulates bladder to contract
         (b) Permits bladder neck and urethra to open
         (c) Relaxation of external urethral sphincter and perineal muscles occurs simultaneous to opening of bladder neck and urethra
9. Factors that contribute to normal micturition
   a. Appropriate bladder sensation during filling
   b. Closed bladder outlet during rest
   c. Absence of involuntary contractions
   d. Absence of anatomic obstruction
   e. Conditions interfering with above may compromise normal micturition
D. Urethra
   1. Description
      a. Hollow muscular tube
      b. Transports urine from bladder to urinary meatus for excretion
   2. Size and position
      a. Females: 4 cm (1½ inches) long; extends from bladder neck (involuntary internal sphincter) to meatus
         i. Voluntary external sphincter surrounds middle third of urethra
      b. Males: 15 cm (6 inches) long
         i. Consists of five portions
            (a) Prostatic (posterior urethra)
            (b) Membranous (posterior urethra)
            (c) Bulbous (anterior urethra)
            (d) Penile (anterior urethra)
            (e) Glandular (anterior urethra)
         ii. Internal and external sphincter surrounds urethra
      c. Purpose of urethra
         i. Final channel for urine excretion
         ii. Emptying
            (a) Female: urethra empties by gravity
            (b) Male: urethra empties by contraction of bulbocavernosus muscle

E. Male genitalia
1. Prostate gland
   a. Encapsulated, three-lobe structure
   b. Size and shape of chestnut
   c. Location
      i.   Base of urinary bladder
      ii. Behind symphysis pubis
      iii. Close to rectal wall
         (a) Easily palpated by rectal exam
         (b) Able to diagnose infections and enlargement of prostate early
         (c) Because of close proximity of prostate to urethra may cause urinary symptoms
   d. Internal structure
      i.   Glandular and muscular
         (a) Glandular tissue
            (i) Secretes thin, milky alkaline fluid into excretory ducts
               a) Acidity protects sperm from acid present in urethra and female vagina
               b) Increases motility of sperm
         (b) Muscular fibers
            (i) Contract during ejaculation
            (ii) Eject prostatic secretion into urethra
               a) Added to semen
2. Seminal vesicles
   a. Two convoluted membrane pouches
   b. Location
      i. Lower part of posterior surface of bladder
      ii. Directly in front of rectum
   c. Secretion
      i.   Is a component of semen
         (a) Protects and nourishes sperm
         (b) Activates motility
      ii. Slightly alkaline fluid with large amount of fructose
      iii. Activation of seminal vesicles depends on adequate levels of testosterone
   d. Each seminal vesicle joins corresponding vas deferens
      i.   Forms an ejaculatory duct
         (a) Two short tubes that pass through prostate gland
         (b) Empty semen containing sperm into urethra
3. Testes (reproductive glands)
   a. Function
      i. Produce sperm
      ii. Produce testosterone (male hormone)
   b. Size and location
      i. Pair of ovoid-shaped organs
      ii. Lie in scrotum
   c. Internal structure
      i.   Seminiferous tubules
         (a) Functional unit of the organ
         (b) Long, convoluted, threadlike structures
         (c) Packed densely in testes
         (d) Converge into a collection of excretory ducts
         (e) Sperm production occurs in seminiferous tubules

4. Epididymis
   a. First portion of paired male genital duct system
   b. Comma-shaped structure
   c. Attached to posterolateral aspect of testis
   d. Divided into three parts
      i. Head
      ii. Central body
      iii. Tapered portion (tail) that is continuous with vas deferens
   e. Site for storage and maturation of sperm cells
5. Vas deferens
   a. Firm, cylindrical tube
   b. Connects epididymis with ejaculatory duct
   c. Consists of thick, muscular walls
      i. Muscular layers assist in propelling sperm through duct system
   d. Allows for storage of sperm for as short as a few hours to as long as 42 days
6. Cowper's glands (bulbourethral glands)
   a. Two small, pea-sized structures
   b. Located on either side of urethra
   c. Secretes mucous through ducts into the urethra
7. Penis
   a. Organ with both excretory and reproductive functions
   b. Composed of a shaft with three sponge-like areas and vascular channels that fill with blood to form an erection
      i. Corpus cavernosum—right and left
         (a) Comprise greater part of the shaft of the penis
      ii. Corpus spongiosum
         (a) Contains the penile urethra
   c. Glans
      i. Tip of penis
      ii. Contains urethral opening
   d. Prepuce
      i. Foreskin covering glans
8. Scrotum
   a. Sac that supports the testes and epididymis
F. Female anatomy
1. Urethra
   a. Shorter than male's
   b. Results in frequent cystitis due to close proximity of the vagina and rectum
2. Periurethral glands
   a. Secrete mucous
      i. Skene
      ii. Bartholin
II. **Assessment Parameters**
A. Preprocedure—emphasize screening for:
1. Urinary habits
2. Level of continence
3. Color and odor of urine
4. Dysuria or inability to void
5. Patient or partner concerns about sexual performance
6. Bleeding dyscrasias; medications affecting coagulation
7. Barriers to learning

B. Postprocedure
    1. Urinary output—amount, character, color
    2. Hematuria, clots
    3. Catheter patency
    4. Swelling
    5. Fever
    6. Scrotal enlargement
       a. May be most evident after pelvic laparoscopy due to insufflation of CO_2
    7. Bladder distention
       a. Important for patient to understand importance of voiding postprocedure
       b. First voiding may be uncomfortable

III. Procedures
  A. Diagnostic
    1. Cystoscopy (cystourethroscopy)
      a. Description
         i.   Direct visualization of urethra, prostatic urethra, and bladder using a lighted tubular telescopic lens
         ii. Can be combined with retrograde pyelograms to examine ureters
      b. Specimens can be obtained
         i.   Saline washings for cytologic examination
         ii. Biopsies of suspicious areas
      c. Indications
         i.   Primary exam for diagnosis and follow-up of bladder tumors
      d. Also used to diagnose urologic disorders such as:
         i.   Prostatism
         ii. Fistulas
         iii. Diverticula
         iv. Congenital abnormalities
         v. Recurrent urinary tract infections (UTIs)
           (a) Contraindicated during active UTIs
         vi. Voiding disorders
    2. Ureteroscopy
      a. Allows endoscopic removal of stones
      b. Allows for maneuvers under direct visualization of the ureters
      c. Indications
         i.   Stones in lower ureter greater than 4 mm in diameter
         ii. Obstruction
         iii. Intolerable pain
         iv. Fever and chills
      d. May be used to remove stones in middle to upper ureter, depending on physician experience
      e. Guide wire in place to ensure proper drainage
    3. Prostate biopsy (three methods)
      a. Transrectal core-needle biopsy
         i.   Core needle (18 gauge) inserted into rectum
         ii. Biopsy of prostatic area
         iii. Procedure may be performed with or without rectal ultrasonography
         iv. Advantages
            (a) Anesthesia not required
            (b) Sepsis and bleeding uncommon
            (c) Patient discomfort minimal

      v. Disadvantages
        (a) Requires antibiotics before and after procedure
        (b) Fleet enema required prior to procedure
        (c) Cost increases with use of ultrasonography
  b. Transrectal fine-needle aspiration
    i. Same as above except using 23-gauge needle
  c. Transperineal core needle
    i. Core needle inserted into perineum (local anesthesia administered)
    ii. Needle goes through perineum into prostate
    iii. Tissue samples obtained
    iv. Performed with or without ultrasonography
    v. Advantages
      (a) No antibiotics required
      (b) Risk for bleeding and sepsis is minimal
    vi. Disadvantages
      (a) Increased cost if performed with ultrasonography
      (b) No longer preferred method of performing prostate biopsy

4. Testicular biopsy
  a. Description
    i. Wedge excision of suspicious tissue

B. Surgical
  1. Biopsy of bladder
    a. Performed during cystoscopy
    b. Use biopsy forceps to obtain specimen
    c. Can also obtain specimens of ureteral or renal pelvic tissue
  2. Biopsy and/or fulguration of bladder tumor
    a. Description
      i. Performed via cystoscopy
      ii. Utilizes electrodes to burn tumor
  3. Circumcision
    a. Description
      i. Excision of the prepuce (foreskin)
    b. Indications
      i. Religious
      ii. Prophylactically in infancy
      iii. Phimosis
        (a) Orifice of prepuce stenosed
        (b) Retraction behind the glans difficult
      iv. Balanoposthitis
        (a) Condition results in inflamed glans and mucous membrane
        (b) May be accompanied by purulent discharge
        (c) May require circumcision
      v. Paraphimosis
        (a) Prepuce not easily reduced from retracted position
  4. Extracorporeal shock wave lithotripsy (ESWL)
    a. Description
      i. Utilizes shock waves through a fluid medium to break up stones
  5. Hematocelectomy
    a. Description
      i. Removal of blood and blood clots from the scrotum
    b. Cause
      i. Trauma from a direct blow
      ii. Complication of scrotal surgery

6. Hydrocelectomy
   a. Description
      i.   Excision of the tunica vaginalis of the testis to remove a hydrocele, or fluid-filled sac
      ii. Hydrocele
           (a) Collection of fluid in the scrotum
           (b) Causes
               (i) Embryonic
               (ii) Imbalance between production and reabsorption of fluid within layers of tunica vaginalis
   b. Treatment
      i.   Aspiration
      ii. Injection of sclerosing agents
      iii. Surgical intervention (hydrocelectomy)
7. Hypospadias repair
   a. Description
      i.   Common urologic defect/deformity of the penis in which the urethral wall is malformed and the urethral opening is on the underside of the penis
      ii. Classifications
           (a) Distal
           (b) Midshaft
           (c) Penoscrotal
           (d) Perineal
      iii. Surgical intervention based on degree of pathologic changes
      iv. Over 300 different types of surgical repair are known
           (a) Surgical correction may require multiple procedures
8. Laser ablation of condyloma
   a. Description of condylomata acuminata
      i.   Caused by human papillomavirus
      ii. Also known as genital warts
      iii. Sexually transmitted
      iv. Lesions
           (a) Soft, fleshy papules
           (b) Found on penis in males
           (c) Found on labia, vulva, vagina, or cervix in females
      v.   Complications
           (a) Hemorrhage
           (b) Penile fistula
   b. Treatment
      i.   Traditional
           (a) Cryotherapy
           (b) Podophyllin 10% in compound tincture of benzoin
      ii. Utilization of a laser beam to remove diseased tissue
           (a) May have less recurrence rate than traditional methods of treatment
      iii. Surgical removal
9. Laser transurethral prostatectomy
   a. Also known as VLAP (visual laser ablation of the prostrate)
      i.   Used to treat benign prostatic hyperplasia (enlargement of the prostate gland)

b. Description
    i.   Laser vaporizes prostatic tissue instead of traditional urethral resection of the prostate (TURP) method
    ii. Advantages
       (a) Patients do not require continuous bladder irrigation, and can be discharged the same day
c. Other technologies available that accomplish the same objective without incurring the cost of laser

10. Meatotomy
  a. Description
    i.   Enlargement of the external urethral meatus to correct stenosis or stricture

11. Orchiectomy
  a. Description
    i.   Surgical removal of one or both testes
  b. Indications
    i.   Control symptomatic metastatic cancer
    ii. Trauma
    iii. Infection
  c. Prostheses may be inserted

12. Orchiopexy
  a. Description
    i.   Suspension of the testis within the scrotum to correct undescended testicles
  b. Cause
    i.   Testis fails to descend into scrotum during gestation

13. Penile prosthesis insertion/removal
  a. Description
    i.   Prosthesis implanted for treatment of sexual impotence
    ii. Serves as a stent to enable vaginal penetration for sexual intercourse
    iii. Various types of implants are utilized to treat impotence

14. Spermatocelectomy
  a. Description
    i.   Removal of spermatocele
       (a) Cystic mass
       (b) Contains white fluid and dead sperm
    ii. Appears behind testicle
    iii. Is separate from testicle
  b. Cause
    i.   Leakage of sperm
       (a) Caused by trauma or infection

15. Testicular detorsion
  a. Description
    i.   Torsion or twisting of testes
    ii. Affects males between birth and young adulthood
    iii. Very painful
  b. Causes
    i.   Not fully understood
  c. Treatment
    i.   Urologic emergency
       (a) To decrease tissue necrosis
    ii. Requires immediate detorsion of testicle and pexis to scrotum
    iii. Involves correction of twisting and vascular supply to the testicle

16. Ureteral stent insertion/removal
    a. Description
       i.   Stents are placed to keep the lumen of the ureter patent
17. Urethral dilatation/internal urethrotomy
    a. Description
       i.   Gradual dilatation of the urethra and lysis of a stricture
18. Varicocelectomy
    a. Description
       i.   Ligation and excision of dilated veins in the scrotum through an inguinal incision or an incision above the superior iliac spine
19. Vasectomy
    a. Description
       i.   Excision of a section of the vas deferens, generally for sterilization purposes
20. Vasovasostomy
    a. Description
       i.   Anastomosis of two segments of the vas deferens to reverse a vasectomy

IV. Intraoperative Issues
A. Types of anesthesia
   1. Local anesthetic, with or without epinephrine
   2. Monitored anesthesia care (MAC), with or without IV conscious sedation
   3. General anesthesia by mask, nasal, or oral endotracheal tube
   4. Regional anesthesia—spinal or epidural block
B. Procedural techniques
   1. Microsurgical
   2. Endoscopic
   3. Laser
   4. ESWL

V. Perianesthesia Priorities Phase I—Preoperative Care
A. Objective
   1. Purpose of the preoperative phase of care
      a. Assess and prepare the patient for the surgical experience
      b. Baseline data is obtained with which to plan and implement nursing care
      c. The educational process that began in the physician's office continues at this time and continues throughout the continuum of care
B. Assessment
   1. Physical—as stated previously
   2. Assess for educational needs related to preoperative care and post-discharge planning
   3. Assess for psychosocial needs
      a. Developmental age needs
      b. Family/responsible adult companion availability
      c. Community resources needed, including home health services
C. Plan of care
   1. Include patient/family/responsible adult companion in developing a plan of care appropriate to the age of the patient
   2. Nursing diagnoses might include:
      a. Anxiety/fear related to knowledge deficit, unfamiliar environment, separation from family, lack of control, potential sexual dysfunction, etc.
      b. Pain related to surgical/procedural intervention
      c. Potential for injury
      d. Potential for infection

D. Interventions
   1. Nursing interventions might include:
      a. Ensure that all laboratory studies are completed as ordered/indicated
      b. Provide information on preoperative preparation (NPO, discontinuation of medications, hygiene, ride/aftercare arrangements, etc.)
      c. Obtain baseline vital signs
      d. Ensure legal authorization is appropriate (informed consent)
      e. Provide orientation to surroundings
E. Evaluation
   1. Evaluation of interventions/patient response might include:
      a. Diagnostic testing results are reviewed, abnormal results reported to appropriate physician, and follow-up completed as indicated
      b. Patient/family/responsible adult is questioned to determine understanding of preoperative instructions and postoperative care needs as indicated
      c. Determine that patient has made arrangements for aftercare

VI. **Phase II—PACU**
A. Objective
   1. The objective of PACU care is to ensure that the patient safely recovers from the immediate effects of surgery and anesthesia
B. Assessment
   1. Routine PACU protocol
   2. Procedure-specific assessment as indicated
C. Plan of care
   1. Plan should be appropriate to the age of the patient
   2. Nursing diagnoses might include:
      a. Anxiety/fear related to knowledge deficit, unfamiliar environment, separation from family, lack of control, potential sexual dysfunction, etc.
      b. Pain related to surgical/procedural intervention
      c. Potential for injury
      d. Potential for infection
      e. Urinary retention
      f. Self-esteem disturbance
      g. Body image disturbance
   3. Be alert for potential complications
      a. Cystoscopic procedures—diagnostic studies, bladder biopsy, insertion of stents
         i.   Severe hematuria
         ii. Urinary tract infection
         iii. Urinary retention
         iv. Dysuria
         v.   Bladder spasms
      b. Scrotal procedures—prostate biopsy, varicocelectomy, orchiectomy, hydrocelectomy, vasectomy, vasovasostomy, torsion repair
         i.   Bleeding—hematoma formation or frank bleeding (common complication)
         ii. Compromise of testicular blood supply
         iii. Torsion of testicle—onset of sudden pain
      c. Penile procedures—circumcision, hypospadias repair
         i.   Bleeding
         ii. Swelling
      d. ESWL
         i.   Hematoma
         ii. Urinary obstruction due to fragments

        iii. Urinary tract infection
        iv. Pain/ureteral colic
        v. Sepsis
        vi. Intractable nausea and vomiting

D. Nursing interventions
  1. General
    a. Routine PACU care per protocol
    b. Monitor vital signs per protocol
    c. Administer medications for pain and nausea as ordered
    d. Observe for bleeding and other complications
    e. Ensure a safe environment
    f. Monitor urinary output
    g. Maintain privacy/dignity
  2. Procedure-specific
    a. Cystoscopic procedures
      i. Catheter care as indicated
    b. Scrotal procedures
      i. Ice packs
      ii. Scrotal support
    c. Penile procedures
      i. Ice pack—avoid placing ice near tip of penis
      ii. Catheter care as indicated
      iii. Frequent dressing checks
    d. ESWL
      i. Increase fluid intake to promote passage of disintegrated urinary calculus
        (a) Prevents development of steinstrasse
          (i) Build up of stone particles in ureter
          (ii) Frequent complication of ESWL
          (iii) Treatment includes laser lithotripsy or stenting to relieve obstruction
      ii. Postural positioning and ambulation
        (a) Greater volume of stone particles more easily passed
      iii. Monitor hematuria
        (a) Normal for some degree of hematuria
        (b) Monitor for:
          (i) Increase in hematuria
          (ii) Change in color
          (iii) Presence of blood clots
        (c) Hematuria begins to resolve in 48 hours
      iv. Strain urine to verify passage of stone fragments

VII. Phase III—Preparation for Discharge
  A. Objective
    1. The objective of Phase III is to ready the patient to return to home, prepared—in conjunction with a caregiver—to successfully manage postoperative care
    2. Education of the patient and caregiver is a critical factor in a successful ambulatory surgery outcome
  B. Assessment
    1. Procedure-specific assessment continues as outlined in Phase II to ensure that postoperative status is stable prior to discharge
  C. Plan of care
    1. Plan should be appropriate to the age of the patient

2. Nursing diagnoses might include:
   a. Anxiety/fear related to knowledge deficit, unfamiliar environment, separation from family, lack of control, potential sexual dysfunction, etc.
   b. Pain related to surgical/procedural intervention
   c. Potential for injury
   d. Potential for infection
   e. Potential for urinary retention
   f. Self-esteem disturbance
   g. Body image disturbance
   h. Knowledge deficit
D. Nursing interventions
   1. Procedure-specific interventions initiated in Phase II continue
   2. The patient and family are also instructed to continue interventions at home as appropriate
   3. Education interventions
      a. Discussion, demonstration, written materials, etc.
      b. Copies of all materials given to patients should be maintained in the medical record or on the unit
E. Evaluation
   1. Evaluation of clinical interventions continues as noted in Phase II
   2. Evaluation of learning
      a. Patient/caregiver verbalization of understanding, demonstrating a skill, etc.
      b. Patient and responsible party should sign that they have been instructed and had the opportunity to have questions answered

VIII. Education Content
A. Preoperative
   1. General
      a. NPO
      b. Preoperative hygiene
      c. Environment
      d. Facility protocols
      e. Aftercare arrangements
      f. Perioperative course
   2. Procedure-specific
      a. Discontinue medications affecting bleeding time per physician order
      b. Antibiotics as ordered
      c. ESWL—avoid skin powders or oils
B. Postoperative
   1. General
      a. Activity
      b. Diet—encourage fluids
      c. Medications
      d. Complications
      e. Follow-up care
   2. Procedure-specific
      a. Cystoscopic procedures
         i. Catheter care as indicated
         ii. Mild hematuria is expected
         iii. Mild dysuria is expected
      b. Scrotal procedures
         i. Dressing/suture site care
         ii. Scrotal support and/or ice packs to decrease swelling

---

BOX 30–1.   Key Educational Patient Outcomes

- Patient describes preoperative care requirements for specific surgical procedure
- Postprocedure, the patient verbalizes understanding of expected and unexpected complications and describes procedure to notify physician
- The patient who has undergone an ESWL procedure can verbalize understanding of the intraoperative and postoperative procedure and can describe the importance of increasing fluid intake
- Patients who have undergone surgical intervention on the urinary system will exhibit normal patterns of urinary elimination postoperatively with little pain or hematuria
- The patient who is discharged home with an indwelling catheter in the bladder can describe routine care of the device

---

   c. Penile procedures
     i.   Dressing/suture line care
     ii. Catheter care as indicated
   d. ESWL
     i.   Strain urine for stones as ordered
     ii. Anticipate discomfort as stones are passed
     iii. Hydrate well
     iv. Mild petechiae and bruising are common

Bibliography

1. Gray, H. (1985). *Anatomy of the Human Body*. Carmine Clemente, ed. Philadelphia: Lea & Febiger.
2. Guyton, A.C. (1991). *Textbook of Medical Physiology*. Philadelphia: Saunders.
3. Jordan, G.H., Schlossberg, S.M. (1996). Complications of interventional techniques for urethral stricture disease: Direct visual internal urethrotomy, stents, and laser intervention. In Carson, C.C., ed. *Topics in Clinical Urology: Complications of Interventional Techniques*. Tokyo: Igaku–Shoin.
4. Karlowicz, K.A. (1995). *Urologic Nursing—Principles and Practice*. Philadelphia: Saunders.
5. Meeker, M.H., Rothrock, J.C. (1995). *Alexander's Care of the Patient in Surgery*, 10th ed. St. Louis: Mosby.
6. Miller, K.M. (1994). Post anesthesia care of the genitourinary surgical patient. In Drain, C., ed., *The Post Anesthesia Care Unit: A Critical Care Approach to Post Anesthesia Nursing*. Philadelphia: Saunders.
7. Monahan, F.D., Neighbors M. (1998). *Medical Surgical Nursing Foundations for Clinical Practice*, 2nd ed. Philadelphia: Saunders.
8. Nagle, G.M. (1993). The Urological Surgical Patient. In Litwack, K., ed. *Core Curriculum for Post Anesthesia Nursing Practice*. Philadelphia: Saunders.
9. Patterson, D.E., Segura, J.W. (1996). Complications of extracorporeal shock wave lithotripsy, ureteroscopic, and percutaneous procedures. In Carson, C.C., ed. *Topics in Clinical Urology: Complications of Interventional Techniques*. Tokyo: Igaku–Shoin.
10. The Surgical Specialties, Part 2. (1993). In Burden, N., ed., *Ambulatory Surgical Nursing*. Philadelphia: Saunders.
11. Winters, J.C., Appell, R.A. (1996). Complications of the use of injectables in the treatment of incontinence and reflux. In Carson, C.C., ed., *Topics in Clinical Urology: Complications of Interventional Techniques*. Tokyo: Igaku–Shoin.

REVIEW QUESTIONS

1. A mass caused by obstruction of the tubular system in the scrotum is a

   A. Hydrocele
   B. Cystocele
   C. Spermatocele
   D. Varicocele

2. Following a hydrocelectomy, the nurse can anticipate postoperative care to include

   A. Application of ice
   B. Application of heat
   C. Observation for inguinal swelling
   D. Observation for hematuria

3. When instructing the patient and family following ESWL, the nurse advises them to

   A. Anticipate significant pain
   B. Report discoloration of urine
   C. Change dressings prn
   D. Increase fluid intake

4. The ESWL patient should anticipate hematuria to resolve

   A. Within 12 hours
   B. Within 18 hours
   C. Within 48 hours
   D. Within 72 hours

5. The patient should be instructed to call the physician post ESWL for

   A. Hematuria 24 hours postprocedure
   B. Passage of stone fragments
   C. Petechiae
   D. Ureteral colic

6. Disadvantages of performing a transrectal core-needle biopsy include all of the following except

   A. Requires antibiotics before and after procedure
   B. Fleet enema required prior to procedure
   C. Sepsis and bleeding commonly occur
   D. Cost increases with use of ultrasonography

7. Indications for circumcision include

   A. Religious
   B. Phimosis
   C. Balanoposthitis
   D. All of the above

8. The most common complication after scrotal procedures is

   A. Infection
   B. Urinary retention
   C. Incontinence
   D. Hematoma

9. Postoperative instructions for the patient discharged with an indwelling urinary catheter should include

   A. Maintenance of closed system and daily irrigation
   B. Daily cleansing with soap and water
   C. Application of topical antibiotic daily
   D. Empty drainage every 12 hours

10. Post varicocelectomy, the surgeon should be notified if the nurse notes

    A. Scrotal edema
    B. Ecchymosis
    C. Hematuria
    D. Inguinal swelling

ANSWERS TO QUESTIONS

1. C
2. A
3. D
4. C
5. D

6. C
7. D
8. D
9. B
10. D

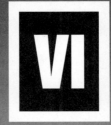

Other Surgical Specialties

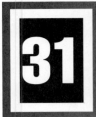

Dental/Oral and Maxillofacial Surgery

Denise O'Brien
University of Michigan Health System
Ann Arbor, Michigan

I. **Anatomy and Physiology**
   A. Mouth and oral cavity include the following structures:
      1. Lips, teeth, gums, buccal mucosa, tongue, palate (hard and soft), tonsils, pharynx, temporomandibular joint (see Figure 31–1)
   B. The oral cavity is bounded by the jaw bones and associated structures (muscles and mucosa) (see Figures 31-2 and 31-3)
      1. Includes the cheek, palate, oral mucosa, the glands whose ducts open into the cavity, the teeth, and the tongue
      2. Except for the teeth, interior of mouth is covered with mucous membrane, lined with salivary glands
         a. Secrete saliva
         b. Aid in the first step of digestion of food
   C. Oral cavity forms the beginning of the digestive system
      1. This is where chewing occurs
      2. The site of the organs of taste
      3. Mouth is entrance to the body for food, occasionally air
      4. Major organ of speech and emotional expression
   D. Associated structures
      1. Buccal: pertaining to or directed toward the cheek
      2. Tooth: hard calcified structure set in the alveolar processes of the mandible and maxilla; for mastication of food

1. Describe anatomy and physiology of oral cavity pertinent to the ambulatory surgery patient undergoing oral/maxillofacial procedures.
2. Identify assessment parameters for patients undergoing oral/maxillofacial operative procedures.
3. Define nursing care priorities in each postanesthesia phase.
4. Identify common reasons for admission following oral/maxillofacial procedures.
5. Describe patient education following oral/maxillofacial procedures related to diet, pain management, oral care, activity, and follow-up.

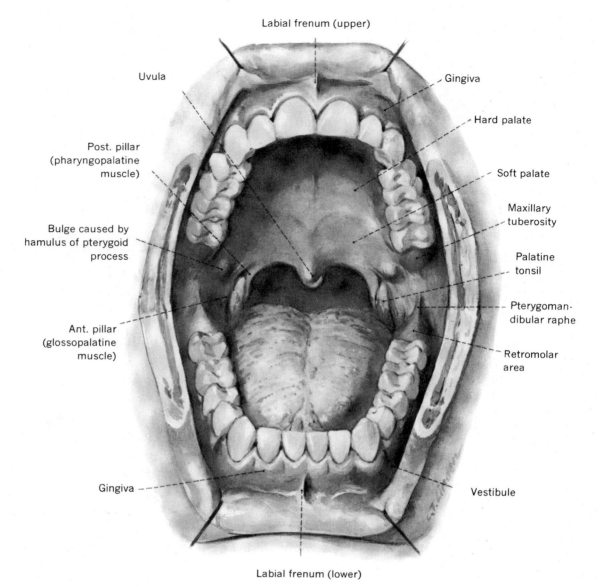

Figure 31–1.   The oral cavity.   (Reproduced from Massler, M., Schour, I. [1958]. *Atlas of the Mouth in Health and Disease*, by permission of the American Dental Association, Chicago.)

 3. Gingiva: mucous membrane (the gum) surrounding the teeth
   a. Covers the tooth-bearing border of the jaw
   b. Overlies crowns of unerupted teeth
   c. Encircles the necks of erupted teeth
   d. Supporting structure for subjacent tissues
 4. Mandible: horseshoe-shaped bone forming the lower jaw; largest and strongest bone of the face; articulates with the skull at the temporomandibular joints
 5. Maxilla: irregularly shaped bone that forms the upper jaw, actually two identically shaped bones that are considered one
   a. Assists in the formation of the orbit, the nasal cavity, and the palate
   b. Supports the upper teeth
   c. Described as the architectural key of the face, touches all facial bones except mandible

6. Palate: the roof of the mouth, consists of:
    a. Hard palate, the rigid anterior portion, hinged to the soft palate
    b. Soft, the posterior, fleshy part of the palate, flanked by tonsils; in the middle of the soft palate is the uvula, a fleshy projection pointing down to the tongue
7. Tongue: movable muscular organ on the floor of the mouth
    a. Location of organs of taste
    b. Aids in chewing, swallowing, and the articulation of sound
8. Nerves (see Figure 31–4)
    a. From the maxillary division of the trigeminal nerve (Cranial Nerve V), posterior, middle and anterior superior alveolar nerves supply sensation to the upper teeth
    b. The mandibular division gives off the lingual nerve (sensation of anterior two thirds of tongue, the floor of mouth, gums), inferior alveolar nerve (sensation of premolar, molar teeth of mandible) and at its terminus—mental nerve (sensation of the lower lip and chin)
9. Temporomandibular joint: bicondylar joint formed by the head of the mandible and the mandibular fossa, and the articular tubercle of the temporal bone

II. Assessment Parameters Specific to Procedures
A. Examination
    1. Inspection and palpation of greatest use
        a. Head and neck
            i.   General appearance

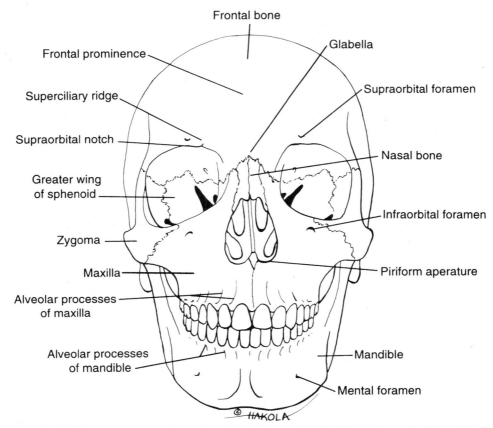

Figure 31–2.   The skull, anterior view.   (Reproduced from Ferraro, J.W. [1997]. *Fundamentals of Maxillofacial Surgery.* New York: Springer-Verlag, by permission.)

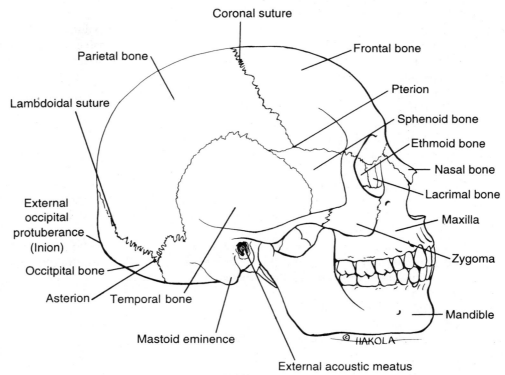

Figure 31–3.   Lateral view of the skull.   (Reproduced from Ferraro, J.W. [1997]. *Fundamentals of Maxillofacial Surgery*. New York: Springer-Verlag, by permission.)

      ii. Facial appearance
      iii. Trismus (limited degree of mouth opening)
      iv. Neck lumps
      v. Gross facial swelling
      vi. Skin color and texture
    b. Intraoral
      i. Tongue: size, mobility, color, and texture
      ii. Oral mucosa (palate, cheeks, labial mucosa, floor of mouth): exam for changes in color, texture, ulcers, lumps
      iii. Alveolar ridges and gingivae: color, texture, gingival recession, ulcers, lumps
      iv. Teeth: number, position, restorations, crowns, caries, cracked/missing teeth, exposed structure
  B. Increased risk associated with history or need to alter perioperative management
    1. Cardiac: may require antibiotic prophylaxis
      a. Endocarditis
      b. Mitral valve prolapse with mitral regurgitation
      c. Valve implants
    2. Implants: antibiotic prophylaxis may be needed
      a. Joints (major replacements)
      b. Grafts of artificial materials
    3. Coagulation and bleeding disorders
      a. Factor VIII deficiency (hemophilia)
      b. Von Willebrand's disease

      i. Factor VIII, Synthetic Factor VIII, ε-Aminocaproic acid (EACA or Amicar), or DDVAP (desmopressin acetate) may be given just before procedure begins

    c. Anticoagulant therapy

      i. Coagulation testing may be required (prothrombin, partial thromboplastin time, platelet count) to determine coagulation status before proceeding with elective surgery

4. Immuno-compromised patient or immune disorders

    a. HIV, AIDS

    b. Patient with history of organ transplant

    c. Universal precautions should be used with every patient

    d. Immuno-compromised patient may require special care (isolation, scheduling, altered medication regimen)

5. Trauma

    a. Edema present

      i. Recent injury

      ii. May delay operative repair until edema diminishes

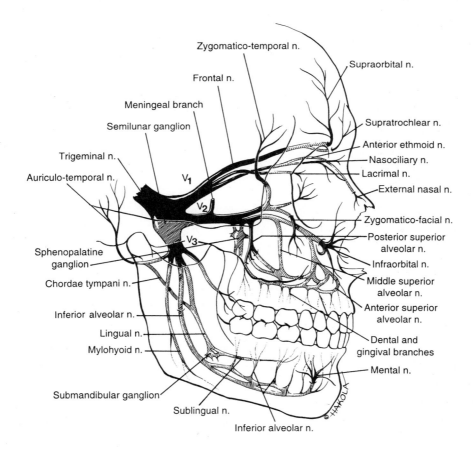

V_1 = ophthalmic division
V_2 = maxillary division
V_3 = mandibular division

Figure 31–4. The trigeminal nerve (Cranial Nerve V). (Reproduced from Ferraro, J.W. [1997]. *Fundamentals of Maxillofacial Surgery.* New York: Springer-Verlag, by permission.)

   b. Disfigurement: may be significant and emotionally disturbing to patient and others

  6. Chronic pain

   a. Pain-tolerance alterations

   b. Chronic analgesic use may alter postoperative analgesic management

  7. Nutritional status changes

   a. Difficulty chewing, swallowing

   b. Pain may interfere with ability to eat and meet caloric demands and nutritional requirements

  8. Developmentally challenged

   a. Potential behavioral problems (combative, disruptive, abusive)

   b. Legal authorization appropriately obtained before treatment commences

 C. Airway status evaluation

  1. Evaluation of airway for ease of intubation in maxillofacial surgery

   a. Mobility of the neck—ability to touch chin to chest and each shoulder; flex and extend

   b. Position of the trachea relative to the mandible—distance from thyroid cartilage to anterior bony chin; at least 6.5 cm acceptable

   c. Ability of the patient to open the mouth—at least 3.6 cm in adults desirable

   d. Structures visualized when the patient opens the mouth and vocalizes "ahh . . . "—see the uvula and surrounding pharyngeal structures

 D. Determine the educational needs of patient and caregiver

  1. Oral care, analgesia, preoperative anxiety

  2. Discharge planning

 E. Nursing diagnoses

  1. Risk for injury

  2. Anxiety

  3. Sensory/perceptual alterations

  4. Pain/discomfort

  5. Risk for infection

  6. Knowledge deficit

  7. Body image disturbance

  8. Fear related to discomfort

  9. Alteration in nutrition

III. Operative Procedures

Common operative procedures and techniques are included. The reader is referred to a comprehensive text on oral and maxillofacial surgery for additional procedures and techniques.

 A. Arch bars

  1. Rigid metal bars used to splint and fix the teeth and/or maxilla or mandible

  2. Wire ligatures attach the bars to the teeth

  3. Used for treatment of avulsed teeth, fractures of the mandible or maxilla

 B. Closed reduction of mandibular (jaw) fracture

  1. Erich-type arch bars ligated to teeth most common method of fixation

  2. Maxillomandibular fixation (MMF) using stainless steel loops or elastics for a minimum of 4 weeks considered best for providing reduction and fixation

  3. MMF acceptable for ambulatory surgery if there is no gross edema and/or bleeding

  4. Used for alignment and stabilization of fractures to allow proper healing

 C. Dental examination: using visual and instrument methods, the oral cavity is inspected and the teeth and supporting structures are probed for defects, lesions, mobility, and infection

D. Dental implant
   1. A prosthetic tooth with an anchoring structure surgically implanted beneath the mucosal or periosteal layer or in the bone
   2. Replace a single missing tooth, lost to injury or other reasons
E. Dental prophylaxis: cleansing of teeth (stains, materia alba, calculus, removal of plaque)
F. Dental restoration
   1. Replacing by artificial means
   2. Reforming lost tooth structure, missing, damaged, or diseased teeth with alloy of silver, gold, or acrylic resin
G. Genioplasty: operative repair of chin deformities (microgenia, macrogenia, asymmetric chin are a few of the defects) by open bone reduction, augmentation with synthetic or natural materials, or osteotomy with plate and screw fixation
H. Gingivectomy:
   1. Excision of all loose infected and diseased gingival tissue
   2. Used to eradicate periodontal infection and reduce the gingival sulcus depth
I. Implants
   1. Used to stabilize or totally support tooth replacements; prostheses may be fixed or fixed/removable
   2. Osseointegration screw technique (Branemark)
      a. Titanium screw inserted into jaw bone, grows into the bone (osseointegrates)
      b. After 3 months (mandible) or 6 months (maxilla) attached to and loaded with a prosthesis
   3. Transmandibular implant (Bosker)
      a. Consists of a base plate, screws to fix the plate to the mandible, and posts that attach to a bar (dolder) in the mouth
      b. Lower prosthesis is attached to the bar; prosthesis started 4 to 6 weeks after surgery
J. Intraoral biopsy: removal of abnormal tissue for histopathological examination
   1. Excisional: complete removal of a lesion with primary closure
   2. Incisional: small representative portion of a lesion is removed if the lesion is large and the defect left from its removal could not be closed primarily
K. Multiple dental extractions
   1. Surgical removal of teeth
   2. May follow trauma, significant or recurring infection, nonrestorable teeth, or in preparation for prosthetic replacement
L. Odontectomy: tooth extraction
M. Open reduction and internal fixation of zygomatic fracture
   1. Using a transconjunctival or lower eyelid subciliary incision with skin muscle flap and orbital floor exploration, the fracture reduced and fixated with wires or microplate system for the infraorbital rim and wires or miniplating fixation of the zygomaticomaxillary buttress
   2. Intent to realign fractured bone fragments and restore facial contour
N. Splint
   1. Made of acrylic resin or metal, used as space maintainer or fixator, hold teeth in alignment; temporarily permanent or removable
   2. Used in orthognathic surgical procedures to stabilize the maxillomandibular position (secured to the maxilla and mandible, interlocked, retain the desired position of the osteotomized units)
   3. Used to reduce and stabilize maxillofacial fractures, may be used in the interim before MMF or plate and screw (rigid) fixation

O. Temporomandibular joint (TMJ) arthroscopy
   1. Direct visual inspection and examination of the interior TMJ structures using an endoscopic instrument
   2. Indications include diagnosis of internal joint pathology, lavage of joint, lysis of adhesions, biopsy of synovial tissue

IV. Intraoperative Priorities

A. Anesthesia choice
   1. General: nasal intubation desired for unobstructed visualization of orofacial structures
   2. Conscious sedation with local anesthesia
      a. Midazolam, ketamine (glycopyrrolate to decrease oral secretions) less risk of respiratory depression; reduced emergence delirium with midazolam
      b. Benzodiazepine with fentanyl: O_2 recommended when used with local anesthesia; may use methohexital or propofol for additional sedation
   3. Local anesthesia used alone for minor oral procedures or used as an adjunct during general anesthesia
      a. Minimize immediate postoperative pain
      b. Minimize bleeding in operative field
      c. Help separate tissue planes to ease dissection
      d. Allow for less anesthetic agent due to reduced surgical stimulus

B. Intraoperative concerns
   1. Hemostasis and intraoral bleeding
      a. Hemostatic agent may be used
      b. Gelfoam, Surgicel, Avitene, topical thrombin, bone wax (for bone bleeders)
   2. Airway
      a. Loss of reflexes with excessive sedation
      b. Positioning of endotracheal tube, potential displacement
      c. Foreign body aspiration

V. Postanesthesia Priorities

A. Phase I
   1. Airway
      a. Spontaneous, unassisted breathing
      b. Adjunct in place: nasal trumpet, oropharyngeal airway
      c. Endotracheal tube: nasal insertion
      d. Observe for respiratory complications
   2. Hemodynamic stability
      a. Vital signs stable, consistent with baseline
      b. Observe for cardiovascular complications
   3. Bleeding
      a. Hemostasis may be difficult to obtain
      b. Risk for hemorrhage
      c. Increases risk of nausea and vomiting: swallowed blood may precipitate nausea/vomiting due to irritating effect of blood in stomach
   4. Report from anesthesia/oral surgeon/perioperative nurse
      a. Implants/prostheses inserted
      b. Splints: location, type
      c. Oral packing: location, plan for removal
      d. Oral sutures: location, extreme care when suctioning
      e. MMF (wired jaws)
         i. Wire cutters/scissors immediately available
         ii. Clear instructions from surgeon when appropriate to cut fixation wires and what wires to cut
         iii. Usually cut for vomit and for respiratory distress

5. Discomfort
   a. Maximum pain intensity occurs about 3 hours after surgery; begin analgesics intraoperatively or immediately postoperatively
   b. Long-acting local anesthetic infiltrated into operative site; usually bupivacaine with epinephrine to provide 8 to 12 hours of analgesia
   c. Opioids: decreasing use in ambulatory oral/maxillofacial surgery due to increased use of NSAIDs
   d. NSAIDs: ketorolac may provide superior analgesia following extractions
6. Drainage from mouth
   a. Position to facilitate drainage of saliva, bloody secretions
   b. Drooling or excessive salivation and unable to swallow (reflex absent or excessive pain)
   c. Suction prn with soft catheter
7. Dressing
   a. No dressing when incisions are intraoral
   b. Internal dressing may be moistened gauze sponge
   c. External dressing
      i. Pressure chin strap (Jobst type)
      ii. Foam tape
8. Edema
   a. Can be significant, especially in longer procedures
   b. Position with head of bed elevated
   c. Administer steroid if ordered, continued controversy regarding effectiveness in reducing inflammatory reaction
   d. Ice packs may help reduce blood flow to operative site and subsequent inflammatory response; check with surgeon before applying, may actually increase blood flow (rebound effect after ice pack removed)
9. Fluids/nutrition
   a. Clear to full liquid high-caloric diet as tolerated and ordered
   b. Do not force fluids especially when nausea/vomiting present
   c. Causes of nausea and vomiting
      i. Narcotic analgesics
      ii. Blood in stomach
      iii. Starvation leading to weakness, low blood sugar levels
   d. Hydrate with IV fluids (replacement and maintenance)
      i. Lactated ringers (Hartmann's)
      ii. Dextrose-containing solutions
   e. When nausea/vomiting are present
      i. Administer antiemetics as ordered; determine if antiemetic prophylaxis given
      ii. Commonly use droperidol, prochlorperazine, metoclopramide, ondansetron (See Chapters 8 and 22 for discussion on antiemetics)
10. Reaction to local anesthetics
    a. What appears to be an allergic reaction to local anesthetic (LA) may actually be a reaction to preservative methylparaben or sulfite
    b. Allergy to LA is rare
    c. Traumatic penetration of a nerve (prolonged numbness), vein (hematoma), or artery (systemic toxic effects)
    d. Systemic (cardiac) reactions to epinephrine (used to minimize bleeding) in LA, rather than LA itself
    e. Toxicity caused by overdose leads to excitation of central nervous system followed by profound CNS depression, cardiovascular collapse, possible death

11. Oral hygiene
    a. Take care to not disrupt clot; gently swab the oral cavity, hold saline rinse for 8 to 12 hours postprocedure
    b. Lubricate lips with petroleum jelly or emollient cream, steroid (0.5% hydrocortisone) lip cream—long procedures expect significant edema of lips
12. Antibiotic as ordered: common following trauma, patients with cardiac valvular disease, history of rheumatic fever or implants
    a. The oral cavity is laden with bacteria; bacteria enter the bloodstream through oral incisions, traumatic lacerations
    b. Infections can lead to loss of bone and teeth, distributive shock (septic), damage to heart valves, endocarditis, loss of implants, scarring, large vessel complications (carotid erosion or venous thrombosis)
13. Provide patient with means of communication while in PACU
    a. Bell
    b. Writing tools
        i. Pen/pencil, paper pad
        ii. Magic slate/stylet
        iii. Dry-erase board/marker
14. Reasons for admission following outpatient operative procedure
    a. Airway obstruction
    b. Unanticipated MMF
    c. Severe PONV
    d. Excessive blood loss
    e. Severe pain
    f. Persistent bleeding from extraction sites
    g. Slow recovery from anesthesia
15. Nursing diagnoses
    a. Risk for injury
    b. Anxiety
    c. Sensory/perceptual alterations
    d. Pain/discomfort
    e. Risk for infection
    f. Knowledge deficit
    g. Body image disturbance
    h. Fear related to discomfort
    i. Alteration in nutrition
B. Phase II
    1. Operative site
        a. Continued bleeding: tamponade by biting saline-moistened gauze for approximately 30 minutes
        b. Epinephrine-soaked gauze or packs not recommended; rebound vasodilation can occur when a vasoconstrictor is used, leading to increased bleeding
        c. Pressure packs may need to be maintained for 2 hours or some specified time postprocedure—determine appropriate time for removal and discharge
    2. Discomfort
        a. Oral analgesic medications initiated in preparation for discharge home
            i. May have started in Phase I
            ii. Determine effectiveness of medication before patient discharged home on same analgesic
            iii. If ineffective may need prescription changed or other follow-up (see Chapter 24 on pain management)
        b. Continue ice pack as ordered

3. Oral care
   a. Oral suctioning initiated by patient when appropriate and patient capable
   b. Begin oral fluids if desired and not already started in Phase I; avoid extremes of heat
4. Education
   a. Includes patient/family/responsible adult companion
   b. Instructions
      i. Oral hygiene
      ii. Avoid temperature extremes in food and beverages
      iii. Care of bands/wires
      iv. For patient with MMF
         (a) How and when to cut wires
            (i) Airway distress
            (ii) Vomiting
      v. Pain-relief alternatives
         (a) Dental wax may be used to protect oral mucosa and decrease irritation and discomfort from protruding wires or metal bands
      vi. TMJ procedures
         (a) Trismus may be problem
         (b) TMJ physiotherapy initiated
         (c) Provide information on jaw-opening exercises
C. Phase III
1. Oral hygiene
   a. Brushing difficult if not impossible due to swelling and pain
      i. Swelling reaches maximum in 2 to 3 days, subsides gradually
      ii. Rinses may help in reducing swelling
   b. Saline rinses (1 tsp. table salt in ½ glass hot water) for 2 minutes, three to six times a day, especially after meals
      i. No rinsing for at least 8 to 12 hours after procedure so as not to disturb clot (surgeon may order up to 24 hours before rinsing begins); disruption of the clot may lead to painful "dry socket" (localized osteitis)
         (a) Most often develops from second to fifth postoperative day
         (b) Chief complaint is pain; also may complain of odor or a bad taste
         (c) Treatment is conservative: gentle warm saline irrigation of site, sedative, dressing over site until patient no longer symptomatic
      ii. Antiseptic mouthwashes may also be prescribed
         (a) Most common is chlorhexidine 0.2%
         (b) Held over surgical site for 1 minute, then expectorated
         (c) This should not be used for more than 1 week as it may stain the teeth
   c. Continued bleeding
      i. Instruct patient to replace gauze sponge over bleeding site and bite firmly for 20 to 30 minutes; if a bleeding tooth socket, a teabag over the socket may be helpful
      ii. If bleeding persists, patient needs to be evaluated by surgeon
2. Nutrition
   a. Instruct patient re: alcohol and smoking avoidance for first 48 hours
   b. Diet/food preparation
      i. Avoid hot foods/liquids for first 48 hours
      ii. Instruct patient to advance to soft foods or pureed diet (nutritional supplement) as tolerated or ordered by surgeon
   c. Encourage fluid intake especially during hot weather

3. Vomiting
   a. Prepare patient and family for possibility of vomiting swallowed blood; suggest adequately sized receptacle for ride home and at home in case of emesis
   b. Caution patient/caregiver to call surgeon/facility
      i. If vomiting persists for >6 hours
      ii. Continuing to swallow blood: may require evaluation to determine source of bleeding
4. Pain
   a. Ice packs, heat application especially for TMJ procedures
   b. Oral analgesics
      i. Suggest contacting surgeon if pain is not relieved by prescribed analgesics, intolerable or increasing
      ii. Unrelieved or increasing pain may indicate infection, retained root, bone, foreign body, maxillary sinus problems
   c. Alternatives
      i. Dental wax may be applied to wires/bands to reduce mucosal irritation
      ii. Explore with patient/caregiver other potential pain-management techniques (see Chapter 24 on pain management)
5. Wound care
   a. See oral hygiene instructions for intraoral incisions
   b. For external incisions
      i. Keep wound clean and dry for minimum of 24 to 48 hours
      ii. May be instructed to remove dressing after 24 to 48 hours and clean incision with saline or half-strength hydrogen peroxide; cover with antibiotic ointment
      iii. Observe incision for signs of infection: redness, swelling, drainage
6. Activity
   a. Rest
      i. Limit activity until pain and swelling subside
      ii. Sleep with head elevated on several pillows to reduce swelling and minimize bleeding
      iii. While taking opioid analgesics, avoid operating machinery, driving automobiles, using sharp or potentially injurious articles, or drinking alcohol
   b. Exercise
      i. For first 24 hours any exercise is discouraged
      ii. Defer vigorous activity, restrict until surgeon allows; may be up to 4 weeks after surgery
         (a) Aerobic activity may increase heart rate and blood pressure, leading to increased bleeding from operative site(s)
7. Follow-up care
   a. Arrange for return visit with surgeon in specified time interval
      i. Patients with drains, MMF, extensive procedures may require return visit on first postoperative day
      ii. Sutures removed in 5 to 7 days postoperatively
   b. Return to work dependent on procedure, patient work
   c. Risk for secondary hemorrhage
      i. Seven to 10 days after surgery
      ii. Often due to an infected wound and poor oral hygiene
   d. Fever: contact surgeon if temperature over 100.4°F to (38°C) or as ordered by surgeon

---

BOX 31-1.   Key Patient Educational Outcomes

Phase I
- Patient will express feelings of lessened anxiety
- Patient will describe minimal to tolerable pain
- Patient will request analgesic to manage pain
- Patient will perform oral suctioning and handle oral secretions unassisted
- Patient will be able to communicate with nurse without using verbal skills

Phase II
- Patient tolerating discomfort following administration of oral analgesics
- Patient/caregiver describe oral hygiene following instruction
- Patient demonstrates use of gauze sponge for tamponade of bleeding
- Patient demonstrates safe, gentle, and effective oral suctioning
- Patient/caregiver verbally describe wire cutting (patients with MMF)
- Patient progressing to upright position with minimal orthostatic effects: dizziness, lightheadedness, nausea

Phase III
- Patient/caregiver describe follow-up required
- Patient/caregiver identify risks associated with operative procedure: infection, hemorrhage, pain, vomiting
- Patient/caregiver describe oral care, activity, medications, and diet
- Patient/caregiver demonstrate knowledge of medications (analgesics, antibiotics, antiemetics, etc.) by describing purpose and administration of each medication prescribed

---

VI. **Future Considerations in Oral and Maxillofacial Surgery**
   A. Expanding and evolving
      1. Facial esthetics
      2. Cosmetic procedures
         a. Traditionally thought to be domain of plastic surgeons
      3. Maxillofacial surgery
   B. Techniques and materials
      1. Advancing
         a. Progression of wires and bands
         b. Maxillomandibular fixation to plates and screws
         c. Rigid internal fixation
   C. Procedures
      1. Continue to be refined as techniques advance
      2. Additional procedures
         a. In the past required extended inpatient stays
         b. Will fall into the realm of ambulatory surgery

BIBLIOGRAPHY

1. Dimitroulis, G. (1997). *A Synopsis of Minor Oral Surgery*. Oxford, England: Reed Educational and Professional Publishing Ltd.
2. Donoff, R.B. (1997). *Massachusetts General Hospital Manual of Oral and Maxillofacial Surgery*, 3rd ed. St. Louis: Mosby.
3. *Dorland's Illustrated Medical Dictionary*, 28th ed, (1994). Philadelphia: Saunders.
4. Ferraro, J.W. (1997). *Fundamentals of Maxillofacial Surgery*. New York: Springer-Verlag.
5. Kaban, L.B., Pogrel, M.A., Perrott, D.H. (1997). *Complications in Oral and Maxillofacial Surgery*. Philadelphia: Saunders.
6. Kwon, P.H., Laskin, D.M. (1997). *Clinician's Manual of Oral and Maxillofacial Surgery*, 2nd ed. Carol Stream, IL: Quintessence Publishing.
7. *Miller-Keane Encyclopedia & Dictionary of Medicine, Nursing, & Allied Health*, 6th ed. (1997). Philadelphia: Saunders.
8. White, P. (1997). *Ambulatory Anesthesia & Surgery*. Philadelphia: Saunders.

REVIEW QUESTIONS

1. Epinephrine added to local anesthetic provides vasoconstriction allowing for diminished bleeding intraoperatively. When the effect of the vasoconstrictor wears off, what may happen?

   A. Arterial spasm
   B. Continued vasoconstriction
   C. No change
   D. Rebound vasodilation

2. The maxilla touches all facial bones except the

   A. Temporal
   B. Mandible
   C. Zygoma
   D. Frontal

3. Trismus results in

   A. Difficulty in opening the mouth
   B. Painful mastication
   C. Difficulty swallowing
   D. Airway obstruction

4. While assessing the patient scheduled to undergo an elective genioplasty, the nurse discovers the patient is taking coumadin (warfarin) for treatment of an embolic episode. What test(s) would be appropriate before proceeding with the operative procedure?

   A. Blood chemistries
   B. Blood typing
   C. Hematocrit and hemoglobin
   D. Prothrombin (PT)

5. The patient arrives in the PACU following multiple dental extractions under general anesthesia. Local anesthesia was injected at the onset of the procedure. What analgesic might be your choice for this patient?

   A. Ketorolac
   B. Morphine
   C. Acetaminophen with codeine
   D. Aspirin

6. Patients undergoing oral or maxillofacial procedures with general anesthesia are best managed with what type of airway?

   A. Oral endotracheal tube
   B. Nasal endotracheal tube
   C. Laryngeal mask airway
   D. Tracheostomy

7. The patient is discharged home following third molar extractions following instructions on oral hygiene, bleeding, diet, pain management, and follow-up care. While at home, the patient experiences bleeding from the operative site. The patient should

   A. Call the surgeon
   B. Return to the facility immediately
   C. Roll up a moistened clean gauze sponge and bite it for 30 minutes
   D. Rinse mouth with warm saline solution, followed by antiseptic rinse

8. Following a mandibular fracture that resulted in placement of arch bars and plating, Ms. S is experiencing bleeding and increasing pain. She is 9 days postprocedure. The most likely cause of her bleeding and pain is

   A. Undiagnosed coagulopathy
   B. Infection
   C. Jaw misalignment
   D. Allergic reaction

9. The patient runs daily. He has just undergone a procedure requiring maxillomandibular fixation. Instructions have been reviewed with the patient and his caregiver. Which statement would indicate the patient does not fully understand his discharge instructions?

   A. "You'll have to drive me home, Mom."
   B. "I can drink as much as I want, right?"
   C. "Great, I can start running again tomorrow afternoon!"
   D. "I guess I won't be going in to work anytime soon."

10. Nerves of the maxillary or mandibu-
    lar divisions of the trigeminal nerve
    can be injured during oral or maxillo-
    facial operative procedures. Among the
    causes are

    A. Dental implants
    B. Local anesthetic injections
    C. Tumor or cyst excision
    D. All the above

ANSWERS TO QUESTIONS

1.	D	6.	B
2.	B	7.	C
3.	A	8.	B
4.	D	9.	C
5.	A	10.	D

Neurosurgery/Neurologic Procedures

Serina Carpenter
Forrest General Hospital
Hattiesburg, Mississippi

I. **Nervous System Anatomy**
   A. Cells
      1. Neuron
         a. Structures
            i.   Dendrite: receives information
            ii. Cell body
            iii. Axon: sends information
               (a) Myelinated (insulated)
               (b) Unmyelinated
         b. Functions
            i.   Sensory (afferent—from)
               (a) Special senses
                  (i)   Smell
                  (ii) Taste
                  (iii) Vision
                  (iv) Auditory
               (b) Pain and temperature
               (c) Proprioception (position sense) and vibration
               (d) Touch
            ii. Motor (efferent—to)
            iii. Other (such as interneurons)
         c. Transmission
            i.   Electrical impulse
               (a) Depolarization—K ion influx, Na ion outflow
               (b) Repolarization—K ion pump, Na ion pump restore membrane potential
               (c) Axonal versus saltatory conduction

        (i)   Axonal: entire axon must be depolarized such as in unmyelinated fibers making conduction slow

        (ii)   Saltatory conduction: only sections of a myelinated axon are depolarized, the current jumping from each node of Ranvier leading to more rapid impulse conduction

  ii. Chemical transmission

    (a) Synapse: vesicles release neurotransmitter (NT) from the presynaptic membrane into the synaptic cleft which attaches to receptor sites on the post synaptic membrane of the target organ (i.e., another neuron, muscle, organ) resulting in the appropriate response (i.e., muscle contraction or relaxation)

    (b) Neurotransmitters (NT): chemicals that inhibit, stimulate, or modulate the response of the target organ (i.e., endorphins, dopamine, acetylcholine, serotonin, substance-P)

2. Support cells

  a. Central nervous system (CNS)

    i.   Astrocytes—form the blood brain barrier and provide structure

    ii.   Oligodendrocytes—form the myelin covering of axons

    iii. Ependymal cells—line the cerebrospinal fluid pathways

    iv. Microglial—scavenger cells

  b. Peripheral nervous system (PNS)

    i.   Schwann cells—form myelin covering of axons

B. Covering (see Figure 32–1)

  1. Central nervous system

    a. Dura mater ("hard mother")

      i.   Tough fibrous covering, more distensible over lumbar region

    b. Arachnoid (weblike)

      i.   CSF circulates through this "web"

      ii.   Arachnoid villi—CSF is absorbed into the venous system

    c. Pia mater ("little mother")

      i.   One cell-layer thick, not visible, in direct contact with brain and spinal cord

  2. Axons

    a. Central nervous system

      i.   Myelin formed by oligodendroglia cells

    b. Peripheral nervous system

      i.   Myelin formed by Schwann cells

C. Central nervous system

  1. Brain

    a. Cerebrum

      i.   Frontal lobes

        (a) Frontal poles

          (i)   Attention span

          (ii)   Goal-directed behavior

        (b) Premotor strip

        (c) Motor strip

        (d) Broca's area (left hemisphere)

          (i)   Expressive speech (producing language)

      ii.   Parietal lobes

        (a) Sensory strip

          (i)   Interpretation of tactile sensation (i.e., soft, hard, smooth, etc.)

        (b) Association area

          (i)   Allows for body/self awareness by associations of sensory information

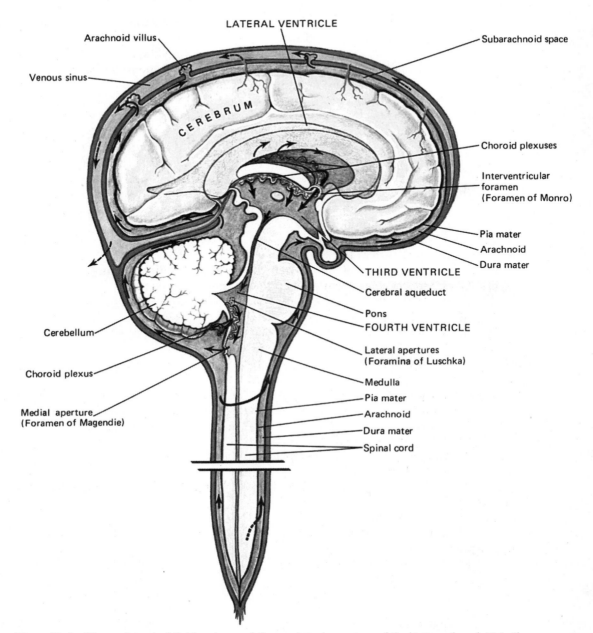

Figure 32–1.   The cerebrospinal fluid system and the meningeal coverings of the brain and cord. Note the directions of flow of cerebrospinal fluid indicated by the arrows.   (From Guyton, A.C. [1991]. *Basic Neuroscience: Anatomy & Physiology*, 2nd ed. Philadelphia: Saunders, p. 36.)

    iii. Temporal lobes
        (a) Wernicke's Area (left hemisphere)
            (i)   Receptive speech (understanding language)
        (b) Sound interpretation (right hemisphere)
        (c) Memory
        (d) Smell
    iv. Occipital lobes
        (a) Visual cortex

b. Basal ganglia (deep cerebral gray matter in cerebral hemispheres)
  i.   Motor system
c. Diencephalon
  i.   Thalamus
       (a) Sensory relay station
  ii. Hypothalamus
       (a) Temperature control
       (b) Appetite
       (c) Hormonal feedback system
       (d) Major interface between endocrine system and autonomic nervous system
  iii. Epithalamus
d. Limbic system (interconnected system involving several areas of cerebral hemispheres)
  i.   Emotions (aggression, anger)
  ii. Sexual drive
e. Brain stem
  i.   Midbrain
       (a) Third cranial nerve (occulomotor)
           (i)   Moves eye up, down, and medially
           (ii) Opens lid
           (iii) Parasympathetic outflow constricts pupil
           (iv) Sympathetic outflow dilates pupil
       (b) Fourth cranial nerve (trochlear)
           (i)   Moves eye down and in
  ii. Pons
       (a) "Bridge" between motor system and cerebellum
       (b) Fifth cranial nerve (trigeminal)
           (i)   Sensation of face (three branches)
           (ii) Sensation to cornea (corneal reflex)
           (iii) Muscles of mastication
       (c) Sixth cranial nerve (abducens)
           (i)   Moves eye out laterally
       (d) Seventh cranial nerve (facial)
           (i)   Movement of face, allows facial expression
       (e) Eighth cranial nerve (auditory)
           (i)   Auditory branch (hearing)
           (ii) Vestibular branch (balance)
  iii. Medulla
       (a) Ninth cranial nerve (glossopharyngeal)
           (i)   Taste—anterior two-thirds of tongue
           (ii) Sensory to tongue and soft palate
       (b) Tenth cranial nerve (vagus)
           (i)   Parasympathetic outflow
           (ii) Sensory to posterior pharynx
       (c) Eleventh cranial nerve (accessory)
           (i)   Shoulder shrug
       (d) Twelfth cranial nerve (hypoglossal)
           (i)   Extends tongue
       (e) Vomiting center
       (f) Respiratory center

  f. Cerebellum
   i. Balance
   ii. Motor gracefulness
  g. White matter connections
   i. Corpus callosum: left and right hemisphere association pathways, allows the hemispheres to "talk" to each other
   ii. Internal capsule: major descending tract from cortex
 2. Spinal cord (see Figure 32–2)
  a. Descending tracts (motor tracts) efferent—to
   i. Corticospinal tract
  b. Ascending tracts (sensory tracts) afferent—from
   i. Spinothalamic (pain and temperature)
   ii. Posterior columns (proprioception)
  c. Gray horns (neurons)
   i. Anterior (motor)
   ii. Posterior (sensory)
   iii. Lateral (sympathetic)
  d. Spinal cord segments
   i. Eight cervical segments
    (a) C4 innervates diaphragm
    (b) C5, 6, 7, and 8 innervate arm and hand
   ii. Twelve thoracic segments
    (a) Intercostal muscle innervation important for strong cough
    (b) Sensory landmarks
     (i) T4—nipple
     (ii) T10—umbilicus
   iii. Five lumbar segments
    (a) Sensory landmark
     (i) Anterior legs

Cutaneous Innervation of the Upper Extremity

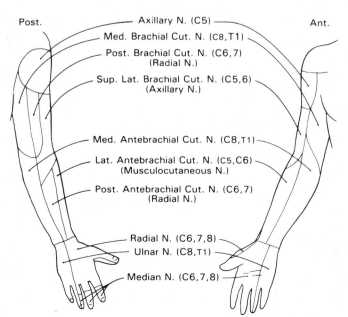

Post.

Ant.

Axillary N. (C5)
Med. Brachial Cut. N. (C8,T1)
Post. Brachial Cut. N. (C6,7)
(Radial N.)
Sup. Lat. Brachial Cut. N. (C5,6)
(Axillary N.)
Med. Antebrachial Cut. N. (C8,T1)
Lat. Antebrachial Cut. N. (C5,C6)
(Musculocutaneous N.)
Post. Antebrachial Cut. N. (C6,7)
(Radial N.)
Radial N. (C6,7,8)
Ulnar N. (C8,T1)
Median N. (C6,7,8)

Figure 32–2. Cutaneous innervation of the upper extremity. (From Wolf, J. with original illustrations by David Factor. [1981]. *Segmental Neurology*. Baltimore: University Park Press, p. 109.)

(b) Motor
  (i) Leg movement
  (ii) Dorsoflexion of foot (L5)
iv. Five sacral segments
  (a) Sensory landmark
    (i) Perineum "saddle area"
    (ii) Posterior legs (S1)
  (b) Motor
    (i) Plantarflexion of foot
    (ii) Sphincters
e. Anatomical features
  i. In the adult, the spinal cord ends at the first lumbar vertebrae
  ii. The nerve roots of the lumbar and sacral segments hang in a cluster to exit the spinal column at each appropriate level and is called the Cauda Equina (horse's tail); therefore, in the adult, during a lumbar puncture the needle is inserted below the spinal cord, although a nerve root may be touched
  iii. The dura at the end of the spinal canal is distensible and allows for shunting of cerebrospinal fluid into this area whenever we strain, thus preventing elevations of intracranial pressure during activities
D. Cerebrospinal fluid (CSF)
  1. Functions
    a. Cushions central nervous system
    b. Allows for normal increases of intracranial pressure as during sneezing, straining, etc.
  2. Pathway (see Figure 32–3)
    a. Lateral ventricles in the cerebral hemispheres exit through the foramina of Monro into the
    b. Third ventricle which exits through the Aqueduct of Sylvius into the
    c. Fourth ventricle which exits through one of the Foramina of Luschka or the Foremen of Magendie to circulate
    d. Down the spinal cord or over the cerebral hemispheres
  3. Production/absorption
    a. Produced by the choroid plexus in the lateral, third, and fourth ventricles at a rate of about 1 cc/3 minutes, approximately 500 cc/day
    b. Produces a continuous flow with approximately 140 to 150 cc in the system
    c. Absorbed via the arachnoid villi over the cerebral hemispheres into the venous system
  4. Characteristics
    a. Clear, colorless
    b. No RBC
    c. 0 to 3 WBC/mm^3
    d. Protein 35 mg/dL
    e. Glucose two thirds of blood glucose
E. Peripheral nervous system
  1. Divisions
    a. Twelve cranial nerves
    b. Thirty-one pairs of spinal nerves (a pair presents at each vertebral level from its corresponding spinal segment)
    c. Characteristics
      i. Motor axons (efferent) exit the spinal cord anteriorly
      ii. Sensory axons (afferent) enter the spinal cord posteriorly
      iii. The groups of motor and sensory axons travel in nerve roots, trunks, and branches

Cutaneous Innervation of the Lower Extremity

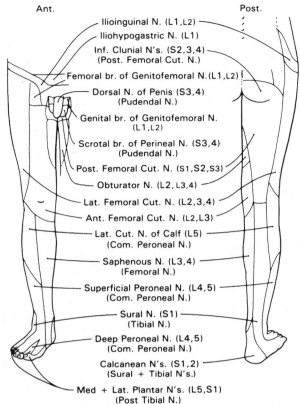

Ant.   Post.

Ilioinguinal N. (L1,L2)
Iliohypogastric N. (L1)
Inf. Clunial N's. (S2,3,4)
(Post. Femoral Cut. N.)
Femoral br. of Genitofemoral N. (L1,L2)
Dorsal N. of Penis (S3,4)
(Pudendal N.)
Genital br. of Genitofemoral N.
(L1,L2)
Scrotal br. of Perineal N. (S3,4)
(Pudendal N.)
Post. Femoral Cut. N. (S1,S2,S3)
Obturator N. (L2,L3,4)
Lat. Femoral Cut. N. (L2,3,4)
Ant. Femoral Cut. N. (L2,L3)
Lat. Cut. N. of Calf (L5)
(Com. Peroneal N.)
Saphenous N. (L3,4)
(Femoral N.)
Superficial Peroneal N. (L4,5)
(Com. Peroneal N.)
Sural N. (S1)
(Tibial N.)
Deep Peroneal N. (L4,5)
(Com. Peroneal N.)
Calcanean N's. (S1,2)
(Sural + Tibial N's.)
Med + Lat. Plantar N's. (L5,S1)
(Post Tibial N.)

Figure 32–3. Cutaneous innervation of the lower extremity. (From Wolf, J. with original illustrations by David Factor. [1981]. *Segmental Neurology.* Baltimore: University Park Press, p. 110.)

d. Major nerves of the upper extremity
   i. Radial nerve
       (a) Sensory
           (i)   Dorsum of hand
           (ii) Individualized, minor sensory role
       (b) Motor
           (i)   Triceps
           (ii) Brachioradialis
           (iii) Extensors of the forearm, wrist, and fingers
   ii. Median nerve
       (a) Sensory
           (i)   Palm surface of the thumb, index, middle, and half of the ring finger
           (ii) Posterior tips of the index and middle fingers
       (b) Motor
           (i)   Pronators of the forearm
           (ii) Thumb opposition
   iii. Ulnar nerve
       (a) Sensory
           (i)   Little finger and half of ring finger
       (b) Motor
           (i)   Thumb and palm abduction/adduction
           (ii) Extension of fourth and fifth fingers

   e. Major nerves of lower extremities
      i.   Sciatic nerve
      ii. Femoral nerve
      iii. Common peroneal nerve

II. Neurological Assessment
   A. Level of consciousness (most important factor in assessment)
      1. Alertness—assess during admission by how well and how quickly questions are answered (avoid terms such as lethargic, drowsy etc.; use description such as falls asleep with 3-stage command)
         a. Eyes open when you enter room, spontaneously
         b. Eyes open when name called
         c. Eyes open when stimulated
         d. Able to stay alert to instructions or requests without falling asleep
      2. Orientation—assess the appropriateness of the conversation to the situation (loss of orientation begins with loss of time, then place, then person)
         a. Time: date, day of week, month, year, recent or upcoming holiday
         b. Place: name of building, floor, city, county, state
         c. Person: identifies you as nurse, knows family/visitors
      3. Memory
         a. Long term: allergy and medical histories
         b. Short term: able to remember nurse's name during length of stay, follows and repeats instructions, able to give history of morning events leading up to admission, reason for admission and preadmit instructions
         c. Recall: immediately able to repeat nurse's name when introduced and instructions given them (deficit most common residual effect of IV conscious sedation)
   B. Motor: observe spontaneous movements and symmetry of movements, positions self for blood pressure or other procedures, turns self, provides self care
      1. Strength scale
         a. 5 points: no deficit/weakness
         b. 4 points: able to lift extremity against gravity and maintain position without wavering
         c. 3 points: able to lift extremity against gravity but wavers and cannot sustain
         d. 2 points: able to slide along support surface such as bed/chair
         e. 1 point: flicker movement
      2. Upper extremities
         a. Grasp: have patient squeeze your first and second fingers, compare right with left
         b. Extension: patient extends arms in front with palms up, eyes closed, observe for arm drift indicating mild weakness
         c. Able to dress self, buttoning, etc.
      3. Lower extremities
         a. Heel and toe walk: able to walk several steps on heels, then on toes
         b. Leg lift: lying in bed, able to lift one leg at a time to clear bed and hold without wavering, compare left with right
      4. Trunk
         a. Able to sit on side of bed independently
         b. Has strong cough
   C. Sensory (always compare right and left sides and test with patient's eyes closed)
      1. Touch: eyes closed, identifies where touched; test opposite side to see if each side "feels the same"
      2. Pain/temperature: eyes closed, identifies if pinprick is sharp and back of pin as dull, or identifies ice chip as cold

3. Proprioception: eyes closed, identifies when finger, extremity, or joint is raised, lowered, bent, or repositioned by examiner
4. Alterations
   a. Pain (refer to Chapter 24 on pain management)
   b. Paresthesia: odd sensations ("creeping, crawling, tingling, pins and needles") whether in response to stimulation or not
   c. Hyperesthesia: increased sensitivity to touch/temperature
   d. Hypesthesia (hypoesthesia): decreased sensitivity to touch/temperature ("numbness")
D. Cerebellar (coordination/balance)
   1. Rapid movements
      a. Tap one foot at a time
      b. Clap hands: left into right/then right into left
      c. Pat leg with palm of hand
   2. Finger-to-nose testing
      a. With arms extended to sides, close eyes, then touch nose alternating left and right in rapid repetitions
   3. Rhomberg test
      a. Able to stand with feet together and eyes closed

III. Neurological Complications
A. Seizures: anything that the brain does normally can surface as a seizure
   1. Classification
      a. Generalized
         i. Generalized tonic/clonic (grand mal)
             (a) Description:
                 (i)   Tonic phase: lasts 1 to 2 minutes; the patient is rigid, with increased muscle tone
                 (ii) Clonic phase: usually lasts 1 to 2 minutes; the patient has jerking movements that gradually slow then stop; usually breathing stops for 30 seconds to 1 minute
                 (iii) Post-ictal phase: patient does not remember seizure, confused, usually wants to sleep, may be combative when stimulated
             (b) Medical emergency: notify physician immediately
                 (i)   No history of epilepsy
                 (ii) Lasts more than 5 minutes
                 (iii) One seizure occurs after another (status epilepticus)
                 (iv) If the seizure began while still under general anesthesia, the only symptom may be that the patient is not waking up; as the brain fatigues the outward motor signs of tonic/clonic movement are lost and the patient will be flaccid; therefore, any patient not awakening from anesthesia should have an EEG to rule out status epilepticus
             (c) Treatment
                 (i)   Do not restrain
                 (ii) Do not force anything into the mouth
                 (iii) Turn to side
                 (iv) Protect from self harm and the environment, pillow under head, remove harmful objects
                 (v)   Padded "BITE" may be placed between molars if patient opens mouth
                 (vi) May use oxygen if available
                 (vii) Suction as needed; do not force into mouth

          (d) Assessment
               (i)   What was patient doing when seizure started
               (ii)   What was the first indication that a seizure had begun (confusion, jerking in any part of the body, etc.)
               (iii) Length of seizure
               (iv) Physical appearance (body position, limb movement)
               (v)   Bowel or bladder incontinence
               (vi) Obtain stat glucose and electrolytes

      ii.   Absence (petit mal): more common in children
         (a) Description
               (i)   Short (several seconds) of blinking spells
               (ii)   May occur 30 or greater times per day
         (b) Medical concern if number of seizures reduces quality of life

  b. Partial
      i.   Complex partial (temporal lobe)
         (a) Description
               (i)   Appears awake, but confused
               (ii)   May turn to examiner when name called
               (iii) Automatisms: repetitive activity, not goal oriented such as rubbing, rocking, pulling at clothes or bed linens
               (iv) Activity is not goal oriented
         (b) Medical emergency: notify physician immediately
               (i)   If no history of epilepsy
               (ii)   If lasts more than 5 minutes
               (iii) If one occurs after another
               (iv) Obtain stat glucose and electrolytes
               (v)   Observe closely for secondary generalization
         (c) Treatment
               (i)   Do not restrain, patient may become hostile and perceive intervention as a threat
               (ii)   Redirect activity or ambulation by placing barriers (i.e., close doors, place chairs in his/her path)
         (d) Assessment
               (i)   What was patient doing just prior to seizure
               (ii)   Length of time seizure lasts
               (iii) Automatisms
               (iv) Was patient able to speak

B. Stroke (cerebrovascular accident [CVA])
  1. Classification
    a. Ischemic
      i.   Thrombotic (most common)
         (a) May progressively worsen over time
      ii.   Embolic
         (a) Sudden onset
    b. Hemorrhagic
      i.   Aneurysm with subarachnoid hemorrhage
      ii.   Intracerebral
  2. Warning signs
    a. Loss of strength and/or sensation usually on one side of the body
    b. Decreased vision, dimness of vision, loss of vision in one eye, double vision
    c. Difficulty talking or understanding speech
    d. Difficulty swallowing

e. Severe headache

f. Sudden dizziness, nausea, and/or vomiting

3. Treatment

a. Stat brain CAT scan uncontrasted

b. Maintain normotension (do not overtreat elevated blood pressure)

c. Neuroassessment q. 15 to 30 minutes

C. Headache

1. Migraine (may be triggered by many factors involved with surgical procedures)

a. Careful history should reveal method of treatment

b. Analgesics/narcotics/serotonin

c. Ice/cool cloth to head/back of neck

d. Treat even mild hypoglycemia

e. Maintain fluid intake (nausea and vomiting may occur)

2. Muscle tension (may be related to surgical position)

a. Neutral head position

b. Massage/topical creams

c. Encourage range of motion of neck and shoulders

d. Relaxation techniques (deep breathing, etc.)

IV. Procedures

A. Carpal tunnel release (example of peripheral nerve entrapment)

1. Disorder

a. Characteristics

i.   Results from pressure on the median nerve

ii.   Associated health factors

(a) Diabetes mellitus

(b) Pregnancy

(c) Premenstrual fluid retention

(d) Obesity

(e) Arthritis

iii. Occupational risks

(a) Carpenters

(b) Piano players

(c) Keyboard operators

(d) Others requiring repetitive wrist movement or wrist pressure

iv.   Most common in females ages 40 to 60

b. Symptoms

i.   Pain, paresthesia ("pins and needles"), numbness in the hand and may radiate up the arm

ii.   Exacerbation of pain upon wrist flexion, often interrupting sleep due to normal wrist flexion during sleep

iii. Weakness in the thumb, first, second, and third fingers

c. Conservative treatment

i.   Wrist splints worn at night

ii.   Ergonomic changes in work area (padded keyboard wrist support)

2. Pathology

a. Carpal ligament—"tent" formed at base of palm which thickens with repetitive trauma

b. The carpal bones form the dorsal and lateral wall of the "tunnel"

c. Median nerve passes through this tunnel and may swell with repetitive trauma

d. Tendons of flexor muscles and bones of the wrist and hand prevent room for expansion

3. Preprocedure
   a. History
      i.   Pain, numbness, paresthesia of hand
      ii.   Weakness of grip
   b. Assessment
      i.   Atrophy of ball of thumb (thenar eminence)
      ii.   Tinel's sign—tingling sensation along the distribution of the median nerve with percussion in the area of the wrist crease
      iii. Forced wrist flexion test—after 1 minute of wrist flexion symptoms exacerbate
      iv.   Phalen's test—wrist hanging off table or chair for 30 seconds to 1 minute exacerbates symptoms
      v.   Electromyography and nerve conduction studies (EMG/NCS)
            (a) Diagnostic in most cases
      vi.   Symptoms may be elicited when blood pressure checked and cuff pressure exceeds systolic pressure; therefore avoid blood pressure checks in affected arm
      vii. Shaking or moving the hand may relieve symptoms
4. Procedure
   a. Anesthesia may be from local infiltration, Bier block, axillary block or general
   b. The carpal ligament is sectioned vertically over the median nerve
   c. Incision
      i.   Along the ulnar or medial side of the thenar grove (most common)
      ii.   Along the median grove
      iii. Endoscopically (½-inch incision)
5. Postprocedure
   a. Assessment: check all fingers but most particularly the thumb, index, and middle fingers q. 15 minutes for 1 hour, then q. 30 minutes for 1 hour, then q. hour until discharged
      i.   Sensation to touch (numbness and paresthesia is common particularly if nerve block used for anesthesia, document resolution)
      ii.   Sensation to pin prick or temperature; this is intact if patient is describing pain (with local anesthesia expect loss for several hours, record the return of this protective mechanism)
      iii. Blanching of fingertips—compare with uninvolved fingertips (normal capillary refill <1 second, greatest accuracy is comparison with other hand)
      iv.   Assess dressing for drainage and increasing tightness
   b. Care
      i.   Keep hand elevated at a level of or higher than the heart
      ii.   If dressing becomes constricting request or have standing order to clip dressing ½ to 1½ inches on back of hand
      iii. Do not take blood pressure in affected arm
   c. Discharge instructions
      i.   Keep elevated on pillows when sitting or lying
      ii.   Use sling for elevation and protection only when ambulating
      iii. Keep elbow free of pressure
      iv.   Exercise the fingers throughout the day
      v.   Check fingers for movement, sensation, and color (compare with uninvolved hand) several times a day (upon arising, at each meal, and at bedtime)
      vi.   Avoid soiling dressing or hand; use unaffected hand or ask for assistance
      vii. To bathe, place large ziplock or other plastic bag over hand and tape securely around arm for protection

        viii. Report to physician or surgery center:

           (a) Drainage, bleeding through dressing

           (b) Pain not controlled by prescribed medications

           (c) Loss of sensation, severe swelling, or skin discoloration

           (d) Soiled or wet dressing that should be changed before physician follow-up appointment

           (e) Fever >101°F

        ix. Physician follow-up appointment

B. Epidural patch

  1. Disorder

    a. Characteristics

      i. Follows a lumbar puncture (LP)

        (a) Postmyelogram

        (b) Post LP for diagnostic tests

        (c) Post intrathecal catheter removal

        (d) Post intrathecal injection of medication

      ii. Most often related to large-bore lumbar puncture needle >20 g

    b. Symptoms

      i. Severe headache

        (a) Worsens when up

        (b) May extend into neck

        (c) Prevents activities

      ii. Nausea and vomiting

    c. Conservative treatment

      i. Bed rest

      ii. Fluid challenge

      iii. Analgesics/antiemetics

      iv. Abdominal binder

  2. Pathology

    a. Mechanical tension on the meninges

      i. Headache

      ii. Neck stiffness (nuchal rigidity)

    b. Mechanical tension of the central nervous system

      i. Nausea/vomiting

      ii. Photophobia

      iii. Irritability

  3. Preprocedure

    a. History

      i. Recent lumbar puncture (2 days to 2 weeks)

      ii. Failed conservative treatment

      iii. Persistent headache, nausea, and vomiting

    b. Assessment

      i. Description of headache (usually frontal and extends over head into neck)

      ii. Pain scale rating

      iii. Level of dehydration

        (a) Fluid intake for past several days

        (b) Amount of vomiting

        (c) When last voided

        (d) Skin turgor

        (e) Venous prominence

        (f) Hypotension

        (g) Tachycardia

        (h) Electrolytes

4. Procedure
   a. Have patient lie down in quiet, dark room with limited visitors
   b. Patient may be too ill to listen to detailed instructions; limit information
   c. Detailed explanations may be given to significant other
   d. Establish at least one intravenous route (two sites may be needed if severely dehydrated)
   e. Prepare to obtain 15 to 20 cc of blood under careful aseptic technique for patch (physician may prefer to obtain blood)
      i. Intermittent IV access for blood retrieval
      ii. Prep site for phlebotomy
         (a) Povodine prep
   f. Place patient prone (pillow under abdomen)
      i. May be done under fluoroscopy
   g. Epidural puncture is performed (best if at previous LP site)
      i. Anesthesia
         (a) Local infiltration
         (b) IV conscious sedation
   h. Assist with LP prep (warm povodine in microwave, for patient comfort)
   i. Obtain or assist with blood for patch
   j. Blood is injected into epidural space
   k. Bandaid applied (remove povodine from LP-prepped area on back)
5. Postprocedure
   a. Assessment
      i. Severity of headache (pain scale)
      ii. Description of headache (observe for changes)
      iii. Observe for nerve root irritation (blood may cross into CSF)
         (a) Symptoms worsen
         (b) Pain in legs or groin area
         (c) Inability to void
   b. Care
      i. Force fluid, caffeinated (IV fluid bolus, if nausea persists)
      ii. Caffeine
         (a) Beverages
         (b) Tablets
         (c) IV (caffeine, sodium benzoate, 500 mg)
      iii. Bed rest with head of bed flat
      iv. Establish ability to void
   c. Discharge instructions
      i. Bed rest with only a small pillow
         (a) Up to bathroom only for 24 hours
         (b) Then gradually increase activity
         (c) If symptoms return, return to bed rest with bathroom privileges
      ii. No straining, no lifting for 1 week
      iii. No exercising for 1 week
      iv. No sexual activity for 1 week
      v. Remove bandaid after 24 hours
      vi. May take short shower in warm (not hot) water after 24 hours if symptoms have improved
      vii. Avoid aspirin-containing products
      viii. Notify physician
         (a) Temp >101°F

      (b) Pain not controlled by prescribed medication
      (c) Nuchal rigidity begins or worsens
      (d) Nausea persists, unable to take in fluids
    ix.   At any point, if symptoms return, bed rest must be resumed (patch procedure may be repeated)
C. Excision of neuroma
  1. Disorder
    a. Characteristics
      i.   Results from trauma to the nerve, particularly the axon
         (a) Surgical or traumatic incision
         (b) Amputation sites
         (c) Repeated trauma
            (i)   Oral from dentures, etc.
            (ii) Wrist/hand from repetitive work injuries, etc.
            (iii) Morton's neuroma from trauma to the digital nerve
            (iv) Any traumatized nerve
      ii. Associated health factors
         (a) Traumatic injuries
         (b) Familial tendency
         (c) Poorly fitted shoes
      iii. Morton's neuroma more common in adult women
    b. Symptoms
      i.   Pain at neuroma site
      ii. Numbness and tingling around neuroma and distally
    c. Conservative treatment
      i.   Injection with various medications and saline
      ii. At operative/amputation sites many methods have been and are currently being tried to prevent neuroma formation
      iii. Morton's neuroma
         (a) Padding in shoes
         (b) Limiting walking/standing
         (c) Proper fitting footwear, avoiding heels >1 inch
  2. Pathology
    a. The traumatized axon degenerates to the next proximal node of Ranvier
    b. Axonal sprouts grow out as the axon repairs itself
    c. When the axonal sprouts do not grow to the end organ, they continue to grow in a random bundle, forming a neuroma
  3. Preprocedure
    a. History
      i.   Pain
      ii. Paresthesia
    b. Assessment
      i.   Pain scale score
      ii. Sensitivity to palpation
      iii. Degree of sensory deficit distal to neuroma
         (a) Morton's neuroma test sensitivity of toes to pain/temperature
         (b) Other sites test as appropriate
      iv. Obtain MRI or CT if completed as part of medical workup
  4. Procedure
    a. Anesthesia may be local infiltration, nerve block, epidural, spinal, or general
    b. The neuroma is excised and the nerve ending may be buried into bone, muscle, or other attempts to prevent reoccurrence

    c. Morton's neuroma
       i.   Incision
          (a) Vertical plantar
          (b) Dorsal

5. Postprocedure
    a. Assessment: check extremity distal to surgical site q. 15 minutes for 1 hour, q. 30 minutes for 1 hour, and q. hour until discharge
       i.   Sensation to touch distal to surgical site (consider type of anesthesia, document resolution)
       ii. Sensation to pain/temperature distal to surgical site, compare preop pain score and description to postop (consider type of anesthesia, document resolution)
       iii. Capillary refill and warmth of digits compare with unaffected extremity (capillary refill <1 second)
       iv. Assess dressing for drainage and increasing tightness
    b. Care
       i.   Keep extremity elevated at level or above heart
       ii. If dressing becomes constricting obtain order or have standing order to clip ½ to 1½ inches on opposite surface of incision
       iii. If upper extremity, avoid taking blood pressure in affected arm
    c. Discharge instructions
       i.   If pain and temperature sensation not in tact distally to surgical site, skin integrity should be checked at least daily; protective devices should be worn to prevent injury
          (a) Morton's neuroma
             (i)   Inspect toes and bottom of foot daily
             (ii) Do not wear open-toe shoes
             (iii) Wear properly fitted shoes with adequate toe box
          (b) Wrist/hand
             (i)   Inspect fingers and hand daily
             (ii) Wear thick gloves for gardening, dishwashing, etc.
             (iii) Avoid tight-fitting rings
       ii. Keep extremity elevated on pillows when sitting or lying
       iii. For upper extremity, may have sling for when up; for lower extremity, ambulation should be limited to bathroom and necessity for 1 week
       iv. Keep elbow free of pressure (upper extremity procedure)
       v.   Exercise fingers or toes throughout the day
       vi. Check fingers or toes for movement, sensation, and color (compare with unaffected extremity) upon arising, at meal times, and at bedtime
       vii. Avoid soiling dressing or extremity
       viii. To bathe, place large ziplock or other plastic bag over extremity and tape securely in place; keep extremity elevated out of bath water
       ix. Report to physician or surgery center
          (a) Drainage, bleeding through dressing
          (b) Pain not controlled by prescribed medications
          (c) Loss of sensation, severe swelling, or skin discoloration
          (d) Soiled or wet dressing that should be changed before physician follow-up appointment
          (e) Fever >101°F
       x.   Physician follow-up appointment
       xi. Neuroma may return, preventive measures/lifestyle changes
          (a) Morton's neuroma

(i)   Properly fitted shoes, ½-inch heels
(ii)   Sit rather than stand, limit walking
(iii)   Low impact exercise, prefer to avoid foot pressure (bicycle rather than step-aerobics, etc.)
(b) Wrist/hand trauma
(i)   Assess work station for improved methods
(ii)   Wear padded protective devices

D. Microendoscopic diskectomy (lumbar disc removal)
1. Disorder
    a. Characteristics
        i.   Ruptured intravertebral disc with resulting pressure on a nerve
        ii.   Associated health factors: no clear indication of a particular risk factor except age; disc rupture in most cases is thought to be due to the weight-loading of an erect posture
            (a) Misuse of back
            (b) Static positions at work
                (i)   Sitting at a desk/workstation
                (ii)   Standing at a workstation
                (iii)   Sedentary lifestyle
            (c) Weight-loading phenomenon
                (i)   Load that is too heavy
                (ii)   Load that is too bulky
        iii.   Occupational risks
            (a) Poor ergonomic conditions
            (b) Little ability to change position at work area
            (c) No particular occupation at risk
        iv.   Age-related phenomenon
            (a) Greatest risk between 30 to 50 years of age
            (b) Peak occurrence in the 40s
    b. Symptoms
        i.   Pain
            (a) Sharp, stabbing, burning
            (b) Radiates into a dermotome and can be fairly accurately traced by the patient
            (c) Pain increases with any straining, Valsalva's maneuver, sneezing, coughing
        ii.   Paresthesia may exist anywhere along the affected dermatome
        iii.   Weakness and atrophy may become evident in the muscles innervated by the specific nerve root
        iv.   Decreased or loss of reflexes specific to the innervation of the involved nerve root
        v.   Specific nerve root involvement (disc rupture at one level may involve more than one root and with individual anatomical variations symptoms may vary)
            (a) Pressure on L4, L5, or S1 nerve root (sciatica)
                (i)   Pain radiating down one buttock, possibly into the ipsilateral posterior thigh, knee, calf, and may extend all the way into the foot
                (ii)   Usually more comfortable with leg flexed
                (iii)   Sitting may be particularly painful
                (iv)   Weakness
                    a) L5—unable to walk on heels due to weakness of dorsoflexion
                    b) S1—unable to walk on toes due to weakness of plantarflexion

(v) L4 and L5—most common areas of disc herniation in the lumbar spine

(b) Pressure on L2 or L3 nerve root (more rare)

(i) Pain radiating into the groin, anterior thigh, and medial calf of affected leg

(ii) Will usually assume a position of knee and hip flexion with lateral rotation of the hip

c. Conservative treatment

   i. Activity restrictions

     (a) Bed rest

     (b) Avoid sitting for >30 minutes at a time

   ii. Steroid or antiinflammatory treatment

     (a) Topical

     (b) Oral medication

   iii. Traction

   iv. Exercise

   v. Heat and massage

   vi. Ice massage or ice application

   vii. Sleeping position/mattress adjustments

   viii. Ergonomic evaluation of work environment

2. Pathology

a. Disc (ruptured disc can be compared with a jelly-filled donut that has been compressed slightly—the jelly exits out of the open rim)

   i. Fibrous outer rim—annulus fibrosa—tear in this rim allows gelatinous nucleus pulposus to herniate out

   ii. Gelatinous center—nucleus pulposus—becomes drier as we age, therefore fewer disc ruptures after age 50, although other aging processes cause low back pain

     (a) Allows for bending of spine

     (b) Hydraulic shock absorber for upright position

b. Vertebrae

   i. Body—in between each body there is a disc

   ii. Laminal arch—the thin bone at the side of the spinous process of which a piece is removed in order to get over the nerve root and ruptured disc

   iii. Spinous process—the bone ridge that you feel when you run your hand down the back

   iv. Spinal foramen—opening in center of vertebra for the spinal cord

   v. Neural foramen—canal on each side of the vertebra for the pair of exiting nerve roots

c. Posterior spinous ligament—thick in the center, weaker edges allows most common disc ruptures to be lateral at the neural foramen

d. The laterally ruptured disc "pinches" the nerve root between it and the bone of the neural foremen, leading to the radiating nerve root pain, paresthesia, numbness, and eventually weakness

e. Individual differences

   i. Not all persons with a ruptured disc are symptomatic

   ii. Not all persons with classic symptoms have a ruptured disc

   iii. Many people with nerve root pain, given time and conservative treatment, can avoid or delay surgery

f. Goals of disc removal (does not stop back pain)

   i. Relieve pain that interferes with the quality of life

   ii. Prevent permanent motor weakness and muscle atrophy

g. Disc degeneration and nerve root symptoms are not life threatening, therefore this is considered an elective procedure by most

3. Preprocedure

a. History

    i.   Failed conservative treatment

    ii. No history of previous back surgery, particularly near the level of anticipated surgery

    iii. Lateral disc herniation (can be performed bilaterally)

b. Assessment

    i.   Pattern and description of pain, paresthesia, and numbness

    ii. Pain scale score

    iii. Preferred position that helps decrease pain

    iv. Any positions that increase pain

    v. Weakness

       (a) Walk on toes

       (b) Walk on heels

       (c) Difficulty with ambulation

       (d) Elimination difficulties

          (i)   Incontinence

          (ii) Difficulty voiding

    vi. MRI, CT, myelogram results (MRI may be diagnostic without myelogram)

    vii. Electromyogram (EMG)/nerve conduction study (NCS) results (may or may not be done)

4. Procedure

a. Patient has Foley catheter inserted (due to length of procedure)

b. Placed over frame

c. A small 15-mm incision is made over the site (left or right of the midline)

d. The endoscope is positioned and verified with X-ray

e. Part of the lamina is removed to allow access to the nerve root

f. The nerve root is identified and protected as the loose pieces of disc are removed

g. The nerve root is verified as being "free" without pressure

h. A foramenotomy may be performed (bone along the neural foramen can be drilled away leaving a slightly larger area for the nerve to pass through)

i. Equipment is removed and a bandaid is placed over the entry site (occasionally a stitch or staple is used to control bleeding)

j. Benefits

    i.   Can be done under local or epidural anesthesia

    ii. Minimal tissue damage to skin, muscle, and other tissue at entry site

    iii. Minimal scarring, therefore less morbidity

5. Postprocedure

a. Assessment

    i.   Description of pain, paresthesia, numbness; compare with preoperative

    ii. Pain scale score; compare with preoperative

    iii. Weakness

       (a) Walk on heels

       (b) Walk on toes

       (c) Difficulty ambulating

    iv. Bandaid intact without bleeding

    v. Able to void

b. Care

    i.   Remove Foley catheter

    ii.   Teach to get out of bed "statue style"
        (a) Turn to unaffected side
        (b) Lower legs off bed, while pushing upper body up with upper
             extremities, keeping back straight
    iii. Ambulate increasing distances and to bathroom, to ensure ambulation
        ability at home

  c. Discharge instructions
    i.   No lifting of anything more heavy than a cup, newspaper
    ii.   No bending, stooping, leaning, straining, or exercise
    iii. Do not stay in bed; being up most of day will help patient rest better at night
    iv. Sleep on a firm mattress
    v.   Listen to your back; if you feel tired, rest; if you feel "stiff," walk
    vi. Do not rest on a boggy couch; if you have a recliner you may recline
        back in it
    vii. Do not stay in one position for an extended period of time; avoid sitting
        for more than 30 minutes to 1 hour without taking a short walk
    viii. No driving, may ride for short distances
    ix. Remove bandaid after 48 hours
    x.   May shower after 48 hours, pat wound dry (may replace bandaid after
        wound is completely dry)
    xi. No sitting in a tub of water with incision under water
    xii. Call physician
        (a) Fever >101°F
        (b) Unusual headache that worsens when up
        (c) Pain not controlled by prescribed medication
        (d) Drainage from or swelling around the operative site
        (e) Persistent nausea or vomiting
    xiii. Physician follow-up visit

E. Muscle biopsy
  1. Disorder
    a. Characteristic (diagnostic of motor disorders)
      i.   Muscular dystrophy
      ii.   Autoimmune diseases
      iii. Metabolic defects
      iv. Genetic disorders
      v.   Differentiation between myopathic verses neurogenic etiology
      vi. Other
    b. Symptoms
      i.   Vary greatly depending on disorder and progression
         (a) Weakness
           (i)   Totally independent, deficits not noticeable
           (ii) Needs minimal assistance
           (iii) Needs moderate assistance
           (iv) Needs maximum assistance
         (b) Involvement
           (i)   Symmetrical (affecting both sides equally)
           (ii) Asymmetrical (one side more affected than the other)
           (iii) Proximal involvement (truncal muscles and muscles closer to the
               body more affected)
           (iv) Distal involvement (hands and feet more greatly affected than
               shoulder and hip)
           (v)   Segmental (upper extremities affected greater or lesser than lower
               extremities)

2. Pathology
   a. Striated muscle tissue involvement
      i. Atrophy
      ii. Necrosis
      iii. Regeneration
      iv. Inflammation
      v. Abnormal number or size of fibers
      vi. Infection
      vii. Parasite infiltration
      viii. Other
3. Preprocedure
   a. History
      i. Weakness
         (a) Areas affected
         (b) Severity
      ii. Pain description/scale score
      iii. Limitation of activities of daily living
      iv. Recent IM injection or EMG of specific muscle precludes biopsy of involved muscle
   b. Assessment
      i. Strength
      ii. Independence/dependence
      iii. Pain
         (a) Description
         (b) Scale score
4. Procedure
   a. Site
      i. Upper extremity
         (a) Biceps
         (b) Deltoids
      ii. Lower extremity
         (a) Quadriceps
         (b) Gastrocnemius (particularly if nerve biopsy is performed at the same time)
   b. Anesthesia
      i. May be avoided due to alteration in results
      ii. Local use of EMLA or other topicals should be considered
      iii. Local skin infiltration
      iv. Nerve block
   c. Technique
      i. Percutaneous—large-bore biopsy needle
      ii. Open biopsy: incision 2 to 8 cm
   d. Tissue preservative
      i. Obtain specific storage, transport, and preservative information and equipment/chemicals
      ii. Improper care can make specimen inadequate for testing
5. Postprocedure
   a. Assessment
      i. Dressing integrity (type of dressing determined by extent of biopsy)
      ii. Pressure dressing with elastic wrap, check for constriction, capillary refill, warmth, and swelling
      iii. Pain description and scale score

b. Care
  i.   Ice may be applied to decrease bruising
  ii. Limit activity of extremity involved
  iii. Elevate extremity
  iv. Elastic pressure dressing may require rewrapping if constricting
c. Discharge instructions
  i.   Keep dressing dry
  ii. Dressing changes
      (a) Percutaneous with bandaid and elastic wrap after 24 hours
      (b) Incision dressing and elastic wrap according to specific physician
          (varies from 48 hours to suture removal at 7 to 10 days postbiopsy)
  iii. Shower after dressing removed
  iv. Do not soak in tub for 1 week or until 24 hours after suture removal
  v.   Limit activities
      (a) Percutaneous—2 days
      (b) Open—1 week
  vi. Call physician
      (a) Fever >101°F
      (b) Redness, swelling, inflammation evident at site
      (c) Drainage from site
      (d) Pain not controlled by analgesics
  vii. Follow-up with physician performing biopsy and/or referral physician
F. Nerve biopsy (controversial due to discomfort and morbidity)
  1. Disorder
    a. Characteristics (diagnosis of motor or sensory pathology)
      i.   Genetic disorders
      ii. Metabolic disorders
    b. Symptoms
      i.   Motor deficits (done in combination with muscle biopsy in order to
           diagnose whether muscle, nerve, or transmission abnormality)
      ii. Sensory deficits
    c. Involvement
      i.   Symmetrical
      ii. Asymmetrical
      iii. Proximal
      iv. Distal
      v.   Segmental
  2. Pathology
    a. Characteristics of specific neuronal disease
  3. Preprocedure
    a. History
      i.   Weakness
      ii. Loss of sensation
      iii. Paresthesia
      iv. Dysesthesia
      v.   Pain
          (a) Description
          (b) Scale score
      vi. Does anything make symptoms worse or improve symptoms
    b. Assessment
      i.   Assess deficits
          (a) Sensory-loss areas
          (b) Motor deficits

      ii. Sensory changes
        (a) Pain (current)
          (i)   Description
          (ii) Scale score
        (b) Paraesthesia
     iii. Information regarding procedure
        (a) Painful when nerve is incised
        (b) Sensory deficit may result
        (c) Neuroma may form at biopsy site

4. Procedure
  a. Site (upper extremities are avoided due to residual deficit following biopsy)
     i.   Sensory-sural nerve
     ii.   Motor
        (a) Deep peroneal nerve
        (b) Accessory deep peroneal nerve
  b. Anesthesia
     i.   Local infiltration
     ii.   Nerve block proximal to biopsy just prior to incision
  c. Technique
     i.   Sural nerve
        (a) 8-cm incision lateral and parallel to Achilles tendon
          (i)   Entire nerve if sensation has been lost
          (ii) Fibers biopsied with attempts to maintain some sensation in
              innervated area
        (b) Distal 1 to 2-cm incision medial to the saphenous vein
     ii.   Peroneal nerve
        (a) Lateral incision from fibular head to the tibia

5. Postprocedure
  a. Assessment
     i.   Pain control as anesthesia resolves
        (a) Description of pain
        (b) Pain scale score
     ii.   Sensory deficits
        (a) Loss of pain and temperature
        (b) Proprioception loss
        (c) Paraesthesia
          (i)   Severity
          (ii) Description (burning, tingling, itching)
        (d) Loss of light touch (numbness)
     iii. Motor deficits
     iv. Assess proximal to site for pressure signs from tourniquet/cuff used
        during surgery to control bleeding
     v.   Integrity of dressing
        (a) Drainage
        (b) Elastic wrap pressure dressing, check for constriction, capillary refill,
          warmth, and swelling
  b. Care
     i.   Limit activity, limit weight bearing on affected leg
     ii.   Elevate extremity except when up to bathroom
  c. Discharge instructions
     i.   Keep dressing dry
        (a) Small incision dressing may be changed after 48 hours

        (b) Large incisions may be wrapped with elastic dressing and physician may prefer to change dressing at return visit—verify physician preferences

    ii. May bathe with involved leg supported out of water

    iii. May shower when pressure dressing removed; dry wound and replace dressing

    iv. Sutures will be removed in 10 to 14 days (7 days for small incision)

    v. If pain and temperature sensation lost, demonstrate to patient and warn of safety concerns

        (a) Inspect area daily

        (b) When wearing new footwear, observe after 2 hours for pressure areas

        (c) Test bath water with uninvolved extremity

    vi. If proprioception lost

        (a) Be alert to increased risk of falls

        (b) Wear low-heeled shoes

        (c) Use a slower pace (using a cane may help remind patient)

        (d) Scan field; use vision to compensate for proprioception loss

    vii. Paraesthesia

        (a) May persist for months

        (b) Becomes intermittent

        (c) Worse upon first arising or after sitting for long periods

    viii. Limit activity, up to bathroom

        (a) Small incision limit for 2 days

        (b) Seven to 10 days for large incisions

    ix. Elevate extremity when not ambulating

    x. Wear cotton or wool socks

    xi. Notify physician

        (a) Temperature >101°F

        (b) Signs of infection

        (c) Drainage from site

        (d) Pain not controlled by prescribed medication

        (e) Pressure dressing resulting in swelling and discomfort of extremity

        (f) Persistent paraesthesia

    xii. If sensory deficits/alterations are severe, refer to foot care clinic for follow-up care

    xiii. Follow-up with surgeon and/or referring physician

G. Ulnar nerve transfers (cubital tunnel syndrome, tardy ulnar palsy, Feindel-Osborne Syndrome)—some controversy exists as to whether transposition is the treatment of choice; several options exist such as decompression of the cubital tunnel

  1. Disorder

    a. Characteristics

      i. Ulnar nerve entrapment

        (a) Following trauma to the elbow

        (b) Due to prolonged pressure

           (i) Leaning on the elbow during telephone use

           (ii) Bed rest related to illness or surgery

        (c) Callus formation in the ulnar groove

    b. Symptoms

      i. Numbness of fifth and lateral aspect of the fourth fingers

      ii. Weakness of abduction and flexion of the fourth and fifth fingers

      iii. Loss of dexterity of hand

      iv. Loss of proprioception

      v. Eventually clawing of the fourth and fifth fingers and wrist

    c. Conservative treatment
       i.   Elbow padding
       ii. Relieve pressure on elbow
       iii. Antiinflammatory agents

2. Pathology
    a. Ulnar nerve arises from the brachial plexus
    b. Travels in the posterior upper arm
    c. Enters the forearm through the cubital tunnel at the elbow (vulnerable and common area of trauma)
       i.   The capacity of the cubital tunnel is minimized during flexion of the elbow, therefore the nerve and tunnel are at greatest risk for damage during flexion
          (a) Pressure
          (b) Trauma
          (c) Overuse
       ii. The capacity of the cubital tunnel is maximized during the extension of the elbow
    d. Continues down the posterior arm into the fourth and fifth fingers

3. Preprocedure
    a. History
       i.   Onset is insidious
       ii. Paraesthesia of fourth and fifth fingers
       iii. Pain may not exist
       iv. Hand clumsiness
       v.   Health risks related to poor recovery
          (a) Advanced age
          (b) Neuropathy
             (i)   Diabetic
             (ii) Alcoholic
             (iii) Renal
          (c) Muscle atrophy in ulnar nerve distribution
          (d) Acute trauma
    b. Assessment
       i.   Pattern and description of paraesthesia
       ii. Pain
          (a) Pain pattern and scale score
          (b) If no pain, test for pain and/or temperature sensation in fourth and fifth fingers and hand
       iii. Grip strength
       iv. Do not take blood pressure in affected arm

4. Procedure
    a. Anesthesia
       i.   Axillary nerve block
       ii. General
    b. Incision between the olecranon process and the medial epicondyle of the humerus
    c. Incision length about 10 cm
    d. The ulnar nerve is brought out of the cubital tunnel and placed anteriorly
    e. Several variations exist
       i.   Subcutaneous
       ii. Submuscular

5. Postprocedure
   a. Assessment
      i. Sensation of fifth and lateral one-half of fourth fingers
      ii. Pain description and scale score
      iii. Motor
         (a) Fourth and fifth fingers
         (b) Grip strength
         (c) Wrist movement
      iv. Capillary refill of fingers <1 second or compare with uninvolved hand
      v. Dressing fit and tightness
      vi. Immobilizer, cast, or splint fit without pressure areas
      vii. Drainage
   b. Care
      i. Keep elbow immobilized at a right angle
         (a) Cast or splint
         (b) Elastic immobilizer
      ii. Active and isometric exercises should be performed prior to discharge
   c. Discharge instructions
      i. Immobilized for several weeks at a right angle
      ii. Removal, replacement, and care of immobilization device
      iii. Inspection of skin for pressure areas due to immobilization
      iv. Active exercises of the fingers, hand, wrist, and shoulder 3 to 4 times/day
      v. Isometric exercises of the forearm and biceps/triceps 3 to 4 times daily
      vi. Dressing changes specific to immobilization device and physician
      vii. Return of function may take months
      viii. Notify physician
         (a) Temperature >101°F
         (b) Pain not relieved by prescribed medication
         (c) Bleeding or drainage
         (d) Pressure area or symptoms of pressure under device
            (i) Unusual odor
            (ii) Drainage on device
      ix. Physician follow-up appointment

BOX 32-1.   Key Patient Educational Outcomes

- The post microendoscopic diskectomy patient will be able to demonstrate proper technique for getting out of bed
- The post carpal tunnel release patient will verbalize the importance of keeping the extremity elevated using a pillow or sling, keeping the elbow free of pressure, exercising fingers frequently, and checking the fingers for movement and sensation
- The post epidural blood patch patient will verbalize the importance of remaining on bed rest for 24 hours postprocedure
- The patient and/or significant other will demonstrate knowledge of medication administration (analgesics, antibiotics, antiemetics, etc.) by describing the purpose and administration of each medication prescribed
- The patient and/or significant other will describe the proper procedure for dressing care per the physicians' instruction
- The patient with a sensory/perceptual deficit will verbalize recognition of the deficit and discuss methods to compensate by using other perceptual modalities

Bibliography

1. Baker, E. (1994). *Neuroscience Nursing.* St. Louis: Mosby.
2. DeMyer, W.E. (1993). *Technique of the Neurologic Examination,* 4th ed. New York: McGraw-Hill.
3. Litwack, K. ed. (1995). *Core Curriculum for Post Anesthesia Nursing Practice,* 3rd ed. Philadelphia: Saunders.
4. Marshall, B.A., Miller, R.H. (1995). *Essentials of Neu-*

rosurgery, A Guide to Clinical Practice. New York: McGraw-Hill.
5. Wall, P.D., Melzack, R. (1994). *Textbook of Pain,* 3rd ed. Edinburgh: Churchill Livingstone.
6. Wilkins, R.H., Rengachary, S.S. (1996). *Neurosurgery,* 2nd ed. Vol III. New York: McGraw-Hill.
7. Wolf, J. (1981). *Segmental Neurology.* Syracuse: University Park Press.

REVIEW QUESTIONS

1. If a patient experiences a generalized tonic clonic seizure (grand mal), the nurse should **not**

   A. Turn the patient on his/her side to prevent aspiration of saliva or vomitus
   B. Put something into the mouth to prevent the tongue from being swallowed
   C. Obtain a stat glucose and electrolytes
   D. Note the time of onset of the seizure

2. To enter the intrathecal sack, the physician has to pass through the

   A. Medulla oblongata
   B. Peripheral nerves
   C. Myelin
   D. Dura

3. Carpal tunnel syndrome results in all except

   A. Paresthesia in the toes
   B. Pain that may radiate up into the proximal limb
   C. Paresthesia in the hands
   D. Symptoms severe enough to awaken the person from sleep

4. During a postoperative assessment, the most important aspect of a neurological assessment is

   A. Memory
   B. Sensation
   C. Level of consciousness
   D. Strength

5. The patient receiving an epidural patch should be instructed to call the physician if symptoms of meningitis exist. These symptoms include
   (1) Worsening headache
   (2) Neck stiffness
   (3) Temperature >101°F
   (4) Nausea/vomiting persists or worsens

   A. All of the above
   B. 1, 2, 3
   C. 2
   D. 3

6. The neurological examination of an extremity should include

   A. Pain/temperature sensation, touch sensation, proprioception, paresthesia, and strength/movement
   B. Pain/temperature sensation and movement
   C. Movement only
   D. Proprioception, paresthesia

7. If sensation to pain/temperature has not returned to an extremity, the patient should be taught to do all of the following except:

   A. Test bath water with unaffected extremity
   B. Check skin integrity daily during bath or prior to bed
   C. Stimulate the area with ice and hot water daily
   D. Wear protective device such as gloves or footwear to prevent injury

8. A neuroma in the peripheral nervous system is a

A. Tumor of glial cells
B. Cluster of axonal sprouts
C. Tumor of nerve bodies
D. Cluster of dendrites

9. The site of a muscle biopsy may be less painful if the nurse does all of the following except

A. Elevate the extremity
B. Encourage exercise
C. Apply ice
D. Restrict activity

10. Nerve entrapment syndromes result from all of the following except

A. Trauma
B. Inflammation of the nerve
C. Neuroma formation
D. Repetitive movements/use

ANSWERS TO QUESTIONS

1. B
2. D
3. A
4. C
5. A

6. A
7. C
8. B
9. B
10. C

Ophthalmologic Procedures

Nancy Saufl
Port Orange Day Surgery
Halifax Medical Center
Daytona Beach, Florida

I. Anatomy of the Eye

Refer to Figure 33–1.

A. Orbit
   1. Two orbital cavities situated either side of midverticle line of skull between cranium and skeleton
   2. A socket for the eyeball and muscles, nerves and vessels necessary for functioning of the eye
B. Eyelids
   1. Movable folds of skin covering the eye
      a. From medial canthus to lateral canthus
   2. Spread lubricating solutions over globe
      a. Keep eyes moist
      b. Prevent evaporation of secretions
   3. Cover eyes during sleep
   4. Protect eyes from excessive light
   5. Protect eyes from injury
   6. Protect eyes from foreign objects
   7. Lined with mucous membrane called palpebral conjunctiva
      a. Covers sclera (visible white portion of eye)
C. Conjunctiva
   1. Thin transparent mucous membrane
      a. Forms a sac that is open in front
      b. Lines back surface of eyelids and front surface of globe
   2. Divided into two parts
      a. Palpebral portion
         i.   Lines back of eyelids

Objectives

1. Describe the anatomy of the eye.
2. Discuss common ophthalmologic surgical procedures.
3. List drugs frequently used for ophthalmologic surgical procedures.
4. Identify possible complications of ophthalmologic surgery.
5. Discuss perianesthesia nursing care for the ophthalmologic surgery patient.

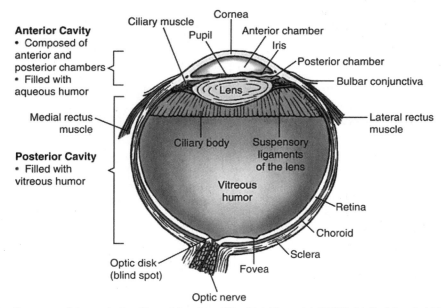

Figure 33–1. Structure of the eyeball. (From Monahan, F.D., Neighbors, M. [1998]. *Medical Surgical Nursing Foundations for Clinical Practice,* 2nd ed. Philadelphia: Saunders, p. 1936.)

      ii.   Contains openings (puncta) of the lacrimal canaliculi
      iii.   Establishes pathway between conjunctival sac and inferior meatus of nose
   b. Bulbar portion
      i.   Transparent; allows sclera to show through
      ii.   Central portion is continuous at limbus with anterior epithelium of cornea
  3. Provides mucous for lubrication
 D. Lacrimal apparatus
  1. Consists of:
   a. Lacrimal gland
      i.   Located in upper outer aspect of each orbit
      ii.   Produces tears
      iii.   Tears empty through lacrimal ducts onto conjunctiva of upper lid
      iv.   Tears are spread across eyeball by blinking
      v.   Tears enter lacrimal puncta
   b. Lacrimal puncta
      i.   Two small openings located in the inner canthus of each upper and lower eyelid
      ii.   Pass into lacrimal canals, lacrimal sac, nasolacrimal duct, and finally into inferior meatus of the turbinate bone of the nose
   c. Lacrimal sac
      i.   Collects tears
   d. Nasolacrimal duct
      i.   Drains tears from lacrimal sac to nose
  2. Tears
   a. Contain water, salts, mucus, lysozyme (bacterial enzyme), and other chemical substances
   b. Purpose
      i.   Clean, lubricate, and moisten eyeball
      ii.   Continually wash surface of eye

c. Increased production of tears when:
- i. Eye exposed to irritating substances
- ii. Emotional stimulus of parasympathetic nervous system triggered

E. Muscles controlling the eye
1. Extraocular muscles (six)
   a. Attached to outside of eyeball and to bones of the orbit
   b. Consist of voluntary skeletal muscle (see Figure 33–2)
      i. Four rectus
         (a) Superior
         (b) Inferior
         (c) Medial
         (d) Lateral
      ii. Two oblique muscles
         (a) Superior
         (b) Inferior
   c. Action
      i. Muscles move eyeball through cranial nerves
         (a) Third (oculomotor)
            (i) Moves eyeball and upper eyelid
            (ii) Size of iris (i.e., constriction and dilation of pupil to regulate amount of light admitted)
            (iii) Control of ciliary muscle to regulate degree of refraction by lens
         (b) Fourth (trochlear)
            (i) Movement of eyeball by superior oblique muscles
         (c) Sixth (abducens)
            (i) Movement of eyeball by lateral rectus muscle
      ii. Muscles work in pairs
      iii. Movement caused by:
         (a) Increase in tone of one set of muscles and a decrease in the tone of the antagonistic (opposite set) of muscles

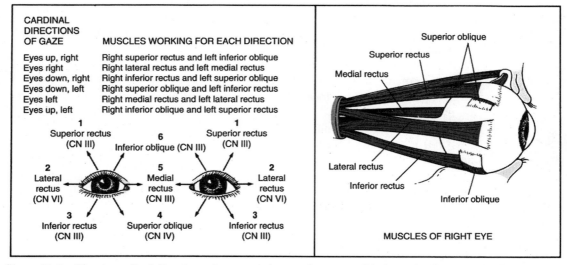

Figure 33–2. The six cardinal directions of gaze and the muscles responsible for each. The six cardinal directions are (1) right, (2) left, (3) up and right, (4) up and left, (5) down and right, and (6) down and left. (From Black, J.M., Matassarin-Jacobs, E. [1997]. *Medical-Surgical Nursing Clinical Management for Continuity of Care,* 5th ed. Philadelphia: Saunders, p. 936.)

2. Movement of upper eyelid
   a. Raised (opened) by levator palpebrae superioris muscle
      i.   Controlled by cranial nerve III and sympathetic nervous system
   b. Closed by orbicularis oculi muscle
      i.   Controlled by cranial nerve VII
3. Iris and ciliary muscles
   a. Smooth, involuntary muscle
   b. Work inside eyeball
      i.   Regulates size of pupil
      ii. Controls shape of lens during accommodation
      iii. Controlled through neural network
           (a) Optic nerve (cranial nerve II)
           (b) Oculomotor nerve (cranial nerve III)
F. Globe (eyeball): supported in orbital cavity on a cushion of fat and fascia; composed of three layers
   1. External, corneal–scleral layer (fibrous, protects other two layers)
      a. Cornea
         i.   Anterior, transparent, avascular part of the external layer
         ii. Serves as a window through which light rays pass to retina
         iii. Supplied by branches of ophthalmic division of fifth cranial nerve
         iv. Composed of five layers
              (a) Epithelium
                  (i)   Cell layers and nerve endings
                  (ii) Account for corneal sensitivity
              (b) Bowman's membrane
                  (i)   Composed of connective tissue fibers
                  (ii) Forms a barrier between trauma and infection
                  (iii) Does not regenerate if damaged
                  (iv) Will leave a permanent scar
              (c) Stroma
                  (i)   Accounts for 90% of corneal thickening
                  (ii) Composed of multiple lamellar fibers
              (d) Descemet's membrane
                  (i)   Thin layer between endothelial layer of cornea and substantia propria (fibrous, tough, and transparent main part of the cornea)
                  (ii) If inflamed, called descemetitis
                  (iii) If protrudes, called descemetocele
              (e) Endothelium
                  (i)   Single layer of hexagonal cells
                  (ii) Does not regenerate
                  (iii) Responsible for proper state of dehydration that keeps cornea clear
                  (iv) Damage causes corneal edema and loss of transparency
      b. Sclera: posterior opaque part of the external layer; tough white outer coat of eyeball
         i.   Portion of sclera can be seen through the conjunctiva as the white of the eye
         ii. Made up of collagenous fibers loosely connected with fascia which receives the tendons of the muscles of the globe
   2. Middle layer: middle covering of the eye comprises the choroid, ciliary body, and iris (referred to as uveal tract)

a. Choroid
   i.   Most posterior portion of middle coat
   ii. Contains many blood vessels; highly vascular
   iii. Deeply pigmented
   iv. Purpose
        (a) Absorbs light rays
        (b) Prevents reflection within eyeball
        (c) Main source of nourishment to retina (through its blood supply)
b. Ciliary body
   i.   Consists of an extension of the choroidal blood vessels, a mass of muscle tissue, and an extension of the neuroepithelium of the retina
   ii. Composed of ciliary muscle and ciliary processes
   iii. Ciliary muscle
        (a) Affects accommodation
        (b) Alters shape of lens as needed to focus light rays from near or distant objects on retina
   iv. Ciliary processes
        (a) Produce aqueous humor
c. Iris
   i.   Colored area of eye
   ii. Anterior portion of the middle layer
        (a) Thin membrane situated in front of the lens
   iii. Peripheral border attached to ciliary body
   iv. Central border is free
   v.   Divides the space between the cornea and the lens
        (a) Anterior and posterior chambers
        (b) Chambers are filled with aqueous humor
   vi. Regulates the amount of light entering the eye
        (a) Muscles contract and relax
        (b) Change size of opening in center (pupil)
        (c) Assists in obtaining clear images
3. Internal layer: innermost layer of neural coat (retina)
   a. Retina
      i.   A thin transparent membrane extending from the ora serrata to the optic disk
      ii. Consists of network of nerve cells and fibers
           (a) Receives images of external objects
           (b) Transfers the impressions via the optic nerve, optic tracts, lateral geniculate body, and optic radiations to the occipital lobe of cerebrum
           (c) Nerve fibers from retina converge to become optic nerve
                (i) Point at which optic nerve enters eyeball is called optic disk (anatomic blind spot)
      iii. Covers choroid
      iv. Found only in back of eye
   b. Retina is composed of layers
      i.   Outer pigment
           (a) Stores vitamin A; needed to produce photopigment rhodopsin
      ii. Inner neural
           (a) Consists of photoreceptor cells (rods and cones)
                (i) Visual receptors that develop generator potentials
                (ii) Relays sensory information to ganglion cells of retina

(b) Rods
  (i)   Located in peripheral retina
  (ii) Allow for vision in dim light
  (iii) Responsible for perception of different shades of light and dark, shapes, and movement
(c) Cones
  (i)   Stimulated by bright light only
  (ii) Responsible for color vision and visual acuity

G. Refractive apparatus (cornea, aqueous humor, lens, and vitreous body)
  1. Cornea
    a. Has greatest refractive power of the ocular structures
    b. Variations in curvature of cornea change its refractive power
  2. Aqueous humor
    a. Fluid responsible for maintaining intraocular pressure
    b. Produced by ciliary processes
    c. Secreted by ciliary body into posterior chamber
    d. Flows from posterior chamber through pupil into anterior chamber
    e. Flows into anterior chamber angle and is filtered out through the trabecular meshwork into Schlemm's canal
    f. Channeled into capillary network and into episcleral veins
    g. Maintenance of normal intraocular pressure
      i.   Occurs as long as there is a balance between:
        (a) Aqueous production **and**
        (b) Aqueous humor outflow
  3. Lens
    a. Suspended behind the iris
    b. Anterior and posterior surfaces are separated by rounded border
    c. Does not shed cells; as it grows the cells compress and harden
    d. Lens expands and retracts through zonular fibers (accommodation)
    e. Accommodation power is lost with aging process
    f. Hardening eventually causes opacity of lens (cataract)
  4. Vitreous body
    a. Glasslike transparent gelatinous mass (vitreous humor)
    b. Composed of 99% water and 1% collagen and hyaluronic acid
    c. Fills the posterior four fifths of the eyeball
    d. Supports the posterior cavity
    e. Keeps the retina in place

H. Nerve and blood supply
  1. Optic nerve (second cranial nerve)
    a. Extends between posterior eyeball and optic chiasma
    b. Carries visual impulses and sensations of pain, touch, temperature from eye to brain
  2. Muscle innervation
    a. Oculomotor (third cranial nerve): primary motor nerve to all rectus muscles (except lateral rectus)
    b. Abducens (sixth cranial nerve) innervates lateral rectus
    c. Trochlear (fourth cranial nerve) innervates superior oblique muscle
  3. Ophthalmic artery
    a. Main arterial supply to orbit and globe
    b. Branch of internal carotid artery

II. Common Ophthalmic Surgical Procedures

A. Blepharoplasty
   1. Description
      a. Repair of the upper or lower eyelid to remove redundant skin
      b. May be cosmetic or therapeutic when the eyelid interferes with vision
      c. Types
         i.   Upper blepharoplasty (upper eyelid only)
         ii. Lower blepharoplasty (lower eyelid only)
         iii. Quadrilateral blepharoplasty (involving all four eyelids)
   2. Preoperative considerations
      a. Patient may be examined by ophthalmologist prior to procedure to rule out ocular symptomatology
   3. Surgical procedure
      a. Excess skin and muscle are resected; periorbital fat is trimmed
      b. Requires meticulous hemostasis
      c. Closed using fine nonabsorbable suture
   4. Postoperative considerations
      a. Iced saline dressings applied immediately to control edema

B. Removal of chalazion
   1. Description
      a. Granulomatous inflammation of a meibomian gland in eyelid
   2. Surgical procedure
      a. Surgical incision and curettage
   3. Most commonly done under local anesthesia in physician's office
   4. Occasionally requires OR setting

C. Repair of entropion
   1. Description
      a. Inward turning, inversion of eyelid
      b. Usually affects lower lid (can affect upper)
      c. Lashes scrape across cornea with each eye blink
      d. Results in corneal ulcer
      e. Seldom seen in persons under 40 years of age
      f. Performed under local or general anesthesia
   2. Intraoperative procedure
      a. Surgical correction of the muscular fibers of the lid, everting the lid margins and eyelashes
      b. Cryotherapy may be used to freeze and remove lashes
         i.   Destroys lash follicle
         ii. Prevents regrowth of lashes
         iii. Preferred method of treatment

D. Repair of ectropion
   1. Description
      a. Outward turning or eversion of eyelid
      b. Caused by relaxation of orbicularis oculi muscle
         i.   Result of normal aging process
         ii. Result of Bell's palsy
      c. Results in exposure of underlying conjunctiva
         i.   Can lead to keratitis (inflammation or infection of the cornea)
      d. Usually bilateral
      e. Common in older persons
   2. Surgical procedure
      a. Shortening of lower lid in a horizontal direction

      b. Mild case can be treated with deep electrocautery 4 to 5 mm from the lid margins

          i.   Resulting scar formation will draw lid to its normal position

E. Ptosis

  1. Description

      a. Drooping of upper eyelid

  2. Three types of ptosis

      a. Congenital

          i.   Caused by failure of levator muscle to develop

          ii.   Weakness of superior rectal muscles

      b. Acquired

          i.   Associated with loss of superior visual field in primary gaze

          ii.   Patient complains of difficulty reading or performing visual tasks in the reading gaze

          iii. Causes

              (a) Mechanical failure

                 (i)   Weight of lid

                 (ii) Trauma

              (b) Myogenic by disease

                 (i)   Muscular dystrophy

                 (ii) Myasthenia gravis

              (c) Neurogenic factors

                 (i)   Caused by laceration of third cranial nerve, the levator, or both

              (d) May be caused by a tumor

          iv. Treatment based on cause and severity

      c. Senile

          i.   Results from poor muscle tone of levator

  3. Surgical procedure

      a. Objective is to create a good upper lid fold with elevation of the lid

      b. Surgical procedures based on advancement of levator muscle, frontalis muscles, or superior rectus muscle

F. Excision of pterygium

  1. Description

      a. Thick triangular growth of epithelial tissue that extends from corner of cornea to the canthus

      b. Appearance may be pale or white

      c. May grow over the pupillary opening

      d. Cause thought to be exposure to constant irritant such as wind, dust, or ultraviolet light

  2. Surgical procedure

      a. Growth is dissected off the cornea and conjunctiva down to the sclera

      b. Low-dose radiation on surgical wound may be used to prevent regrowth

      c. Regrowth rate is 20 to 40%

G. Lacrimal duct disorders

  1. Dacryocystorhinostomy (DCR)

      a. Description

          i.   Establishment of a new tear passageway for drainage directly into the nasal cavity

      b. Surgical procedure

          i.   Nasal cavity is anesthetized topically with cocaine preoperatively

          ii.   Usually performed under general anesthesia

          iii. Lacrimal sac is probed and opened

      iv.   A stent is placed through lacrimal duct drainage system to keep system open until epithelium forms around it and creates a new opening; stent generally removed in 6 weeks

  2. Conjunctivodacrocystorhinostomy

    a. Description

      i.   Variation of DCR

      ii. Necessary if lacrimal sac has been destroyed, must be recreated, or the canaliculi are absent

    b. Surgical procedure

      i.   After completion of DCR, conjunctiva taken from lower lid and sutured to nasal mucosa to form lacrimal sac

      ii. If canaliculus cannot be kept open or is absent:

        (a) Permanent stent (Pyrex tube) is placed

        (b) Patient teaching includes

          (i)   How to place tube back in if it falls out

          (ii) How to clean tube

          (iii) How to hold tube in case of sneezing

  3. Endoscopic DCR

    a. Uses endonasal laser to open pathway into lacrimal sac

    b. Uses endoscopic equipment

    c. Benefits

      i.   Eliminates external incision and scar

      ii. Decreases amount of postoperative discomfort

      iii. Provides hemostasis

      iv. Increases healing time

      v.   Decreased cost

H. Surgery for strabismus

  1. Description

    a. The inability to direct the two eyes at the same object because of lack of coordination of extraocular muscles

    b. Misalignment of the axes of the eyes in which one or both eyes is turned inward or outward

    c. Often accompanied by amblyopia (normal vision fails to develop despite absence of disease or refractive error)

    d. Normally done on children less than 6 years of age

    e. May be done for cosmetic reasons for children older than 6 years of age

    f. Indications for performing procedure on adults

      i.   Bell's palsy

      ii. Muscular dystrophy

      iii. Traumatic injury

      iv. Untreated or unsatisfactory treatment of childhood strabismus

      v.   Muscular paralysis resulting from stroke

  2. Surgical procedure

    a. Corrective surgery is performed to change the relative strength of individual muscles and therefore improve coordination

      i.   May require resection: the removal of a portion of muscle and attachment of cut ends

      ii. May require recession: severance of the muscle from its original insertion with reattachment more posteriorly on the sclera

      iii. May require transplanting a muscle to improve rotation of paralyzed muscle

  b. Intraoperative consideration
    i. Manipulation of rectus muscle will cause transient bradycardia
      (a) Treated with atropine
      (b) If severe, surgeon may have to stop manipulation of rectus muscle
        until heart rate returns to normal
    ii. Bradycardia caused by innervation of branch of vagus nerve

I. Removal of globe
  1. Exenteration
    a. Entire contents of orbit are removed
    b. Requires extensive plastic reconstruction
  2. Evisceration
    a. Removal of the contents of the globe
    b. Preserves sclera and muscular attachments
    c. Prosthesis inserted to maintain shape of eye
      i. Sclera is closed over prosthesis
      ii. Conjunctiva closed over sclera
      iii. Conformer placed under eyelids to maintain space until swelling subsides
        and artificial eye is created
    d. Advantages
      i. Natural attachment of eye muscles
      ii. Normal eye movement
  3. Enucleation
    a. Removal of the diseased globe and a portion of the optic nerve
    b. General anesthesia usually administered
    c. Prosthesis may be inserted

J. Corneal transplant (keratoplasty)
  1. Description
    a. Grafting of corneal tissue from one human eye to another
    b. Performed when patient's cornea is thickened and opacified
    c. Transparency of cornea may be impaired due to infection, burns, or certain
      diseases
    d. Corneal transplant performed to improve vision when basic visual structures
      of eye (optic nerve and retina) are functioning properly
  2. Types
    a. Penetrating keratoplasty (full-thickness)
      i. Most common
      ii. Performed with microscope
    b. Lamellar keratoplasty (partial-thickness)
      i. More difficult than penetrating keratoplasty
      ii. Higher success rate
        (a) Success due to layered cellular arrangement of corneal tissue and
         avascularity
    c. Keratectomy (peeling of the cornea)
    d. Tattooing (simulation of a pupil)
      i. Rarely done
  3. Postoperative considerations
    a. Eye patch and shield remain in place
    b. Usually removed by surgeon day after surgery
    c. Diet and activity as tolerated
    d. Healing of cornea is very slow
      i. Recovery of vision longer than after cataract surgery

4. Potential complications
    a. Rejection of corneal transplant
        i.   Cornea becomes opaque
        ii. Treated with steroids
        iii. May require repeated keratoplasty

K. Radial keratotomy
  1. Description
    a. Used to reduce myopia in adults
    b. Series of precise, partial-thickness radial incisions in the cornea
    c. Results in scar tissue that forms pulls and results in a flattening of the cornea, reducing refractive error
  2. Usually performed under local and topical anesthesia
  3. Potential complications
    a. Glaring from scars
    b. Permanent scarring
    c. Infection resulting in loss of vision
    d. Cataract formation due to injury to lens
    e. Variations in the level of correction
  4. Correction with excimer laser
    a. Ablates top of cornea
    b. Fewer complications
        i.   Minimal glare sensitivity problems
        ii. No chance of perforation
    c. Performed with topical anesthesia
    d. Complications
        i.   Overcorrection
        ii. Undercorrection
        iii. Hazing
    e. Postprocedure treatment
        i.   Instillation of tobramycin dexamethasone suspension drops and 5% homatropine hydrobromide
        ii. Placement of disposable soft contact lens for first three weeks
           (a) Promotes epithelial growth

L. Cataract extraction
  1. Description
    a. Cataract: gradual developing opacity of the lens of the eye
        i.   Can occur at any time
           (a) Etiology in infants
              (i)   Heredity
              (ii) Developmental abnormalities
              (iii) Infection
              (iv) Traumatic eye injury
              (v)   Chemical imbalances (galactosemia and diabetes)
           (b) Etiology in adults
              (i)   Same as infant
              (ii) Prolonged exposure to ultraviolet light
              (iii) Medications (those used to treat glaucoma)
              (iv) Normal part of aging process
    b. Cataract extraction is the removal of the opaque lens from the interior of the eye
  2. Types of procedures
    a. Intracapsular cataract extraction (ICCE)

      i.   Removal of lens, as well as the anterior and posterior capsule, the cortex, and nucleus

      ii. Method has largely been replaced by the extracapsular cataract extraction

      iii. Risk of vitreous humor loss

  b. Extracapsular cataract extraction (ECCE)

      i.   Anterior portion of the capsule is first ruptured, then removed

      ii. Lens cortex and nucleus are expressed from the eye, leaving the posterior capsule behind intact (posterior capsule is excellent support for intraocular lens implantation)

  c. Phacoemulsification

      i.   Removal of lens by fragmenting it with ultrasonic vibrations

      ii. Simultaneously there is irrigation and aspiration of the fragments without the loss of the lens capsule

      iii. Very small incision needed

3. Correction of aphakia (absence of lens)

  a. Patient sees objects larger than normal

  b. Objects appear blurred and without detail

  c. Options available for correction

      i.   Glasses

         (a) Aphakia spectacles

         (b) Fitted 6 to 8 weeks after lens extraction

         (c) Acceptable only for binocular aphakia

         (d) Distorts peripheral vision

         (e) Produces change in image size

         (f) Clear image only in direct center of glasses

      ii. Contact lens

         (a) Excellent option for vision correction

         (b) Can be used for monocular aphakia

         (c) Patient has complete field of vision

      iii. Epikeratophakia

         (a) Procedure considered for patients with low endothelial cell counts

         (b) Form of refractive keratoplasty

         (c) Description of procedure

            (i)   Piece of donor corneal tissue is shaped to specific diopter on a cryolathe

            (ii) Tissue sutured to recipient's cornea

            (iii) Changes corneal curvature

            (iv) Results in change of refractive power of cornea

      iv. Placement of intraocular lens (IOL)

         (a) Most commonly used procedure today

         (b) Description of lens

            (i)   Made of plexiglas or polymethyl methacrylate (PMMA)

            (ii) Center can be either biconvex or convexoplano and two haptics (spring-hook appendages)

               a) Polypropylene haptics break down over time

               b) Should not be used on young patients

            (iii) Lens cannot adjust anterior to posterior dimensions

               a) Provides only myopic (nearsighted) or hyperopic (farsighted) vision

               b) Patient decides on need of glasses for distance or reading

      v.   Advantages of IOL

         (a) Shorter rehabilitation period

         (b) Lens used for monocular aphakic correction

  vi. Lens placement
   (a) Anterior chamber
    (i) Used after ICCE
    (ii) Used for secondary lens implantation
   (b) Iris plane
   (c) Posterior chamber
    (i) Only when cataract removed by ECCE or phacoemulsification
    (ii) Most physiologic position for artificial lens
  vii. Sutureless cataract technique
   (a) Increasingly popular
   (b) Rapid visual rehabilitation
 4. Preoperative considerations
  a. Inquire as to patient's use of anticoagulants, nonsteroidal, and anti-inflammatory drugs (Motrin or aspirin); can cause increase in bleeding intraoperatively
  b. Identify adequate home support system; implement referrals if necessary
  c. Review preoperative instructions with patient; provide instructions in large type; use off-white paper to reduce glare
  d. Administer mydriatics and/or additional medications as ordered

M. Procedures to treat glaucoma
 1. Iridectomy
  a. Description
   i. Removal of a section of iris tissue
   ii. Peripheral iridectomy done in the treatment of acute, subacute, or chronic angle-closure glaucoma
    (a) Extensive peripheral anterior synechiae not yet formed
   iii. Reestablishes communication between posterior and anterior chambers
   iv. Relieves pupillary block
   v. Facilitates movement of aqueous humor from posterior to anterior chamber
 2. Trabeculectomy
  a. Description
   i. Creation of a fistula between anterior chamber of eye and subconjunctival space
   ii. Portion of the trabecular meshwork surgically excised
   iii. Facilitates drainage of aqueous humor from the posterior chamber to the anterior chamber for treatment of glaucoma
  b. Adjunctive medical therapy may be utilized to decrease postoperative fibrosis by applying 5-fluorouracil (5-FU) or mitomycin C under the conjunctival flap for 3 to 5 minutes

N. Vitrectomy
 1. Description
  a. Removal of all or part of vitreous gel
 2. Indications (anterior segment)
  a. Vitreous loss during cataract extraction surgery
  b. Anterior segment opacities
  c. Miscellaneous causes
 3. Indications (posterior segment)
  a. Vitreous opacities
  b. Advanced diabetic eye disease
  c. Severe intraocular trauma

        d. Retained foreign bodies
        e. Endophthalmitis
    4. Procedural considerations
        a. Procedure varies according to location of pathologic condition
            i.   Anterior
            ii. Posterior
        b. Requires use of operating microscope, illuminations system, and cutting–suction–infusion system
    5. Intraoperative considerations
        a. Procedure time varies from 1 hour to 6 hours
        b. Protect pressure area on patient
        c. May use elastic stockings
    6. Postoperative considerations
        a. May experience more postoperative pain than is generally associated with ophthalmologic surgeries
            i.   Strong analgesics may be necessary
            ii. Ice packs may help reduce pain
O. Retinal detachment
    1. Description
        a. Separation of a portion of the retina from the choroid
        b. Goal of treatment aimed at repairing tears and returning retina to normal anatomic position
    2. Causes
        a. Intraocular neoplasms
        b. Associated with injury (blow to head)
        c. Normal aging process
        d. Severe myopia
        e. Congenital
        f. Inflammatory process
    3. Signs and symptoms
        a. Patient may experience sudden onset of floaters (floating spots in front of eye)
        b. Loss of vision without pain
        c. Slow decrease in visual field (described as if someone was pulling a curtain in front of eye)
    4. Types
        a. Primary detachment—hole in retina permits fluid to enter space between retina and choroid
        b. Secondary detachment—fluid or tissue builds up between choroid and retina with no hole in retina
    5. Treatment
        a. Diathermy
            i.   Traditional method
                (a) Insertion of microneedles or needle tip of a probe into sclera
                (b) Shortwave radiofrequency energy delivered through needles
                (c) Causes thermal changes in tissue
                (d) Results in scar formation and retinal reattachment at points of adhesion
                (e) Procedure rarely used anymore
            ii. Cryotherapy
                (a) More popular method; less invasive than diathermy
                (b) Application of −80°C cryoprobe to scleral area of detachment
                (c) Inflammation causes adhesion and reattaches retina
                (d) Less complications than diathermy

        b. Pneumoretinopexy
           i.   Injection of air or expansile gases into vitreous cavity
           ii.   Usually done in physician's office
           iii.   Crymotherapy may be used to close and seal hole before gas is injected
           iv.   Patient may be instructed to hold head in certain position until retina reattaches (usually 2 weeks)
        c. Laser therapy
           i.   Used to "spot weld" retina
           ii.   Done in physician's office
           iii.   Can be done in OR in conjunction with vitrectomy
        d. Scleral buckling
           i.   Description
           ii.   A procedure developed to create indentation in the retina so that adherence between the detached area and underlying tissues will result in permanent reattachment
        e. Posterior vitrectomy
           i.   Description
              (a) Objective is to remove vitreous humor without pulling on retina; permits surgeon to work directly on retina
              (b) Can be performed with all techniques for reattaching retina
     6. Preoperative considerations
        a. Instruct patient regarding activity limitations prior to surgery (reduces stress on area of detachment)
        b. Inform patient and family of potential for lengthy surgery (decrease anxiety level)
     7. Postoperative considerations
        a. Patient usually on cycloplegic agents (atropine or cyclopentolate) to dilate pupil and rest muscles of accommodation
        b. May be on antibiotic and steroid eyedrops
        c. Assess patient's ability to instill eyedrops
  P. Laser therapy
     1. Description
        a. Noninvasive ambulatory procedures where a slit lamp is used to deliver the laser beam
        b. May eliminate the need for more invasive procedures
        c. Argon or YAG lasers are utilized in a procedure room
        d. Topical anesthetic drops are instilled
     2. Procedures
        a. Laser trabeculoplasty
           i.   Treatment for open-angle glaucoma
        b. Laser iridotomy
           i.   Treatment for acute or chronic angle-closure glaucoma
        c. Laser posterior capsulotomy
           i.   May be required when patients experience decreased vision within 2 years after ECCE
           ii.   YAG laser used to create a window in the posterior capsule
           iii.   Patients may have pupils dilated
           iv.   Iopidine may be used to prevent increased intraocular pressure

III. Anesthetic Considerations

  A. Types (overview)
     1. Topical
        a. Topical anesthetic eyedrops may be used
        b. Rapid onset with moderate duration of action

2. Local anesthesia block
   a. Used frequently
   b. Contraindications
      i.   Patients who have difficulty lying still
      ii. Children
      iii. Patients who have frequent cough
3. Intravenous conscious sedation used in conjunction with block
4. General anesthesia

B. Topical anesthetic drops
   1. Used frequently
      a. Proparacaine hydrochloride 0.5%
      b. Tetracaine hydrochloride 0.5%
      c. Lidocaine hydrochloride 2%

C. Eye block
   1. Types
      a. Retrobulbar block
         i.   Injection of anesthetic solution into base of eyelids at level of orbital margins or behind the eyeball to block the ciliary ganglion and nerves
      b. Peribulbar block
         i.   Local anesthetic is deposited beside the globe instead of behind it
   2. Performed in two stages
   3. Stage I—blocks eyelid
      a. Three methods
         i.   Van Lint method—blocks peripheral branches of cranial nerve VII in the orbicularis oculi muscle
         ii. Atkinson method—blocks temporal arborization of cranial nerve VII to the orbicularis muscle
         iii. O'Brien method—blocks the main trunk of cranial nerve VII near the temporomandibular joint
   4. Stage II—retrobulbar block
      a. Provides anesthesia to globe and muscular attachments
      b. Blocks branches of cranial nerves III, IV, V, and VI
      c. Common medications used:
         i.   Lidocaine hydrochloride 2% or 4%; mixed with equal parts of 0.75% bupivacaine hydrochloride with hyaluronidase (used for diffusing local anesthetic to surrounding tissue)
         ii. May add epinephrine hydrochloride to prolong effectiveness of agents
         iii. May use as much as 6 ml for retrobulbar block and 10 ml for peripheral tissue
      d. Nursing considerations
         i.   Inform patient of possible burning sensation
         ii. Inform patient of possible feeling of pressure behind eye during injection of medication
         iii. Inform patient that physician may massage eye after injection of medication
              (a) Decreases intraocular pressure
              (b) Aids in diffusing agents
         iv. Patient frequently given intravenous sedation to decrease discomfort during the injection; administer medications per protocol
         v.   Monitor vital signs per protocol
         vi. Patient may be awake during procedure
              (a) Monitor noise level

  e. Nursing care following eye block
    i.   Patient will not have blink reflex; must keep eyelid closed to protect the cornea
         (a) Tape the eyelid closed
         (b) Reassure patient that it is normal to be unable to open the eyelid
  f. Effectiveness of eye block
    i.   Generally very effective
    ii. Occasionally a block may be incomplete and patient will experience pain
    iii. Instruct patient to use hand signal during surgery if he/she experiences pain or discomfort
  g. Potential complications; cancellation of surgical procedure strongly advised for any of the following complications
    i.   Retinal detachment (caused by insertion of needle through globe)
    ii. Injection of anesthetic into optic nerve (irreparable damage)
    iii. Retrobulbar hemorrhage (most common)
         (a) Controlled by pressure to globe
  D. General anesthesia
    1. Indications
      a. Children
      b. Patients unable to tolerate local anesthetic with sedation
      c. Extremely anxious patients
      d. Patients with certain systemic diseases
      e. Patients undergoing prolonged operations
    2. Postanesthesia care
      a. Same as any patient who has undergone general anesthesia
 IV. **Drugs Frequently Used for Ophthalmologic Surgery**
  A. Mydriatics
    1. Action
      a. Blocks cholinergic stimulation of sphincter muscle of iris (dilation of pupil)
      b. Blocks accommodative ciliary muscle of lens (paralysis of accommodation)
    2. Types
      a. Phenylephrine hydrochloride (Alconefrin, Neo-synephrine, Prefrin)
      b. Hydroxyamphetamine (Paredrine)
  B. Cycloplegics
    1. Action
      a. Dilate pupils and paralyze accommodation by acting on ciliary muscles (parasympatholytics)
    2. Types
      a. Atropine
      b. Homatropine (homatrocel, isoptophomatropine)
      c. Cyclopentolate (cyclogyl)
      d. Scopolamine (isoptohyoscine, mydramide)
      e. Tropicamide (Mydriacyl)
  C. Miotics
    1. Action
      a. Used to constrict the pupil (parasympathomimetics)
    2. Types
      a. Cholinergics
        i.   Pilocarpine hydrochloride
        ii. Carbachol (Miostat, Carbacel)
        iii. Acetylcholine chloride (Miochol)
      b. Anticholinesterase
        i.   Physostigmine (Eserine)

   ii. Isoflurophate (Floropryl)

   iii. Echothiophate iodide (Phospholine Iodide)

 D. Osmotic agents

  1. Action

   a. Parenteral agents used to lower intraocular pressure through the blood-ocular gradient

  2. Types

   a. Mannitol (Osmitrol)

   b. Glycerin (glycerol, glyrol, osmoglyn)

 E. Viscoelastic agents

  1. Action

   a. Used to maintain the intraocular chamber during surgery

  2. Types

   a. Sodium hyaluronate (healon, amvisc)

 F. Carbonic anhydrase inhibitors

  1. Action

   a. Parenteral agent used to decrease intraocular pressure; used for glaucoma

  2. Types

   a. Acetazolamide (Diamox)

   b. Methazolamide (Neptazane)

 G. Corticosteroids

  1. Action

   a. Antiinflammatory agents

  2. Types

   a. Hydrocortisone (Solu-Cortef)

   b. Dexamethasone (Decadron)

   c. Prednisolone (Pred-Forte)

 H. Topical antibiotics

  1. Action

   a. Used for prophylaxis of or treatment of infections; may be used in solutions or ointments

  2. Types

   a. Bacitracin, neomycin, erythromycin, tetracycline, gantrisin, tobramycin, gentamycin

   b. Chloramphenicol

V. Preoperative Considerations

Refer to Chapter 7 for complete information.

 A. Assessment

  1. Patient/family's understanding of:

   a. Eye disorder

   b. Goal of surgery

   c. What to expect before, during, and after surgery

  2. Assess in detail patient's understanding of intraoperative procedure; especially in cases where local anesthesia and sedation only is used

  3. Identify patient's reaction to scheduled surgery

   a. Unrealistic expectations regarding improved vision

   b. Anxiety over potential loss of vision

  4. Identify current visual status

   a. May need additional safety precautions if severely impaired

   b. May need additional support postoperatively if visual status of unoperative eye is limited

B. General health assessment per routine protocol
1. Identify illnesses that can cause sneezing, coughing, or increase in intraocular pressure
    a. Patient may not be a candidate for local anesthesia with sedation
    b. May require general anesthesia
C. Preoperative care
1. Relieve anxiety related to impending surgery (the eyes are very sensitive to pain and pressure)
    a. Allow patient time to verbalize concerns
        i. Patient may have misconceptions regarding eye surgery
        ii. Clarify misconceptions
        iii. Some patients may think they will actually see the procedure through the operative eye
    b. Involve the patient in the plan of care
        i. Provide clear written instructions in large type
        ii. Reinforce physician's orders regarding pre- and postoperative medications and eyedrop schedules
    c. Provide emotional support
        i. Convey positive realistic attitude
        ii. Acknowledge validity of patient concerns
2. Verify correct surgical eye
    a. Confirm with patient correct eye for surgery
        i. Document correct eye prior to preoperative sedation
        ii. Keep in mind many patients may be unable to accurately identify the operative eye due to age or mental status
    b. Document correct operative eye
        i. Verify the surgical consent and the history and physical with the scheduled procedure
        ii. Investigate any discrepancy
    c. Clearly identify surgical eye with skin marker
        i. Visual marking should not be the sole way of identifying the correct surgical eye
        ii. Every perianesthesia nurse caring for the patient should verify the patient's understanding, the consent, and the scheduled procedure before proceeding with care
3. What to expect
    a. Length of time (preoperatively, intraoperatively, postoperatively)
    b. Eye patch (depending on surgical procedure)
    c. Reinforcement that improved vision may require a period of time
4. Demonstrate proper method of eyedrop instillation
    a. Explain ways to avoid contamination of eye medications
    b. Reinforce need to follow prescription instructions accurately
    c. Teach proper technique for instillation of eyedrops
        i. Confirm on bottle that drops are for ophthalmic use
        ii. Note the expiration date and discard if outdated
        iii. Wash hands prior to using eyedrops
        iv. Confirm proper eye
        v. Tilt head back for instillation
        vi. Keep eyes open and look upward
        vii. Gently pull down tissue below the lower lid
        viii. Place correct number of eyedrops into the conjunctival sac
        ix. Close eyes and try to avoid excessive blinking or squeezing for several minutes

      x. Gently blot any excess solution from beneath the eye
      xi. Wait 5 minutes before instilling a different type of eyedrop
      xii. Do not touch tip of eye medication dispenser to the eyelid or with hands
  D. Review postoperative routine
    1. Include family/significant other as appropriate
    2. Things to avoid postoperatively
      a. Quick movements
      b. Bending over from the waist
      c. Rubbing eyes
      d. Moderation in activity
      e. Avoid heavy lifting
      f. Proper hand washing before caring for the eye
  E. Nursing considerations
    1. Visually impaired patient
      a. Approach from unaffected or least affected side
      b. Identify self
      c. Speak in normal tone
      d. Provide method for patient to obtain immediate assistance (call bell in reach)
      e. Keep visual aids in close proximity
      f. Allow patient to keep assistive devices as long as possible
      g. Keep walking area clear of obstructions
    2. Administer preoperative medications as ordered
      a. Mydriatics to dilate pupil
      b. Notify physician if expected dilation does not occur
    3. Allow patient to void prior to procedure
      a. Patient will become restless in OR if he/she has a full bladder
  F. Overall assessment of patient's ability to tolerate anesthesia plan
    1. Procedure usually performed under local anesthesia with sedation (adults)
    2. Assess patient's ability to lie still under drapes for long period of time (1 to 3 hours)
    3. Factors influencing decision include:
      a. Chronic cough
      b. Airway difficulties
      c. Claustrophobia
      d. Involuntary motions

VI. Postoperative Considerations

Refer to Chapter 8 for complete information.

  A. Assessment
    1. Routine assessment per protocol
  B. Positioning
    1. Assist patient to chair or recliner
      a. Avoid bumping or jarring
    2. Orient patient to surroundings
    3. Certain operations (vitreoretinal surgery) may require special positioning
      a. Surgeon should provide specific instructions as to positioning
      b. Patient may need to be on side or back
    4. Patient may have decreased pain with head of bed elevated
  C. Drainage
    1. Type and amount; document
    2. Notify physician per protocol

D. Pain and discomfort level
   1. Varies with each procedure
      a. Usually uncommon after most eye surgeries
   2. Varies with type of anesthesia administered
   3. Patient may feel stiff and sore
      a. Results from lying still and flat intraoperatively
   4. Pain usually relieved by acetaminophen, propoxyphen hydrochloride, or similar analgesics
   5. May experience significant pain after vitreoretinal surgery
      a. Administer narcotic analgesic as indicated
      b. Apply ice pack
      c. Notify ophthalmologist if pain not relieved by analgesics

E. Nausea
   1. Caused by manipulation of eye and eye muscles during surgery
   2. May be due to sedation
   3. Medicate immediately to prevent potential vomiting
      a. Vomiting results in increased intraocular pressure
      b. Instruct patient to notify nurse immediately if he/she begins to feel nauseous so that antiemetics may be given
   4. To avoid potential for nausea and vomiting, oral fluids may be held for a while if patient underwent general anesthesia

F. Visual impairment due to surgery
   1. Ensure patient safety at all times
   2. Requires assistance at home
   3. Verify arrangements prior to discharge

G. Eye shields/dressings
   1. Dressing or eye shields usually remain in place until the patient's first postoperative appointment at the physician's office
      a. Instruct patient not to disturb or remove shield/dressing
   2. Alteration in depth perception may be expected when one eye is bandaged
      a. Evaluate patient for adequate balance before allowing him/her to ambulate unassisted
   3. Provide clear written instructions for postoperative care at home
      a. Wash hands before caring for eye
      b. Do not rub eye
      c. Surgeon will remove eye patch/shield during postoperative appointment
      d. Wear glasses or shield at all times to protect the eye
      e. Wear shield at night for sleeping
      f. Do not bend at the waist
      g. Avoid heavy lifting
      h. Do not drive until after first postoperative appointment
      i. Do not drive at all if experiencing double vision
      j. Take all eye medications as ordered
      k. Notify physician if any of the following occur:
         i.   Pain not relieved by acetaminophen
         ii. Sudden loss of vision
         iii. Increasing double vision following surgery
         iv. Temperature greater than 100°F
         v. Significant swelling or redness about the eye
         vi. Unexpected drainage from the eye

H. Discharge instructions (refer to Table 33–1)

Table 33–1 • DISCHARGE INSTRUCTIONS AFTER EYE SURGERY

Use strict aseptic technique when caring for the eye.

Change eye dressing and keep eye shield in place as per the physician's orders.

Use eye medication as directed. (Be certain that the patient knows the name, dose, route, frequency, and expected effect of all medications, and can correctly instill topical ophthalmic preparations.)

Avoid activities that increase intraocular pressure: sudden, jarring movements; bending; coughing; sneezing; forceful nose blowing; and sexual intercourse.

Avoid straining at stool: drink at least 2000 ml of fluid daily (unless contraindicated), eat a high-fiber diet, and take stool softeners as ordered.

Wear dark glasses for photophobia.

Avoid use of eye makeup until otherwise instructed.

Report any increased pain, decreased vision, or purulent drainage.

Return for follow-up visit on (specify date).

From Donovan Monahan, F., Neighbors, M. (1998). *Medical-Surgical Nursing Foundations for Clinical Practice,* 2nd ed. Philadelphia: Saunders, p. 1953.

VII. Possible Complications of Ophthalmologic Surgery

- A. Pain
  1. Minimal in most ophthalmologic surgeries
  2. Causes: increased intraocular pressure; surgical manipulation; pressure from dressing
  3. Treatment: mild analgesic; be aware that the need for stronger medication may indicate possible complications
- B. Bleeding
  1. Minimal for all ophthalmologic surgeries
  2. Cause: dressing too loose
  3. Treatment: apply or reinforce dressing, notify physician
- C. Nausea and vomiting
  1. Usually minimal following ophthalmologic surgery
  2. Causes: oculocardiac reflex; surgical manipulation; general anesthesia
  3. Treatment: antiemetic; avoid potential vomiting
- D. Oculocardiac reflex (nervous response elicited by manipulation of extraocular muscles or surrounding ocular tissue)
  1. Causes: decreased heart rate, blood pressure, and level of consciousness
  2. Is seen immediately to 20 minutes postoperatively
  3. May be seen with all types of ophthalmologic surgeries
     a. Risk increases with vitreoretinal and eye muscle surgeries
     b. May be stimulated by retrobulbar block
  4. Treatment: IV atropine

BOX 33–1.   Key Patient Educational Outcomes

- Patient demonstrates proper method of instilling eyedrops
- Patient verbalizes importance of not disturbing integrity of suture line
- Patient avoids activities known to increase intraocular pressure
- Patient wears eye shield, sunglasses as instructed
- Patient identifies a plan to meet activities of daily living if he/she is unable to perform activities independently
- Patient verbalizes proper procedure for aseptically instilling of eyedrops
- Patient lists signs and symptoms requiring immediate notification of physician

Bibliography

1. Black, J.M., Matassarin-Jacobs, E. (eds). (1997). *Medical-Surgical Nursing Clinical Management for Continuity of Care,* 5th ed. (pages 935–979). Philadelphia: Saunders.
2. Burden, N. (1993). *Ambulatory Surgical Nursing.* Philadelphia: Saunders.
3. *Dorland's Illustrated Medical Dictionary,* 28th ed. (1994). Philadelphia: Saunders.
4. Gruendemann, B.J., Fernsebner, B. (1995). *Comprehensive Perioperative Nursing, Vol 2—Practice,* (pages 21–51). Boston: Jones and Bartlett.
5. Maes, K.S., Britton, T., Bell, B. (1995). The ophthalmic surgical patient. In Litwack, K. ed. *Core Curriculum for Post Anesthesia Nursing Practice,* 3rd ed. (pages 590–601). Philadelphia: Saunders.
6. Monahan, F.D., Neighbors, M. (eds). (1998). *Medical-Surgical Nursing Foundations for Clinical Practice,* 2nd ed. (pages 1935–1993). Philadelphia: Saunders.
7. Spires, R. (1996). The ophthalmic ambulatory surgery patient. *J Post Anesth Nursing,* 11(2):78–79.
8. Thompson-Keith, E. (1995). Ophthalmic surgery. In Meeker, M.H., Rothrock, J.C. (eds): *Alexander's Care of the Patient in Surgery,* 10th ed. (pages 572–635). St Louis: Mosby.
9. Zehren, C. (1994). Post anesthesia care of the ophthalmic surgical patient. In Drain, C.B., ed. *The Post Anesthesia Care Unit—A Critical Care Approach to Post Anesthesia Nursing,* 3rd ed. (pages 343–349). Philadelphia: Saunders.

REVIEW QUESTIONS

1. All of the following are true regarding repair of entropion except

   A. Can result in corneal ulcer
   B. Usually affects upper lid
   C. Lashes scrape across the cornea
   D. Seldom seen in persons under 40 years of age

2. All of the following are true regarding ectropion except

   A. Results in exposure of underlying conjunctiva
   B. Usually occurs bilaterally
   C. Results in inward turning of eyelid
   D. Can be a result of normal aging

3. Surgery to correct strabismus repair

   A. Is normally done on children less than 6 years of age
   B. May be done for cosmetic reasons on children over 6 years of age
   C. May be performed on an adult who has Bell's palsy
   D. All of the above

4. Potential complications of radial keratotomy include all of the following except

   A. Glaring from scars
   B. Cataract formation due to injury of lens
   C. Permanent scarring
   D. Aphakia

5. When reviewing preoperative instructions with the post cataract patient, the nurse would

   A. Instruct patient to continue all medications on the day of surgery
   B. Identify adequate home-support network
   C. Provide written instructions on glossy white paper
   D. Relieve the patient's anxiety level by not going into details

6. For the patient undergoing a vitrectomy, the nurse would

   A. Apply elastic stocking preoperatively
   B. Apply ice to the eye postoperatively
   C. Ensure pressure points are protected intraoperatively
   D. All of the above

7. The patient who exhibits loss of vision without pain or floaters in front of the eye may be showing signs and symptoms of

   A. A cataract
   B. Retinal detachment
   C. Glaucoma
   D. Aphakia

8. The patient is about to undergo a retro-bulbar eye block. Nursing interventions include all of the following except

   A. Informing the patient that there will be absolutely no pain or sensation
   B. Informing the patient that the physician may massage the eye after the injection
   C. Reassuring the patient that it is normal not to be able to open the eyelid
   D. Informing the patient that the eyelid will be taped closed

9. Which of the following is not a potential complication caused by insertion of a retrobulbar block?

   A. Retinal detachment
   B. Absence of blink reflex
   C. Injection of anesthetic into optic nerve
   D. Retrobulbar hemorrhage

10. Carbonic anhydrase inhibitors are used to

    A. Maintain intraocular pressure during surgery
    B. Dilate pupils and paralyze accommodation
    C. Decrease intraocular pressure in patients with glaucoma
    D. Constrict the pupil

ANSWERS TO QUESTIONS

1. B
2. C
3. D
4. D
5. B

6. D
7. B
8. A
9. B
10. C

Orthopedic Surgery

Gayle Miller
St. Luke's Hospital
Jacksonville, Florida

I. Anatomy and Physiology
  A. Tissue of musculoskeletal system
    1. Connective tissue
    2. Muscle
  B. Connective tissue
    1. Development
      a. Develops from mesenchymal cells
      b. Later differentiates into specialized connective tissue cell types
    2. Types (three)
      a. Collagenous tissue
        i.   Derived from dense fibrous connective tissue
        ii. Constructed primarily of collagen fibers
        iii. Includes tendons, ligaments, and fascia
        iv. Tendons
            (a) Dense fibrous connective tissue strands at the ends of muscles that attach muscles to bone
        v.   Ligaments
            (a) Dense connective tissue bands that attach bone to bone and provide stability to joints
        vi. Tendons and ligaments can withstand pulling forces
            (a) Activity
            (b) Joint motion largely affects ligaments
            (c) Muscle contraction largely affects tendons
        vii. Fascia can withstand stretching in all directions
            (a) Suitable for enveloping limbs and muscle compartments

Objectives
1. List common ambulatory orthopedic procedures.
2. Discuss assessment parameters pertinent to the preoperative ambulatory orthopedic patient.
3. Discuss nursing diagnoses related to the care of orthopedic patients.
4. Describe techniques for assessing neurovascular status in the postoperative orthopedic patient.
5. Discuss nursing interventions appropriate to the care of the orthopedic patient.
6. Describe complications of various orthopedic procedures.
7. Discuss the educational needs of the orthopedic patient.

   b. Cartilage: nonvascular tissue composed of collagenous and elastic fibers; the proportion of each type of fiber determines the three types of cartilage
      i.   Hyaline cartilage—very elastic, found in the trachea, in synovial joints, in the larynx, nasal septum, and ribs
            (a) Tends to get calcified in old age
      ii.   White fibrocartilage—thick, shock absorbing, found in symphysis pubis, between vertebrae, and in synovial joints
            (a) Interarticular fibrocartilage—flattened fibrocartilaginous plates between articular surfaces of joints, such as the menisci of the knee
                (i)   Found in temporomandibular, sternoclavicular, acromioclavicular, wrist, and knee joints
            (b) Connecting fibrocartilage—found in joints with limited mobility, such as the intervertebral discs
            (c) Circumferential fibrocartilage—rims surrounding sockets of articular surfaces such as the glenoidal labrum of the hip and the shoulder
            (d) Stratiform fibrocartilage—forms a coating on osseous groove that tendons pass through
      iii. Yellow or elastic cartilage—dense, more flexible and pliant than hyaline cartilage; strong
            (a) Found in the outer ear, epiglottis, and eustachian tube
   c. Bone
      i.   Osseous connective tissue
      ii.   Predominantly made up of a fibrous component called collagen and an amorphous component called calcium phosphate
      iii. Highly porous and vascular
C. Skeletal muscle
   1. Accounts for half the body weight in humans
   2. Has ability to contract
      a. Produces or prevents movement of body and its parts
D. Joints: articulations where bones or two bone surfaces come together
   1. Diarthroses—freely movable, synovial
      a. Uniaxial—move in one axis and only one plane
         i.   Hinge—knee, elbow, finger
         ii.   Pivot—radial head
      b. Biaxial—moves around two perpendicular axes, in two perpendicular planes
         i.   Saddle—base of the thumb
         ii.   Condyloid—distal radius/wrist bones
      c. Multiaxial—moves in three or more planes and around three or more axes
         i.   Ball and socket—hip, shoulder
         ii.   Gliding—vertebral joints
   2. Amphiarthroses—limited movement
      a. Symphysis pubis, intervertebral
   3. Synarthroses—immovable
      a. Sutures—fibrous tissue between skull bones
      b. Syndesmoses—ligaments connecting bones' distal radius/ulna, distal tibia/fibula
      c. Gomphoses—fibrous membrane connects to bone, tooth/mandible or maxilla
      d. Range of motion—degree of movement of a joint (refer to Figure 34–1)
         i.   Angular—changes the size of angles between articulating bones
               (a) Flexion—shortens the angle by bending forward
               (b) Extension—lengthens the angle by bending backwards
               (c) Abduction—movement away from the midline

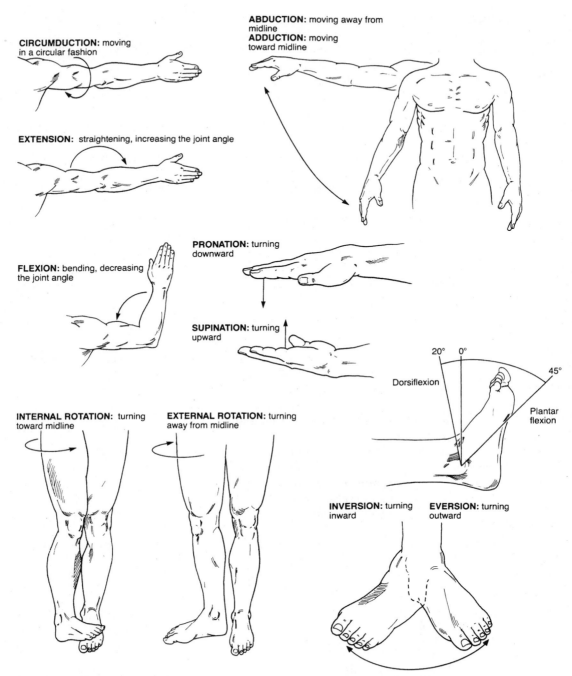

Figure 34–1. Joint movements. (From Maher, A.B., Salmond, S.W., Pellino, T.A. [1998]. *Orthopaedic Nursing.* Philadelphia: Saunders, p. 178.)

    (d) Adduction—movement toward the midline

    (e) Plantar flexion—increases the angle between the foot and the front of the leg by bending the foot and toes down and back

    (f) Dorsiflexion—decreases the angle between the foot and the back of the leg by bending the toes and foot upward

    (g) Hyperextension—stretching a part beyond its normal anatomic limits

    ii. Circular—movement around an axis

      (a) Rotation—moving or pivoting a bone around its axis (side to side of the head)

      (b) Circumduction—movement that resembles a cone shape; the distal part is a wider circle (winding up to throw)

      (c) Supination—palm turns upward while forearm rotates outward

      (d) Pronation—palm turns downward while forearm rotates inward

    iii. Gliding—moving one joint surface over another with no circular or angular movement

    iv. Miscellaneous movements

      (a) Elevation—moving upward, lifting

      (b) Depression—moving downward, lowering

      (c) Inversion—sole of the foot turns inward

      (d) Eversion—sole of the foot turns outward

      (e) Protraction—moving a part forward, such as the jaw or shoulder

      (f) Retraction—moving a part backward

      (g) Opposition—moving parts together (finger and thumb)

E. Compartment

  1. Description

    a. Areas where nerves, muscles, and blood vessels are confined by inelastic structures

      i. Skin, epimysium, fascia, or bone

      (a) 46 anatomic compartments within body

      (b) 36 compartments located in the extremities

  2. Compartment syndrome

    a. Definition

      i. Occurs in an area in the body where muscles, nerves, and blood vessels are encompassed within tissue (e.g., bone or fascia)

      ii. Characterized by high pressure in muscle compartment in closed fascial space

      iii. Causes capillary blood perfusion to be reduced below level necessary for tissue viability

      iv. Compartments most prone to compartment syndrome are the deep posterior, superficial posterior, lateral and anterior compartments of the lower leg, and the volar and dorsal compartments of the forearm

    b. Types

      i. Acute

      (a) Most severe

      (b) Requires surgical intervention

      (c) Common causes—external compression

        (i)   Dressings, casts, braces applied too tightly

        (ii)   Pneumatic antishock garment

        (iii) Surgical positions

        (iv) Automatic blood pressure monitoring devices

      (d) Common causes—increase in compartment contents

        (i)   Bleeding; bleeding disorders

        (ii)   Contusions

        (iii) Trauma

        (iv) Burns

        (v)   Exercise

        (vi) Venous obstruction

            (vii) Ischemia

            (viii) Infiltrated intravenous

            (ix) Frostbite

  ii. Chronic

      (a) Results from increased pressure in compartment from exercise

  iii. Crush

      (a) Results from crush injuries that externally compress the compartment

c. Assessment

  i. Nursing history

      (a) Cause of injury

      (b) Position of extremities after injury

      (c) Position during surgery

      (d) Exercise patterns

  ii. Signs and symptoms—acute

      (a) Increasing pain

      (b) Pain greater than normal for injury

      (c) Pain unrelieved with analgesics

      (d) Patient complaint that pain is continually worse

      (e) Patient describes pain as:

            (i)   Deep

            (ii)   Throbbing

            (iii) Pressure

      (f) Pain on passive stretch

      (g) Complaints of paresthesia ("pins and needles" or "asleep")

      (h) Signs and symptoms occur 6 to 8 hours after injury

            (i)   May take as long as 2 days to occur

d. Diagnosis

  i. Specially designed pressure monitor

      (a) Inserted via large-bore needle into compartment

            (i)   Normal compartment pressure: 0 to 8 mm Hg

            (ii)   Pressure greater than 30 mm Hg results in nerve damage

e. Treatment

  i. Relieve source of pressure

      (a) Loosen external constrictive device

            (i)   Loosen dressing

            (ii)   Bivalving cast

            (iii) Remove tight stockings

            (iv) If unsuccessful in relieving pressure, patient may need fasciotomy

      (b) Treatment for increase in contents of compartment

            (i)   Keep limb at heart level

                a) If above heart level causes decrease in local arterial perfusion

                b) Results in further compromise of local blood flow

            (ii)   Maintain adequate hydration to preserve mean arterial blood flow

            (iii) May require fasciotomy

f. Nursing interventions

  i. High risk for peripheral neurovascular dysfunction

      (a) Assess neurovascular status every 1 to 2 hours

            (i)   Instruct patient on how to assess neurovascular function after discharge

      (b) Assess pain level

            (i)   Notify physician immediately if signs and symptoms of compartment syndrome appear

ii. Treatment
   (a) Notify physician
   (b) Remove restrictive devices (per physician's order)
   (c) Keep affected limb at heart level
   (d) Remove ice
   (e) Ensure adequate hydration
   (f) Prepare for possible intracompartmental monitoring
iii. Assessment
   (a) Pain level
      (i)   Location
      (ii)   Severity
      (iii) Duration
      (iv)   Quality
      (v)   Medicate as ordered
   (b) Alteration in sensation
      (i)   Assess for presence of insensate skin
      (ii)   Educate patient on how to assess self
      (iii) Educate patient regarding safety issues (checking water temperature with unaffected limb prior to immersion, avoiding sharp objects, etc.)
   (c) Potential for infection
      (i)   Assess wound for signs of infection
      (ii)   Monitor temperature
      (iii) Sterile technique for dressing changes

II. Assessment Parameters
A. Overview
   1. Routine assessment per protocol
   2. Operative site
      a. When assessing an extremity, it is helpful to compare the function/sensation of the operative extremity with the function/sensation of the unoperative extremity
      b. For patients with casts and other orthopedic devices
         i. Assess neurovascular status of operative extremity
            (a) Color, capillary refill, temperature, sensation, and movement
            (b) Assess skin around cast
      c. Position
         i. Patient position and position of affected extremity dependent on patient's condition, surgery, and anesthetic technique used
   3. Assessment parameters should be adjusted to individualized procedure
B. Upper extremity procedures
   1. Assess and protect cast/splint:
      a. Cast should be kept dry
         i. Fiberglass casts will dry quickly; plaster casts are slow to dry
         ii. While plaster cast is still damp, take care to prevent indentations or rough edges
      b. Observe for cast defects such as indentations or rough edges that could lead to tissue compression damage
   2. Check neurovascular status (see Table 34–1)
      a. Nerve function
         i. Radial—check sensation at the thumb–index finger web; have the patient hyperextend thumb or wrist

Table 34–1 • **NERVE ASSESSMENT**

COMPARTMENT	NERVES INVOLVED	SIGNS AND SYMPTOMS
Anterior leg	Deep peroneal	Decreased dorsiflexion of foot and toes Tense and tender lateral to tibial crest Anterior pain with toe, foot, or ankle plantarflexion
Lateral leg	Superficial peroneal Deep peroneal	Decreased foot and ankle eversion Sensory deficit over dorsum of foot and perhaps first web space
Superficial posterior leg	Tibial Sural	Decreased plantarflexion of ankle Posterior calf pain with active plantarflexion and passive ankle dorsiflexion Sensory deficit over lateral aspect of foot
Deep posterior leg	Tibial Saphenous	Tenseness hard to detect Passive pain with dorsiflexion of toes or foot, everting foot Paresis in toe flexors and foot invertors
Foot (medial, lateral, central, interosseous)	Digital	Difficult to separate four compartments Tense and swollen Decreased motions Passive stretch pain
Gluteal (3) (tensor, medius/minimus, maximus)	Sciatic	Buttock tenderness and tenseness Decreased extension and abduction of hip Gluteal stretch pain with hip adduction or flexion Paresthesias along distal sciatic
Iliacus (inner wall of pelvis)	Femoral	Very rare, occurs with hemorrhage in pelvis Hip held in flexion Pain with hip extension Tenderness along inguinal ligament Dysesthesia around knee and distally in saphenous nerve
Thigh		
Anterior	Femoral	Decreased knee extension Keeps knee in extended position Passive flexion of knee leads to pain in anterior thigh Active quadriceps contraction leads to pain Paresthesia over knee and medial aspect of leg and foot Tense and tender over anterior thigh
Posterior	Obturator Sciatic	Decreased knee flexion Passive knee extension leads to posterior thigh pain Sensory and motor deficits of distal sciatic if significant pressure elevation Tender and tense over medial thigh Paresthesia and paresis along obturator
Forearm		
Volar	Median Ulnar Anterior interosseous	Sensation and motor function on flexor or palmar surface of the hand Decreased strength in finger and thumb flexors Passive extension of the fingers causes pain in volar forearm Paresis of intrinsic muscles Tenseness and tenderness over volar forearm
Dorsal	Posterior interosseous	Decreased wrist and finger extension Hand may assume extended position Passive finger or wrist flexion leads to pain in dorsal forearm Sensory deficit usually minimal

From Maher, A.B., Salmond, S.W., Pellino, T.A. (1998). *Orthopaedic Nursing,* Philadelphia: Saunders, p. 217.

ii. Median—check sensation on the distal surface of the index finger; have patient oppose thumb and finger

iii. Ulnar—check sensation at distal end of small finger; have patient abduct all fingers

b. Vascular status

   i. Note presence and quality of pulses

   ii. Assess capillary refill

     (a) Normal capillary refill 3 seconds or less

     (b) Perform blanch test

       (i) Compress and release nail bed quickly

       (ii) Compare capillary refill to unaffected extremity

       (iii) Rapid filling may indicate venous congestion

       (iv) Sluggish filling is a sign of arterial insufficiency

   iii. Note color, comparing to unaffected extremity

     (a) Blanching or pallor indicates arterial insufficiency

     (b) Cyanosis indicates insufficient venous return

     (c) Mobility

       (i) Within limitations of the cast/splint, etc., have patient wiggle fingers; this should be easy and not painful

C. Lower extremities

1. Assess and protect cast/splint as above

2. Check neurovascular status frequently

a. Nerve function—peroneal

   i. Check sensation at lateral surface of great toe and medial surface of second toe

   ii. Have patient dorsiflex ankle and extend toes

   iii. Peroneal nerve damage results in foot drop

b. Nerve function—tibial

   i. Check sensation at the medial and lateral surfaces of the sole of the foot

   ii. Have patient plantar flex the ankle and flex the toes

   iii. Signs and symptoms of nerve damage include: pain that is increasing, persistent and localized; paresthesia; hyperesthesia; numbness; motor weakness; or paralysis

c. Vascular status

   i. Assess as noted above

d. Mobility

   i. Within limitations of casts/splints, etc., have patient wiggle toes; this should be easy and not painful

   ii. Severe pain on dorsiflexion of the toes, loss of sensation, or tightness in the calf can indicate compartment syndrome

III. Common Operative Procedures

A. Upper extremity

1. Carpal tunnel release—decompression of the median nerve by dividing the transverse carpal ligament

2. Finger amputation and revision—generally for traumatic injuries, infection, or vascular compromise

3. Joint replacement—small joints of the finger, hand, or wrist; performed to improve function in patients with rheumatoid arthritis or other degenerative diseases

4. Olecranon bursectomy—excision of bursal wall and calcifications

5. Open reduction, internal fixation—surgical placement of hardware such as pins, screws, or plates to maintain position of bones for healing

6. Release of deQuervain's hand—decompression of the dorsal compartment of the hand to treat stenosing tenosynovitis of the wrist at the base of the thumb
7. Release of Dupuytren's contracture—fasciotomy or fasciectomy to treat contracture in the palmar surface of the hand
8. Rotator cuff repair—repair of tendons of the muscles of the rotator cuff
9. Synovectomy—removal of part or all of the synovial lining of a joint to retard progression of rheumatic destruction of the joint

B. Lower extremity
1. Anterior cruciate ligament reconstruction—replacement of damaged ligament with autograft, allograft, or synthetic ligament to return stability to the knee following ligament tear
2. Arthroscopic meniscectomy—removal of a part of the meniscus (cartilage) of the knee using arthroscopic technique
3. Osteotomy—cutting a bone to change its position for weight bearing, or to correct an abnormal curvature
4. Prepatellar bursectomy—excision of bursal wall and calcifications

C. Miscellaneous
1. Arthroscopy: shoulder, wrist, knee, ankle
   a. Diagnostic arthroscopy can be performed in a variety of joints
   b. It involves insertion of a fiberoptic instrument into a joint in order to visualize the interior
   c. Multiple procedures can be performed through a scope, including but not limited to debridement, biopsy, meniscectomy, ligament repair, and removal of loose bodies
2. Bone biopsy—arthroscopic or open
3. Cast change
4. Closed reduction of fractures
5. Cyst removal
6. Debridement—arthroscopic or open
7. Excision of bone spurs—commonly formed as a result of osteoarthritic changes
8. Excision of ganglion—removal of a cystic mass found over a joint or tendon sheath
9. Excision of lesion
10. Hardware removal
11. Joint manipulation, e.g., following knee arthroplasty
12. Muscle biopsy
13. Removal of foreign body
14. Simple tendon repair

IV. **Perianesthesia Priorities: Phase I, Preoperative**
A. Objective
1. The purpose of the preoperative phase of care is to assess and prepare the patient for the surgical experience
2. Baseline data is obtained with which to plan and implement care
3. The educational process continues
   a. Should begin in physician's office at time procedure is scheduled
   b. is continued at this time and throughout the continuum of care
   c. A clinical pathway may be utilized to guide the preparation of the patient
4. Begin discharge planning

B. Assessment
1. General history and assessment; emphasize screening for:
   a. Neurovascular status of involved extremity
   b. Gait and mobility
   c. ADL (activities of daily living) limitations

2. Assess for educational needs
3. Assess for psychosocial needs
   a. Family/responsible adult companion availability
   b. Community resources needed
   c. Impact on employment
4. Initiate discharge planning

C. Plan of care
   1. Include patient/family/responsible adult companion in developing plan of care
   2. Plan should be appropriate to the age of the patient
   3. Nursing diagnoses might include:
      a. Anxiety/fear related to knowledge deficit, unfamiliar environment, separation from family, lack of control, potential for pain
      b. Potential for injury
      c. Potential for infection
      d. Impaired physical mobility
      e. Knowledge deficit
      f. Acute pain or chronic pain
      g. Peripheral neurovascular dysfunction

D. Interventions
   1. Nursing interventions might include but are not limited to:
      a. Ensure legal authorization is appropriate (consent)
      b. Ensure that all laboratory studies are completed as ordered/indicated
      c. Provide information on preoperative preparation (NPO, discontinuation of medications, hygiene, site preparation, ride/home care arrangements, etc.)
      d. Obtain baseline vital signs
      e. Provide orientation to surroundings
      f. Explain postoperative care needs to patient/family/responsible adult companion
      g. Facilitate obtaining assistive devices as needed
      h. Facilitate/provide instruction on gait, crutch walking, etc.
         i. Crutch walking
         (a) Gaits (three)
             (i) Gait pattern determined by patient's diagnosis, weight-bearing status, overall condition, age, and balance
             (ii) Two-point gait
                  a) Opposite arm and leg move simultaneously
                  b) Sequence
                     (1) Right crutch, left foot, left crutch, right foot
                     (2) Used for bilateral partial weight-bearing
             (iii) Three-point gait
                  a) Affected lower extremity and both crutches are moved at the same time
                  b) Used for partial or nonweight-bearing on affected lower extremity
             (iv) Four-point gait (alternate crutch gait)
                  a) Movement of one crutch or one extremity at a time
                  b) Sequence
                     (1) Right crutch, left foot, left crutch, right foot
                     (2) Used when weight-bearing permitted
                     (3) Allows for stability; three points of support are always on the floor

(b) How to sit in a chair
- (i) Walk up to the chair
- (ii) Turn around and back up until chair is felt on back of knees
- (iii) Hold handgrips of both crutches with one hand
- (iv) Place other hand on arm or seat of chair
- (v) Lower self into chair; place weight on handgrips of crutches and on chair arm or seat
- (vi) Slide affected lower extremity forward while lowering self to sitting position

(c) Getting out of chair
- (i) Place both crutches on one side; hold handgrips as above
- (ii) Place other hand on arm or seat of chair
- (iii) Push up until in standing position
- (iv) Be sure chair is strong enough to support weight of pushing and will not tip
- (v) Place one crutch under each arm

(d) Going up stairs (two crutches)
- (i) Walk close to bottom stair
- (ii) Place all weight on handgrips
- (iii) Sequence
  - a) Place unaffected lower extremity on next step
  - b) Move body, affected leg, and crutches
- (iv) Stay in center of steps
- (v) Be sure crutches are centered on step to avoid loosing balance
- (vi) Repeat above sequence

(e) Going up stairs (handrail present)
- (i) Walk close to bottom stair
- (ii) Place both crutches under arm opposite handrail
- (iii) Hold both handgrips in hand opposite handrail
- (iv) Hold handrail with hand on side of handrail
- (v) Put all weight on hands
- (vi) Lift unaffected lower extremity up to next step
- (vii) Move crutches, body, and affected lower extremity up to same step at same time
- (viii) Repeat above sequence

(f) Going down stairs (two crutches)
- (i) Proceed to edge of top step
- (ii) Bend at hips
- (iii) Sequence
  - a) Place both crutches, then affected lower extremity on the next lower step
  - b) Put weight on crutches
  - c) Bring unaffected leg down to same step
  - d) Repeat above sequence

(g) Going down stairs (handrail present)
- (i) Proceed to edge of top step
- (ii) Place both crutches under arm opposite handrail
- (iii) Grasp handrail with hand on side of handrail
- (iv) Sequence
  - a) Move affected lower extremity and crutches to next lower step
  - b) Note: do *not* place weight on affected lower extremity if there is to be no weight bearing

              c) Put weight on hands and wrists on crutches and handrail

              d) Step down with unaffected leg

              e) Repeat above sequence

        (h) Additional safety precautions

           (i)   Do not rest with shoulders leaning on top of crutches

              a) Prolonged pressure under axillary area can result in nerve damage and decreased circulation to arms

              b) Rest with weight on handgrips and unaffected lower extremity

           (ii)   Use care when walking on slippery floors

           (iii) Avoid throw rugs

           (iv) Keep crutch tips clean (dirt buildup can increase slipperiness of crutches)

        (i) Refer to Table 34–2

  E. Evaluation

    1. Evaluation of interventions/patient response might include:

      a. Laboratory results are reviewed, and follow-up completed as indicated

      b. Patient/family/responsible adult companion are questioned to determine understanding of preoperative instructions

      c. Determine that patient has made arrangements for home care

      d. Determine that patient can use assistive devices safely and properly

V. Perianesthesia Priorities: Phase II, PACU

  A. Objective

    1. Ensure that the patient safely recovers from the immediate effects of surgery and anesthesia

  B. Assessment (procedure-specific)

    1. Pulse

    2. Capillary refill

    3. Color

    4. Sensation

    5. Temperature

    6. Motion

  C. Plan of care

    1. Plan should be appropriate to the age of the patient

    2. Nursing diagnoses might include:

      a. Anxiety/fear related to knowledge deficit, unfamiliar environment, separation from family, lack of control, etc.

      b. Pain related to surgical/procedural intervention

      c. Alteration in mobility

      d. Potential for injury

      e. Peripheral neurovascular dysfunction

      f. Potential for infection

      g. Altered peripheral tissue perfusion

      h. Knowledge deficit

    3. Be alert for potential complications

      a. Neurovascular compromise

        i.   Numbness, tingling

        ii. Edema

        iii. Pallor, altered capillary refill

      b. Excessive pain

      c. Pulmonary embolism

      d. Compartment syndrome

Table 34-2 • PATIENT PATHWAYS: CASTS, SPLINTS, IMMOBILIZERS

	DURING CAST/IMMOBILIZER APPLICATION	WHILE CAST IS DRYING	DURING CAST/IMMOBILIZER USE	DURING AND AFTER CAST REMOVAL/AFTER IMMOBILIZER USE
Activity	Need to maintain position during cast application	Use the palms of your hands, not your fingers, to support the cast when moving Reposition your extremity or yourself every 2 hours Do not put weight on your casted extremity until after it is dry (you will be instructed how much weight you are allowed to bear)	Do not use the cast or immobilizer or its parts to turn Learn to apply and remove immobilizer and when it needs to be worn Use your uninvolved arm(s) and leg(s) often Actively exercise joints above and below cast or immobilizer Your weight-bearing and activity parameters are: Change position(s) at least every 2 hours	Exercises to decrease joint stiffness Muscle-strengthening exercises Activity restrictions Methods to avoid reinjury
Tests and Treatments	X-rays May be limited for body casts or if sedation is to be used		X-rays	X-rays
Diet			Drink plenty of fluids Eat well-balanced meals Include roughage and bulk in your diet Call your health-care provider if you have any nausea or vomiting	

Teaching		
Purpose of cast or immobilizer Area to be enclosed Type of casting material Special equipment to be used Use of premedication or sedation May feel very warm and constricting, then cold May need to be casted for mold for immobilizer It may take 48–72 hours for a plaster cast to dry; synthetic casts usually dry in about 30 minutes Keep cast uncovered until it is dry Do not put casted area on a plastic-covered area; this could cause increased heat and skin damage If icebags are used, they should be only ½ to ¾ full and should be positioned to avoid identations Do not use lamps, fans, or hairdryers to dry your cast; they may burn the skin or cause the cast to crack from too rapid drying; fans may increase a feeling of coldness as the cast dries	Check cast for cracks, softening, or flaking every day Do not get plaster casts wet; for any type of cast or immobilizer, use plastic to protect the edges, especially around the perineum; commercially available urine and stool collection devices may be needed Avoid humidifiers Cleanse soiled plaster with mild, white, powdered cleanser and slightly damp cloth Immerse synthetic casts only with physician order; if allowed to get wet, hairdryers set on low heat may be allowed for drying Do not place any foreign objects under your cast or immobilizer Report any changes in sensation or movement to your health-care provider	The cast cutter is a vibrating saw; the padding under your cast will protect your skin from being scratched The skin under your cast or immobilizer will be very dry, flaky, and paler than normal Use gentle skin care with oils The muscles under your cast or immobilizer will be smaller and have less tone than normal

From: Maher, A.B., Salmond, S.W., Pellino, T.A. (1998). *Orthopaedic Nursing*, 2nd ed. Philadelphia: Saunders, p. 306.

D. Nursing interventions (procedure-specific)
1. Upper extremity procedures
    a. Position the hand above the heart
    b. Provide a sling if ordered
    c. Assess and protect cast/splint
        i.   Cast should be kept dry as noted above
        ii. Observe for cast defects that could lead to tissue compression damage (see Table 34–2)
    d. Apply ice packs as ordered
    e. Check neurovascular status (see Table 34–1)
        i.   Nerve function
            (a) Radial—check sensation at the thumb–index finger web; have the patient hyperextend thumb or wrist
            (b) Median—check sensation on the distal surface of the index finger; have patient oppose thumb and finger
            (c) Ulnar—check sensation at distal end of small finger; have patient abduct all fingers
        ii. Vascular status—assess capillary refill
            (a) Normal capillary refill 3 seconds or less
            (b) Perform blanch test
                (i)   Compress and release nail bed quickly
                (ii) Compare capillary refill to unaffected extremity
                (iii) Rapid filling may indicate venous congestion
                (iv) Sluggish filling is a sign of arterial insufficiency
            (c) Note color, comparing with unaffected extremity
                (i)   Blanching or pallor indicates arterial insufficiency
                (ii) Cyanosis indicates insufficient venous return
        iii. Mobility
            (a) Within limitations of casts/splints, etc., have patient wiggle fingers; this should be easy and not painful
2. Lower extremities
    a. Position the extremity above the heart
    b. Assess and protect cast/splint
        i.   Cast should be kept dry
        ii. Observe for cast defects that could lead to tissue compression damage
    c. Apply ice packs/cooling device as ordered
    d. Check neurovascular status frequently
        i.   Nerve function—peroneal
            (a) Check sensation at lateral surface of great toe and medial surface of second toe
            (b) Have patient dorsiflex ankle and extend toes
            (c) Peroneal nerve damage results in foot drop
        ii. Nerve function—tibial
            (a) Check sensation at the medial and lateral surfaces of the sole of the foot
            (b) Have patient plantar flex the ankle and flex the toes
            (c) Signs and symptoms of nerve damage include: pain that is increasing, persistent and localized; paresthesia; hyperesthesia; numbness; motor weakness; or paralysis
        iii. Vascular status
            (a) Perform blanch test
                (i)   Compress and release nail bed quickly

          (ii)   Compare capillary refill with unaffected extremity
          (iii)   Rapid filling may indicate venous congestion
          (iv)   Sluggish filling is a sign of arterial insufficiency
       (b) Note color, comparing with unaffected extremity
          (i)   Blanching or pallor indicates arterial insufficiency
          (ii)   Cyanosis indicates insufficient venous return
       (c) Signs and symptoms of nerve damage include loss of pulse, sluggish or absent capillary refill, pallor, cyanosis, blanching, temperature decrease, paresthesia, or hyperesthesia

    iv. Mobility
       (a) Within limitations of casts/splints, etc., have patient wiggle toes; this should be easy and not painful
       (b) Severe pain on dorsiflexion of the toes can indicate compartment syndrome

VI. Perianesthesia Priorities: Phase III, Preparation for Discharge
  A. Objective
    1. The objective of Phase III is to ready the patient to return to home, prepared—in conjunction with a caregiver—to successfully manage postoperative care
    2. Education of the patient and caregiver is a critical factor in a successful ambulatory surgical outcome
    3. If education was begun preoperatively, reinforcement is done at this time
  B. Assessment
    1. Procedure-specific assessment continues as outlined in Phase II to ensure that the postoperative status is stable prior to discharge
  C. Plan of care
    1. Plan should be appropriate to the age of the patient
    2. Nursing diagnoses might include but are not limited to:
      a. Pain related to surgical/procedural intervention
      b. Alteration in mobility
      c. Potential for infection
      d. Altered peripheral tissue perfusion
      e. Peripheral neurovascular dysfunction
      f. Knowledge deficit
    3. Be alert for potential complications as noted above
  D. Education interventions/methods
    1. Discussion, demonstration, written materials, etc.
    2. Copies of all materials given to the patient/caregiver should be maintained in the medical record or on the unit
  E. Evaluation
    1. Evaluation of clinical interventions continues as noted in Phase II
    2. Evaluation of learning
      a. Patient/caregiver verbalization of understanding, demonstrating a skill, etc.
      b. Patient and responsible party should sign that they have been instructed and had the opportunity to have questions answered

VII. Education Content
  A. Preoperative
    1. General
      a. NPO
      b. Aftercare arrangements
      c. Preoperative hygiene and/or scrubs
      d. Environment of surgical suite

    e. Facility protocols

    f. Anticipated perioperative course

    g. Wear loose, comfortable clothing to accommodate casts/splints/dressings

    h. Anticipated ADL modifications

  2. Procedure-specific

    a. Cast care

      i.   Alert for signs and symptoms of infection (drainage, foul smell, etc.)

    b. Dressings

    c. Positioning—elevation of extremity

    d. Use of assistive devices

      i.   Slings

      ii. Crutches

      iii. Walker

      iv. Cane

      v.   Splints

      vi. Braces

B. Phase III, preparation for discharge

  1. General

    a. Activity

    b. Diet

    c. Medications

    d. Complications

    e. Follow-up care

    f. Emergency notification parameters

  2. Procedure-specific

    a. Elevate extremity to decrease edema and pain

    b. Keep dressings dry

    c. Report any signs of bleeding or infection to the physician

    d. Cast/splint care (see Table 34–2)

    e. Use of ice packs/cooling device as ordered

    f. Use of assistive devices

    g. Signs of neurovascular compromise

BOX 34–1. Key Patient Educational Outcomes

- Patient is able to identify signs and symptoms of complications related to immobility of extremity and seeks necessary medical intervention
- Patient is able to identify early signs and symptoms of infection and seeks appropriate medical intervention
- Patient is able to identify appropriate safety measures to follow when using assistive devices in order to prevent injury
- Patient is able to perform activities of daily living using assistive devices as appropriate
- The patient with a cast is free of complications caused by compromised circulation to extremity and can verbalize potential complications such as change in color, temperature, movement, sensation, and edema
- Patient verbalizes accurate information regarding prescribed analgesic, proper method of administration, and potential side effects
- Patient verbalizes nonpharmacologic interventions to decrease pain, e.g., elevation of extremity, application of ice, immobilizer properly applied

Bibliography

1. Clark, S., Strommen, K. (1994). Disorders of the hand. In Maher, A.B., Salmond, S.W., Pellino, T.A., eds. *Orthopaedic Nursing*. Philadelphia: Saunders.
2. Dunwoody, C.J. (1994). Modalities for immobilization. In Maher, A.B., Salmond, S.W., Pellino, T.A., eds. *Orthopaedic Nursing*. Philadelphia: Saunders.
3. Folman, D.A. (1994). Anatomy and physiology of the musculoskeletal system. In Maher, A.B., Salmond, S.W., Pellino, T.A., eds. *Orthopaedic Nursing*. Philadelphia: Saunders.
4. Folman, D.A., Maher, A.B. (1994). Assessment of the musculoskeletal system. In Maher, A.B., Salmond, S.W., Pellino, T.A., eds. *Orthopaedic Nursing*. Philadelphia: Saunders.
5. Gray, H. (1985). *Anatomy of the Human Body*. Clemente, C. (ed.). Philadelphia: Lea & Febiger.
6. Guyton, A.C. (1991). *Textbook of Medical Physiology*. Philadelphia: Saunders.
7. Kull, L. (1995). The orthopedic surgical patient. In Litwack, K., ed. *Core Curriculum for Post Anesthesia Nursing Practice*. Philadelphia: Saunders.
8. Maher, A.B., Salmond, S.W., Pellino, T.A. (1998). *Orthopaedic Nursing*, 2nd ed. Philadelphia: Saunders.
9. Pellino, T.A., Polleck, L.A. (1994). Complications of orthopaedic disorders and orthopaedic surgery. In Maher, A.B., Salmond, S.W., Pellino, T.A., eds. *Orthopaedic Nursing*. Philadelphia: Saunders.
10. Rivellini, D. (1994). Perioperative considerations for the orthopaedic patient. In Maher, A.B., Salmond, S.W., Pellino, T.A., eds. *Orthopaedic Nursing*. Philadelphia: Saunders.
11. Ross, D. (1991). Acute compartment syndrome. *Orthopaedic Nursing*. March/April vol. 10(2).
12. Ross, D. (1996). Chronic compartment syndrome. *Orthopaedic Nursing*. May/June Vol 15(3).
13. Schrefer S. (ed.) (1995). *Mosby's Patient Teaching Guides*. St. Louis: Mosby.
14. The surgical specialties—part 2: Gynecologic and obstetric, urologic, orthopedic and podiatric, general, and cardiovascular surgical procedures. (1993). In Burden, N., ed. *Ambulatory Surgical Nursing*. Philadelphia: Saunders.

REVIEW QUESTIONS

1. To assess the function of the radial nerve, the nurse should ask the patient to

   A. Hyperextend the wrist
   B. Dorsiflex the thumb
   C. Abduct all fingers
   D. Adduct all fingers

2. When performing a blanch test postoperatively, the nurse notes sluggish filling. This is a sign of

   A. Venous insufficiency
   B. Venous congestion
   C. Arterial insufficiency
   D. Arterial dilatation

3. A classic sign of compartment syndrome is severe pain on

   A. Eversion of the foot
   B. Dorsiflexion of the toes
   C. Inversion of the hip
   D. Plantar flexion of the foot

4. To assess the sensory function of the peroneal nerve, the nurse will

   A. Prick the medial lateral surface of the sole of the foot
   B. Have the patient flex his/her toes
   C. Prick the web space between the great and second toes
   D. Have patient dorsiflex the ankle

5. In preparing the patient to go home with a plaster cast, the nurse instructs the patient to

   A. Refrain from weight-bearing for 12 hours
   B. Report any foul odors to physician
   C. Use powder to keep skin dry under the cast
   D. Keep the extremity elevated at heart level

6. Mr. Smith was admitted to the PACU following a left arthroscopic ACL repair. On assessment the nurse compares both extremities and notes that Mr. Smith has complaints of tingling in the right leg. The nurse attributes this to

   A. Hanging the right leg over the edge of the OR bed
   B. Placing the right leg in a stirrup
   C. Maintaining 90-degree flexion of the left leg
   D. Elevating the left leg higher than the right

7. In teaching the patient about crutch walking to be used postoperatively, the nurse instructs the patient to

   A. Put both crutches in the hand on the side of the strong leg when getting up from a chair
   B. Adjust the handpieces so that the elbow maintains a 45-degree angle
   C. Go up stairs with the stronger leg first
   D. Adjust the height of the crutches so that there are four finger widths of space between the crutches and underarms

8. Compartments most prone to compartment syndrome include all of the following except

   A. Deep posterior of lower leg
   B. Superficial posterior of lower leg
   C. Medial anterior of lower leg
   D. Volar and dorsal of forearm

9. To check the nerve function of the ulnar nerve, the nurse would

   A. Check the sensation on the distal surface of the index finger; have patient oppose thumb and finger
   B. Check the sensation at distal end of small finger; have patient abduct all fingers
   C. Check the sensation at the thumb–index finger web; have the patient hyperextend thumb or wrist
   D. Check the sensation on the proximal surface of the index finger; have patient oppose thumb and finger

10. When positioning the patient postoperatively, proper patient position will be dependent on all of the following except

   A. Operative procedure performed
   B. Analgesics administered
   C. Anesthetic technique used
   D. Patient's condition

ANSWERS TO QUESTIONS

1. A
2. C
3. B
4. C
5. B

6. A
7. C
8. C
9. B
10. B

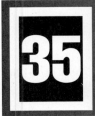

Otorhinolaryngologic Surgery

Gayle Miller
St. Luke's Hospital
Jacksonville, Florida

I. Anatomy and Physiology

Refer to Figure 35–1.

A. Ear
  1. Outer ear
    a. Pinna (auricle)
      i.   Yellow elastic cartilage covered by skin
      ii. Collects sound waves
      iii. Directs sound waves to external acoustic meatus
    b. Auditory canal—external acoustic meatus
      i.   Extends to the tympanic membrane
    c. Tympanic membrane (eardrum)
      i.   Thin, transparent, pearly gray, cone-shaped membrane
      ii. Stretches across the ear canal
      iii. Separates the middle ear (tympanic cavity) from the outer ear
    d. Nerve supply
      i.   Auriculotemporal branch of the trigeminal nerve
        (a) General sensory
        (b) Innervates tympanic membrane, external acoustic meatus, anterior auricle
  2. Middle ear
    a. Structure
      i.   Ossicles
        (a) Malleus

Objectives

1. Describe common ear–nose–throat (ENT) procedures performed in the ambulatory setting.
2. Discuss potential complications of ear procedures.
3. Describe assessment of the cranial nerves following ENT procedures.
4. Describe the rationale for positioning of patients following ear surgery.
5. Discuss methods of decreasing nausea and vertigo.
6. List precautions patients should be informed of in postoperative teaching.

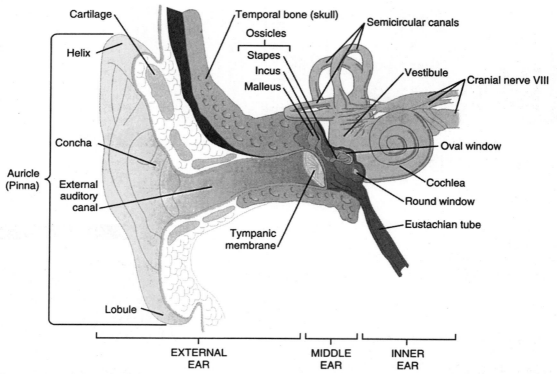

Figure 35–1. Anatomy of the ear. (From Black, J.M., Matassarin-Jacobs, E. [1997]. *Medical-Surgical Nursing Clinical Management for Continuity of Care,* 5th ed. Philadelphia: Saunders, p. 981.)

        (i)   Hammer
        (ii) Largest of the three ossicles
    (b) Incus
        (i)   Anvil
        (ii) Middle ossicle
    (c) Stapes
        (i)   Stirrup
        (ii) Inner-most ossicle
  ii.   Eustachian tube
    (a) Channel connecting the tympanic cavity and the nasal part of the pharynx through which air reaches the middle ear
  b. Function
    i.   Ossicles form a chain from tympanic membrane to the oval window
    ii. Transmits vibrations to inner ear, conducting sound to the inner ear
3. Inner ear
  a. Cochlea—spiral-shaped, forms the anterior part of the labyrinth of the inner ear; contains three compartments
    i.   Scala vestibuli
    (a) Part of the cochlea above the spiral lamina which divides the canal
    ii. Scala tympani
    (a) Part of the cochlea below the spiral lamina
    iii. Cochlear duct (scala media)
    (a) Canal between the scala tympani and scala vestibuli
  b. Organ of Corti
    i.   Organ lying against the basilar membrane in the cochlear duct

        ii. Contains special sensory receptors for hearing

        iii. Consists of neuroepithelial hair cells that respond to vibration from the ossicles, converting mechanical energy to electrochemical impulses

   c. Vestibular labyrinth—controls equilibrium

        i. Utricle

           (a) Larger of the two divisions of the membraneous labyrinth of the inner ear

        ii. Sacule

           (a) Smaller of the two divisions of the membraneous labyrinth of the vestibule

           (b) Communicates with the cochlear duct by way of the ductus reuniens

        iii. Semicircular canals

           (a) Description

               (i) Three canals—anterior, lateral, and posterior

               (ii) Passages in the inner ear

               (iii) Located in the bony labyrinth

           (b) Functions

               (i) Control sense of balance

               (ii) Respond to movement of head

               (iii) Can cause feeling of dizziness or vertigo after spinning

               (iv) Motion sickness results from unusual movements of the head which result in stimulation of the semicircular canals

B. Nose

  1. External

    a. Upper—formed by nasal bones and maxilla

    b. Lower—formed by connective tissue

    c. Nares—separated by columella, formed from nasal cartilage

    d. Nasal septum

        i. Nasal cartilage

        ii. Vomer bone

        iii. Perpendicular plate of ethmoid bone

  2. Internal—nasal cavity

    a. Nares (nostrils)

        i. External opening of the nasal cavity

    b. Choanae

        i. Paired openings between nasal cavity and oropharynx

    c. Nasopharynx

        i. Part of the pharynx above the soft palate

    d. Eustachian tube

        i. Narrow channel that connects tympanum with nasopharynx

    e. Paranasal sinuses

        i. Arranged in four pairs

           (a) Maxillary

           (b) Frontal

           (c) Sphenoid

           (d) Ethmoid

    f. Nasal duct

        i. Extends from the lower part of the lacrimal sac to the inferior meatus of the nose

        ii. Channel through which tear fluid is conveyed into the cavity of the nose

    g. Turbinate bones

        i. Extend horizontally along the lateral wall of the nasal cavity

        ii. Separates the middle meatus of the nasal cavity from the inferior meatus

    h. Nasal septum
      i. Separates the nasal cavity into two fossae
    i. Nerve supply
      i. Trigeminal nerve
        (a) Cranial nerve V
        (b) General sensory, motor
        (c) Face, teeth, mouth, nasal cavity
      ii. Cranial nerve I (olfactory)
        (a) Special sensory
        (b) Nerve of smell
    j. Other nerves to consider
      i. Cranial nerve II (optic)
        (a) Special sensory
        (b) Nerve of sight
        (c) Can be damaged in endoscopic sinus surgery
    k. Blood supply
      i. Internal maxillary
      ii. Anterior ethmoid
      iii. Sphenopalatine
      iv. Nasopalatine
      v. Pharyngeal
      vi. Posterior ethmoid
  C. Throat
    1. Mouth
      a. Lips
      b. Buccal cavity
      c. Lingual cavity
        i. Tongue
        ii. Hard palate
        iii. Soft palate
    2. Pharynx (see Figure 35–2)
      a. Throat
        i. Nasopharynx
          (a) Lies posterior to the nose and above the level of the soft palate
          (b) Provides passageway for air
          (c) Contains opening of the eustachian tubes
        ii. Oropharynx
          (a) Extends from soft palate to the hyoid bone
          (b) Provides passageway for both air and food
        iii. Laryngopharynx
          (a) Extends from the hyoid bone to the lower border of the cricoid cartilage
          (b) Continues with the esophagus
          (c) Anterior entrance of the larynx is the epiglottis
    3. Tonsils
      a. Types
        i. Palatine tonsils
          (a) Pair of oval-shaped structures
          (b) Size of almonds
          (c) Partially imbedded in mucous membrane
          (d) One on each side of the throat

ii. Lingual tonsils
    (a) Below palatine tonsils
    (b) At base of tongue
iii. Pharyngeal tonsils (adenoids)
    (a) Located in upper rear wall of oral cavity
    (b) Fair size in childhood, shrink after puberty
b. Functions
   i. Part of the lymphatic system
   ii. Help to filter the circulating lymph of bacteria and other foreign material that may enter body through mouth or nose

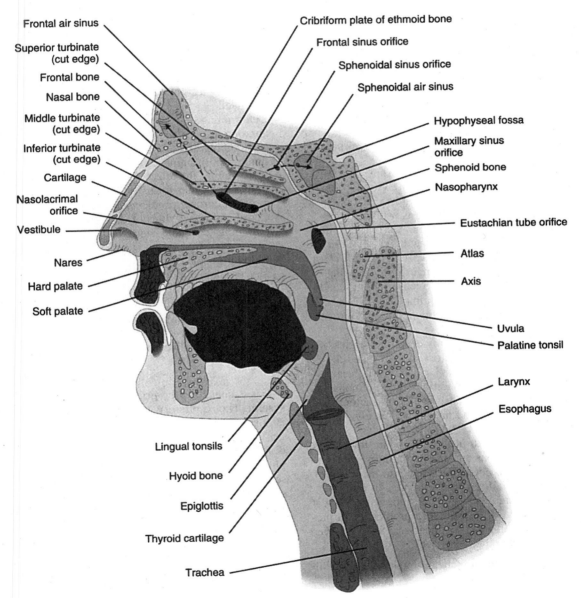

Figure 35–2. Structures of the upper airway. (From Black, J.M., Matassarin-Jacobs, E. [1997]. *Medical-Surgical Nursing Clinical Management for Continuity of Care*, 5th ed. Philadelphia: Saunders, p. 1022.)

       c. Nerve supply
         i.   Middle and posterior branches of the maxillary and glossopharyngeal nerves
         ii. Cranial nerve X (vagus)
            (a) Parasympathetic, visceral, afferent, motor, general sensory
            (b) Supplies sensory fibers to ear, tongue, pharynx, and larynx
            (c) Supplies motor fibers to pharynx, larynx, esophagus
       d. Blood supply
         i.   External carotid branch (ascending palatine branch of facial artery)
    4. Larynx
       a. Thyroid cartilage
         i.   Shield-shaped cartilage
         ii. Produces prominence on neck ("Adam's apple")
       b. Hyoid bone
         i.   Horse-shaped bone
         ii. Situated at the base of the tongue, just below the thyroid cartilage
       c. Cricoid cartilage
         i.   Ring-like cartilage
         ii. Forms lower and back part of larynx
       d. Epiglottis
         i.   Lid-like cartilage structure
         ii. Hangs over the entrance to the larynx
       e. Arytenoid cartilages
         i.   Jug-shaped cartilage of the larynx
       f. Corniculate cartilages
         i.   Two small conical nodules of yellow elastic cartilage
         ii. Articulate with the arytenoid cartilages
       g. Cuneiform cartilage
         i.   Elongated yellow elastic cartilage in the aryepiglottic fold
       h. Glottis
         i.   Vocal apparatus of the larynx
         ii. Consists of true vocal cords (vocal folds) and opening between them
       i. Nerve supply
         i.   Superior laryngeal nerve
            (a) Motor, general sensory, visceral afferent, parasympathetic
           (b) Cricothyroid muscle and inferior constrictor muscles of the pharynx, mucous membrane of back of tongue and larynx
         ii. Recurrent laryngeal nerve
            (a) Parasympathetic, visceral afferent, motor
           (b) Tracheal mucosa, esophagus, cardiac plexus

II. Assessment Parameters
  A. Preoperative
    1. Emphasize screening for:
      a. Bleeding disorders in patient or family
      b. Medications affecting clotting
      c. Sensory or motor deficits
      d. Airway compromise
  B. Postoperative
    1. General airway status—can be compromised by swelling, bleeding, reactive airway disorder, or packings
    2. Procedure-specific assessment should include:
      a. Ear procedures

    i.   Facial nerve function—assess facial symmetry by asking patient to:
         (a) Smile enough to show teeth
         (b) Wrinkle forehead
         (c) Pucker lips
         (d) Wrinkle nose
         (e) Squeeze eyelids shut
         (f) Stick out tongue
    ii. Nausea—places patient at high risk for aspiration
    iii. Vertigo
  b. Oropharyngeal procedures
    i.   Packs in place—check security of packs, assess for interference with airway
    ii. Presence of edema—leads to airway compromise
    iii. Nausea
    iv. Frequent swallowing—can indicate presence of bleeding
  c. Sinus/nasal procedures
    i.   Packs in place
    ii. Frequent swallowing
    iii. Assess for visual disturbance, particularly with endoscopic sinus
         procedures
    iv. Assess for CSF leak
    v.   Remind patient of need to breathe through mouth

III. Operative Procedures
  A. Ear
    1. Foreign body removal—common in pediatrics
    2. Mastoidectomy—removal of diseased bone of the mastoid; related to infection or cholesteatoma
    3. Myringotomy with or without tubes—incision of the tympanic membrane to treat otitis media
    4. Stapedectomy—removal of the stapes to treat otosclerosis, and replacement with a prosthesis
    5. Tympanoplasty—procedure performed on the middle ear to improve hearing and prevent recurrent infection
    6. Myringoplasty—surgical restoration of perforated tympanic membrane by grafting
  B. Sinus
    1. Caldwell-Luc antrostomy—creates a large opening in the antral wall to remove diseased sinus tissue and promote drainage
    2. Endoscopic sinus surgery—less radical than Caldwell-Luc; utilizes an endoscope to remove diseased tissue, promote ventilation and drainage
    3. Ethmoidectomy—removal of diseased middle turbinate, reduces the ethmoidal labyrinth to one large cavity, promoting drainage
    4. Nasal antral window—creates an opening in the lateral wall of the nose under the middle turbinate, relieves edema or infection of the membrane lining, decreases sinus headaches
  C. Nasal
    1. Closed or open reduction of nasal fracture
    2. Nasal polypectomy—removal of polyps that cause obstruction to air flow
    3. Rhinoplasty—reconstruction of the shape of the nose, sides, tip, or hump
    4. Septoplasty/submucous resection—removal of osseous or cartilaginous portions of the septum to repair congenital or traumatic deformities that interfere with normal respiratory function or nasal drainage

D. Oropharyngeal
1. Adenoidectomy
2. Biopsies
3. Laryngoscopy with or without polypectomy
4. Pharyngoscopy
5. Tonsillectomy with or without adenoidectomy or myringotomy
IV. **Perianesthesia Priorities: Phase I, Preoperative**
A. Preoperative objectives
1. Assess and prepare for the surgical experience
2. Obtain baseline data
a. Used to plan and implement nursing care
3. Initiate the educational process
a. Continues throughout the continuum of care
B. Assessment
1. General history and assessment; emphasize screening for:
a. Bleeding disorders in patient or family
b. Medications affecting clotting
c. Airway compromise
d. Sensory or motor deficits
2. Assess for educational needs
3. Assess for psychosocial needs
a. Developmental-age needs
b. Family/responsible adult companion availability
c. Community resources needed
C. Plan of care
1. Include patient/family/responsible adult companion in developing a plan of care appropriate to the age of the patient
2. Nursing diagnoses might include but are not limited to:
a. Anxiety/fear related to knowledge deficit, unfamiliar environment, separation from family, lack of control, etc.
b. Pain related to surgical/procedural intervention
c. Potential for injury
d. Potential for infection
D. Interventions
1. Nursing interventions might include, but are not limited to:
a. Ensure that all laboratory studies are completed as ordered/indicated
b. Provide information on preoperative preparation (NPO, medications, hygiene, ride/aftercare arrangements, etc.)
c. Obtain baseline vital signs
d. Ensure legal authorization if appropriate (informed consent)
e. Provide orientation to surroundings
E. Evaluation
1. Evaluation of interventions/patient response might include:
a. Laboratory results are reviewed, and follow-up completed as indicated
b. Patient/family/responsible adult companion are questioned to determine understanding of preoperative instructions
c. Determine that patient has made arrangements for aftercare
V. **Perianesthesia Priorities: Phase II, PACU**
A. Objective
1. Ensure that the patient safely recovers from the immediate effects of surgery and anesthesia

B. Assessment
   1. General—per protocol
      a. Airway status—patient is at high risk for airway compromise
      b. Vital signs
      c. Bleeding
      d. Discomfort
      e. Toxic reactions to local anesthetic
      f. Effects of medications, including cocaine if used
   2. Procedure-specific—see assessment parameters noted previously
C. Plan of care
   1. Include patient/family/responsible adult companion in developing a plan of care appropriate to the age of the patient
   2. Nursing diagnoses might include those listed above
   3. Be alert for potential complications
      a. Ear procedures
         i.   Nausea
         ii. Vertigo
         iii. Graft/prosthesis compromise
         iv. Facial nerve damage
      b. Sinus procedures
         i.   CSF leakage
         ii. Visual disturbances
         iii. Hematoma
         iv. Tooth pain
         v.   Cardiac dysrhythmias from cocaine or epinephrine
      c. Nasal procedures
         i.   Swelling
         ii. Bleeding
         iii. Cardiac dysrhythmias
      d. Oropharyngeal procedures
         i.   Bleeding
         ii. Edema
         iii. Airway obstruction
D. Nursing interventions
   1. General
      a. Monitor vital signs per protocol
      b. Administer medications for pain and nausea as ordered
      c. Observe for bleeding and other complications
      d. Ensure a safe environment
   2. Procedure-specific
      a. Ear procedures
         i.   Positioning should be clarified by physician
              (a) Operated ear upward prevents graft displacement; downward promotes drainage
              (b) Head of bed elevation >30-degrees decreases edema
         ii. Prevent or treat nausea
              (a) Avoid sudden, rapid head motion and excessive movements
              (b) Administer antiemetic as ordered
              (c) Encourage slow deep breathing
              (d) Administer IV fluids as ordered to maintain hydration
         iii. Assess facial nerve function as noted above

        iv. Avoid pressure on dressing; do not disturb inner dressing

        v. Avoid coughing or sneezing

           (a) Instruct patient to do so with mouth open to avoid pressure in the inner ear

           (b) Do not allow patient to blow nose forcefully

  b. Sinus and nasal procedures

     i. Position to prevent aspiration and reduce edema

     ii. Change mustache dressing prn

     iii. Apply ice to increase vasoconstriction and reduce swelling

  c. Oropharyngeal procedures

     i. Position to prevent aspiration and reduce edema

     ii. Observe for bleeding; note swallowing of blood

     iii. Offer cool or tepid fluids

E. Evaluation

  1. Response to interventions are evaluated continually throughout the patient's stay

  2. Alterations to plan of care are made as indicated

  3. Examples might include:

    a. Pain medication effectiveness

    b. Effectiveness of measures to prevent nausea

VI. Perianesthesia Priorities: Phase III, Preparation for Discharge

A. Objective

  1. Ready the patient to return to home, prepared—in conjunction with a caregiver—to successfully manage postoperative care

  2. Education of the patient and caregiver is a critical factor to a successful ambulatory-surgery outcome

B. Assessment

  1. Procedure-specific assessment continues as outlined in Phase II to ensure that postoperative status is stable prior to discharge

C. Plan of care

  1. Plan should be appropriate to the age of the patient and developed in conjunction with the patient and family/caregiver

  2. Nursing diagnoses established previously are still pertinent

  3. Be alert for potential complications as noted previously

D. Nursing interventions

  1. Procedure-specific interventions initiated in Phase II continue

  2. The patient and family are also instructed to continue interventions at home as appropriate

  3. Education interventions

    a. Discussion, demonstration, written materials, etc.

    b. Copies of all materials given to patients should be maintained in the medical record or on the unit

E. Evaluation

  1. Evaluation of clinical interventions continues as noted above

  2. Evaluation of learning

    a. Patient/caregiver verbalization of understanding, demonstrating a skill, etc.

    b. Patient and responsible party should sign that they have been instructed and had the opportunity to have questions answered

VII. Education Content

A. Phase I, Preoperative

  1. General

    a. NPO

    b. Preoperative hygiene and/or scrubs, shampoos

c. Environment
d. Facility protocols
e. Aftercare arrangements
f. Perioperative course

2. Procedure-specific
a. Avoid nose blowing and sneezing, bending, or pressure-creating activities
b. Dressings and packings to anticipate
c. Positioning restrictions
d. Anticipate a feeling of fullness with oropharyngeal procedures
e. Mouth breathing for nasal and sinus procedures
f. Swallowing blood may result in brown/red emesis and nausea

B. Postoperative
1. General
a. Activity
b. Diet
c. Medications
d. Complications
e. Follow-up care

2. Procedure-specific
a. Ear procedures
   i. Positioning per physician
   ii. Keep dressings dry
   iii. Limit sudden or excessive movements to decrease nausea and vertigo
   iv. Report any signs of bleeding or infection to the physician
   v. Avoid coughing and nose blowing
b. Sinus and nasal procedures
   i. Avoid sneezing and nose blowing
   ii. Leave packing in place
   iii. Change mustache dressing prn
   iv. Maintain head elevation
   v. Ice packs as ordered
   vi. Report any increase in bloody drainage or signs of infection
c. Oropharyngeal procedures (tonsillectomy/adenoidectomy)
   i. Diet—progress from cool/tepid liquids to soft foods to normal diet
   ii. Avoid excessive talking, throat clearing, coughing, smoking, spicy or mechanically hard foods, thermal extremes in food and beverages, aspirin or products containing aspirin, and physical exertion
   iii. Oral hygiene—rinse gently frequently for bad breath
   iv. Notify physician for bright red bleeding
   v. Expect dark stools from swallowed blood
   vi. For late bleeding (days 5–10 postoperatively, when eschar separates)—lie down quietly and remain calm; notify physician if bleeding persists
   vii. Expect some neck stiffness or rhinitis

C. Documentation must include:
1. Assessment and planning for meeting educational needs
2. Interventions—discussion, demonstration, written materials, etc.
3. Copies of all materials given to patients should be maintained in the medical record or on the unit
4. Evaluation of learning—verbalization of understanding, demonstrating a skill, etc.
5. Patient and responsible party should sign that they have been instructed and had the opportunity to have questions answered

---

BOX 35–1.   Key Patient Educational Outcomes

- The patient who has undergone an ear procedure verbalizes precautions to remain free of infection; avoids water in ears, uses ear plugs
- The patient who has undergone a nasal procedure is able to verbalize measures to decrease dry mouth, secondary to mouth breathing; frequent mouth care performed, oral mucous membranes are moist
- Patient verbalizes measures to decrease pain after sinus surgery; application of ice, administration of analgesics
- The tonsillectomy and adenoidectomy patient or caregiver verbalizes the appropriate diet following surgery
- The patient who has undergone nasal surgery is able to describe the typical postoperative events
- The patient is able to list precautionary measures to prevent new nasal bleeding

---

Bibliography

1. Black, J.M., Matassarin-Jacobs, E. (1997). *Medical-Surgical Nursing—Clinical Management for Continuity of Care*, 5th ed. Philadelphia: Saunders.
2. Burden, N. (ed) (1993). *Ambulatory Surgical Nursing*. Philadelphia: Saunders.
3. Drain, C.B. (1994). *The Post Anesthesia Care Unit: A Critical Care Approach to Post Anesthesia Nursing*. Philadelphia: Saunders.
4. Gray, H. (1985). *Anatomy of the Human Body*. Clemente, C., ed. Philadelphia: Lea & Febiger.
5. Guyton, A.C. (1991). *Textbook of Medical Physiology*. Philadelphia: Saunders.
6. Litwack, K., ed. (1995). *Core Curriculum for Post Anesthesia Nursing Practice*, 3rd ed. Philadelphia: Saunders.
7. Meeker, M.H., Rothrock, J.C. (1991). *Alexander's Care of the Patient in Surgery*, 9th ed. St. Louis: Mosby.

REVIEW QUESTIONS

1. Disturbances in equilibrium can be related to disease processes in the

   A. Cochlea
   B. Scala vestibuli
   C. Auricle
   D. Vestibular apparatus

2. To prevent graft displacement following ear surgery, the nurse should position the patient with

   A. Operated ear down
   B. Head of the bed up
   C. Operated ear up
   D. Head of the bed flat

3. After ear surgery, the nurse avoids sudden rapid motion in order to prevent

   A. Pain
   B. Nausea
   C. Dyspnea
   D. Bleeding

4. To assess nerve function following a mastoidectomy, the nurse should ask the patient to

   A. Open the mouth
   B. Blink the eyes
   C. Wrinkle the forehead
   D. Lift the head

5. Postoperatively, the patient who has undergone an ENT surgical procedure can have a compromised airway due to

   A. Swelling
   B. Bleeding
   C. Reactive airway disorder
   D. Packings
   E. All of the above

6. During the preadmission assessment, emphasize screening for all of the following except

   A. Bleeding disorders in patient and family
   B. Sensory and motor deficits
   C. Socioeconomic status
   D. Developmental age needs
   E. Medications affecting clotting

7. Potential complications following ear procedures include all of the following except

   A. Vertigo
   B. CSF leakage
   C. Facial nerve damage
   D. Graft/prosthesis compromise
   E. Nausea

8. All of the following are true regarding the palatine tonsils except

   A. They lie one on each side of the throat
   B. They are the size of almonds
   C. They are located at the base of the tongue
   D. They are partially imbedded in mucous membrane

9. Potential complications of ear procedures include

   (1) Nausea
   (2) Vertigo
   (3) Graft/prosthesis compromise
   (4) Facial nerve damage

   A. 1, 2
   B. 2, 3
   C. 2, 3, 4
   D. All of the above

10. To prevent or treat nausea in the postoperative ENT patient, the nurse should

    A. Avoid sudden, rapid head motion and excessive movements
    B. Administer antiemetic as ordered
    C. Encourage slow deep breathing
    D. Administer IV fluids as ordered to prevent dehydration
    E. All of the above

ANSWERS TO QUESTIONS

1. D
2. C
3. B
4. C
5. E

6. C
7. B
8. C
9. D
10. E

Plastic and Reconstructive Surgery

Lisa Peck Glazier
Mercy Hospital
Portland, Maine

I. **Anatomy of the Skin**
   A. The largest organ of the body
   B. Structure of the body
   C. Structure of the skin
      1. Epidermis
         a. Outer layer
         b. Varies in thickness—thickest over soles of feet and thinnest over eyelids
      2. Dermis—true skin
         a. Contains nerve endings, capillaries, and the lymph system
         b. Composed of connective tissue and collagen
      3. Subcutaneous tissue—contains adipose tissue and connective tissue; attached to dermis by collagen
      4. Deep fascia—surrounds muscle and bone; connects periosteum to bone
      5. Skin also includes hair, nails, and sweat and sebaceous glands
   D. Physiology of skin
      1. Protective barrier against physical, chemical, and bacterial agents
      2. Maintains body temperature
      3. Functions as a sensory organ—pressure, touch, temperature, and pain
      4. Prevents loss of body fluid
      5. Excretes waste from sweat glands
      6. Contributes to self-concept and body image

Objectives

1. Describe the anatomy of skin.
2. Describe the physiology of wound healing.
3. Discuss the impact of plastic surgery on body image.
4. Describe preoperative preparation of the plastic and hand surgical patient.
5. List common ambulatory plastic and reconstructive surgeries.
6. Discuss the nursing care for the individual surgical procedures outlined.
7. Discuss expected educational outcomes for each surgical procedure.

II. Wound Healing
  A. Wound
    1. A disruption of the integrity and function of tissues in the body
  B. Process of wound healing
    1. Inflammatory—hemostasis and epithelialization occur, WBCs cleanse wound; stage lasts up to four days
    2. Proliferative—collagen synthesis occurs giving strength to the wound, granulation tissue forms; stage lasts up to three weeks
    3. Remodeling—collagen fibers are remodeled and scar matures
      a. Becomes flat, thin, silver in color
      b. Stage lasts 1 to 2 years
  C. Factors influencing wound healing
    1. Age
      a. Children heal rapidly
      b. Geriatrics heal slower due to decreased circulation
    2. Nutrition—malnutrition, dehydration, and vitamin deficiency slow healing process
    3. Nicotine—causes poor healing due to oxygen deprivation and vasoconstriction
    4. Endocrine function—steroids decrease inflammatory response
    5. Presence of foreign body—slows healing due to inflammatory response
    6. Infection—slows healing due to prolonged inflammatory response
    7. Dead space—accumulation of air or fluid slows healing, promotes infection
III. Preanesthesia Assessment: Body Image Considerations of the Plastic Surgery Patient
  A. Body image—the mental picture we possess of our own body
    1. Body image is a changing dynamic entity influenced by internal and external factors
    2. Body image is a component of how we feel about ourselves
  B. Motivation for plastic surgery
    1. Internal motivation—surgery to change physical appearance of oneself
    2. External motivation—surgery to change physical appearance at recommendation of others
    3. Patients internally motivated are most pleased with surgical outcomes
  C. Preoperative assessment related to body image
    1. Understand patient's perception of body deformity
    2. Understand patient's expectation of surgical outcome
    3. Explore significant other's feelings regarding procedure
    4. Assess postoperative support and coping mechanisms
  D. Integration of surgical changes into body image
    1. Patients may progress through the stages of grieving
    2. Changed physical appearance slowly integrates into body image and then self-concept
    3. Some patients never integrate changes into body image; may request more surgery or require counseling
  E. Nursing care related to body image
    1. Encourage patient to verbalize feelings
    2. Reassure patient that it is normal to desire physical attractiveness
    3. Support the stages of grieving
    4. Be nonjudgmental with verbal and nonverbal communication
IV. Preoperative Teaching for the Plastic and Reconstructive Patient
  A. Specific instructions
    1. Discuss bruising and swelling that will be present postoperatively
    2. Encourage patient to prepare caregivers for postoperative appearance
    3. Refer to an aesthetician for camouflage makeup as indicated

    B. Head and neck surgery
      1. Instruct patient to bring sunglasses and scarves on day of surgery
      2. Have a supply of ice ready at home
    C. Laser resurfacing
      1. Explain postoperative skin and dressing care regime
      2. Include list of needed supplies
      3. No hair spray or makeup the day of surgery
      4. Physician may prescribe preoperative antibiotic, antiviral, Retin A, or Solaquin Forte
      5. Should discontinue Accutane for at least 6 months
    D. Breast surgery
      1. Wear front buttoning shirt on day of surgery to decrease pain when dressing
    E. Abdominoplasty and suction lipectomy
      1. Instruct patient to have extra pillows available for splinting and positioning
      2. Encourage patient to set up a living area to include minimal stair climbing
    F. Hand surgery
      1. Wear clothing with large sleeve openings
      2. Prepare the home for living with one upper extremity
      3. Pillows needed for elevation of affected extremity

V. Postanesthesia: Phase I Considerations
    A. Airway management
      1. Maintain patency
      2. Suction prn
      3. Provide oxygen as needed
      4. Assess frequently for hematoma formation that may cause airway obstruction, i.e., facelift, neck liposuction (refer to Table 36–1)
      5. Assist with smooth extubation to decrease risk of bleeding at operative site
    B. Maintain cardiac stability
      1. Keep blood pressure within normal limits
      2. Control pain with medications
      3. Use antihypertensives if pain control ineffective for elevated blood pressure
      4. Monitor cardiac rhythm
    C. Monitor surgical site
      1. Assess dressing frequently
      2. Observe for hematoma formation
      3. Maintain patency of drains
      4. Monitor amount of drainage
    D. Maintain normothermia
      1. Apply warm blankets
      2. Use available warming techniques
      3. Warm fluids
      4. Check temperature frequently

Table 36–1 • HEMATOMA RECOGNITION

Increasing pain not effected by higher medication doses
Severe ecchymosis or pallor
Increasing firmness of tissue surrounding the operative site
More swelling on one side than the other
Difficulty breathing or swallowing (face lift)
Loss of vision or pressure behind the eye (blepharoplasty)

E. Pain management
1. Implement pain-assessment tools to monitor pain
2. Administer pain medications using the multimodal approach
   a. Narcotics
   b. Nonsteroidal antiinflammatories (NSAIDs)
   c. Local anesthesia in wounds
F. Nausea and vomiting
1. Prevention
   a. Pretreat with antiemetics for effective approach
2. Untreated pain and narcotics may cause nausea
3. Vomiting should be avoided to prevent tension on suture lines and hematoma formation
4. Administer antiemetics prn
G. Fluid management
1. Evaluate for signs of hypovolemia
2. Administer fluids to replace blood loss
H. Positioning
1. Elevate surgical site to prevent swelling
2. Position to prevent tension on suture lines
3. Position to decrease pain
I. Neurovascular status
1. Assess for nerve damage
2. Monitor tissue perfusion of affected area
J. Comfort measures
1. Maintain calm, reassuring environment
2. Allow for ventilation of feelings
3. Provide reassurance for cosmetic patients
   a. Desire for physical attractiveness is normal

VI. Operative Procedures
A. Abdominoplasty
1. Description
   a. Surgical removal of redundant tissue of the abdomen
   b. Involves skin, fascia, and adipose tissue
   c. May include closure of abdominal wall muscles
2. Purpose
   a. To improve body shape
   b. Correct muscle wall deformity
3. Postanesthesia care, Phase II considerations
   a. Anesthesia—general
   b. Patient selection important for ambulatory abdominoplasty
      i.   Must stay within close proximity to surgicenter
      ii. Patient must be motivated
      iii. Home support must be adequate
   c. Maintain good pain control so patient can ambulate, cough, and deep breathe
   d. Control nausea so pain medications will be tolerated
   e. Maintain correct positioning
      i.   Head of bed elevated
      ii. Pillow under knees
      iii. Use pillow splint for coughing and moving
      iv. Walk in stooped position for 1 week

    f. Empty drains as needed
        i.   Two Jackson Pratt drains not unusual
        ii. Empty and record drainage
        iii. Maintain patency of drains
            (a) Clots can be a sign of hematoma formation
    g. Patient will wear a compression girdle for two to three weeks
  4. Patient education
    a. Review instructions with patient and caregiver
        i. Demonstration for positioning and moving
        ii. Activity restrictions
    b. Drain-emptying demonstration
    c. Hematoma assessment
    d. Pain-management techniques
B. Surgery of the breast
  1. Reduction mammoplasty/mastopexy
    a. Description
        i. Surgical excision of redundant breast tissue and skin with recontouring of
           breast shape
    b. Purpose
        i. Reduction—to decrease neck, back, and shoulder pain
        ii. Mastopexy—aesthetic procedure to lift breasts
    c. Postanesthesia care, Phase II considerations
        i.   Patient selection important for outpatient reduction
            (a) Home care must be adequate
        ii. Anesthesia—general
        iii. Assess for hematoma
            (a) Palpate superior aspect of pectoralis muscle over the third rib to the
                clavicle
        iv. Drains may be used postoperatively for mastopexy or breast reduction
            (a) Monitor drainage
            (b) Reinforce to keep clothing and bedding dry
        v.   Treat pain
            (a) Usually described as moderate
                (i) May need IV narcotic on emergence
            (b) Control with strong narcotics at home (i.e., oxycodone for first day
                or two)
        vi. Patient will have on compression bra
            (a) Tube gauze over the bra assists in holding reinforcement ABDs
                in place
        vii. Prevent and treat nausea and vomiting
            (a) Vomiting can cause hematoma formation
        viii. Provide aggressive fluid replacement for blood loss
            (a) Usual blood loss 400 cc
            (b) Replace with crystalloid or colloid as needed
            (c) Some patients may require hospitalization if symptomatic after blood
                loss and fluid replacement
    d. Patient education
        i. Observe for hematoma formation
        ii. Activity
            (a) No heavy lifting or strenuous activity for 1 month
            (b) No pushing self up with arms
                (i) Instruct patient and caregiver on how to make position changes

          (c) Usually a return appointment in 24 hours for drain removal

          (d) Steristrips or sutures may be removed in one week

          (e) Compression bra for 2 to 3 weeks

          (f) Demonstration on how to reinforce dressing

2. Augmentation mammoplasty
   a. Description
      i. To increase the breast size or improve breast shape with the use of a prosthesis
      ii. Prosthesis placed under the pectoral muscle or mammary tissue through an inframammary, axillary, areolar incision or endoscope
   b. Purpose
      i. To improve body image and self confidence
   c. Postanesthesia care, Phase II considerations
      i. Anesthesia—general or local with MAC
      ii. Assess for hematoma
         (a) Palpate superior aspect of pectoralis muscle over the third rib to the clavicle
         (b) Breast size should remain equal
      iii. Assess for signs of pneumothorax
         (a) More common with axillary incision
         (b) Have chest tube and drainage setup available
         (c) Auscultate lung sounds
      iv. Provide pain relief
         (a) Pain is moderate to severe
         (b) Prosthesis beneath chest muscle is more painful
         (c) Multimodal drug therapy effective
            (i) Narcotics IV and oral, Toradol
            (ii) Local anesthesia in wounds
            (iii) Muscle relaxants for spasm
            (iv) Ice may be helpful for pain control
      v. Prevent and treat nausea so oral pain medications can be tolerated
   d. Patient education
      i. Observe for hematoma
      ii. Ace wrap or soft-support bra may be worn for one week
      iii. Observe for capsule formation
      iv. May occur months after surgery
         (a) Massage instructions per physician preference
         (b) Massage usually begins 2 weeks postoperatively
            (i) Massage keeps prosthesis mobile in pocket
      v. Activity
         (a) Restrict arm activity for three to four weeks

3. Breast reconstruction
   a. Description
      i. Replacement of breast with the use of tissue expansion and placement of prosthesis postmastectomy
   b. Purpose
      i. To replace a lost body part
      ii. Usually due to cancer
   c. Postanesthesia care, Phase II considerations
      i. Ambulatory care may include initial insertion of tissue expander or replacement of ruptured expander
      ii. Modified mastectomy usually done in hospital with placement of expander

        iii. Flap reconstruction of breast presently done in hospital setting
        iv. Anesthesia—general
        v. Nursing care same as augmentation mammoplasty
        vi. Psychological support crucial as patients have had multiple procedures and cancer diagnosis
        vii. Patients come back when expansion complete
            (a) Prosthesis inserted
            (b) Nipple reconstruction done
            (c) Nipple tattoo or graft reconstruction
        viii. Pain can be severe with initial insertion of expander
            (a) Treatment same as augmentation
    d. Patient education
        i. Observe for hematoma formation
        ii. Report deflation of tissue expander
        iii. Could mean rupture
        iv. Limit arm activity for 1 month
        v. Frequent appointments required for inflation of expander with saline
  4. Gynecomastectomy
    a. Description
        i. Removal of excessive breast tissue in male patient
    b. Purpose
        i. To improve self confidence and body image
    c. Postanesthesia care, Phase II considerations
        i. Anesthesia—general or local (for small excision)
        ii. Assess for hematoma formation
        iii. Maintain patency of drains (Jackson Pratts not unusual)
        iv. Pain usually described as moderate
    d. Patient education
        i. Observe for hematoma
        ii. Provide instruction and demonstration of drain care
            (a) Usually removed after 48 hours
        iii. Arm activity limited for one month
        iv. ACE wrap or compression vest usually worn for compression
C. Surgery of the face and neck
  1. Description
    a. Rhytidectomy—facelift
        i. Tightening of all tissue of the face and neck with excision of redundant tissue
    b. Coronal browlift
        i. Tightening the tissue of the forehead and brow with excision of redundant tissue
    c. Endoscopic surgery of the head and neck
        i. Face, neck, and brow lift may be performed with the endoscopic technique when redundant tissue excision is not required
        ii. Postoperative assessment and intervention remain the same as for open techniques
  2. Purpose
    a. To remove wrinkle and facial laxity giving a more rested, youthful appearance
  3. Postanesthesia care, Phase II considerations
    a. Patient selection and home care very important for outpatient facial surgery
    b. Anesthesia—MAC or general

    c. Assess for hematoma formation
       i.   Palpate neck, forehead, and check frequently
       ii.   Bulky dressings common
          (a) Assess for absence of increasing tightness, difficulty breathing, or swallowing
       iii. If any question of hematoma, notify surgeon so dressing can be taken down
       iv. Maintain patency of drains
          (a) May have Jackson Pratts or Penrose
    d. Maintain normal blood pressure
       i.   To prevent hematoma formation
       ii.   Manage pain before it increases blood pressure
       iii. Treat uncontrolled hypertension with antihypertensives if pain management not the cause
       iv. Prevent nausea and vomiting
       v.   Provide calm, reassuring environment to decrease anxiety
    e. Maintain comfort
       i.   Pain can be considered moderate to severe for facelift
       ii.   Browlift pain usually described as severe headache
       iii. Begin medications before all local anesthesia has resolved
       iv. Combination of oral and IV narcotics may be required
       v.   Toradol very effective but contraindicated by some physicians due to bleeding potential
       vi. Ice effective for brow pain
    f. Positioning
       i.   Elevate head of bed to decrease swelling
       ii.   Avoid activities that increase blood pressure
       iii. Avoid turning head side to side or nodding
       iv. Assess cranial nerve VII
       v.   Ask patient to smile, frown, wrinkle forehead and nose
       vi. Assess facial symmetry
       vii. Assess sensation of earlobes
       viii. If facial nerve is damaged it will regenerate with time

4. Patient education
    a. Activity
       i.   Avoid strenuous activity for 1 month
    b. Elevate head and torso with two pillows at bedtime
    c. Observe for hematoma formation
       i.   Drain care demonstration
       ii.   If drains are present they are usually removed in 24 hours
    d. Hair washing per physician
       i.   Usually after sutures are removed in 1 week
    e. Soft diet with little chewing
    f. Appropriate use of pain medications and ice for pain control

D. Blepharoplasty
  1. Definition
    a. Surgical removal of redundant skin and adipose tissue with shortening of muscles of the upper and lower eyelids
    b. Surgical incisions may be done with laser or scalpel
  2. Purpose
    a. To provide patient with a more youthful and less fatigued look
    b. To improve vision fields

   3. Postanesthesia care, Phase II considerations
     a. Anesthesia—local
     b. Assess for signs of retrobulbar hematoma formation
       i. Medical emergency
       ii. Signs
         (a) Pressure behind eye
         (b) Loss of vision
       iii. Observe for:
         (a) Pallor, ecchymosis, firmness, or complaints or pain or tightness around eyes
         (b) Proptosis
           (i) Forward displacement or bulging eye
     c. Maintain normal blood pressure
       i. Retards hematoma formation
       ii. Avoid straining, lifting, bending at least 1 week
       iii. Elevate head of bed
     d. Pain usually described as mild to moderate
       i. Control with moderate strength narcotics (codeine or hydrocodone usually effective)
       ii. Ice packs provide pain control and decrease swelling
  4. Patient education
     a. Activity
       i. Avoid activities that will increase blood pressure
       ii. Limit reading and television
         (a) Observe for hematoma formation
       iii. Use ice as ordered
         (a) Keep cloth between ice bag and skin
         (b) Frozen peas in the bag works well
       iv. Eyes may be dry and lashes crusty with bloody drainage
         (a) Mild blurring is expected
         (b) Call immediately for loss of vision or pressure behind eye
         (c) Use sterile saline drops to moisten eyes and separate lashes
       v. Sutures usually removed in 5 days or surgeon preference
 E. Laser resurfacing
  1. Definition
     a. Removal of rhytids (wrinkles) and other skin irregularities with the ultrapulse carbon dioxide laser
  2. Purpose
     a. To remove signs of aging and give a youthful appearance
  3. Postanesthesia care, Phase II considerations
     a. Anesthesia—local or general
     b. Provide comfort measures
       i. Medicate with narcotics as needed
         (a) NSAIDs helpful
       ii. Pain can be mild to severe
         (a) Ice to affected area or cold gel mask decreases discomfort and swelling
     c. Elevate head of bed
     d. Continue prophylactic antibiotics and antiviral agents as ordered
     e. Provide nourishment through a straw
       i. Full face resurfacing will cause swelling around the mouth
     f. A child's toothbrush can assist with mouth care

g. Skin care will vary according to physician preference
    i.   Open technique (no dressing)
        (a) Cool saline compresses on the face for the first night
        (b) On day one, q.i.d. vinegar and water soaks with gentle removal of crusts
        (c) Frequent application of petroleum jelly, antibiotic ointment, Aquaphor, or Preparation H
        (d) Goal is to keep skin soft, pink, and free of crusts
        (e) Soaks are continued until the crusting ceases (7 to 10 days), then a moisturizer is used
h. Closed technique
    i.   Flexan (biomembrane dressing) is applied to the affected area
        (a) Any exposed areas are treated with the open technique
        (b) Flexan dressing is changed according to the physician's preference
    ii.   N-terface dressing can be applied to affected areas
        (a) It is held in place with tube gauze and 4×4's to absorb drainage
        (b) Soaks may be done through the dressing and application of petroleum jelly or other lubricant is put on over the dressing
        (c) N-terface is changed according to physician's preference
i. Laser resurfacing patients require reassurance and reinforcement of skin care instructions
    4. Patient education
      a. Activity
        i.   Elevate head of bed
      b. Skin and dressing care per physician's preference
      c. Continue antiviral and antibiotic agents as ordered
      d. Observe and report any signs of infection
      e. Encourage patient to call office with any questions on skin care
      f. Instruct patient to avoid sun while skin is healing
        i.   When healed, use at least a 15 sunscreen
      g. Instruct patient to notify physician if any hyperpigmentation changes are noted
      h. Face will remain pink for 4 to 6 weeks
        i.   Camouflage makeup is helpful
F. Rhinoplasty
    1. Description
      a. Excision of fat, cartilage, and skin with fracturing of nasal bones to reshape the nose
    2. Purpose
      a. To improve body image and self confidence
    3. Postanesthesia care, Phase II considerations
      a. Anesthesia—general or MAC with local anesthesia
      b. Provide comfort measures
        i.   Pain usually described as moderate but may be severe
        ii.   Medicate with oral or IV narcotics prn
            (a) NSAIDs can be helpful
            (b) Begin medications before local anesthesia resolves
            (c) Ice mask to reduce swelling and pain
      c. Provide calm, reassuring environment
        i.   Patient may have packing in both nares
        ii.   Inability to breathe through nose can be anxiety-producing
            (a) Provide reassurance

        iii. Mouth will be very dry
            (a) Give frequent mouth care
        iv. Position patient with head of bed elevated
        v. Prevent postoperative nausea and vomiting
            (a) Encourage patient to expectorate any postnasal bloody secretions
            (b) Medicate with antiemetics prn

4. Patient education
  a. Activity
    i. No strenuous activity for 1 month
    ii. No flexing from waist
    iii. No flexing head
  b. Nasal packing usually removed in 24 to 72 hours
  c. Continue ice mask at home
    i. Swelling and bruising may be worse on second or third postoperative day
  d. Use humidifier at home to prevent drying of mucous membranes
    i. Force fluids

G. Otoplasty
  1. Description
    a. Reshaping of the cartilage and skin of the outer ear
  2. Purpose
    a. To correct prominent or malformed ears
    b. To improve body image and self confidence
  3. Postanesthesia care, Phase II considerations
    a. Anesthesia—local or general depending on age of patient
    b. Frequently a procedure for school-age children
    c. Assess for hematoma formation
      i. Use severe pain as an indicator because of bulky head dressing
    d. Medicate for pain with oral narcotics
      i. Usually described as moderate pain
    e. Children have usually suffered teasing due to ears
      i. Assure them that surgical outcome is good
  4. Patient education
    a. Activity
      i. Elevate head with two pillows
      ii. No strenuous activity for 2 to 4 weeks
    b. Ears will be sensitive to cold and swell in heat for 3 to 6 months
    c. Observe for hematoma
    d. Bulky head dressing usually worn for 1 week

H. Suction lipectomy
  1. Description
    a. Removal of adipose tissue with suction-assisted device from face, neck, abdomen, thighs, buttocks, flanks, and extremities
  2. Purpose
    a. To remove pockets of adipose tissue for body contouring
  3. Postanesthesia care, Phase II considerations
    a. Anesthesia—general or local
    b. Medicate for pain
      i. Usually described as mild to moderate
    c. Maintain fluid balance
    d. Observe for hypovolemia
      i. Replace fluids as indicated by clinical signs and symptoms
      ii. Autologous blood should be available when high blood loss is expected

    iii. EBL will be decreased with the tumescent technique versus the nontumescent technique

        (a) Tumescent technique

            (i) Involves infusion of saline, lidocaine, and epinephrine into area to be suctioned

            (ii) Lipolysis is improved and blood loss is decreased

            (iii) Third spacing can occur with removal of large volumes of adipose tissue

    e. Assess for hematoma formation

    f. Compression applied with compression garment or ACE wraps

    g. Keep dressings flat and smooth for even contouring

    h. See Table 36–2

4. Patient education

    a. Instruct patient to push fluids to cover third space fluid shifts

    b. Compression garment will be worn for 24 hours to several weeks (physician preference)

    c. Activity

       i. Rest; minimal activity for first week

       ii. Avoid strenuous activity for 1 month

    d. Observe for hematoma formation

    e. Bruising and swelling are expected

    f. Female urinal can aid in elimination while compression garment is worn

    g. Instruct patient to protect bedding the first 24 hours as drainage is not unusual

    h. Sponge bathing may be required while patient is restricted to compression garment

I. Excision of lesions

1. Description

    a. Lesions to be excised will be benign or malignant

    b. Benign skin lesions

       i. Nevus

          (a) Most common skin lesion

          (b) Round

          (c) Brown or black in color

          (d) Flat or raised

          (e) With or without hair

       ii. Three types

          (a) Intradermal

          (b) Junctional

          (c) Compound

       iii. Most need no treatment unless a change is noted or if there is constant irritation

---

Table 36–2 • LIPOSUCTION COMPLICATION RISK ASSIGNMENT BY VOLUME

1500 ml or less of fat aspirate	Low risk
1500 ml–2500 ml of fat aspirate	Moderate risk
2500 ml or greater of fat aspirate	High risk (requires close supervision at home or hospitalization)

From Murrary, J.A. (1996). *Core Curriculum for Plastic and Reconstructive Surgical Nursing*, 2nd ed., Pitman, NJ: Anthony Jannetti.

        iv.   Junctional may convert to malignant melanoma

        v.   Treatment

           (a) Simple excision

    c. Malignant skin lesions

        i.   Basal cell carcinoma

           (a) Definition

               (i)   Most common skin cancer

               (ii) May be nodular with an ulcerated center or crusted, dermatitis-like

           (b) Treatments

               (i)   Surgical excision

               (ii) Possible flap graft, radiation, topical chemotherapy, or cryosurgery

        ii.   Squamous cell carcinoma

           (a) Definition

               (i)   Begins as a red papule

               (ii) Progresses to an area that ulcerates, then crusts

               (iii) Invades underlying tissue

           (b) Treatment

               (i)   Surgical excision

               (ii) Treatments may also include:

                   a) Node dissection (for recurrent or large lesions)

                   b) Chemotherapy

                   c) Radiation

        iii.   Malignant melanoma

           (a) Suspicious lesions with:

               (i)   Change in size

               (ii) Change in color (brown to black)

               (iii) Change from smooth to rough

               (iv) Irregular borders

               (v)   Change in sensation

               (vi) Satellite lesions

           (b) Treatment

               (i)   Surgical excision

               (ii) Wide margins

               (iii) Graft may be required

               (iv) Prognosis determined by size and depth of lesion

           (c) Other treatment may include:

               (i)   Wide excision

               (ii) Node dissection

               (iii) Radiation

               (iv) Chemotherapy

2. Postanesthesia care, Phase II considerations

    a. Anesthesia—local

    b. Provide reassurance and allow patient time to verbalize

    c. Can be very anxious regarding biopsy results

    d. Elevate extremities

    e. Monitor dressings

3. Patient education

    a. Instruct patient to keep incision dry per physician orders

    b. Protect incision from sun

    c. Use 15 sunscreen or greater

    d. Reduce activity of affected body part for 1 to 2 weeks

J. Surgeries of the hand
1. Description
   a. Ganglionectomy
      i. Definition—excision of a painful fluid-filled cyst attached to joint capsule or tendon
   b. Palmar fasciectomy
      i. Definition—release of a flexion contracture of the metacarpophalangeal joints
   c. Carpal tunnel release
      i. Definition—decompression of the carpal tunnel releasing pressure on median nerve; may be done with endoscope
   d. Trauma—can include:
      i. ORIF of fractures
      ii. Microsurgery to repair nerves, vessels, and tendons
2. Postanesthesia care, Phase II considerations
   a. Anesthesia—local, axillary, bier block, or general
   b. Assess extremity for circulation and neurologic status
      i. Include sensory, motor, color, and capillary refill
   c. Apply temporary sling for discharge home after axillary block
   d. Elevate extremity above level of heart using pillows
   e. Provide adequate analgesia for discharge home
      i. Consider multimodal treatment for very painful procedures (i.e., narcotics, local and NSAIDs)
         (a) Ganglionectomy—moderate to severe pain
         (b) Palmar fasciectomy—moderate pain
         (c) Carpal tunnel release—can be mild to severe pain; endoscopic repair usually more painful first postoperative night
         (d) ORIF and nerve repairs—usually moderate to severe pain
         (e) Tendon repairs—moderate pain
      ii. Pain is very individual but should not be underestimated in hand surgery
   f. Maintain drain patency—palmar fasciectomy
3. Patient education
   a. Activity
      i. No lifting or working with affected hand for 1 week
   b. Keep extremity elevated
   c. Observe circulation and neurological status of extremity
   d. Drain-emptying demonstration

VII. Phase III Care
A. Postoperative telephone call elicits information to assess:
1. Hematoma formation, patency of drains, and drainage on dressings
2. Pain assessment and medication usage

BOX 36-1.   KEY PATIENT EDUCATIONAL OUTCOMES

- Patient will describe signs of hematoma
- Patient will describe dosing of pain medications and report uncontrolled pain
- Patient will report uncontrolled nausea and vomiting
- Patient will report excessive drainage on dressing or in drainage collection system
- Patient will report signs and symptoms of infection
- Patient will report any impairment of circulation or neurological deficit
- Patient will understand activity and any limitations or restrictions

   3. Signs of infection
   4. Level of activity
   5. Presence of nausea and vomiting (try to determine cause)
   B. Reinforce postoperative teaching
   C. Provide reassurance
   D. Instruct patient to call with any questions or concerns

Bibliography

1. Burden, N. ed. (1993). *Ambulatory surgical nursing.* Philadelphia: Saunders.
2. Fowler, M. (1994). Body contouring surgery. In Black, J., ed. *Nurs Clin North Am,* 29(4):753–761.
3. Fritsch, D. (1995). The plastic surgery and burn patient. In Litwack, Kim, ed. *Core curriculum for post anesthesia nursing practice,* 3rd ed. Philadelphia: Saunders.
4. Gabriel, S., O'Fallon, M., Kurkland, L. (1994). Risk of connective-tissue diseases and other disorders after breast implantation. *N Engl J Med,* 330:1697.
5. Goodman, T. ed. (1996). *Core Curriculum for plastic and reconstructive surgical nursing,* 2nd ed. Pitman, NJ: Anthony Jannetti.
6. Gutek, P., Fowler, M., Heeter, C. (1993). The forehead lift. *Plast Surg Nurs,* 13:4.
7. Mangan, M. (1994). Current concepts in breast reconstruction. In Black, J., ed. *Nurs Clin North Am,* 29(4):763–776.
8. Moncada, G. (1994). Traumatic injuries of the face and hands. In Black, J., ed. *Nurs Clin North Am,* 29(4):777–789.
9. Pettis, D., Vogt, P. (1992). Complications after suction-assisted lipoplasty. *Plast Surg Nurs,* 12:4.
10. Pitman, G. (1993). *Liposuction and aesthetic surgery,* St. Louis: Quality Medical Publishing.
11. Pruzinsky, T. (1993). Psychological factors in cosmetic plastic surgery: Recent developments in patient care. *Plast Surg Nurs,* 13(2):65–71.
12. Seckel, B. (1996). *Aesthetic laser surgery.* Boston: Little, Brown.
13. Sieggreen, M. (1987). Healing of physical wounds. *Nurs Clin North Am,* 22(2):439–447.
14. Sipos, D. (1995). Carpal tunnel syndrome. *Orthop Nurs,* 14(1):17–20.
15. Spencer, K. (1994). Selection and preoperative preparation of plastic surgery patients. In Black, J., ed. *Nurs Clin North Am,* 29(4):697–709.
16. Stotts, N. (1993). Wound healing. In Kinney, M., Packa, D., Dunbar, S., eds. *AACN's Clinical Reference for Critical Care Nursing,* 3rd ed. St. Louis: Mosby.
17. Williams, L. (1994). Facial rejuvenation. In Black, J., ed. *Nurs Clin North Am,* 29(4):741–751.

REVIEW QUESTIONS

1. Symptoms of hematoma formation post-rhytidectomy would include all except:

   A. Increasing pain
   B. Tightness of the skin
   C. Difficulty breathing or swallowing
   D. Nausea

2. Factors that inhibit wound healing would include all except:

   A. Proper nutrition
   B. Chronic illness
   C. Smoking
   D. Steroids

3. The symptoms of carpel tunnel syndrome are created by pressure on which nerve?

   A. Radial
   B. Median
   C. Ulnar
   D. Digital

4. The correct positioning for the abdominoplasty patient is:

   A. Prone
   B. Lateral Sims
   C. Supine with a pillow under the knees
   D. Flexed semifowlers

5. Postoperative fluid demand will be highest after which procedure?

   A. Liposuction
   B. Tumescent technique of liposuction
   C. Endoscopic carpal tunnel release
   D. Otoplasty

6. Symptoms of a retobulbar hematoma after a lower lid blepharoplasty include all except:

   A. Mild blurring
   B. Eye pain
   C. Proptosis
   D. Pressure behind eye

7. Which agent would be inappropriate for multimodal pain control postaugmentation mammoplasty with placement of prosthesis under the pectoral muscle?

   A. Narcotic
   B. Ice
   C. Aspirin
   D. Oral muscle relaxant

8. A complaint of a frontal headache is most common after which procedure?

   A. Rhytidectomy
   B. Blepharoplasty
   C. Browlift
   D. Otoplasty

9. Changes in a lesion that would be indicative of cutaneous malignant melanoma would include all except:

   A. Change in color from brown to black
   B. Irregular edges
   C. Decrease in size
   D. Change in surface from smooth to rough

10. All of the following are true regarding the inflammatory process of wound healing except:

   A. WBCs cleanse the wound
   B. Granulation tissue forms
   C. Hemostasis and epithelialization occur
   D. Process lasts up to 4 days

ANSWERS TO QUESTIONS

1. D
2. B
3. B
4. D
5. A

6. A
7. C
8. C
9. C
10. B

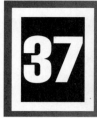

Podiatric Surgery

Brenda S. Gregory Dawes
AORN
Denver, Colorado

I. **Anatomy and Physiology of the Skeletal Structure of the Foot**
   A. Bony structure
   1. Tarsals
       a. Talus
           i. Located between bimalleolar fork and tarsus
           ii. Ligament attachments, no tendons
       b. Calcaneus
           i. Largest bone in foot
       c. Cuboid
           i. Wedge-shaped
       d. Scaphoid (navicular)
           i. Bound with ligaments
       e. Cuneiforms—three
           i. Interposed between scaphoid, first three metatarsals, and cuboid
           ii. Wedge-shaped
   2. Metatarsals—five
       a. First toe (great toe)
       b. Four lesser toes
       c. Articulates with three cuneiforms
       d. Form tarsometatarsal or Lisfranc's joint
   3. Phalanges
       a. Great toe, proximal, and distal
       b. Lesser toes (2, 3, 4, 5) proximal, middle, distal
   4. Sesamoids
       a. Small, round bones
       b. Embedded (partially or totally) in substance of corresponding tendon
       c. Pressure-absorbing mechanism

Objectives

1. Identify the skeletal structure of the foot.
2. Incorporate specific physical and psychosocial changes in the assessment of persons with foot disease.
3. Understand operative procedures of the foot.
4. Prioritize postanesthesia care to be provided following surgical procedures on the foot.

B. Arches
   1. Formed by bony structure
   2. Longitudinal (lengthwise) arches
      a. Medial longitudinal arch
         i.   Formed by calcaneus, talus, navicular, three cuneiforms, and first three metatarsals
      b. Lateral longitudinal arch
         i.   Formed by calcaneus, cuboid, and fourth and fifth metatarsals
   3. Transverse—across the ball (top) of the foot
C. Muscles, ligaments and tendons, nerves (multiple structures)

II. Assessment Parameters (Procedure-specific)
A. Structural disorders
   1. Causes
      a. Weakness of muscles, ligaments, and tendons
      b. Imbalance between bone support and supporting structure
      c. Constant wear, rub
B. Identified disorders
   1. Hallux valgus (hallux abducto valgus)
      a. Lateral angulation of great toe
      b. Progresses, resulting in medial deviation of first metatarsal
      c. Often accompanied by multiple disorders and symptoms; commonly affects lesser toes
      d. Adults—chief complaint is dull ache over medial eminence
      e. Adolescent—chief complaint is unrelated to pain; cosmesis desired, family history prevalent
   2. Hallux varus
      a. Medial angulation of the great toe at the metatarsal joint
   3. Hallux rigidus
      a. Painful stiffness of first metatarsalphalangeal joint of the toes
      b. Caused by arthritis
   4. Corns
      a. Conical thickening of skin in areas of constant irritation
   5. Bursal hypertrophy
      a. Inflammation of the joint
   6. Digital deformity
      a. Mallet toe
         i.   Flexion posture of the distal interphalangeal joint
         ii. Most commonly affects second toe
         iii. Associated with a long digit
         iv. Caused by pressure at tip of toes
         v.   Occurs in persons with peripheral neuropathy, no known reason
      b. Varus toes
         i.   Curly or overlapping toes
         ii. Flexion and varus rotation
         iii. Commonly affects 3, 4, 5
      c. Hammertoe deformity
         i.   Affects one of the lesser four toes (commonly second toe)
         ii. Hyperextension at metatarsophalangeal joint, flexion at proximal interphalangeal joint
         iii. Etiology unknown

    d. Clawtoe
      i. Hyperextension of metatarsophalangeal joint with flexion of the proximal interphalangeal joint
      ii. Associated with cavus foot deformity and neuromuscular conditions
  7. Interdigital deformity (Morton's neuroma)
    a. Benign enlargement of third common digital branch at site of bifurcation of interdigital nerves (medial plantar nerve)
    b. Frequently between and distal to third and fourth metatarsal heads
    c. Symptoms/common findings
      i. Pain in plantar forefoot area (sharp, dull, throbbing, or burning sensation)
      ii. Swelling of plantar metatarsal
      iii. Affects females more than males
      iv. Overweight person
  8. Pes planus (flat foot)
    a. Loss of normal medial longitudinal arch
    b. Initial treatment is conservative therapy with shoes, arch supports
    c. Surgical treatment with onset of disabling pain
    d. Correction procedures include Miller, Durham flatfoot plasty, triple arthrodesis, calcaneal displacement osteotomy
  9. Pes cavus (hollowfoot, clawfoot)
    a. Occurs with neuromuscular conditions as spina bifida, cerebral palsy, muscular dystrophy, congenital clubfoot
    b. Muscular weakness in foot
    c. Several procedures required for repair
      i. Soft tissue release, decrease contracture
      ii. Tendon transfer to correct muscle imbalance
      iii. Osteotomy
      iv. Arthrodesis

III. Elective Operative Procedures
  A. Treatment of disorders
    1. Determined by the degree of involvement
    2. Goals toward alignment, shortening, stabilization
    3. Multiple procedures may be indicated
  B. General intraoperative care
    1. Tourniquet application
    2. Operative site cleansing (including hair removal and cleaning toenails)
    3. Provision of sterile instruments, supplies
    4. Availability of implants including joint replacement, K-wire (pins), screws
  C. Procedures
    1. Arthrodesis
      a. Excision of bone wedges with fusion
      b. Indicated for severe compromise of muscle function; digital and metatarsophalangeal joint stability inadequate
      c. Treatment for hallux valgus
        i. Method: divide tendon, resect cartilage, provide stability to joint with K-wire or other means
      d. Triple arthrodesis—subtalar joint, talonavicular joint, tarsometatarsal joint
        i. Treatment for equinis deformity, cavus deformity, flat foot, or forefoot cavus
    2. Arthroplasty
      a. Resection or replacement of bony structure of joint
      b. Indicated for alleviation of pain and correction of digits with flexor to rigid deformity as:
        i. Inflammatory arthritis

      ii. Degenerative arthrosis

      iii. Congenital deformity

      iv. Flail toes

      v. Revision of previous surgery

  c. Keller resection arthroplasty: tissues released around the joint, expose articular surface, resect medial eminence, implant (K-wire) seated, capsulorrhaphy completed

3. Bunion procedures

  a. Revision of soft tissue structures and/or bone to correct deformity

  b. Soft tissue procedures correct muscle imbalance: McBride, DuVries, Mann, Silver

  c. Soft tissue and bone procedure: Keller resection arthroplasty, Chevron osteotomy, Akin procedure

  d. Purpose: simple treatment of hallux valgus causing impaired function and/or pain; cosmetic improvement

  e. Satisfactory for older adult, less mobile

4. Capsulotomy

  a. Incision of capsule

  b. Treatment of equinovarus foot

  c. Performed in conjunction with other procedures

  d. Method: incision through superficial fascia, expose joint, incise capsule

5. Endoscopic plantar fasciotomy

  a. Operative tissue repair using a less-invasive procedure

  b. Completed using fluroscopy

  c. Procedure: stab incision, blunt dissection to create a channel, pass a trocar, release the plantar fascia

  d. Open procedure more invasive; appropriate procedure for fascia release

6. Exostectomy

  a. Resection of lateral prominences (callus) of toes

  b. Commonly fifth toe

7. Hammertoe repair

  a. Abnormal flexion posture of the proximal interphalangeal joint of one of the lesser four toes

  b. Second toe most frequently affected

  c. Metatarsophalangeal joint

  d. Stage of deformity depends on joint involvement and degree of contracture

  e. Treatment

      i. Soft tissue procedures: Girdlestone, Taylor, Parrish, Mann, Coughlin

      ii. Soft tissue and bone procedures

8. Mallet toe repair

  a. Flexion posture of the distal interphalangeal joint

  b. Second toe most frequently affected

  c. Etiology:

      i. Pressure at tip of toes, possibly caused by shoes

      ii. Persons with peripheral neuropathy, no known reason

  d. Treatment:

      i. Flexor tenotomy at distal interphalangeal flexion crease

      ii. Subtotal or total resection of middle phalanx

9. Osteotomy

  a. Removal or addition of a bone wedge

  b. Extraarticular or intraarticular

  c. Extraarticular most commonly in the calcaneus for cavo-varus heel

        d. Metatarsal osteotomy for plantar calluses, hallux valgus: many types including wedge resection, Chevron, "Z," Reverdin, Mitchell

        e. Mitchell osteotomy: capsular incision, medial eminence removed, drill holes offset and suture passed; double osteotomy completed with excision of bone between, capital fragment displaced and suture tied, medial capsulorrhaphy completed

    10. Tenotomy

        a. Incision of tendon; eliminates tendon function; relieves contracture

        b. Completed in conjunction with other procedures

IV. Postanesthesia Priorities

  A. Phase I

    1. Predisposing factors

        a. Congenital, acquired, or traumatic

        b. Older adult and children included in the spectrum

        c. Existing conditions—neuromuscular disease, effect on other systems, neuropathy, diabetes, arthritis

        d. Previous procedures or anticipated future procedures (bilateral treatment needs)

    2. Condition of foot

        a. Appearance and sensation

           i. Soreness, tenderness, edema

           ii. Temperature equal on each foot

    3. Color

        a. Blanching of nail beds

    4. Vascular status

        a. Presence of dorsalis pedis pulse on dorsal center of metatarsal area of each foot

        b. Poor vascularity may impede healing

    5. Goals of procedure

        a. Pain relief

        b. Return or improvement of mobility

        c. Cosmetic improvement

        d. Extent of procedure influences outcome

    6. Support system

        a. Available assistance

        b. Impaired mobility related to other disease processes

    7. Awareness of procedure and expected outcomes

        a. Procedure to be performed

        b. Anesthetic type

           i. General anesthetic

           ii. Ankle block with IV conscious sedation

               (a) Procedure for block

               (b) Sensory deficit—length and precautions

        c. Complications

           i. Loss of function, muscular imbalance

           ii. Neurovascular compromise, swelling

  B. Phase II

    1. Neurovascular status

        a. Sensation in affected and opposite extremity

        b. Pulses

        c. Coloration, blanching of nail beds

    2. Preventive measures

        a. Elevation of extremity

        b. Ice pack

BOX 37-1. KEY PATIENT EDUCATIONAL OUTCOMES

- Patient will demonstrate proper use of supportive devices (crutches, walker, walking shoe)
- Patient will describe proper dosing procedure for prescribed analgesic medication(s) and report uncontrolled pain
- Patient will report excessive drainage on dressings
- Patient will describe signs and symptoms of infection and report findings to physician immediately
- Patient will report any neurological or circulatory impairment
- Patient will describe understanding of need for limited mobility for 6 to 8 weeks

---

C. Phase III
   1. Ambulation/mobility
      a. Home care availability
      b. Sensory deficit with use of ankle block up to 8 hours
      c. Support devices—crutches, walker, walking shoe
         i. Proper fit
            (a) Walking shoe long enough to protect toe; short enough to prevent tripping
         ii. Return demonstration of use
      d. Nonweight-bearing ambulation 3 to 5 days
      e. Limited mobility 6 to 8 weeks (longer depending upon procedure)
   2. Wound care
      a. Incision site clean, dry
         i. Report bleeding, discharge
         ii. Protect K-wire(s) if used
            (a) Clean around site with alcohol daily
            (b) Removal time depends on procedure; possibly 6 to 8 weeks
      b. Dressings remain intact, clean, dry (no showering)
      c. Soft tissue procedures
         i. Bulky, soft dressing for support
         ii. Three to 6 weeks with bandages in place (more involved procedures, longer bandage remains)
         iii. Compression dressing after 2 to 4 weeks
      d. Soft tissue and bone procedures
         i. Six to 8 weeks with bandages in place, guarded ambulation
         ii. External support several additional weeks
         iii. If bone graft used, may immobilize 3 to 6 months
      e. Skin care beneath cast, dressing
   3. Return of function
      a. Pain relief
         i. Nonsteroidal antiinflammatory medications (NSAIDs)
            (a) Pain following foot surgery intense
            (b) Evaluate medication interactions
         ii. Elevation of extremity
         iii. Ice packs
      b. Ambulation to tolerance
      c. Preventive measures
         i. Eliminate pressure, rub on toes from footwear

BIBLIOGRAPHY

1. Fulkerson, J.P. (1996). Arthroscopy of the foot and ankle. In Cooper, P.S., Murray, T.F., eds. *Clinics in Sports Medicine.* Philadelphia: Saunders.
2. Gregory, B. (1994). *Orthopaedic Surgery.* St. Louis: Mosby.
3. Laurin, C.A., Riley, L.H., Roy-Camille, R. (1991). *Atlas of Orthopaedic Surgery,* Volume III. Paris: Masson.
4. McGlamery, E.D., Banks, A.S., Downey, M.S. (1992). *Comprehensive Textbook of Foot Surgery,* 2nd ed., Baltimore: Williams & Wilkins.
5. Mourad, L.A. (1991). *Orthopedic Disorders.* St. Louis: Mosby.
6. Richardson, E.G. (1992). Surgical techniques, disorders of the hallux, pes planus, lesser toe abnormalities. In Crenshaw, A.H., ed. *Campbell's Operative Orthopaedics,* 8th ed. St. Louis: Mosby.

REVIEW QUESTIONS

1. The most frequent cause of foot disorders is

   A. Incorrect muscular structure for activity-type of person
   B. Standing for long hours
   C. Imbalance between bone structure, muscle, and ligament
   D. Poor foot care

2. Hallux valgus, or lateral angulation of the great toe

   A. Causes sharp, burning pain in the sole of the foot
   B. Is commonly the only complaint of the patient
   C. Is associated with neuropathy or neuromuscular diseases
   D. Is accompanied by other disorders such as deviation of first metatarsal

3. The surgical procedure(s) associated with hallux valgus is

   A. Triple arthrodesis
   B. Arthrodesis or osteotomy
   C. Extosectomy
   D. Plantar fasciotomy

4. An abnormal flexion posture of the proximal interphalangeal joint, with hyperextension of the metatarsophalangeal joint of one of the lesser four toes, is

   A. Hammertoe
   B. Hallux rigidis
   C. Exostosis
   D. Interdigital deformity

5. The most frequent indication for a bunionectomy is

   A. Mallet toe
   B. Equinovarus foot
   C. Deformity of great and lesser toes
   D. Simple treatment for pain, poor function

6. Patients with soft tissue and bone cuts can expect to be fully ambulatory after

   A. 2–3 weeks
   B. 4–5 weeks
   C. 6–8 weeks
   D. 9 weeks

7. Activity levels for the first 3 to 5 days following foot surgery includes

   A. Complete bed rest
   B. Nonweight-bearing ambulation
   C. Return to routine activities
   D. Dependent upon tolerance level of the patient

8. Postoperative care of the patient undergoing foot surgery with K-wire insertion includes

   A. Ice packs directly to the area of K-wire insertion
   B. Expose K-wire for healing
   C. Removal within 3 to 5 days
   D. Clean K-wire site daily with alcohol

9. Pain experienced following foot surgery is

   A. Described as intense
   B. Relieved with nonsteroidal antiinflammatory agents and use of ice packs
   C. Benefited by elevation of the extremity as much as possible
   D. All of the above

10. Multiple surgical podiatric procedures, requiring longer length of rehabilitation, would be included for correction of

   A. Pes cavus (clawfoot)
   B. Excision of callus
   C. Plantar fasciotomy
   D. Removal of Morton's neuroma

ANSWERS TO QUESTIONS

1. C
2. D
3. B
4. A
5. D

6. C
7. B
8. D
9. D
10. A

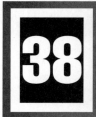

Special Procedures

Gayle Miller
St. Luke's Hospital
Jacksonville, Florida
Linda Boyum
The Outpatient Center of Boynton Beach, LTD
Boynton Beach, Florida

Due to the extensive number of procedures that can be classified as "special procedures," emphasis of this chapter will include only those procedures commonly encountered in the ASC or outpatient unit. This includes endoscopic procedures, radiologic procedures, and electroconvulsive therapy.

  I. **Overview**
   A. Definition
      1. Variety of procedures performed throughout facility may be termed "special procedures"
      2. May include nonsurgical diagnostic procedures as well as invasive procedures
      3. May be performed in special unit (endoscopy, radiology), on nursing unit, or in PACU
      4. Examples include:
         a. Endoscopy
         b. Radiologic exams
         c. Electroconvulsive therapy (ECT)
   B. Involvement of PACU, ASC staff
      1. May or may not be involved in:
         a. Preprocedure preparation of patient
         b. Intraprocedure assessment and monitoring
         c. Postprocedure recovery and discharge
      2. Varies according to facility protocols
 II. **Anatomy and Physiology**
   A. Gastrointestinal (GI) procedures (refer to Figure 38–1)

1. Anatomy of GI tract
   a. Mouth (oral or buccal cavity)
      i.   Teeth, tongue, hard and soft palates, cheeks, lips, pharynx
      ii. Salivary glands
           (a) Parotid
           (b) Sublingual
           (c) Submandibular

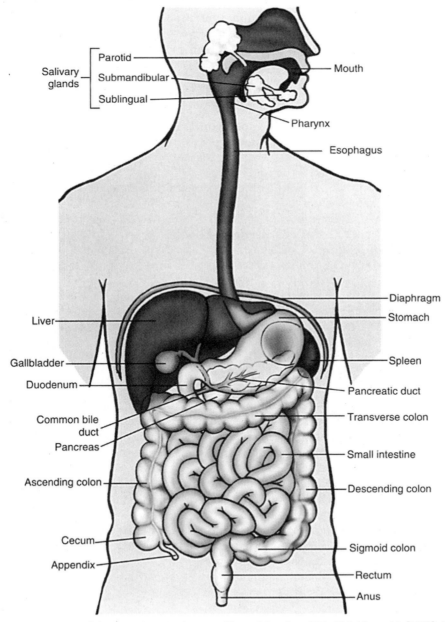

Figure 38–1.   Basic anatomy of the gastrointestinal tract.   (From: Monahan, F.D., Neighbors, M. [1998]. *Medical surgical nursing foundations for clinical practice,* 2nd ed. Philadelphia: Saunders.)

  b. Esophagus
   i. Muscular tube
   ii. Approximately 2.5 cm in diameter
   iii. Approximately 25 cm long
   iv. Extends from pharynx to stomach
   v. Positioned posterior to trachea and anterior of vertebral column
   vi. Sphincters
    (a) Upper pharyngoesophageal
    (b) Lower esophagogastric (cardiac)
  c. Stomach
   i. Located in left upper quadrant of abdomen
   ii. Consists of:
    (a) Fundus, body, pylorus (antrum), and cardiac region
   iii. Sphincters
    (a) Esophagogastric (cardiac)
     (i) Prevents backward reflux of stomach contents
    (b) Pyloric
     (i) Works with duodenum to create pressure gradient which allows emptying of stomach
  d. Small intestine
   i. Tube-shaped structure
   ii. Approximately 18 feet long; 1 inch in diameter
   iii. Three sections
    (a) Duodenum
     (i) C-shaped; first section
    (b) Jejunum
     (i) Middle section
    (c) Ileum
     (i) Last section
   iv. Properties
    (a) Circular folds increase absorptive surfaces of small intestines
  e. Large intestines
   i. Tube-shaped structure approximately 6 feet long and 2 inches in diameter
   ii. Consists of:
    (a) Cecum
     (i) Positioned at junction of ileum and colon
     (ii) Contains ileocecal valve and appendix
    (b) Ascending colon
     (i) Portion from cecum to hepatic flexure
    (c) Transverse colon
     (i) Segment from hepatic flexure to splenic flexure
     (ii) Transverses abdominal cavity
    (d) Descending colon
     (i) Segment from splenic flexure to iliac crest
     (ii) Located on left side of abdomen
    (e) Sigmoid colon
     (i) S-shaped segment
     (ii) Ends at rectum
    (f) Rectum
     (i) Last portion of large intestine
     (ii) Approximately 5 inches long
     (iii) Segment after sigmoid colon
     (iv) Connects to anal canal

2. Nerve supply—occurs two ways
  a. Neural transmission to smooth muscle
    i. Stimulates movement of food through GI tract
    ii. Occurs as a result of distention of myenteric plexus or submucosal plexus
  b. Autonomic nervous system
    i. Sympathetic
      (a) Thoracic and lumbar splenic nerves
        (i) Inhibit secretions and movement
        (ii) Cause contraction of sphincters
    ii. Parasympathetic
      (a) Vagus nerve
        (i) Causes increase in motor activity
        (ii) Causes increase in secretions
        (iii) Causes sphincters to relax
        (iv) Results in peristalsis
3. Function of GI system
  a. Ingestion
  b. Transport
  c. Digestion
  d. Absorption
  e. Elimination

III. Common Procedures
  A. Endoscopy—overview
    1. Visualization of the inside of a body cavity
    2. Usually performed with lighted flexible fiberoptic scope
    3. Provides undistorted image of body cavity
    4. Illumination provided by external light source
    5. Scope designed to allow for passage of instruments
      a. Allows for:
        i. Pictures to be taken
        ii. Biopsies to be obtained
        iii. Polyps to be removed
        iv. Foreign objects to be removed
        v. Bleeding areas to be cauterized
  B. Abdominal paracentesis
    1. Removal and drainage of ascitic fluid in the peritoneal cavity
    2. Diagnostic tool to examine ascitic fluid
    3. Palliative measure to relieve abdominal pressure that may be interfering with respiratory function
  C. Anoscopy
    1. Examination of the anal canal with an anoscope
  D. Anal manometry
    1. Used to assess:
      a. Anal and rectal muscles
      b. Sphincter problems
        i. Can be associated with several disorders, especially fecal incontinence
      c. Chronic constipation
  E. Colonoscopy
    1. Direct visualization of the large intestine from the rectum
    2. Used to evaluate for malignancy, polyps, inflammatory bowel disease, diverticulitis, strictures, or bleeding

F. Endoscopic retrograde cholangiopancreatography (ERCP)
    1. Invasive radiologic exam to visualize the pancreatic ducts, hepatic ducts, and common bile ducts
    2. Uses a flexible fiberoptic duodenoscope
    3. Contrast material is injected
    4. May include removal of stones, sphincterotomies, or dilatation
G. Esophageal dilatation
    1. Enlargement of the lumen of the esophagus
    2. Accomplished by forcing a series of increasingly larger dilators through a narrowed area (axial force)
    3. May use a balloon dilator to accomplish opening of a narrowed area (radial force)
H. Esophagogastroduodenoscopy
    1. Direct visualization of esophagus, stomach, and proximal duodenum
    2. Flexible fiberoptic endoscope passed through mouth
    3. Used to diagnose esophageal or gastric lesions, hiatus hernia, esophageal varices, esophagitis, ulcer disease, polyps, strictures (achalasia), bleeding, or motility disorders
I. Percutaneous endoscopic gastrostomy (PEG)
    1. Placement of feeding tube via endoscopy for enteral nutrition
    2. Procedure:
        a. Lighted endoscope inserted into stomach
        b. Light shines against abdominal wall
            i.   Allows visualization of tube placement site
        c. Large-gauge needle and suture passed through abdominal wall and stomach wall
            i.   Snare or biopsy forceps used to bring inner end of suture up through patient's mouth (via endoscope)
        d. PEG tube is tied to suture
            i.   Pulled through mouth into stomach
            ii. Pulled out abdominal wall
        e. Tube is anchored using internal and external rubber bumpers or internal retention balloon and outer disk
    3. Advantages
        a. Less risk than surgical gastrostomy
        b. Procedure done under sedation rather than general anesthesia
        c. Faster recovery
        d. Feedings can begin within 24 hours
        e. Can be performed in endoscopy suite or at bedside
        f. Less costly
J. Percutaneous endoscopic jejunostomy
    1. Tube is passed into jejunum through opening in abdominal wall
    2. Approach can be surgical or percutaneous
    3. Procedure
        a. Small tube passed through percutaneous endoscopic gastrostomy tube
        b. Guided via endoscope into duodenum
        c. Tube propelled by peristalsis into jejunum
        d. Placement confirmed by X-ray
            i.   Contrast medium injected
    4. Considerations
        a. Small diameter of tube predisposes it to clogging
        b. Tube can migrate back to stomach due to vomiting
        c. Feedings are continuous due to jejunum not being a normal reservoir for nutrients

K. Polypectomy
   1. Removal of a protruding growth or mass of tissue that protrudes from a mucous membrane; usually performed via endoscope
      a. Pedunculated—attached to mucous by a slender stalk or pedicle
      b. Sessile—broad-based polyp
L. Proctosigmoidoscopy
   1. Endoscopic exam of distal sigmoid colon, rectum, and anal canal
   2. Performed to evaluate rectal bleeding, polyps, tumors, persistent diarrhea, fissures, fistulas, abscesses, and inflammatory bowel disease
   3. Performed as an initial colorectal cancer screen
   4. Advantages
      a. Better tolerated than rigid proctosigmoidoscopy
      b. Allows for examining more of colon than possible with proctoscope
M. Other diagnostic or therapeutic procedures
   1. Blood transfusion
      a. Types
         i.   Whole blood
         ii.   Packed red cells
         iii. Frozen red blood cells
         iv.   Platelets
         v.   Granulocytes
         vi.   Plasma
         vii. Albumin
         viii. Coagulation factor concentrates
         ix.   Prothrombin complex
         x.   Cryoprecipitate
         xi.   Immune serum globulins
      b. Collected from:
         i.   Donor (homologous)
         ii. Recipient (autologous)
         iii. Donor designated by recipient (designated direct blood)
   2. Bronchoscopy
      a. Direct visualization of walls of trachea, the main-stem bronchus, and the major subdivisions of the bronchial tubes through a bronchoscope
      b. Indications
         i.   Diagnosis
              (a) Lesions, bleeding sites
              (b) Obtain biopsies, bronchial brushing, bronchial washing
         ii. Treatment
              (a) Destroy or remove lesions
              (b) Clear airway
                  (i) Retained secretions
                  (ii) Foreign body
         iii. Evaluation of disease progression
         iv. Evaluation of effectiveness of therapy
   3. Electroconvulsive therapy
      a. Application of brief electrical stimulus to induce a cerebral seizure
         i.   Used to treat major psychiatric disorders, e.g., severe depression
   4. Thoracentesis
      a. Withdrawal of fluid or air from the pleural space
         i.   Amount of removal limited to 1 to 2 liters at one time to avoid mediastinal shift and impaired venous return

      b. Indications
         i.   Diagnostic
            (a) Obtain specimens
         ii.   Therapeutic
            (a) Relieve respiratory distress
            (b) Instill medication into pleural space

IV. Education Content
  A. Preprocedure
    1. General
      a. NPO instructions as appropriate
      b. Hygiene
      c. Environment
      d. Facility protocols
      e. Aftercare arrangements
      f. Amnesic effects of conscious sedation
      g. Medication—discontinue or dose as usual
    2. Procedure-specific
      a. GI
         i.   Bowel prep as appropriate
         ii.   Course of procedure
         iii. Expectations
         iv. Recovery period
      b. ECT
         i.   Preprocedure emphasis includes screening for
            (a) Baseline mental status
            (b) Confusion
            (c) Disorientation
            (d) Cardiovascular disease
            (e) Cerebral pathology and/or suspected increased intracranial pressure
         ii.   Instruct patient to wash hair night before procedure to remove hair products that may interfere with conduction
      c. Blood transfusion
         i.   Patient's level of understanding regarding procedure
         ii.   History of transfusion reactions

V. General Assessment Parameters

For detailed information on preprocedure assessment, the reader is referred to Chapter 7. For detailed information on postprocedure assessment, refer to Chapter 8.

  A. GI procedures
    1. Preprocedure
      a. Preprocedure emphasis on screening for:
         i.   Bleeding disorders in patient or family
         ii.   Medications affecting clotting
         iii. Bowel activity
         iv. Swallowing ability
      b. Ensure understanding of preprocedure preparation (NPO status, diet, enema, etc.)
    2. Postprocedure
      a. General
         i.   Airway/respiratory status
         ii.   Vital signs
         iii. Level of consciousness

3. Procedure-specific
   a. Upper GI tract
      i.   Swallowing ability
      ii. Pain
      iii. Bleeding
      iv. Reaction to local anesthetic
   b. Lower GI tract
      i.   Pain
      ii. Flatus
      iii. Bleeding
B. Electroconvulsive therapy
   1. Preprocedure assessment per routine protocol
   2. Postprocedure
      a. Assess for hypotension and bradycardia
      b. Orientation to time, place, and person
C. Blood transfusion
   1. Preprocedure
      a. Ensure informed consent and/or specific transfusion consent form is complete
      b. Obtain baseline vital signs, including temperature
      c. Assess patient history of transfusion reactions
      d. Educate patient to signs and symptoms of potential reactions
         i. Inform patient to immediately report any unusual feelings
   2. Administration
      a. Ensure blood has been typed and crossmatched and that ABO group and Rh factor match patient's
      b. Check blood for abnormal color or cloudiness (indicates hemolysis)
      c. Check for presence of gas bubbles (indicates bacterial growth)
      d. Check expiration date on blood bag
      e. Confirm information with another professional
      f. Document confirmation
      g. Administration of unrefrigerated blood should begin within one hour
      h. Total administration time should generally not exceed four hours
   3. Nursing interventions during procedure
      a. Assess vital signs per protocol
      b. Be alert for signs of transfusion reaction (see Table 38–1)
      c. Types of reactions
         i.   Acute hemolytic
              (a) Caused by infusion of ABO-incompatible blood
              (b) May cause most severe symptoms
         ii. Febrile, nonhemolytic
              (a) Most common
              (b) Treat symptomatically
         iii. Mild allergic
              (a) Rash, itching, low-grade fever
              (b) May administer antihistamines
         iv. Anaphylactic
              (a) Mild to severe symptoms
         v.   Circulatory overload
              (a) Rare
              (b) Caused by rapid infusion in patient unable to accommodate volume
              (c) Patient may have history of cardiac disease

Table 38–1 • PATIENTS WITH A BLOOD TRANSFUSION REACTION

Assessment Findings:	Patient experiences dyspnea, chest pain, feeling of tightness in chest, increased pulse and respirations, hypertension, chills, fever, facial burning within 15 minutes after transfusion begins, low back pain, headache or full feeling in the head, hematuria, anorexia, oliguria, apprehension, neck vein distention, and shock.
Nursing Diagnosis:	Risk for injury related to antigen-antibody incompatibility.

PATIENT OUTCOMES	NURSING INTERVENTIONS	RATIONALE

Patient's vital signs are within normal range for patient.
Patient indicates that chills, back pain, and headache are absent.
	Monitor vital signs.
	If vital signs change or other untoward symptoms appear, discontinue blood transfusion.
	Also complete the following:
	  Notify physician stat.
	  Keep intravenous line open with saline.
	Draw client's blood for hemoglobin (Hgb), culture, and retyping; obtain urinalysis; and observe voidings.
	Return remaining blood and tubing to blood bank for repeat typing and culture.
	Reassure patient.
	Cover patient with blanket.
	Administer diuretics and colloids as ordered.
	If there is a history of previous reactions, may administer diphenhydramine (Benadryl) prophylactically.
		Although the nurse may not prevent a transfusion reaction, appropriate nursing interventions are important to minimize the trauma of the reaction to the patient.
		The blood is rechecked for errors in typing and cross-matching.

Evaluation:	Compare the patient's status with the expected outcomes. If the outcomes are not met, reassess the patient and revise the plan.
Assessment Findings:	Patient experiences weakness, fatigue 1 to 2 weeks after transfusion, decreased Hgb, and positive Coombs' test results.
Nursing Diagnosis:	Altered health maintenance related to lack of knowledge of delayed antigen-antibody incompatibility.

PATIENT OUTCOMES	NURSING INTERVENTIONS	RATIONALE
Patient states accurate information about the reaction and potential for a delayed reaction.	Inform patient that this reaction is not dangerous and that subsequent transfusions may cause an acute hemolytic reaction.	By knowing to expect a reaction, the patient will be alert to early signs of problems.
Patient states the signs and symptoms of a delayed reaction.	Instruct patient in signs and symptoms of a delayed reaction.	A transfusion reaction can be delayed by up to 2 weeks after the infusion.
Patient verbalizes the need to contact medical personnel if symptoms of a reaction become apparent.	Instruct patient to notify the nurse or physician if signs or symptoms are evident. Check Hgb levels if patient experiences signs or symptoms.	Immediate intervention reduces the risk of complications.

Table continued on following page

Table 38–1 • PATIENTS WITH A BLOOD TRANSFUSION REACTION *Continued*

Evaluation:	Compare the patient's status with the expected outcomes. If the outcomes are not met, reassess the patient and revise the plan.	
Assessment Findings:	Patient is experiencing fever, chills, headache, flushing, tachycardia, palpitations, nausea, vomiting, diarrhea, malaise, and lumbar pain.	
Nursing Diagnosis:	Risk for infection related to bacterial pyogens transfused through blood.	

PATIENT OUTCOMES	NURSING INTERVENTIONS	RATIONALE
Patient remains free of signs and symptoms of a pyogenic reaction. Patient's vital signs are within normal ranges for the patient.	Discontinue blood transfusion. Notify physician stat. Keep vein open with saline. Monitor vital signs. Reassure patient and family. Premedicate with antipyretic.	Appropriate nursing interventions reduce risk of further complications. Changes in vital signs may indicate complications.

Evaluation:	Compare the patient's status with the expected outcomes. If the outcomes are not met, reassess the patient and revise the plan.	
Assessment Findings:	Patient is experiencing dyspnea, nausea, vomiting, urticaria, rash, itching, hives, facial flushing, wheezing, hypotension, shock, diarrhea, tight chest, and anxiety, but no fever.	
Nursing Diagnosis:	Risk for injury related to allergic reaction.	

PATIENT OUTCOMES	NURSING INTERVENTIONS	RATIONALE
Patient remains free of signs and symptoms of an allergic reaction.	Discontinue transfusion. Keep vein open with saline. Notify physician stat. Resume transfusion slowly if the only symptoms are itching, hives, urticaria, rash, and anxiety.	Although the nurse may not prevent an allergic reaction, appropriate nursing interventions are important to minimize the trauma of the reaction.
Vital signs remain within normal range for patient.	Administer antihistamines and monitor vital signs.	Vital sign changes may indicate complications.
Patient indicates that symptoms of a reaction are absent.	If symptoms progress, discontinue transfusion, obtain urinalysis, draw patient's blood, notify blood bank, and return remaining blood and tubing. Administer diphenhydramine 15 to 20 minutes before the transfusion, as ordered, if the patient is suspected to have allergies. Give epinephrine, vasopressors, and crystalloids, if ordered.	The blood is rechecked for proper typing and cross-matching if the reaction continues.

Evaluation:	Compare the patient's status with the expected outcomes. If the outcomes are not met, reassess the patient and revise the plan.	
Assessment Findings:	Patient is experiencing dyspnea, dry cough, rales in lungs, crackles at base of lungs, tightness in chest, bounding pulse, increased blood pressure, orthopnea, cyanosis, tachycardia, neck vein distention, anxiety, coughing of pink, frothy sputum, cold, clammy skin, and restlessness.	
Nursing Diagnosis:	Fluid volume excess related to circulatory overload from blood transfusion.	

Table continued on following page

Table 38–1 • **PATIENTS WITH A BLOOD TRANSFUSION REACTION** *Continued*

PATIENT OUTCOMES	NURSING INTERVENTIONS	RATIONALE
Patient's skin color remain's pink, and skin is dry to touch.	Position patient upright. Check the skin for edema, color, and integrity, especially in the extremities.	Fluid pooling, especially in the extremities, is a sign of fluid overload.
Patient's vital signs remain within normal range for patient.	Monitor vital signs and venous pressure.	Vital sign changes, such as increasing pulse rate and blood pressure, may indicate fluid overload. Adventitious breath sounds may result from pulmonary edema from the fluid overload.
Patient's lungs remain clear upon auscultation.	Monitor lung sounds.	
Patient denies respiratory or circulatory distress.	Apply rotating tourniquets if ordered.	
Peripheral and pulmonary edema are absent.	Administer diuretics, oxygen, morphine, vasodilators, and aminophylline if ordered.	
Evaluation:	Compare the patient's status with the expected outcomes. If the outcomes are not met, reassess the patient and revise the plan.	

From Monahan, F.D., Neighbors, M. (1998). *Medical surgical nursing foundations for clinical practice*, 2nd ed. Philadelphia: Saunders.

    vi. Septic reaction
       (a) Caused by contaminated blood
       (b) Symptoms are immediate
       (c) Fever, chills, hypotension, shock
       (d) Treat with intravenous antibiotics
    vii. Delayed
       (a) Can occur several days to two weeks following transfusion
  D. Bronchoscopy
    1. Preprocedure
      a. NPO for 6 hours prior to procedure
        i. Decrease risk of aspiration
        ii. Remove dentures
    2. Postprocedure
      a. Assess for return of swallow and gag reflex
      b. Assess and prepare to treat potential complications
        i. Bronchospasm
        ii. Hypoxemia
        iii. Bleeding
        iv. Perforation
        v. Aspiration
        vi. Cardiac dysrhythmias
        vii. Infection
        viii. Reaction to local anesthetic
      c. Blood-streaked sputum is expected for several hours postprocedure
      d. Frank bleeding is indicative of hemorrhage
  E. Other diagnostic or therapeutic procedures
    1. Routine assessment per protocol

VI. General Perianesthesia Priorities
   A. Phase I, preprocedure
      1. Objectives
         a. Assess and prepare patient for procedure
         b. Obtain baseline data
         c. Allow for development and implementation of nursing care
         d. Initiate educational process
            i.   Continues throughout the continuum of care
      2. Nursing process
         a. Assessment parameters
            i.   Physical assessment as noted above
            ii. Assess for educational needs
            iii. Assess for psychosocial needs related to developmental age including:
                 (a) Availability of family member or responsible adult companion
                 (b) Community resources needed
      3. Plan of care
         a. Include patient/family/responsible adult companion in developing plan of
            care appropriate to the age of the patient
         b. Nursing diagnoses might include:
            i.   Anxiety/fear related to knowledge deficit, unfamiliar environment,
                 separation from family, lack of control, etc.
            ii. Pain related to procedural intervention
            iii. Potential for injury
            iv. Potential for infection
      4. Interventions
         a. Nursing interventions might include:
            i.   Ensure that all laboratory studies are completed as ordered/indicated
            ii. Provide information on preprocedure preparation (NPO status, medica-
                 tions, hygiene, discharge arrangements [ride, aftercare], etc.)
            iii. Obtain baseline vital signs
            iv. Ensure legal authorization is appropriate (informed consent)
            v.   Provide orientation to surroundings
            vi. For ECT patients:
                 (a) Have patient void immediately prior to procedure
                 (b) Helps prevent incontinence and bladder distention
            vii. Apply monitoring devices as indicated
                 (a) ECG
                 (b) Pulse oximetry
                 (c) EEG according to facility policy
                 (d) Nerve stimulator
      5. Evaluation
         a. Evaluation of interventions/patient response might include:
            i.   Laboratory results are reviewed, and follow-up completed as indicated
            ii. Patient/family/responsible adult companion is questioned to determine
                 understanding of preoperative instructions
            iii. Determine that patient has made arrangements for aftercare as
                 appropriate
   B. Phase II, PACU
      1. Objectives
         a. Ensure that the patient safely recovers from the immediate effects of procedure
            and anesthesia
         b. Patient may or may not receive care in PACU, depending on facility policy

    c. Patient may be transported directly to PACU Phase II, depending on facility policy

2. Nursing process
   a. Assessment parameters
      i. General
         (a) Routine PACU protocol
         (b) Airway status—patient is at high risk for airway compromise
         (c) Vital signs are monitored frequently during and after procedure
         (d) Effects of medications administered
         (e) IV conscious sedation protocol

3. Plan of care
   a. Include patient/family/responsible adult companion in developing a plan of care appropriate to the age of the patient
   b. Nursing diagnoses might include those listed above
   c. Provide for patient safety
   d. Be alert for potential complications

4. Nursing interventions
   a. Monitor vital signs per protocol
   b. Administer medications as ordered
   c. Observe for potential complications
   d. Ensure a safe environment

5. Evaluation
   a. Response to interventions are evaluated continually throughout the patient's stay
   b. Alterations to plan of care are made as indicated

6. For ECT patients (patient may have procedure performed in PACU setting)
   a. Assessment parameters
      i. Airway status
         (a) Patient is at high risk for airway compromise
      ii. Vital signs are monitored frequently (per protocol) during and after ECT procedure
      iii. Effects of medications
      iv. IV conscious sedation protocol
   b. Plan of care
      i. Include patient/family/responsible adult companion in developing a plan of care appropriate to the age of the patient
      ii. Nursing diagnoses might include those listed above
      iii. Provide for safety
      iv. Be alert for potential complications
   c. Nursing interventions
      i. Monitor vital signs per protocol
      ii. Administer medications as ordered
      iii. Observe for complications
         (a) Dysrhythmias
         (b) Aspiration
         (c) Hypotension
         (d) Prolonged seizure
      iv. Ensure a safe environment
         (a) Bite block to prevent damage to teeth and oral cavity during seizure
   d. Evaluation
      i. Response to interventions are evaluated continually throughout the patient's stay
      ii. Alterations to plan of care are made as indicated

7. Blood transfusion
   a. Vital signs per protocol
   b. Assess for latent reaction
C. Phase III, preparation for discharge
   1. Objective
      a. Ready the patient to return to home
      b. Patient and caregiver adequately prepared to successfully manage postprocedure care
      c. Education of patient and caregiver is critical to success of ambulatory procedure outcome
   2. Nursing process
      a. Assessment parameters
         i. General
            (a) Airway/respiratory status
            (b) Bleeding
            (c) Vital signs
            (d) Discomfort
            (e) Reactions to local anesthetics
            (f) Level of consciousness
   3. Plan of care
      a. Include patient/family/responsible adult companion in developing plan of care
      b. Plan should be appropriate to the age of the patient
      c. Nursing diagnoses might include:
         i. Anxiety/fear related to knowledge deficit, unfamiliar environment, separation from family, lack of control, etc.
         ii. Alteration in comfort level
         iii. Ineffective breathing patterns related to sedation
         iv. Potential for infection
      d. Be alert for potential complications
         i. GI
            (a) Bleeding
            (b) Perforated viscus
               (i) Signs include increased temperature, abdominal distention and/or pain, shortness of breath, subcutaneous emphysema
            (c) Respiratory depression
            (d) Vasovagal reaction
         ii. Other
            (a) Blood transfusion
               (i) Transfusion reaction
                  a) Instruct patient/family of signs and symptoms of delayed transfusion reaction
                     (1) Integumentary: itching, rashes, swelling, cyanosis, excessive perspiration
                     (2) Respiratory: tachypnea, dyspnea, apnea, wheezing, cyanosis, rales
                     (3) Urinary: pain on or during urination, oliguria
                     (4) Circulatory: chest pain, increased heart rate, palpitations, headache, fever, chills, muscle aches, tingling, numbness
               (ii) Fluid overload
            (b) Liver biopsy
               (i) Hemorrhage
               (ii) Fluid leakage

     (iii) Subcutaneous emphysema
     (iv) Perforation of viscus
    (c) Bronchoscopy
     (i) Bronchospasm or laryngospasm
     (ii) Hypoxia
     (iii) Bleeding
     (iv) Pneumothorax
    (d) Thoracentesis
     (i) Hemothorax
     (ii) Pneumothorax
     (iii) Air embolism
     (iv) Subcutaneous emphysema
     (v) Bleeding
    (e) ECT
     (i) Bradycardia
     (ii) Tachycardia
     (iii) Hypotension
     (iv) Hypertension
     (v) Airway management problems

  4. Nursing interventions
   a. General
    i. Monitor vital signs per protocol
    ii. Administer medications for pain and nausea as ordered
    iii. Observe for bleeding and other complications
    iv. Ensure a safe environment
   b. Procedure-specific
    i. GI
     (a) Withhold fluid until gag reflex intact
     (b) Observe for complications
    ii. Other
     (a) Observe for complications
     (b) Activity restriction per physician orders
   c. Educational interventions
    i. Discussion, demonstration, written materials, etc.
    ii. Copies of all materials given to patient should be maintained in medical record or on unit

  5. Evaluation
   a. Evaluation of clinical interventions is ongoing until patient is stable and ready for discharge
   b. Evaluation of learning
    i. Patient/caregiver verbalize understanding
    ii. Patient/caregiver able to demonstrate skill
    iii. Patient and responsible adult companion should sign that they have been instructed and had the opportunity to have questions answered

VII. Education content
 A. Postprocedure
  1. General
   a. Activity
   b. Diet
   c. Medication
   d. Complications
   e. Follow-up care
   f. Emergency contact information

BOX 38–1.   Key Patient Educational Outcomes

- Patient undergoing a blood transfusion will be able to accurately relate information regarding the transfusion and the signs and symptoms of a latent reaction
- Patient with a feeding tube in place and/or family member will verbalize understanding of the care of the feeding tube
- Patient undergoing ECT treatment will verbalize understanding of the procedure and comply with preprocedure instructions
- Patient who has undergone IV conscious sedation will verbalize postprocedure requirements, e.g., not to drive or operate machinery, adult companion to drive patient home, etc.

Bibliography

1. Black, J.M., Matassarin-Jacobs, E. (1997). *Medical-Surgical Nursing—Clinical Management for Continuity of Care*, 5th ed. Philadelphia: Saunders.
2. Brandt, B., Ugarizza, D.N. (1996). Electroconvulsive therapy and the elderly client. *J Gerontological Nursing.* December 14–20.
3. Enns, M.W., Reise, J.P. (1992). Canadian Psychiatric Association Position Paper on Electroconvulsive Therapy.
4. *Gastroenterology Nursing, A Core Curriculum.* (1993). Society of Gastroenterology Nurses and Associates. St. Louis: Mosby.
5. Gregoratos, G. (1997). Cardiac catheterization: Basic techniques and complications (1997). In Peterson, K.L., Nicod, P. ed. *Cardiac Catheterization: Methods, Diagnosis, and Therapy.* Philadelphia: Saunders.
6. Meeker, M.H., Rothrock, J.C. (1995). *Alexander's Care of the Patient in Surgery*, 10th ed. St. Louis: Mosby.
7. Monahan, F.D., Neighbors, M. (1998). *Medical Surgical Nursing—Foundations for Clinical Practice*, 2nd ed. Philadelphia: Saunders.
8. O'Brien, D., Burden, N. (1993). The ASC as a special procedures unit. In Burden, N., ed. *Ambulatory Surgical Nursing.* Philadelphia: Saunders.
9. Stuart, G. (1995). Somatic therapies. In Stuart, G., Sundeen, S., eds. *Principles and Practice of Psychiatric Nursing.* St. Louis: Mosby.

REVIEW QUESTIONS

1. The primary indication for electroconvulsive therapy is

   A. Obsessive compulsive disorder
   B. Major depression
   C. Schizophrenia
   D. Panic disorder

2. In preparing for the ECT procedure, the nurse should anticipate monitoring modalities to include

   A. Pulse oximetry and EMG
   B. ECG and EMG
   C. Nerve stimulator and EEG
   D. EEG and CVP

3. Parasympathetic stimulation during ECT may cause

   A. Bradycardia
   B. Tachycardia
   C. Hypertension
   D. Premature ventricular contractions

4. Which drug is used to reverse narcotic-induced respiratory depression?

   A. Epinephrine
   B. Narcan
   C. Physostigmine
   D. Midazolam

5. To treat vasovagal reaction, the nurse should

   A. Provide a quiet environment
   B. Medicate the patient for discomfort
   C. Position the patient with the head level with or lower than the rest of the body
   D. Administer oxygen

6. Complications from a thoracentesis include

   A. Pulmonary edema
   B. Pneumothorax
   C. Hemoptysis
   D. Abdominal bleeding and cramping

7. Potential complications of a liver biopsy include all of the following except

    A. Hemorrhage
    B. Air embolism
    C. Pneumothorax
    D. Bile leakage

8. Post-bronchoscopy assessment should include

    A. Bilateral breath sounds
    B. Urinary output
    C. Return of gag reflex
    D. Pain level

9. The function of the GI system includes

    A. Ingestion
    B. Transport
    C. Digestion
    D. All of the above

10. Signs of lower GI perforation include all of the following except:

    A. Sudden, severe abdominal pain
    B. Abdominal distention
    C. Decreased tympany
    D. Bloody or mucopurulent drainage

ANSWERS TO QUESTIONS

1. B
2. C
3. A
4. B
5. C

6. B
7. B
8. C
9. D
10. D

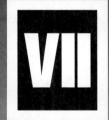

VII

Management

Policies and Procedures

Donna M. DeFazio Quinn
Elliot 1-Day Surgery Center
Manchester, New Hampshire

Objectives

1. Identify and discuss five important functions for policies and procedures.
2. Discuss the proper format of the page layout of policies and procedures.
3. Identify and discuss ten important policies and procedures related to the PACU.
4. Describe the process for obtaining administrative approval of policies and procedures.
5. Discuss the process for revising policies and procedures.

I. Policies

A. Definition
1. Guidelines to assist in decision making
   a. Increases likelihood of consistency in decisions and actions
   b. Means to ensure practice is in compliance with standards
2. Defines responsibility
3. Element of the organization that is an extension of the mission statement
4. Provides order and stability so unit can work as a coordinated group
5. Directs action for thinking about and solving recurring problems related to the objectives of the organization

B. Developed by:
1. Nursing executive
2. RNs
3. Designated nursing staff members
4. Input from ancillary staff members

C. Functions
1. Promotes teamwork
2. Provides clarity and uniformity
   a. Identifies what is expected in a specific manner
   b. Encourages consistency in practice
3. Defines limits of authority and responsibility
4. Aids in delegation
5. Serves as a resource for accreditation and regulatory agencies
   a. Accrediting bodies

             i. Joint Commission for Accreditation of Healthcare Organizations (JCAHO)

             ii. Accreditation Association for Ambulatory Health Care (AAAHC)

        b. State licensing agency

        c. Regulating agencies

             i. Medicare

             ii. Medicaid

             iii. Health Care Financing Administration (HCFA)

6. Provides a basis for change
   a. If current practice is not known, it is difficult to know what needs to be changed
7. Establishes a mechanism for consistent treatment of staff and a framework for staff assignments
8. Provides a safeguard for nursing personnel when legal action ensues
   a. Nurses are held accountable for practice consistent with existing policies at the time of the action
   b. Adherence to policies provides a defense for actions taken
9. Establishes a consistent level of expectation of staff members
   a. Orientation clearly identifies individual's responsibility to know and adhere to policies
10. Process neverending
    a. Continually need to update policies and procedures based on:
       i. Changes in practice
       ii. Changes in regulatory requirements
       iii. Changes in standards
       iv. Changes in technology
    b. Staff members need to be involved in process
       i. Annual review of policies as a whole
       ii. Ongoing review of various policies throughout the year

II. Procedures

A. Definition

1. Instructions that detail steps necessary to complete a task
2. Includes
   a. Necessary steps/process
   b. Supplies
   c. Equipment
   d. Personnel
   e. Documentation

B. Functions

1. Reminder for tasks performed infrequently
2. Resource for orienting new staff members
3. Facilitates cost containment
   a. Identifies necessary supplies
   b. Reduces unnecessary waste
4. Increases productivity
   a. Decreases time lost seeking answers
5. Provides a means to measure quality and appropriateness of care when auditing nursing practice

III. Format of Policies and Procedures

A. Page layout

1. Title
2. Number

3. Authorizing signatures/approving body
4. Review date
5. Revision date
B. Common divisions
  1. Administration
  2. Anesthesia
  3. Environment of care
  4. Employee health
  5. Infection control
  6. Materials management
  7. Medical records
  8. Patient care
  9. Personnel
  10. Pharmacy
  11. Quality management
  12. Registration
  13. Risk management
  14. Safety

IV. **Overview of Policies and Procedures Needed**

The following content outline suggests general required policies and procedures. It is not the intent of this chapter to provide an all-inclusive list of possible policies and procedures.

A. Table of contents
B. Facility/unit philosophy and objectives
C. Mission/vision/values statements
D. Administrative organizational chart
  1. Chain of command
    a. Governing body
    b. Job descriptions
    c. Staffing patterns
    d. Standards of care
  2. Medical staff
    a. Physician privileges
    b. Physician credentialing procedure
    c. Medical advisory committee
E. Patient rights
  1. Rights and responsibility statement
  2. Ethical treatment
  3. Patient grievance process
  4. Advance directives
F. Admission
  1. Criteria
  2. Approved procedure list
  3. Appropriateness of patients
  4. Population served
  5. Testing requirements
  6. Preoperative assessment
G. Discharge
  1. Criteria
  2. Instructions
  3. Responsible adult escort

H. Anesthesia requirements
   1. Consents for anesthesia
   2. Monitoring of patients receiving anesthesia
I. Charges
   1. Self-pay patients
   2. Discounts
   3. Collection notices
J. Consents
   1. Informed consent
   2. Minors
   3. Power of attorney
   4. Sterilization
   5. Administration of blood and blood products
   6. Release of information
K. Emergency procedures
   1. Emergency transfer procedure
   2. Emergency eye wash station
   3. CPR/BCLS/ACLS standards
   4. Malignant hyperthermia crisis
L. Equipment
   1. Operative
   2. Emergency
   3. Preventative maintenance program
   4. Repairs
   5. Medical device reporting requirements
M. Facilities management
   1. Emergency generator
   2. Maintenance of fire warning system
   3. Preventative maintenance program
N. Infection control
   1. Universal precautions
   2. Personal protective equipment
   3. Disposal of contaminated needles/sharps
   4. Handwashing
   5. OR attire
   6. Traffic patterns
   7. Restricted areas
O. Information systems
   1. Description and use of systems
   2. Systems backup and retention policy
   3. System access and password policy
P. Employee health
   1. Annual physical
   2. TB-testing requirements
   3. Sick time
   4. Worker's compensation
Q. Patient care
   1. OR standards of care
   2. PACU standards of care
   3. National, state, and facility standards of care
   4. Nurse:patient ratios
   5. Preoperative testing requirements

      6. Intraoperative monitoring procedures

      7. Postoperative monitoring procedures

      8. Patient education requirements

  R. Physician orders

      1. Standing postoperative orders for PACU

      2. Standing orders for ophthalmology patients

  S. Quality management

      1. Overview of quality management program

      2. Goals of quality management program

      3. Description of indicators/benchmarks

  T. Patient records

      1. Consents

      2. Confidentiality

      3. Order of medical record

      4. Release of information

  U. Safety

      1. Fire safety

      2. Hazardous material training

      3. Emergency preparedness training

      4. Glutaraldehyde exposure monitoring

      5. Waste-gas monitoring

      6. Bomb threat

      7. Violence in the workplace

      8. Body mechanics

  V. Staff member rules and responsibilities

      1. Orientation

      2. Confidentiality

      3. Competency requirements

      4. Performance appraisals

      5. Required education

      6. Conflict-of-interest statement

  W. Supplies

      1. Procurement/ordering

      2. Sterilization

      3. Storage

V. Approval Process for Policies and Procedures

  A. Varies according to individual institutional structure and policy

  B. May be approved by one or a combination of the following:

      1. Individual department

      2. Director of nursing

      3. Nursing leadership committee

      4. Surgical committee (if applicable to facility)

      5. Anesthesia department

      6. Medical executive committee

      7. CEO

      8. Governing board

VI. Use of Manuals

  A. Readily available to staff members

      1. Staff members familiar with contents of manual

      2. Staff members identify needed policies and procedures

  B. Used as reference

VII. Revision of Manuals
  A. Annual reviews
  B. Reviewed with staff
  C. Legal issues
  1. Maintain accurate file noting revisions
    a. Include reason for revision
    b. Date
    c. Potential need exists to provide specific policy in place on specific past date for litigation purposes
      i. Old policies kept on hand for 7 years
      ii. Old policies clearly marked with beginning and end dates

Bibliography

1. Burden, N. (1993). *Ambulatory Surgical Nursing.* Philadelphia: Saunders.
2. Drain, C.B. (1994). *The Post Anesthesia Care Unit.* Philadelphia: Saunders.
3. Huber, D. (1996). *Leadership and Nursing Care Management.* Philadelphia: Saunders.
4. *1996 Comprehensive Accreditation Manual for Ambulatory Care.* Joint Commission for Accreditation of Healthcare Organizations, Oakbrook Terrace, IL; 1995.
5. Phippen, M.L., Wells, M.P. (1994). *Perioperative Nursing Practice.* Philadelphia: Saunders.

REVIEW QUESTIONS

1. A policy

   A. Increases likelihood of inconsistencies
   B. Is designed to discourage order and stability
   C. Is not an extension of the mission statement
   D. Is a guideline to assist in decision making
   E. Is not intended to ensure compliance with standards

2. Policies provide all of the following except

   A. A mechanism for consistent treatment of staff
   B. Clarity and uniformity
   C. A detailed step-by-step instruction of a task
   D. A resource for accreditation and regulatory agencies
   E. Establishing a consistent level of expectation of staff members

3. Procedures function as
   (1) Reminders for tasks performed infrequently
   (2) A resource for orienting new staff
   (3) A means to measure quality and appropriateness of care
   (4) A method to facilitate cost containment
   (5) A means to increase productivity

   A. 1, 2
   B. 1, 3
   C. 1, 2, 3
   D. 1, 2, 4
   E. All of the above

4. The page layout for policies and procedures includes all of the following except

   A. Title
   B. Signatures
   C. Date of revision
   D. Date of JCAHO visit
   E. Date of review

5. Policies and procedures are approved by

   A. Department directors
   B. CEO of facility
   C. Chief executive nurse
   D. Medical director
   E. Any of the above

ANSWERS TO QUESTIONS

1. D
2. C
3. E

4. D
5. E

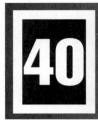

Total Quality Management in the Ambulatory Setting

Nancy K. King
The Surgery Centers
Cleveland, Ohio

I. **Total Quality Management (TQM)**
   A. A philosophy that quality is a responsibility shared by all and applicable to all levels of organization
   B. Works to enhance the performance of important processes involved in the delivery of health care having as much to do with achieving greater organizational efficiency and cost savings as improving quality of care
   C. Continuous improvement focusing on the customer, within and external to the institution, to identify root causes of problems and opportunities for improvement to achieve greater quality and efficiency
   D. Focuses on practices nonclinical as well as clinical aspects of care
   E. Views quality as an entity subject to measurement, the scientific method, and data-driven problem solving
II. **Dimensions of Quality**
   A. Effectiveness
      1. The power of a particular procedure or treatment to improve health status improvement
   B. Efficiency
      1. The delivery of a maximum number of comparable units of health care for a given unit of health resources used
   C. Accessibility
      1. The ease with which health care can be reached in the face of financial, organizational, cultural, and emotional barriers

   D. Acceptability
     1. The degree to which health care satisfies patients
   E. Provider competence
     1. The provider's ability (including technical and interpersonal skills) to use the best available knowledge and judgment to produce the health and satisfaction of customers

III. TQM History

   A. Evolved from Japanese industry after World War II by W. Edward Deming
     1. Dr. Deming developed sampling and data quality improvement strategies and assisted the Japanese in developing high-quality merchandise
     2. His philosophy for quality improvement was adapted by U.S. auto makers in the 1980s
   B. Evolved as a formal process in health care in the late 1980s
   C. Has become a cornerstone and guiding force in businesses, public agencies, and health-care industry in 1990s
   D. Is essential in today's changing health-care marketplace and resultant need for health-care providers to deliver more cost-effective care so that they may survive an increasing competitive environment

IV. Measuring Quality

   A. Traditional ways of measuring quality
     1. Structure standards
       a. Education and training of providers including drugs, equipment, ORs, and other associated aspects of the physical plant comprising the facility in which the care is provided
     2. Process
       a. The set of activities that go on within and between practitioners and patients
         i. Deficiencies in quality and failure to meet customers' needs are viewed as the result of defective processes used by workers, rather than failure of the workers to do their job properly
     3. Outcomes
       a. The end result of care including complication rates, functional capacity and performance, cost effectiveness, and patient satisfaction
         i. Is the number one competitive factor next to cost in health care
         ii. Survey target areas for JCAHO and AAAHC
         iii. One of the most crucial expectations of managed care and third-party payers

V. Changes in the Health-Care Marketplace

   A. Since 1990, insurers have been directing patients to providers within managed-care entities, such as health maintenance organization (HMOs) and preferred provider organizations (PPOs)
   B. Insurers seek low-cost providers, based on a prenegotiated payment for entire sets of services, such as an ambulatory procedure
   C. To support their decision making, insurers rely on claims' data bases that facilitate identification of quality of care and cost-effective providers
   D. Currently insurers are adopting capitation, a financing mechanism in which an annual payment is made to a set of providers who contract to provide specified benefits package for each insured individual during the contract year

VI. Outcomes

   A. Objective measurements
     1. Patient satisfaction
     2. Efficiency
     3. Cost effectiveness
     4. Results of service

  B. Need to measure to stay competitive in health-care industry
  C. The most important concerns are:
    1. Positive patient outcomes
    2. Cost-effective delivery of quality care
  D. Measure against established standards
    1. Benchmarking—defining competitors' best features from both internal and external customers' perspectives, and then adopting the best practices of these organizations to your operations
  E. Focus on results of performance or nonperformance of a function or process
VII. **Customers**
  A. Managing quality requires improving the capability and reliability of processes to meet the needs of the customers who depend on those processes; quality improvement is "customer centered"
    1. In health care, the patient is the most important customer
    2. Other customers include the patient's family and friends, surgeons, and other physicians, nurses, technicians, assistants, administrators, insurers, and vendors both internal and external to workplace
VIII. **Gathering Data and Analysis**
  A. Define current practice
  B. Define customer needs and expectations in ambulatory setting ("What do those who depend on us really want?")
  C. The initial step in improving a process is the adoption of appropriate definitions and the identification of the key measures that should be tracked
  D. Clearly define problem statement so all team members are thinking about the same problem; identify changes needed in process or area to be improved
  E. Collect and analyze data in a uniform fashion
  F. Patterns or trends can be identified with:
    1. Checksheet
    2. Flowchart
    3. Histogram
    4. Control chart
    5. Pareto chart
    6. Cause-and-effect diagram
    7. Scatter diagram
  G. Evaluate data and validate current practice or identify opportunities for improvement
  H. Implement changes with pilot program
  I. Change process as indicated by deficiencies
  J. Evaluate effectiveness
  K. Start process again from beginning
IX. **Sources of Data Collection**
  A. Surveys/questionnaires
    1. Should be consumer oriented
  B. Phone call or written survey
    1. Postoperative phone call is an important tool for evaluating patient's postoperative condition, reinforcing teaching, and obtaining performance feedback
    2. Mail-back questionnaires tend to generate low response rate (20–40%)
    3. Sources of gathering data
      a. Physician
      b. Payer
      c. Patient
      d. Employee

e. Patient records
f. Observation
g. Variance reports
h. Infection control reports

X. Indicators

A. Monitor the quality of all aspects of care
B. May include clinical criteria, clinical standards, practice guidelines
C. Stated in objective terms
D. Are measured
E. Based on current knowledge or structure and projected needs, standards or industry changes
F. Classified as outcome, process, or structure

XI. Collecting Data

A. Numerator identification
   1. Number of times the behavior or condition is met
B. Denominator identification
   1. Total number of patients, cases, medical records, or other variables surveyed or studied
C. Compliance rate
   1. Calculated by dividing the numerator by the denominator

XII. Frequency of Data Collection

A. Related to frequency of activity monitored
   1. Significance of event or activity monitored
   2. Common cause variation:
      a. Inevitable, inherent variation in the system
   3. Special cause variable:
      a. Variation resulting from sources outside the system, unplanned events, freak occurrences, human error
   4. Essential consideration to decide which episode of the process is the most important to address
   5. Designated time or length of study

XIII. Unique Issues for Ambulatory Care

A. Low incidence of severe adverse events
B. Transient but disturbing side effects, such as postoperative pain, nausea and vomiting, and dysphagia may influence a patient-based assessment for quality of care
C. Short length of stay
   1. Brief window to obtain desired outcomes
   2. Families or significant others share responsibility for postop care of patient at home
   3. Cross-training of nurses and support personnel reduces number of different persons treating a patient as well as enhances continuity of care
   4. Simplified paperwork and documentation leaves more time for direct care
D. Payment structure
   1. Fixed or "packaged" fees for standard surgical procedures (PPO/HMO)
   2. Complications or unplanned admissions to the hospital may incur more expenses
   3. Timeliness of care
   4. Convenience
E. Wellness-oriented and family-centered
   1. Teaching
      a. Encompasses all ages of patient
      b. Thorough postoperative instructions to patient and family member/significant other

2. Nurses must consider:
   a. Educational background of patient, family member/significant other
   b. Literacy
   c. Language barriers
   d. When and where to obtain follow-up care documented
   e. What to do in case of emergency documented
   f. Patient and family compliance
   g. Patient safety
F. Traditional outcomes
   1. Have historically been assessed in terms of surgical and anesthesia-related complications
      a. Unplanned hospital admissions
      b. Prolonged recovery time after anesthesia
      c. Unscheduled postop physician or emergency room visit
      d. Mortality
      e. Major morbidity
   2. More recent outcomes focus on patient experience
      a. Incidence of postop nausea and vomiting
      b. Pain or surgical discomfort
      c. Dizziness
      d. Sore throat
      e. Return to usual activities
      f. Patient satisfaction

Bibliography

1. Berk, J., Berk, S. (1993). A total quality management overview, everyone has a customer. *Total Quality Management, Implementing Continuous Improvement.* New York: Sterling Publishing.
2. Crosby, P.B. (1995). A quality carol, the first absolute: The definition of quality conformance to requirements, the quality vaccine. *Quality Without Tears, The Art of Hassle-Free Management.* New York: McGraw-Hill.
3. Kleinpell, R.M. (1997). Improving telephone follow-up after ambulatory surgery. *J PeriAnesth Nursing,* 12(5):336–340.
4. McGoldrick, K.E. (1995). *Ambulatory Anesthesia: A Problem-Oriented Approach.* Baltimore: William & Wilkins.

REVIEW QUESTIONS

1. Deficiencies in quality and failure to meet customers' needs are viewed as the result of

   A. Failure of workers to do their job properly
   B. Defective processes used by the workers
   C. Influence of insurers to cut costs
   D. Lack of outcome data to identify customer needs

2. The most important customer in health care is the

   A. Surgeon
   B. Insurers
   C. Patient's immediate family
   D. Patient

3. The initial step in improving a process is

   A. Identification of key measures that should be tracked
   B. Collecting data
   C. Define expected outcome
   D. Implement change with a pilot program

4. In data analysis, the compliance rate is

   A. Number of times the behavior or condition are met
   B. Total number of variables surveyed or studied
   C. Calculated by subtracting the numerator from the denominator
   D. Calculated by dividing the numerator by the denominator

5. Which statement best describes TQM?

   A. Quality is an ongoing responsibility shared by every employee and applicable to all levels of an organization
   B. Mainly focuses on clinical aspects of care
   C. Views quality as an entity subject to measurement with data-driven problem solving, without a scientific method
   D. Functions mainly to achieve greater organizational efficiency

6. Which of the following is **not** a dimension of quality?

   A. Effectiveness
   B. Accountability
   C. Accessibility
   D. Acceptability
   E. Efficiency

ANSWERS TO QUESTIONS

1. B
2. D
3. A

4. D
5. A
6. B

Personnel Selection, Management, and Staff Development

Donna M. DeFazio Quinn
Elliot 1-Day Surgery Center
Manchester, New Hampshire

PERSONNEL SELECTION

I. Qualifications of Nursing Staff
  A. Characteristics
   1. Goal-oriented
   2. Ambitious
   3. Organized
      a. Good time-management skills
   4. Independent thinker
   5. Excellent communication skills
      b. For patient teaching
         i. Assess, implement, and evaluate teaching effectiveness
      c. For interactions with patients, family members, visitors, coworkers, physicians, business office personnel, and other health-care professionals
      d. Establishing effective nurse–patient relationship quickly
      e. For all age groups, socioeconomic backgrounds and educational levels
         i. Pediatric patients
         ii. Geriatric patients
         iii. Patients with language barriers
            (a) Access to interpreters
         iv. Physically and mentally challenged
   6. Patient advocate

740

7. Self-confident
    a. Ability to handle emergencies
    b. Confidence in coworkers' abilities to handle emergencies
8. Experienced
    a. Solid medical/surgical experience
    b. Specialty clinical background beneficial
        i.   Pediatrics
        ii. Geriatrics
        iii. Critical care
            (a) Especially valuable in freestanding ASC where support personnel may not be readily available during emergencies
9. Positive attitude
    a. Caring
    b. Compassionate
    c. Empathetic
    d. Respectful
    e. Shows true concern and respect for patient, family, and employer
10. Flexible
    a. Willing to cross-train/float based on unit needs
    b. Willing to work additional/less hours based on unit needs
11. Team-spirited
    a. Ability to work together with other health-care professionals
    b. Work toward common goal of safe and efficient patient care
12. Able to set priorities
    a. Detail oriented
    b. Institutes measures to correct identified deficiencies
13. Able to make quick and accurate assessments

B. Job descriptions
    1. Purposes
        a. Clearly defines role and responsibility of particular position
        b. Used as a tool to recruit employees
        c. Used for employees requesting internal transfers to department
        d. Basis for developing performance appraisals, evaluations, competency statements
            i. Serves as a standard to rate employee
        e. Identifies health and safety regulations
    2. Includes:
        a. Reporting structure
        b. Specific job duties and responsibilities
        c. Standards of performance
        d. Educational requirements
            i. Prior experience
            ii. Required certifications (BCLS, ACLS, etc.)
        e. Ability to use specialized equipment
        f. Ability to function independently
        g. Ability to communicate effectively
        h. Confidentiality of information
        i. Physical requirements
        j. Number of employees the position directly supervises (if applicable)
        k. Working conditions and potential health hazards
            i. Exposure to:
                (a) Heat, cold, noise, odors, chemical, fumes, etc.

   3. Revisions
      a. Revise periodically
      b. Reflect current practice standards
   4. Accessibility
      a. Accessible to employees
II. The Interview Process
   A. Purpose
      1. Obtain information
      2. Give information
      3. Determine if applicant meets requirements for position
   B. Interviewer
      1. Utilize interview skills to:
         a. Establish rapport with interviewee
         b. Provide exchange of information through communication
      2. Introductions
      3. Acquaint applicant with position
         a. Provide with job description
         b. Provide with performance appraisal tool
      4. Share information with applicant
         a. Policies and procedures
            i.   Facility/department "mission/vision/values" statement(s)
         b. Overview of function of unit
         c. Relationship of unit to others (e.g., PACU Phase I to PACU Phase II)
         d. Anticipated work schedule
         e. Facility
         f. Benefits/salary range
         g. Decision-making process for selection of applicants
      5. Assess applicant for:
         a. Dependability
         b. Willingness to assume responsibilities of job
         c. Willingness to work with others
         d. Interest in job
         e. Adaptability
         f. Flexibility
         g. Consistency of goals with available opportunities
         h. Appearance to job requirements
      6. Ask open-ended questions
         a. Situation-based questions will elicit the applicant's ability to handle clinical situations
         b. Elicit applicant's technical skills
            i.   How do you keep abreast of new technologies, standards, or products?
            ii. Have you ever developed a method to make a certain technical task easier to perform? Describe it.
         c. Elicit applicant's ability to analyze a problem, situation, or process
            i.   Describe a difficult problem that you have had to solve in the past. How did you come up with a solution?
         d. Elicit the applicant's credibility
            i.   Have you ever had to compromise your standards in order to get a job done?
            ii. What was the situation? How did you resolve it?
         e. Elicit applicant's communication skills

  i. Can you describe a situation in which you had to confront and resolve an issue with a person you did not have a good relationship with?

  ii. What different approaches do you use when communicating with peers? Physicians?

f. Elicit applicant's approach to customer service

  i. How can you provide value to your patients?

  ii. Can you describe an instance where you took it upon yourself to make sure a patient's problem was resolved?

g. Elicit applicant's initiative

  i. Describe an instance where you did more than was required in your job

  ii. Have you ever identified a problem and corrected it before anyone else did? Describe the situation.

  iii. Have you ever devised a more cost-efficient manner to perform a task? What did you do?

h. Elicit applicant's leadership ability

  i. Can you describe a circumstance where you had to successfully motivate others to do things they were unwilling to do?

i. Elicit applicant's ability to plan and organize

  i. How do you establish priorities for patient care?

  ii. Have you ever been in a situation where you had to deal with a lot of patients at one time? How did you do it?

j. Elicit applicant's ability to work with others

  i. Describe a situation when you felt you truly collaborated with other members of the team to get a particular job done

  ii. Describe a situation in which you had to work closely with someone who you didn't particularly get along with. How did you handle it? Why was it so difficult to get along with this person?

k. Do not violate employment laws

  i. Title VII of the Civil Rights Act of 1964 as amended by the Civil Rights Act of 1991

   (a) Prohibits discrimination based on race, color, sex, religion, or national origin

   (b) Covers all areas of employment including hiring, discharge, classification and pay practices, and promotion

  ii. Age Discrimination in Employment Act of 1967

   (a) Bans discrimination against employees and applicants over age 40

  iii. Rehabilitation Act of 1973

   (a) Applies only to federal government contractors or to employers who receive "federal financial assistance" (including Medicare funds)

   (b) Requires employers to take "affirmative action" to employ and advance qualified handicapped individuals

  iv. Americans With Disabilities Act

   (a) Prohibits discrimination against individuals with disabilities

   (b) Protects the qualified individual with a disability with regards to job application procedures, hiring, advancement or discharge of employees, employee compensation, job training, and other terms, conditions, and privileges of employment

   (c) Cannot refuse to hire based on disability

  v. Federal Pregnancy Discrimination Act

   (a) Discrimination on the basis of pregnancy constitutes illegal sex discrimination in violation of Title VII

       vi. Equal Pay Act
        (a) Prohibits discrimination on the basis of sex in the payment of wages
        (b) Requires equal pay for equal work
   7. Listen to applicants' responses
   8. Ask follow-up questions if more information is needed
   9. Be consistent with all applicants
  10. Allow applicant to ask questions
     a. Answer questions
     b. Obtain additional information for applicant if needed
  11. Closing
     a. Clarify any questions
     b. Inquire if current employer can be contacted for reference
     c. Identify time frame for final selection of applicant
  12. Provide contact information should applicant have additional questions
     a. Name, address
     b. Telephone number
  13. Summarize interview
     a. Write up synopsis of candidate
     b. Include strengths and weaknesses
C. Interviewee
  1. Pre-interview preparation
    a. Prepare list of questions
  2. Dress in professional manner for interview
  3. Arrive promptly at appointed time
  4. Present good first impression
    a. Projected through total image
      i. Appearance
      ii. Behavior
     iii. Communication skills
       (a) Verbal
       (b) Nonverbal
  5. Listen to interviewer
  6. Answer questions openly and honestly
    a. Respond to the question at hand only
    b. Keep on track
  7. Express positive qualities when situation presents itself
    a. Team-player attitude
    b. Past relevant experience
    c. Personal values
      i. Pride in work
      ii. Commitment to quality patient care
     iii. Accountability
     iv. Motivation
      v. Role model
     vi. Organized
    vii. Ability to:
       (a) Admit mistakes and take corrective action
       (b) Set priorities
       (c) Negotiate situations
       (d) Implement productive measures towards conflict resolution
  8. Send follow-up letter confirming continued interest in position

D. Final selection of applicant
 1. Rule out unqualified applicants
 2. Check references of qualified applicants
 3. Evaluate applicant's behavior, skills, and knowledge against the job requirements
 4. Evaluate applicant's motivation and interest in position
 5. Use caution if any of the following are present:
  a. History of moving from job to job
  b. History of continued conflict with peers
  c. Applicant expresses concern regarding work hours
  d. Applicant does not have any questions during interview process
  e. Applicant does not display characteristics of typical ambulatory perianesthesia nurse
 6. Select the best candidate
 7. Offer position

MANAGEMENT AND STAFF DEVELOPMENT

III. Orientation

A. Definition
 1. Provides professional education
 2. Includes expected roles and responsibilities
 3. Provides socialization
 4. Allows person to acquire necessary knowledge and skills to fulfill expectations of job description
 5. Places person in state of information dependency
B. Learning role
 1. Process of internally reorganizing thought patterns, perceptions, assumptions, attitudes, feelings, and skills
 2. Tests reorganization of above in relation to new work setting
 3. Can only take place effectively when:
  a. Atmosphere in teaching–learning interaction reduces threats and defensiveness
  b. Atmosphere provides support during the process of changing patterns of thought and behavior
 4. Affected by climate
  a. More positive learning in warm and friendly atmosphere
  b. Produce more and feel more secure if environment is businesslike and work-centered
 5. Outcomes of positive learning experience
  a. Growth
  b. Change in behavior
  c. Change in learner
  d. Change in interpersonal self-actualization
C. Teaching role
 1. Expert clinician
  a. Desires to share expertise
  b. Provides learner with broad knowledge base
  c. Certification in specialty desirable
   i. Affirms nurse models consistent application of nursing process and adheres to identified standards
  d. Understands the needs of the adult learner
  e. Understands the principles of adult education

D. Methods
    1. Teacher-centered learning
        a. Traditional approach to learning
        b. Learner unable to identify own learning needs
        c. Teacher decides what should be learned
    2. Learner-centered approach
        a. Learner identifies own learning needs
        b. Teacher identifies appropriate learning experience
        c. Requires creativity on part of the teacher

IV. Orientation Program
  A. Formal (written) program
    1. Identifies facility/unit philosophy
    2. Clarifies program
    3. Identifies goals and objectives of program
        a. Gives generalized direction to teacher and learner regarding philosophy
        b. Describes how roles and responsibilities contribute collectively to philosophy
  B. Types of programs
    1. Traditional
        a. Focus on acquisition of knowledge
        b. Does not include direct application of knowledge learned
    2. Competency-based orientation (CBO)
        a. Focus on acquisition of knowledge **and**
        b. Application of knowledge in workplace
  C. Contents (see Table 41–1)
    1. Learning objectives of orientation program
        a. Individualized
        b. Describe how educational needs will be met
        c. Two types of objectives
            i.   Program-related
                (a) Describe broad behavior changes
                (b) Occur as result of participating in orientation program
            ii.   Learner-related
                (a) Describe changes learner will achieve relating to new role and responsibilities
                (b) Describe how individual behaviors will change as result of participating in orientation program
        d. Identify measurable criteria
            i.   Behaviors that identify how learner will progress from basic competency to excellence
    2. Necessary skills
    3. Documentation forms
    4. Pertinent department policies and procedures
  D. Length of orientation program
    1. Individualized to meet learner's needs
    2. Generally 3 months if no previous PACU experience
        a. Individual should work full time during orientation period
        b. Works closely with preceptor (experienced PACU nurse) for entire orientation period
  E. Evaluation
    1. Provide ongoing evaluation completed by:
        a. Manager
        b. Preceptor
        c. Orientee (self-assessment)

Table 41–1 • CONTENT OF ORIENTATION PROGRAM

Review of anatomy and physiology of the cardiorespiratory system:
  Pathophysiologic processes of the cardiorespiratory system
  Factors altering circulatory or respiratory function following surgery and anesthesia
  Monitoring techniques
  Cardiac dysrhythmias
  Airway maintenance, equipment, and techniques
  Ventilatory support, equipment, and procedures
  Cardiorespiratory arrest and its management
  Treatment of hypotension and hypertension
  Interpretation of laboratory values
  Identification and treatment of malignant hyperthermia
Review of other physiologic considerations:
  Neurologic system
  Musculoskeletal system
  Genitourinary system
    Fluid and electrolyte balance and imbalance
  Gastrointestinal system
  Integumentary system
  Pediatric–adolescent physiology
  Geriatric physiology
  Physiology of pregnancy
Anesthesia:
  General concepts
  Administration and properties of selected agents (include all agents routinely used in facility)
  Nursing implications
Care of the PACU patient:
  Physical assessment of the postoperative patient
  General PACU care
  Specific care required following procedures (include all specialty procedures routinely performed in facility)
  Postoperative medications
  Patient teaching
    Preoperative
    Postoperative
  Department specifics

The above list represents suggested content for a basic PACU orientation program. Additional materials appropriate to the practice setting should also be included.

Adapted from: Drain, C.B. (1994). *The Post Anesthesia Care Unit*, 3rd ed. Philadelphia; Saunders, pp. 21–22.

    2. Evaluation is formal (written)
    3. Purpose
      a. Acquire and process evidence needed to improve learning–teaching process
      b. Determine if goals and objectives are being met
      c. Determine if teaching plan needs to be revised
V. Continuing Education
  A. Mandatory education
    1. Depends on requirements of facility, state health department, board of nursing, or other regulatory or accrediting agencies
    2. Program may include:
      a. Fire/safety
      b. BCLS/ACLS

  c. Infection control/universal precautions
  d. Hazardous material management
  e. Disaster training
B. Inservice education
  1. Activities intended to assist the nurse to acquire, maintain, and/or increase competence
  2. Reflects employer's goals and service commitments
  3. Includes but is not limited to review of previously learned skills
  4. Focus is on peer learning activities
  5. May develop specialty nursing knowledge, skill, or attitudes
  6. Emphasis of inservice education
    a. Patient care aspects
    b. Nursing practice implications
C. Continuing education
  1. Definition
    a. Planned educational activities
    b. Intended to build on educational and experiential bases of the nurse
  2. Includes current and emerging concepts, principles, practices, theories, and/or research in or related to nursing
  3. Includes immediate or futuristic application to meet nursing practice needs or goals of the learner
  4. Contact hours are granted (usually)
D. Educational files
  1. Maintained for all employees
  2. Attendance at programs/outside conferences is documented
  3. Includes copies of:
    a. BCLS/ACLS certification
    b. Specialty certification
    c. Competency checklists
VI. Nursing Competency
A. Definition
  1. A principle of professional practice
  2. Identifies the ability of the provider to administer safe and reliable care on a consistent basis (O'Toole, 1997)
  3. Competency-based education
    a. Is based on sound adult education principles
    b. Allows individual opportunity to properly demonstrate ability to perform skills and activities
    c. Allows individual to apply knowledge and skills to "real world" situations
    d. Can be incorporated into an orientation program
    e. Can be incorporated into yearly performance appraisal to validate staff members' competency
    f. Allows deficiencies to be addressed in a timely manner
B. JCAHO standard
  1. HR.3: The competence of all staff members is continually assessed, maintained, demonstrated, and improved (JCAHO, 1998)
    a. Facility measures employees' ability to perform duties and meet expectations as defined in job description
    b. Facility defines the process
    c. Assessment of staff competence
      i.   Maintained through ongoing assessment and educational activities

Table 41–2 • PURPOSE OF KNOWLEDGE-BASED OBJECTIVES AND NURSING CARE COMPETENCIES

1. Provide a standard for safe pre- and postanesthesia nursing practice
2. Direct the activity of nursing knowledge and skill specific to pre- and postanesthesia care
3. Direct the individual nurse toward a professional practice by providing guidelines for pacing the acquisition of knowledge, thereby taking a joint responsibility in his/her own development
4. Direct the clinical instructor in providing adequate orientation and ongoing inservice
5. Provide the nurse managers with guidelines for performance appraisals
6. Provide the pre- and postanesthesia nurse with guidelines for his/her own self-evaluations, thereby making the evaluation process a joint effort

From Zickuhr, M., Atsberger, D. (1995). *Pre- and Postanesthesia Nursing Knowledge Base and Clinical Competencies.* Philadelphia: Saunders.

    ii. Periodic and objective measurement of:
       (a) Job performance
       (b) Current competencies
       (c) Skills
  C. Purpose of competency assessment (see Table 41–2)
    1. Set standards
    2. Ensure adequate orientation
    3. Provide basis for performance appraisal
  D. Levels of nursing practice pre- and postanesthesia (see Table 41–3)
    1. Level I (beginner postanesthesia nurse)
    2. Level II (postanesthesia nurse)
    3. Level III (senior postanesthesia nurse)
    4. Level IV (advanced postanesthesia nurse)
  E. Assessing competency
    1. Perianesthesia competencies include, but are not limited to:
      a. Assessing the physiological health status of the patient
      b. Complying with safety and emergency protocols as identified in policies and procedures
      c. Administering medications as prescribed
      d. Monitoring the patients physiologically pre- and postprocedure as required
      e. Anticipating potential patient problems; initiating interventions to prevent them
      f. Respecting the patient's right to privacy

Table 41–3 • LEVELS OF NURSING PRACTICE FOR PRE- AND POSTANESTHESIA NURSING

Level I	General practitioner; needs direct supervision in pre- and postanesthesia nursing
	Identifies and evaluates nursing interventions with assistance
Level II	Beginner charge and teacher 1:1; needs general supervision
	Identifies and evaluates nursing interventions
Level III	Experienced charge and teacher 1:1; needs little supervision
	Manages and coordinates nursing staff for a specific shift
Level IV	Manager of patient care, nursing administration; researcher
	Participates in unit development

From Zickuhr, M., Atsberger, D. (1995). *Pre- and Postanesthesia Nursing Knowledge Base and Clinical Competencies.* Philadelphia: Saunders.

      g. Maintaining accountability for nursing actions

      h. Measuring effectiveness of nursing interventions

      i. Monitoring patient outcomes

      j. Continually assessing all aspects of patient care and modifying interventions as necessary to meet patient needs

      k. Participating in preoperative and postoperative patient teaching, including family members/significant others as appropriate

      l. Documenting nursing actions as identified in policies and procedures

   F. Frequency of competency assessment

     1. Initial orientation to unit

     2. Yearly thereafter

     3. Includes documentation in personnel file

VII. Performance Appraisals

   A. Job evaluation

     1. Reflects criteria contained in job description

     2. Purpose

      a. To maintain, improve, and motivate employee behaviors

      b. Participative process

      c. Ensures effective two-way communication

     3. Measures efficiency against standards

     4. Determines competence

     5. May include peer review

     6. Readily available to employee

      a. Allows employee to know expectations, role, and responsibilities

      b. Assists employee to improve job performance

   B. Completion

     1. Three months after beginning employment

     2. Annually

      a. Maintain in personnel file

      b. Employee keeps a copy

   C. Benefits of performance appraisal

     1. See Table 41–4

   D. Performance appraisal tools

     1. Types

      a. Narrative regarding employee performance

      b. Checklist

      c. Rating scale

      d. Criteria-based, reflecting job description

Table 41–4 • BENEFITS OF PERFORMANCE APPRAISALS

- Improve performance
- Improve communication
- Reinforce positive behavior
- Be one method employed to communicate about and ultimately to correct negative or less than optimal behavior
- Provide a basis for rewards, which also is a basis for motivation
- Provide a basis for termination if necessary
- Identify learning needs and develop personnel

From Huber, D. (1996). *Leadership and Nursing Care Management*, Philadelphia: Saunders, p. 535.

2. Standardized form
   a. Objective
   b. Consistent and fair
3. Employee performs self-assessment
   a. Employee and manager review together
   b. Discuss differences
4. Needs to be objective
5. Should assess knowledge, skills, and activities of employee
6. Should enhance staff development

E. Content of performance appraisal includes but is not limited to:
1. Assessment skills
2. Communication skills
   a. Peer interactions
   b. Physician interactions
   c. Patient and family interactions
   d. Interactions with other health-care professionals
3. Technical skills
4. Clinical skills
5. Autonomy in decision making
6. Accountability
7. Patient teaching activities
8. Quality management activities
9. Professional growth and development
10. Behavioral characteristics
    a. Flexibility
    b. Leadership

F. Staff performance issues
1. Counseling and direction occurs throughout the year, not just at time of performance appraisal
2. Plan for improvement identified and agreed on
3. Documented
4. Issue reevaluated in specified period of time

Bibliography

1. Burden, N. (1993). *Ambulatory Surgical Nursing.* Philadelphia: Saunders.
2. *Competency Based Orientation Credentialing Program,* 1997 edition. Thorofare, NJ: ASPAN.
3. Drain, C.B. (1994). *The Post Anesthesia Care Unit.* Philadelphia: Saunders.
4. Huber, D. (1996). *Leadership and Nursing Care Management.* Philadelphia: Saunders.
5. Loraine, K. (1997). Orientation is as simple as 1-2-3. *Nurs Manage,* 28(1):35–36.
6. *1998–1999 Comprehensive Accreditation Manual for Ambulatory Care.* (1998). Joint Commission for Accreditation of Healthcare Organizations, Oakbrook Terrace, IL.
7. O'Toole, M.T., ed. (1997). *Miller-Keane Encyclopedia & Dictionary of Medicine, Nursing, & Allied Health,* 6th ed. Philadelphia: Saunders.
8. Peratino, B.A. (1997). Common mistakes to avoid when interviewing. *OR Manager,* 12(11):22–24.
9. Phippen, M.L., Wells, M.P. (1994). *Perioperative Nursing Practice.* Philadelphia: Saunders.
10. Schramm, C.A., Hoshowsky, V.M. (1995). Developing competency-based perioperative orientation programs. *AORN J,* 62(4):579–590.
11. Shaffer, F., Kobs, A. (1997). Measuring competencies of temporary staff. *Nurs Manage,* 28(5):41–45.
12. Speers, A.T., Gilberg, K.M., Koch, F.A. (1995). Competency-based orientation for registered perioperative nurses. *AORN J,* 62(4):567–578.
13. Voorhees, M. (1996). Using competency-based education in the perioperative setting. *Nurs Manage,* 27(8):35–38.
14. Ward, M.J., Price, S.A. (1991). *Issues in Nursing Administration.* St. Louis: Mosby.
15. Wells, M.M.P. (1987). *Decision Making in Perioperative Nursing.* Toronto: B.C. Decker.

REVIEW QUESTIONS

1. The purpose of a job description is
   (1) To clearly define the role and respon-
       sibility of a particular position
   (2) To serve as a standard for rating an
       employee
   (3) To use it as a recruiting tool
   (4) To serve as a basis for performance
       appraisals

   A. 1, 4
   B. 2, 4
   C. 1, 2, 4
   D. 1, 2, 3
   E. All of the above

2. A job description should include all of
   the following except

   A. The reporting structure
   B. Standards of performance
   C. Educational requirements
   D. Supervisor's name
   E. Work conditions

3. The orientation of an individual to a unit
   (1) Provides the opportunity for profes-
       sional education
   (2) Provides for socialization
   (3) Provides the individual with the
       ability to acquire necessary knowl-
       edge and skills to fulfill the expecta-
       tions of the job description
   (4) Places the individual in a state of
       information dependency

   A. 1, 3
   B. 1, 2, 3
   C. 3, 4
   D. All of the above
   E. None of the above

4. Outcomes of positive learning experiences include all of the following except

   A. Growth
   B. Change in behavior
   C. No change in the learner
   D. Change in interpersonal self-
      actualization
   E. Change in the learner

5. The teacher-centered learning method

   A. Involves the learner identifying his/
      her own learning needs
   B. Involves a nontraditional approach
      to learning
   C. Involves the teacher deciding what
      should be learned
   D. Involves the student deciding what
      should be learned

6. Contents of a PACU orientation program
   generally include all of the following
   except

   A. Review of anatomy and physiology
      of the cardiorespiratory system
   B. Monitoring techniques
   C. General concepts of anesthesia
   D. Administration of anesthetic agents
   E. Physical assessment of the pre- and
      postoperative patient

7. Inservice education activities

   A. Are intended to assist the nurse to
      acquire, maintain, and/or increase
      competence
   B. Reflect the employer's goals and
      service commitments
   C. Focus on peer learning activities
   D. May develop specialty nursing
      knowledge, skill, or attitudes
   E. All of the above

8. Competency-based education

   A. Allows individuals to apply
      knowledge and skills in role-playing
      situations
   B. Cannot be incorporated into an
      orientation program
   C. Does not allow deficiencies to be
      addressed in a timely manner
   D. Allows the individual to properly
      demonstrate his/her abilities to
      perform designated skills and
      activities
   E. Is unable to validate staff member's
      competency

9. Performance appraisals

   A. Are used to measure efficiency against standards
   B. Ensure effective two-way communication
   C. May include peer review
   D. Reflect criteria as established in the job description
   E. All of the above

10. Performance appraisal tools

    (1) Should always be in the narrative form
    (2) Should be consistent and fair
    (3) May be criteria based reflecting the job description
    (4) Should assess knowledge, skills, and activities of the employee
    (5) Are only completed by the manager

    A. 1, 2, 4
    B. 2, 3, 4
    C. 1, 3, 5
    D. 1, 2, 5
    E. All of the above

ANSWERS TO QUESTIONS

1. E
2. D
3. D
4. C
5. C

6. D
7. E
8. D
9. E
10. B

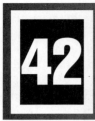

Conflict Management and Team-Building

Patricia Muller-Smith
Saint Francis Health System
Tulsa, Oklahoma

Objectives

1. Identify five sources of conflict.
2. List five key components of successful conflict resolution.
3. Identify the five styles of conflict management and discuss two situations in which each style is used.
4. Discuss three types of teams and the problems associated with them.
5. List the four stages of team development and discuss how members feel in each stage.

I. Conflict

A. Definition
   1. An opposition of wills, principles, or forces
   2. The tension generated by differences of opinion

B. Sources of conflict
   1. Scarce or undisturbed resources
      a. Limited money
      b. Limited staff
      c. Limited time
      d. Downsizing
   2. Differences (thoughts, feelings, ideas, perceptions)
      a. Expectations
      b. Previous experience
      c. Self concept
      d. Sentiments
   3. Role
      a. Goals/objectives
      b. Demands
      c. Responsibilities
   4. Work flow/design
      a. Reengineering
   5. Specialization versus generalization
      a. Cross-training
      b. Multi-skilled workers

C. Stages of conflict
   1. Anticipation: unfocused anxiety—a "feeling" that a problem exists
   2. Suppressed: known but unexpressed differences
   3. Discussion: differences expressed openly but are not resolved

4. Open dispute: conflict acknowledged and individuals begin to take positions
5. Open conflict: rigid positions are assumed and communication is difficult and unproductive

D. Areas where conflict occurs
   1. Interpersonal—inside one's self
      a. Values
      b. Discomfort with change
      c. Feeling threatened
   2. Interpersonal—between two individuals
      a. Goals and objectives seen as incompatible
      b. Power struggle
   3. Intra group—within an established group
      a. Clicks
      b. Shifts
   4. Inter group—between two or more established groups
      a. Units are integrated as reengineering or redesign takes place
      b. Both groups are downsized and asked to assume increased workload

E. Categories of conflict
   1. Facts—differences about data
      a. Information is not clear, consistent, or shared
      b. Individuals do not have all the facts
   2. Methods—differences about how something is or should be done
      a. Constant change created by restructuring
      b. No clear or singular way to change in order to be effective
   3. Goals—differences about desired outcomes
      a. Quality patient care versus financial viability
   4. Values—differences in belief systems
      a. Individuals value different things
      b. Individuals act in ways that serve their personal values system
      c. Values are non-negotiable and do not change

F. To resolve conflict, the following must be present:
   1. Trust
      a. Among the individuals and/or groups
      b. Intent of all participants is a good outcome for all individuals in the group
   2. Communication
      a. Effectively identifies issues
      b. Allows for honest feedback
   3. Commitment
      a. To continue discussion until a mutually agreed-upon solution is reached

G. Key components of successful conflict resolution
   1. All parties are aware of the conflict and understand the issues involved
   2. Ongoing communication among the involved parties until everyone is satisfied that a statement of the issues is clear and valid
   3. Behavior is the focus of attention and not the underlying motive
   4. The environment supports open nonjudgmental discussion and humor is used to break the tension
   5. Confrontation is frequent but is used to clarify or problem-solve
   6. Agreement of those involved to withdraw from the conflict when tensions are too high, but commit to reestablishing the communication in the near future
   7. Role-play the opposing point of view—walk a mile in the other's shoes
   8. Look for areas of agreement first; not areas of discord
   9. Project the impact of all possible solutions
   10. Allow experimentation as a natural process in the search for the best solution

H. Positive conflict supports growth and progress by:
   1. Arousing feelings and energy in individuals
   2. Stimulating greater feelings of identity with the group
   3. Increasing motivation to perform group tasks
   4. Calling attention to problems that exist
   5. Serving to diffuse feelings about larger problems
   6. Serving as a means for groups to test and adjust to the existing balance of power
I. Negative conflict depletes individual energy and limits both individual and group effectiveness by:
   1. Creating feelings of frustration, hostility, and stress
   2. Impairing judgment and ability to perform
   3. Increasing pressure to conform within the group
   4. Decreasing problem-solving
   5. Diffusing energy that is needed for productive work
   6. Refusing to cooperate with one another; group begins blocking activities
   7. Distorting communications
   8. Developing stereotypes—"they" becomes the "enemy"
J. Seven principles for maintaining positive relationships during conflict
   1. Build winners through consensus; voting builds losers
   2. Declare a moratorium when emotions are high
   3. Encourage equal participation
   4. Actively listen
   5. Separate fact from opinion
   6. Separate people from problem
   7. Divide and conquer
K. Five "don'ts" during conflict
   1. Don't get in a power struggle
   2. Don't become detached from the conflict
   3. Don't let conflict establish the agenda
   4. Don't be caught "awfulizing"
   5. Don't be fooled by projection
L. Develop a win-win philosophy
   1. Focus on mutually beneficial outcomes
   2. Define problem in terms of meeting each other's needs
   3. Entertain many possible solutions
   4. Maintain a positive attitude

II. Conflict-Management Styles

A. Avoiding (hiding)
   1. Differences are external, inevitable, unchangeable
   2. Differences are harmful
B. Competing (forcing)
   1. Differences are black and white
   2. Some are right
   3. Differences need to be erased
C. Accommodating (smoothing)
   1. Differences drive people apart
   2. Conflict calls for sacrifice and yield
D. Collaborating (confronting)
   1. Differences are natural and provide opportunity for creative problem-solving
E. Compromise
   1. Differences should be aired, followed by give and take

III. Choosing the Correct Style
  A. Avoiding; use when:
    1. The quality of the outcome is not important
    2. The level of the individual or group commitment is not important
    3. The levels of power among individuals is not equal
  B. Competing; use when:
    1. The levels of power are clear
    2. Group commitment is not important
    3. Quality of the decision is important
  C. Accommodating
    1. There is no power struggle
    2. Group commitment is important
    3. Quality of outcome is moderately important
    4. Desire to build up credits and markers is strong
  D. Compromising
    1. Power is equal among individuals and group
    2. Mutually satisfying outcomes can be achieved in both quality and acceptance
  E. Collaborating
    1. Quality is important to both parties and cannot be compromised
    2. Both parties must accept the agreed-upon solution
    3. Both parties see the problem as a means of learning and working through feelings

IV. Teams/Teamwork
  A. Types of teams
    1. Problem-solving
    2. Project focused
    3. High performance
  B. Problems with teams
    1. Made up of individuals with different values and goals
    2. Often looking for ways to reallocate scarce resources
    3. Few team members have adequate training in group management
  C. How teams develop
    1. Stage 1—Forming; members feel:
      a. Excitement, anticipation, and optimism
      b. Pride in being chosen for project
      c. Initial tentative attachment to the team
      d. Suspicion, fear, and anxiety about the job ahead
    2. Stage 2—Storming; members feel:
      a. Resistance to the task and to quality-improvement approaches
      b. Uncomfortable with using new methods
      c. Sharp fluctuations in attitude about the team
      d. Doubtful of project's chance for success
    3. Stage 3—Norming; members feel:
      a. A new ability to express criticism constructively
      b. Acceptance of membership in the team
      c. Relief that everything seems to be working out
    4. Stage 4—Performing; members feel:
      a. They have insight into personal and group processes
      b. They understand each other's strengths and weaknesses
      c. Satisfied at group's process
  D. Signs of trouble
    1. Cannot easily describe the team's mission
    2. Meetings are formal, stuffy, or tense
    3. Great deal of participation but little is accomplished

    4. Lots of talk, no communication

    5. Disagreements are aired in private conversations after meetings

    6. Decisions tend to be made by the formal leader with little involvement of other team members

    7. Confusion exists about roles and work assignments

    8. Individuals in other departments who are necessary to project success are not cooperating

    9. Too many people have the same style of conflict resolution

    10. The team has been together three months and is still unsure of its function

E. How to build a successful team

    1. Get to know the members

    2. Define the team purpose

    3. Clarify roles

    4. Establish norms

    5. Develop a game plan

    6. Encourage questions

    7. Share the limelight

    8. Be participatory

    9. Celebrate accomplishments

    10. Assess team effectiveness

F. Leadership behaviors during team development

    1. Stage 1—Forming

      a. Provide structure, assurance, and direction

      b. Clarify goals and reinforce as necessary

      c. Provide clear agenda

      d. Keep group focused

      e. Don't expect high productivity

    2. Stage 2—Storming

      a. Allow for difference

      b. Focus on problems, not people

      c. Discuss the underlying beliefs and values

      d. Lead and involve members

      e. Expect to be challenged

      f. Keep realistic goals

      g. Don't expect high productivity

    3. Stage 3—Norming

      a. Talk about norms

      b. Talk about how team is doing

      c. Clarify roles and responsibilities

      d. Begin to take a stab at real issues

    4. Stage 4—Performing

      a. Let team manage issues

      b. Encourage collaborative decision

      c. Allow flexibility

      d. Focus on self-learning

Bibliography

1. Fisher, R., Ury, W. (1991). *Getting to Yes.* New York: Penguin.
2. Parker, G.M. (1991). *Team Players and Teamwork.* San Francisco: Jossey Bass.
3. Thomas, K., Kilmann, R. (1979). *Conflict Mode Instrument.* New York: Xicom.
4. Ury, W. (1993). *Getting Past No.* New York: Bantam Books.

REVIEW QUESTIONS

1. Sources of conflict include all of the following except

   A. Scarce or undistributed resources
   B. Differences of thoughts, feelings, ideas, and perceptions
   C. Trust among members of the group
   D. Specialization versus generalization

2. Key components of successful conflict resolution include
   (1) All parties involved being aware of the conflict and understanding the issues involved
   (2) Ensuring ongoing communication among the parties involved until everyone is satisfied that a statement of the issues is clear and valid
   (3) Looking for areas of discord first, then identifying areas of agreement
   (4) Identifying the impact of all possible solutions
   (5) Agreeing to withdraw from the conflict when tension becomes too high and not committing to resume communication again in the future

   A. 1, 2, 3
   B. 2, 4, 5
   C. 1, 4, 5
   D. 1, 2, 4

3. Negative conflict depletes individual energy and limits both individual and group effectiveness through all of the following except

   A. Creating feelings of frustration, hostility, and stress
   B. Increasing pressure to conform within the group
   C. Stimulating greater feelings of identity with the group
   D. Diffusing energy that is needed for productive work

4. The five conflict-management styles include

   A. Avoiding, competing, contending, collaborating, and compromise
   B. Competing, accommodating, coordinating, collaborating, and compromise
   C. Accommodating, collaborating, coordinating, competing, and compromise
   D. Avoiding, competing, accommodating, collaborating, and compromise

5. Which conflict-management style is used when (1) power is equal among the individuals in the group and (2) mutually satisfying outcomes can be achieved in both quality and acceptance?

   A. Competing
   B. Compromising
   C. Collaborating
   D. Coordinating

6. The four stages of team development include

   A. Bonding, norming, forming, and collecting
   B. Forming, norming, performing, and collaborating
   C. Performing, bonding, collecting, and norming
   D. Forming, storming, norming, and performing

7. Signs of trouble within a team include all of the following except

   A. Cannot easily describe the team's mission
   B. Meetings are informal, inconsequential, and tense
   C. There is lots of talk with no communication
   D. There is confusion regarding roles and work assignments

8. In order for a team to be successful, in which stage should leadership provide: (1) structure, assurance, and direction, (2) clarification of goals and reinforcement as necessary, (3) clear agendas, and (4) measures to keep the group focused?

   A. Forming
   B. Storming
   C. Performing
   D. Collaborating

ANSWERS TO QUESTIONS

1. C
2. D
3. C
4. D

5. B
6. D
7. B
8. A

Certification Concepts and Testing Strategies

Kathy Carlson
Abbott Northwestern Hospital
Minneapolis, Minnesota

I. **Certification: Examination Concepts**
   A. Purposes of perianesthesia certification
      1. Consumer protection
         a. Demonstrate personal accountability to the health-care consumer for one's own professional nursing practice
         b. Document to consumers and employers that a perianesthesia nurse has mastered a core of knowledge about the specialty
      2. Quality
         a. Promote delivery of quality care
         b. Define a minimum level of competence
      3. Excellence
         a. Commit to clinical and professional excellence
         b. Demonstrate ongoing responsibility for educational growth
      4. Personal growth
         a. Enhance personal and professional satisfaction through voluntary effort
         b. Earn a credential beyond licensure
   B. Excelling personally, excelling professionally
      1. Increase personal gratification
      2. Promote professional growth
      3. Document mastery of a core of specialty
II. **Programs in Perianesthesia Nursing Certification**
   A. American Board of Perianesthesia Nursing Certification (ABPANC)
      1. Develops, constructs, and evaluates the certification examinations

Objectives

1. State two purposes of certification.
2. Name each domain that delineates the role of the ambulatory surgery nurse.
3. Describe four key elements of the process to create CAPA examinations.
4. List five strategies to mentally prepare for testing.
5. Identify six cues or techniques to read examination questions (items) and select the most correct response.

2. Coordinates and administers the certification program through the Professional Examination Services (PES)
3. Monitors *re*certification programs
4. Offices in New York; contact 1-800-6-ABPANC

B. Certification options
1. CAPA: Certified Ambulatory Perianesthesia Nurse
    a. Established 1994
    b. Examination derives from a separate role delineation than the CPAN examination
2. CPAN: Certified Postanesthesia Nurse
    a. Established 1986
    b. Examination based upon a role delineation by practicing postanesthesia nurse
    c. Role delineation is regularly reevaluated

C. Establishing certification candidacy
1. Obtain and comprehend the *most current edition* of *Perianesthesia Nursing Certification Examination Handbook and Application* from: ABPANC Program Director, Professional Examination Service (PES), 475 Riverside Drive, New York, New York 10115; (212) 367-4200; fax (212) 367-4266
2. Determine eligibility; candidates must document:
    a. Minimum of 1,800 hours of direct nursing care in a *postanesthesia* **or** *ambulatory surgery* setting within the most recent three years
    b. Leadership, education, research, and patient care in a postanesthesia setting (CPANs) **or** perianesthesia setting (CAPAs)
    c. Current, valid licensure as a registered nurse, granted through the N-CLEX format
3. Select your test date and site
    a. Each autumn
        i.   First Saturday in November
        ii. Several cities in all geographic locations
    b. Each spring
        i.   Sunday morning prior to ASPAN's national conference
        ii. Host city for national conference and other selected cities
4. Complete application and submit by deadlines established by ABPANC, generally:
    a. 8–10 weeks before autumn administration
    b. 6 weeks before spring administration
    c. Contact the current certification handbook for specific dates, locations and deadlines

III. **A Certification Examination: Key Elements and Creation**
A. Role delineation—the examination's blueprint
1. Specific statements that establish the boundaries, or scope, of the nurse's role
2. States core tasks, knowledge, and skills within the delineated practice
3. Defined by nurses in current perianesthesia practice
4. Established while planning any new examination
5. Examination questions developed to measure the candidate's knowledge of concepts related to the role delineation
6. Role is redelineated periodically to monitor changes in practice
7. CAPA and CPAN examinations arise from *separate* role delineations
B. Domains: perianesthesia nurse's primary responsibilities in practice
1. Primary categories in role delineation
2. Identified domains of CAPA exam
    a. Direct care
    b. Education
    c. Leadership

3. Ethics and research are viewed as aspects of each practice domain
4. Specific knowledge concepts and measurable skills are identified within each domain

C. Validation—confirming the importance of each domain
   1. Practicing registered nurses assign a *weight* to the knowledge and skill statements within each domain
   2. This process considers the importance of task, knowledge or skill, and potential outcomes if a specific knowledge or skill is not mastered
   3. Validators ask "Just how critical *is* this item of knowledge or skill to safe practice?"
   4. Validators focus on the candidate who meets minimum of the qualifications for certification

D. Creating examination questions—an approach to an exam item
   1. Multiple-choice format and careful phrasing
      a. Scenario: may be inserted before a set of questions to provide background for a question and "set the clinical stage"
         i. Provides details: age, health, type of anesthetic, surgery, setting, etc.
         ii. Exam candidate can imagine this situation when reading stem
         iii. *Example:* "Twenty minutes after PACU admission following a knee arthroscopy with repair of a torn anterior cruciate ligament (ACL), Mr. Hobble Weakly's pulse oximeter reads 90%. He is alert, rates his pain as a 6 (scale 0–10) and blood pressure is 106/76 with heart rate 96 beats per minute in a sinus rhythm."
      b. Stem: sentence that begins the test item (see Table 43–1)
         i. Poses a problem to solve
         ii. Written as a question or incomplete phrase
         iii. Find word hints: notice phrasing and use of key words, such as *except, most likely, always, never, least*
      c. Distractor: three incorrect choices to complete stem (see Table 43–1)
         i. Read critically: are you asked to plan? prioritize? evaluate outcomes? determine best or worst intervention?
         ii. Next, use reason to eliminate unlikely, implausible options
      d. Answer: correct response to complete stem (see Table 43–1)
         i. Continue to critically reason the most correct response
         ii. Reconsider the rationales used to eliminate other distractors (as in choices a, b, and c, above)
         iii. Ask again: does this option make the most sense in practice?
         iv. Does your intutition agree?
   2. Who crafts these items?
      a. Certified perianesthesia nurses (CAPAs and CPANs)
      b. Workshop participants working with mentors
      c. Members of ABPANC committees or the Board of Directors
   3. Process: how does a writer develop an item?
      a. Consider a critical piece of knowledge or identify a skill that each perianesthesia nurse must know to practice competently
      b. Obscure facts or practices relating to a single geographic region are not appropriate for a national certification examination
      c. Develop the idea into a multiple-choice question with a stem, three distractors, and *only* one absolutely correct answer
      d. Apply reasoning skills similar to the exercise in Table 43–1 to verify that the item is practice-based, logical, and applies to the established domains of perianesthesia nursing

Table 43–1 • CRITICAL REASONING: DERIVING THE ITEM'S MOST CORRECT ANWSER

Item 153.*	
Stem	*Patient education priorities for Ms. I.P. Sorely following her extracorporeal shockwave lithotrypsy (ESWL) focus primarily on the importance of:*
Distractors × 3 &	A. Hematuria prevention
Correct answer × 1	B. Limited oral fluids
	C. Antiobiotic complications
	D. Forced hydration
Reasoning process:	To reason an answer to this item, the CAPA candidate must understand the ESWL procedure and the principles of postoperative care.
	Distractors in Item 153 are plausible and could fit Ms. Sorely, *except:*
Re: distractor a:	Hematuria is a likely and expected result following Ms. Sorely's procedure; teaching her can't *prevent* mild hematuria, though she does need to report overt bleeding. **Decision:** *Choice "a" is probably incorrect*
Re: distractor b:	The nurse must know that Ms. Sorely has to force, not limit, fluids postoperatively; since she will return home, the nurse will teach and document I.P.'s tolerance of oral fluids. **Decision:** *Choice "b" opposes appropriate postoperative care after ESWL and is clearly incorrect*
Re: distractor c:	Ms. Sorely does need to learn about reportable side effects related to her antibiotic. The nurse includes this information with her discharge instructions, though perhaps with less emphasis than for a "primary" educational focus as asked in the stem. **Decision:** *Choice "c" is a plausible, but probably not so high priority as choice "d."*
Re: distractor d:	To purge stone fragments from her kidneys after ESWL, Ms. I.P. Sorely requires at least 2,000 ml of fluid each day. Fluids also help prevent infection, colic, and possible ureteral reobstruction. **The CAPA candidate knows that of all the distractors given in the item, noncompliance with forced hydration has the greatest risk of negative postoperative outcomes.** Hydration becomes a primary educational priority for nurses because of the high medical priority after ESWL. **Decision:** *Choice d is the most correct of these distractors.*

Mark the answer sheet: The candidate marks "d" next to #153 on the answer form.

*Imitation item: #153 is from an imitation exam

    e. Review the item—often with another writer—for accuracy, clarity, grammar, and a comment about whether the answer too obviously "stands out" among the distractors

    f. Revise, often more than once; review again, revise again

    g. Reference the item to content in current literature

    h. Submit to ABPANC through PES

  4. Process: where does the item go after submission to ABPANC?

    a. Each item is critiqued by ABPANC committees and directors

      i.   Is item's focus relevant to its domain in the role delineation?

      ii. Is content relevant and important?

      iii. Are style and format correct?

      iv. Is specified answer correct?

      v.   Are distractors absolutely incorrect?

      vi. Is phrasing clear?

      vii. Is item referenced to *current* literature?

      b. During this critique, the item may again be revised

      c. Each item is assigned a level of difficulty to reflect the cognitive skill required to answer question

         i.   Level I item requires knowledge recall

         ii.   Level II item requires candidate to relate facts or ideas

         iii. Level III item requires candidate to apply concepts to resolve a situation

E. The item bank—a question storehouse

   1. Secure, central location to house accepted items for a future examination

   2. *Separate* item banks for CAPA and CPAN exams

   3. Maintained at PES

   4. Regularly reviewed by ABPANC to reassess current relevance of specific items

   5. PES compiles statistics to critique each item's performance on the exam

F. Constructing an examination—blending the questions

   1. Items selected by computer from item bank

   2. Validated role delineation, or exam "blueprint," specifies the number of items to appear on the CAPA exam for each domain

      a. Direct care domain: 108 items (54%)

      b. Education domain: 48 items (28%)

      c. Leadership domain: 44 items (22%)

   3. Each exam is composed of 200 multiple-choice items

   4. ABPANC reviews each draft of an exam to consider the mix of questions selected by the computer, item readability, content accuracy, and grammar

G. Passing point—establishing the minimum required score

   1. Determined by psychometric criteria

   2. Currently established by ABPANC using the Angoff method

   3. Reevaluated for each new examination version

IV. Preparing to Certify: Personal Planning

A. Self assessment

   1. Attitude: who am I? why do I want to certify?

      a. Identify your motivation to certify

      b. View as an educational opportunity, not an imposed requirement

   2. Available time and tools: what can help? when?

      a. For the months until examination date

      b. To schedule regular study periods

      c. To attend a review course

      d. To rest and reflect

   3. Study habits and testing approach: be honest—what's my style?

      a. Distractible or focused?

      b. Prefer independent or group study?

      c. Need a review course to refresh ideas?

      d. Anxious or calm?

      e. Past success with multiple-choice style

      f. Personality: how do I cope with test stress?

   4. Identify clinical strengths: what do I know?

      a. Areas and knowledge I feel *most* confident about

      b. Content needing additional review

      c. Honest appraisal!

   5. Create a support system: who, what can help me?

      a. Affirmations

      b. Family, friends, and colleagues

B. Set study priorities and implement a plan
   1. Decide what to learn, then sharpen thinking
      a. Determine essential *"must know"* content
         i.   Ambulatory surgery scope of practice
         ii. Scan specialty resources for critical concepts
              (a) ASPAN-sponsored publications
              (b) Anesthesia-specific texts
              (c) Journals
         iii. Register for a certification review course
         iv. Conduct a literature search for newest medications and practices
      b. Learn and understand principles
         i.   Relate relevant facts to clinical situations
         ii. Reconsider minor details—"what do I *really* need to know" to practice?
         iii. Ask questions about a situation
              (a) Make up stories
              (b) Brainstorm possible answers about the story, both sensible and
                  nonsensical; ask:
                  (i)   "Why is this man restless?"
                  (ii) "How does this drug work?"
                  (iii) "What are the nurse's priorities?"
                  (iv) "Can I explain the physiology?"
         iv. Develop long-term memory: create your personal database
              (a) A process of accumulating tidbits of knowledge and creating levels of
                  understanding over time
              (b) These come together to apply to a situation when needed
   2. Know your knowledge gaps
      a. Locate or create pretests
      b. Review texts and literature
      c. Converse with other nurses
      d. List familiar and less "secure" concepts
   3. Manage your time, maximize fun!
      a. *Never* cram!
         i.   Only creates a mishmash of unrelated, jumbled facts
         ii. Saturates short-term memory
         iii. Less likely to recall on command
      b. Schedule blocks of study time on calendar
      c. Concentrate first on knowledge deficits
      d. Study material in manageable chunks
         i.   For example: fluid concepts today, electrolytes next week
      e. Arrange study groups
         i.   Assign topics for members to present
         ii. Dialogue, debate
      f. Respect the established study schedule
         i.   Shun interruptions by phone, family
         ii. Set long- and short-term study goals
         iii. Maintain the pace and monitor progress
   4. Involve your body senses to reinforce learning
      a. Use your voice: teach a concept
         i.   In the locker room while changing into scrubs at work
         ii. Walking through the park with a friend
         iii. To calm a squirming youngster (who needn't comprehend!)
         iv. To your pet (who will sit with raptured attention!)

  b. Simulate situations
   i.   Role-play asthmatic breathing
   ii.   Practice listening to breath sounds on the cat's chest
   iii.   Model Phase I care of a patient with a regional arm block
   iv.   Write cue (flash) cards
  c. Apply high-level critical thinking to clinical situations
   i.   Repeat a pretest and smile when you improve your score
   ii.   Write ten test items, then reason answers with your study group
   iii.   Mentally create a picture of a situation or clinical syndrome
      (a) Envision osmosis in hyperglycemic serum
      (b) Imagine how a patient looks while you review the effects of
          inadequately reversed muscle relaxants
      (c) Draw the electrocardiogram associated with a potassium of 6.6 mEq/L
   iv.   Write a lesson plan for age-appropriate discharge education for a
        5-year-old
   v.   Compare and contrast assessments and interventions to treat septic and
        hypovolemic shock
  d. Infuse humor for fun and memory
   i.   Sing a memorable acronym to remember cranial nerves
   ii.   Clap rhythms of heart sounds
   iii.   Set electrolyte imbalances into limerick form
 5. Monitor your educational growth
  a. Periodically quiz yourself on difficult content
  b. Consciously use new knowledge in clinical setting, and smile
  c. Ask for and listen to verbal reinforcement by peers about your new knowledge
  d. Practice nursing with newfound confidence
  e. Celebrate successes
  f. During a quiet second between patients, practice quick recall of memory cues
     you created to retain information
C. Certification day: time to show your stuff!
 1. Plan ahead, then show up early, rested, relaxed, prepared
  a. Rehearse: wear a confident, positive manner
   i.   Imagine success: see your name followed by CAPA
   ii.   Eat, sleep, and dress for success
      (a) Comfortable clothes, in layers to accommodate varied room
          temperatures
      (b) Show your colors: wear positive, optimistic reds, yellows, bright pink
      (c) Avoid drugs (alcohol, excess caffeine, sugar)
   iii.   Drive or walk to test site before test day; locate parking
   iv.   Assemble required materials for easy access on exam day
      (a) *Photo* identification
      (b) Exam admission information
      (c) Several #2 soft-lead pencils
      (d) Your concentration
   v.   Rehearse your breathing and muscle relaxation techniques to reduce
        tension during the exam
  b. During the exam:
   i.   Mild anxiety is a benefit: increases focus, performance, and concentration
   ii.   Listen carefully to proctor's instructions
   iii.   Remember your affirmations
   iv.   Concentrate; ignore room distractions
   v.   Take periodic deep breaths

    vi. Focus: you've mastered this exam content
       (a) Read each item carefully
       (b) Don't rush—you have 4 hours
       (c) Plan 30–45 seconds per question
          (i)   Less for memory recall items
          (ii) More for detailed analytic items
          (iii) It's okay to jot notes or memory cues in test booklet
    vii. Use systematic approach to reason each question
       (a) Look for hints, key words in question
       (b) Rule out obviously incorrect options
       (c) Apply the nursing process and nursing practice models
       (d) Use context to identify best answers
       (e) Rule out bizarre or professionally inappropriate options
       (f) Don't "read in" any unstated meaning
       (g) Guess when uncertain of answers—there's no penalty
       (h) Trust your intuition—it's often correct
    viii. Review your exam
       (a) Correlate each item number on test with number on answer form
       (b) Continue this cross-check through entire exam
       (c) *Completely* erase stray marks
       (d) Review *all* your answers
       (e) Change answers when logically appropriate
          (i) One often selects a correct response on second look
          (ii) May improve test result

Bibliography

1. ABPANC: Perianesthesia Nursing Certification Examination Handbook and Application. New York: Professional Examination Service.
2. Carlson, K. (1995). *Certification Review for Perianesthesia Nurses* Philadelphia: Saunders.
3. Dickenson-Hazard, N. (1990). Develop your thinking skills for improved test taking. *Pediat Nurs,* 16(53):480–481.
4. Elkins, S.G. (1989). Personality of a test taker. *Plast Surg Nurs,* 9(2):90.
5. Highfield, M.E., Wong, G. (1992). How to take multiple-choice tests. *Nursing,* 22(10):117, 121–122, 125–126.
6. Kortbawi, P.A. (1990). Test-taking skills: Giving yourself an edge. *Nursing,* 20(6):95–96, 98, 199.
7. Litwack, L. (1994). Test-taking techniques. In Litwack, K., ed. *Core Curriculum for Post Anesthesia Nursing Practice,* 3rd ed. Philadelphia: Saunders, pp. 672–679.
8. Litwack, L. (1995). Test-taking techniques. *J Post Anesth Nurs,* 10(5):277–279.
9. Nugent, P.M., Vitale, B.A. (1993). *Test Success: Test-Taking Techniques for Beginning Nursing Students.* Philadelphia: FA Davis.
10. Sides, M.B., Korchek, N. (1994). *Nurse's Guide to Successful Test-Taking,* 2nd ed. Philadelphia: Lippincott.
11. Smith, S.F. (1993). Coping with test anxiety. *Healthcare Trends & Transition,* 5(2):18–19.
12. Waddell, D.L., Blankenship, J.C. (1994). Answer changing: A meta analysis of the prevalence and patterns. *J Cont Educ in Nurs,* 25(4):155–158.
13. Yee, J.W., Highfield, M.E. (1995). Tackling tests confidently. *Nursing,* 25(3):86.

REVIEW QUESTIONS

1. A perianesthesia nurse might seek a certification for any of the following purposes except to

   A. Enhance the nurse's professional and personal satisfaction

   B. Demonstrate interest in consumer safety and protection

   C. Document mastery of specialty knowledge

   D. Comply with licensure and credentialing standards of a specialty nursing organization

2. The candidate for the Certified Ambulatory Perianesthesia Nurse (CAPA) credential prepares for certification by reviewing the domains of ambulatory surgical nursing which, as delineated, include any of the following concepts except

    A. Recognizing corticosteroid effects
    B. Skill in qualitative research design
    C. Knowledge of leadership concepts
    D. Teaching wound-drain concepts

3. Methods to stimulate thinking skills when preparing for certification might include any of the following except

    A. Creating questions from clinical scenarios
    B. Memorizing physiologic effects of neuromuscular blockers on examination eve
    C. Constructing acronyms to recall child development facts
    D. Imagining nursing actions related to care of a woman unresponsive after 5 hours of enflurane

4. On a certification examination, an item that **most** challenges critical thinking might ask the candidate to

    A. Compare fluid requirements of a young adult with needs of an elderly woman
    B. Recall facts about properties of inhalation anesthetics
    C. Plan care priorities for a pregnant and hypotensive patient after cholecystectomy
    D. Analyze arterial blood gas measures for a mechanically ventilated patient

5. When reading an item on the certification examination, the candidate chooses the most plausible answer by

    A. Assessing each distractor separately to reason whether it is correct or not
    B. Always considering distractors that include the word "never" or "all of the above" as correct

    C. Never guessing, trusting that no answer reduces the test score less than an incorrect response would
    D. Choosing one distractor as correct because another distractor confirms the choice by expressing a similar idea

6. When creating a certification-level examination, a role delineation is conducted to

    A. Specify the scope of the nurse's role
    B. Identify consumer expectations
    C. Validate the relative importance of a skill
    D. Establish candidate eligibility criteria

7. Strategies to increase success during the certification examination include

    A. Focus energy on the most difficult questions first
    B. Imagine other, unstated factors that could influence the answer to a question
    C. Regularly correlate numbers between answer-and-question form to verify position
    D. Set a pace to answer 75 questions in the first 2½ hours of the exam

8. When considering whether to change an answer on the certification examination, the candidate considers research results about test-taking behavior that conclude

    A. The changed response is based on an impulsive guess that is wrong as often as correct
    B. Changing answers improves test scores
    C. A change to a correct answer correlates low stress in the test-taker and moderate item difficulty
    D. Most often, examinees change a correct answer to a wrong response

9. Test anxiety is a phenomenon that

   A. Can be redirected to improve performance
   B. Is best ignored by focusing on learning
   C. Must be eliminated before the examination
   D. Is enhanced by caffeine, biofeedback, and sugar

10. The CPAN and CAPA certification examinations are constructed as 200-question, multiple-choice tests in which

   A. Carefully "reading into the question" best guides the candidate to determine the correct response
   B. The candidate reasons one correct answer from a field of plausible, but absolutely incorrect distractors
   C. Leaving unknown questions blank will significantly increase the candidate's score
   D. The correct answer may be an obscure detail based upon clinical practices in one area of the country

ANSWERS TO QUESTIONS

1. D	6. A
2. B	7. C
3. B	8. B
4. C	9. A
5. A	10. B

Index

Note: Page numbers in *italic* refer to illustrations; those followed by t refer to tables.